Clinical Biochemistry in Diagnosis & Management

A.S. Saini
M.B.B.S., M.Sc., Ph.D.
Professor of Biochemistry,
SBMN Dental College, Asthal Bohar, Rohtak
Former Director, Professor & Head,
Department of Biochemistry,
PG Institute of Medical Sciences, Rohtak

J. Kaur
M.B.B.S., D.G.O., M.D. (Biochemistry)
Reader, Department of Biochemistry,
Government Medical College, Chandigarh

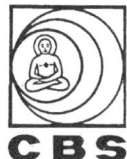

CBS

CBS Publishers & Distributors Pvt. Ltd.

New Delhi • Bengaluru • Chennai • Kochi • Kolkata • Mumbai
Bhubaneswar • Hyderabad • Jharkhand • Nagpur • Patna • Pune • Uttarakhand • Dhaka

ISBN: 81-239-0759-1

First Edition: 2001
Reprint: 2004, 2009, 2011, 2015, 2020

Published by **Satish Kumar Jain** and produced by **Varun Jain** for
CBS Publishers & Distributors Pvt. Ltd.,
4819/XI Prahlad Street, 24 Ansari Road, Daryaganj, New Delhi - 110002
delhi@cbspd.com, cbspubs@airtelmail.in • www.cbspd.com
Ph.: 23289259, 23266861, 23266867 • Fax: 011-23243014

Corporate Office: 204 FIE, Industrial Area, Patparganj, Delhi - 110 092
Ph: 49344934 • Fax: 011-49344935
E-mail: publishing@cbspd.com • publicity@cbspd.com

Branches:
• *Bengaluru:* 2975, 17th Cross, K.R. Road, Bansankari 2nd Stage,
  Bengaluru - 70 • Ph: +91-80-26771678/79 • Fax: +91-80-26771680
  E-mail: cbsbng@gmail.com, bangalore@cbspd.com
• *Chennai:* No. 7, Subbaraya Street, Shenoy Nagar, Chennai - 600030
  Ph: +91-44-26681266, 26680620 • Fax: +91-44-42032115
  E-mail: chennai@cbspd.com
• *Kochi:* Ashana House, 39/1904, A.M. Thomas Road, Valanjambalam,
  Ernakulum, Kochi • Ph: +91-484-4059061-65
  Fax: +91-484-4059065 • E-mail: cochin@cbspd.com
• *Kolkata:* 6-B, Ground Floor, Rameshwar Shaw Road, Kolkata - 700014
  Ph: +91-33-22891126/7/8 • E-mail: kolkata@cbspd.com
• *Mumbai:* 83-C, Dr. E. Moses Road, Worli, Mumbai - 400018
  Ph: +91-9833017933, 022-24902340/41 • E-mail: mumbai@cbspd.com

Representatives:

• Hyderabad: 0-9885175004	• Nagpur: 0-9021734563
• Patna: 0-9334159340	• Pune: 0-9623451994
• Jharkhand: 0-9811541605	• Uttarakhand: 0-9716462459

Printed at:
Neekunj Print Process, Delhi

Foreword

The emphasis in the usual text books of clinical subjects is more on the clinical diagnosis and treatment of diseases without going into the details of pathophysiological basis of biochemical alterations. Similarly texts of Biochemistry describe in detail the biochemical changes without laying adequate emphasis on the clinical and applied aspects of such alterations. The present book bridges the gap between these two approaches. This book describes the pathophysiological basis of biochemical alterations in various disease states. The processes have been described in simple and easily understood language. Liberal use of figures, charts and tables further help in grasping the core points of the text. Case histories have been included to illustrate how biochemical alteration help in reaching at a correct clinical diagnosis. *Such a book will be useful to the clinicians (residents of most clinical departments) for understanding the biochemical basis of various biochemical laboratory investigations. At the same time it will also help the residents of biochemistry and other investigative departments to understand the clinical and applied aspects of the biochemical alterations in a patient.* For self evaluation of the reader, the authors have given objective type questions at the end of each chapter. These questions have been so designed as to assess the application of the knowledge in certain clinical situations. The authors have done a remarkable job in producing such a book which should be immensely useful both to inquisitive clinicians including practising doctors as well as sensitive biochemists.

DR. O.N. BHAKOO
MD.DCH.FIAP. FAMS.

FORMER :
− PROF. & HEAD, DEPTT. OF PEDIATRICS &
  NEONATOLOGY PGI, CHANDIGARH
− HON. CONSULTANT, HAMMERSMITH HOSPITAL, LONDON.
− FELLOW NEONATOLOGY, MCMASTER UNIVERSITY, CANADA.

About the Authors

Dr. A.S. Saini, formerly, Director and Professor and Head, Deptt. of Biochemistry Post Graduate Institute of Medical Sciences, Rohtak, is one of the very senior medical graduates opting for Biochemistry as his career. He guided a large number of MD/PhD Biochemistry students and post graduates of other departments and supervised a large number of ICMR and CSIR projects, publishing about 100 research and review papers, six of which have been reported as recommended methods in different books. He served as member National Executive Nutrition Society of India, and Medical Council of India also as a member of some of their Expert Groups. He was President of Indian Association of Medical Biochemists for the year 1994-95. He has already authored 'A Textbook of Biochemistry' published by C.B.S. Publishers, New Delhi.

Dr. (Mrs.) J. Kaur, after graduating and obtaining D.G.O. from Mahatma Gandhi Institute of Medical Sciences Sevagram, subsequently opted for Biochemistry as her career. Presently, she is working as Reader in Biochemistry at Government Medical College Chandigarh. She has about a score of research publications and is trained in Endocrinological and DNA (PCR) techniques and presently her field of interest is Clinical Endocrinology. She is also a co-author in the Textbook of Biochemistry referred above.

Preface

With advances in pathophysiological understanding of disease processes and investigative methodologies, management of different diseases has greatly improved. At the same time, however, the list of possible investigations in different diseases has also greatly increased. It has now become imperative that the biochemical tests should be judiciously selected during disease diagnosis and management. This is the essence of the use of test algorithms and the probability approach in the disease diagnosis process. In the present scenario of confusing array of available laboratory tests (which are not pleasant to the pocket of the patient), two important implications emerge. Firstly, there is need for better understanding of the pathophysiological processes of different diseases and specificity and sensitivity of different tests used for their diagnosis, to enable proper selection of the laboratory tests. Secondly, the Biochemistry Departments must play an active role in choice and interpretation of these tests. The present deplorable state of affairs has been summed up in the innocent but well-meaning remarks of Dr. O.N. Bhakoo (see the foreword)".....such a book should be immensely useful both to *inquisitive* clinicians................ as well as *sensitive* biochemists....."

The present book is an attempt of the authors to sensitize both the residents of the Biochemistry Departments as well as budding clinicians, to the need made out in the above paragraph.

The main stress of the book is on disease diagnosis for which both clinical findings and the laboratory tests have their own importance, (although, neither of the two has 100% predictability value, for the purpose). Thus desired stress has been laid on the clinical presentations of patients. Brief mention of pathophysiological mechanisms should facilitate both, grasp of clinical presentations as well as selection of suitable tests for the problems of the patients. The biochemical tests have been discussed in context of the demand of the clinical situation. The reason for the choice of the test has amply been explained. The analytical and theoretical details about the tests have been avoided. At many places, relative importance of the clinical features or results of other investigations to the bio-chemical test, in a clinical situation, has been defined.

In order to limit the size of the book the text has been kept brief and easily understood and lot of information has been incorporated into tables and figures which need to be carefully studied. Appendix B also contains some useful information besides the reference values. The objective type questions are meant to highlight certain points of the text. Some of these, however, provide independent pieces of information. The case histories are meant to illustrate the manner in which the information in a chapter will be required to be used. These are only illustrative and not taken out of the case files of actual patients.

Inspite of our best efforts the book is bound to have deficiencies. We will be grateful if the readers kindly make reference to these as well as send their valuable suggestions to improve utility of the book.

A.S. SAINI
J. KAUR.

Acknowledgements

We are extremely grateful to Dr. O.N. Bhakoo former Prof. and Head Deptt. of Pediatrics and Neonatology, P.G.I. Chandigarh for his interest and help in preparing of manuscript of Chapter 18 of this book and also for kindly agreeing to write foreword to this book, comprising no less than 400 pages. We are obliged to him for sparing so much of his valuable time.

A number of other senior clinicians also graciously accepted to review different chapters of the manuscript. Dr. R.J. Dash Prof. & Head Deptt. of Endocrinology P.G.I. Chandigarh read through the text of all the chapters on endocrinology (except Chapter 10) and made extensive useful observations. We are obliged for his kind help. Dr.(Mrs.) Sushila Rathee former Prof. and Head Deptt. of Obstetrics and Gynecology P.G.I.M.S. Rohtak read part of Chapter 18 at an early stage of the manuscript and made useful suggestions. She also kindly made available some useful literature from her personal library. Dr. S.C. Srivastva former Prof. and Head Deptt. of Medicine P.G.I.M.S. Rohtak read through Chapter 9 and found time from his busy practice to discuss the management part of lipid disorders with one of us. His suggestions were extremely useful. Other Professors of Medicine from the same Institute who graciously agreed to offer observations included, Dr. K.C. Malhotra (Chapter 7 & 14), Dr. S.N. Khosla (Chapter 6), Dr. S.K. Mahajan (Chapter 4) and Dr. Nitya Nand (Chapter 15). Kind guidance and help of Dr. I.B. Singh, former Professor of Anatomy PGIMS, Rohtak and Professor Emeritus M.D. University, Rohtak is also gratefully acknowledged. Dr. R.K. Marya Professor of Physiology Al-Arab Medical University, Benghazi (Libya) made useful suggestions about general plan of the book. Dr. N.K. Saini Reader Department of SPM and Dr. (Mrs.) Ashuma Sachdeva a Resident of Biochemistry Deptt., rendered valuable help in proof reading. Contributions of all these colleagues are gratefully acknowledged.

The present teaching assignment of one of us (A.S. Saini) at S.B.M.N. Dental College Asthal Bohar has been extremely conducive for the tough task of completing this book. For that we are grateful to the President of Institution Mahent Chand Nath Yogi and the Director Dr. Markandy Ahuja. The authors also thankfully acknowledge the cooperation extended by Prof. V.K. Kak Director Principal and Secretary Med. Education, Govt. Med. College Chandigarh.

We would also like to thank, M/s. CBS Publishers and Distributors, New Delhi for their interest and cooperation in publication of this book.

A.S. SAINI
J. KAUR

Contents

and dibucaine number (P.86): • Enzymes in diagnosis of myocardial infarction (P.86): • Early diagnosis of myocardial infarction for thrombolytic therapy (P.87): • Indications of multi-organ failure in cardiogenic shock (P.105): • Enzymes in diagnosis of liver and muscle diseases (P.87): • Specific plasma proteins, in diagnosis of clinical disorders (P.90): • Immunonephlometry, immunoturbidometry and immunoelectrophoresis (P.91,P.97): • Evaluation of serum/plasma proteins (P.90,P.96,T.5.11): • Serum albumin in clinical diagnosis (P.91,T.5.7): • Differentiating hemoglobin from myoglobin in a red coloured biological solution (P.94): • Monitoring intensity of a chronic inflammation (P.95,P.97): • Polyclonal gammopathy (P.96): • Primary immune-deficiency disorders (P.93,T.5.8,T.5.10): • AIDS (P.94,T.5.8): • Evaluation of the immune system (P.95): • Multiple myeloma (97): • MGUS (P.98,T.5.14): • Waldenstroms macroglobinemia (P.98): • Heavy chain disease (P.99): • Amyloidosis (P.98): • Tumor markers (P.99): • Screening procedures for certain malignancies (P.101): • Tumor markers for germ cell tumors (P.101): • CSF (P.102): 29. Transudates and exudates (P.103).

Case histories (P.104)
CH 1. A case of multiple myeloma: **CH 2.** A case of myocardial infarction: **CH 3.** A case of hepatic metastases.

Objective type questions (P.106)
CSF examination (15): Diagnostic use of specific proteins (5): Electrophoresis (6,7): Immunodeficiency (8,9): Myeloma (10,11,12): Myocardial infarction (1,2): Plasma proteins (4): Transaminases (3): Tumor markers (14).

CHAPTER 6 GASTROINTESTINAL TRACT INCLUDING LIVER AND PANCREAS.......... 109
• Bilirubin metabolism and bile pigmant based tests to differentiate the three types of jaundice (P.109): • Different parameters useful in diagnosis of liver disorders (P.111,T.6.1): • In born errors of bilirubin transport, conjugation and secretion in liver (P.111,F.6.2): • Physiological jaundice (P.115): • Diagnosis of hemolysis and haemolytic jaundice (P.113,F.6.3): • Acute viral hepatitis (P.115): • Use of serological markers in viral hepatitis (P.115,F. 6.4, T.6.2). • Liver function tests during the course of viral hepatitis (P.115,F.6.4,T.6.2): • Significance of bilirubin in acute viral hepatitis (P.116,F.6.5): • Hepatitis caused by drugs/toxins (P.117): • Cirrhosis and pathophysiology of clinical features and complications (P.118,T.6.4): • Wilson's disease (P.120); • Diagnostic criteria (P.121): • Hemochromatosis (P.121): • α_1-Antitrypsin deficiency (P.121): • Hepatic encephalopathy (P.121): • Panhepatic necrosis and microvasicular steosis (P.122,F.6.6): • Reye's syndrome (P.122,F.6.6): • Biliary obstruction (P.122): • Extrahepatic; intrahepatic,restricted and widespread cholestasis (P.123,T.6.5): • Primary biliary cirrhosis (P.123): • Passive congestion of liver (P.124): • Gastric function assessment (P.125): • Zollinger Ellison syndrome (P.126): • Acute pancreatitis (P.126); • A scheme for interpretation of increased amylase (P.127): • About amylase and lipase (P.128): • Chronic pancreatitis (P.128): • Pancreatic cancer (P.128).

Case histories (P.128)
CH 1. A case of acute viral hepatitis: **CH 2.** A case of cirrhosis: **CH 3.** A case of gall stones: **CH 4.** A case of chronic hepatitis: **CH 5.** A case of primary biliary cirrhosis: **CH 6.** A case of acute pancreatitis.

Objective type questions (P.131)
Acute pancreatitis (15,16): α_1 Antitrypsin deficiency (13): Chronic hepatitis (8,9): Fulminant hepatic failure (4): Gall stones (14): Hepatic encephalopathy (10,11): Hepatitis viral (2,3): Hepatitis drug toxicity (1): Hepatorenal syndrome (7): Macrovasicular hepatic steotosis (5): Pancreatic disorders (17): Reye's syndrome (6): Wilson's disease (12).

CHAPTER 7 DIABETES MELLITUS AND HYPOGLYCEMIA 135
• Classification of primary diabetes mellitus (P.135): • Relation of insulin resistance and insulin secretion in type II disorder (P.136,T.7.3): • Biochemical basis of clinical features (P.137): • Type II disease and syndrome X (P.137,F.7.1): • Diabetic ketoacidosis (P.138,140): • Metabolic differences in complete loss

hypertensive for pheochromocytoma (P.320,T.15.11): • Liddle syndrome, Bartter's syndrome (P.317): • Gordon's syndrome (P.317).

Case histories (P. 321)
CH 1. A case of Addison's disease. **CH 2.** A case of Cushing's syndrome: **CH 3.** A case of congenital adrenal hyperplasia.

Objective type questions (P. 323)
Addison's disease (7,8): Adrenal androgen hypersecretion (11): Adrenal cortical tumor (6): Bilateral adrenal hyperplasia (4): CRH test (13): Function tests (3): Hypoaldosteronism (12): Hyporeninemic hypoaldosteronism (15): Incidentaloma (9): Pheochromo-cytoma (10): Primary aldosteronism (14): Pseudo-Cushing's syndrome (5): Steroids,rennin angiotensin system (2): Stimulation tests (1).

• Paraneoplastic manifestations of tumors (cachexia,endocrine and others) (P.327): • MEN type I (P.328): • MEN type II (P.329): • PGA syndromes (P.330): • Biochemical changes in cancer (P.331): • Tumor lysis syndrome (P.331): • Some considerations of geriatric endocrinology (thyroid disorders, diabetes mellitus, calcium metabolism, hyperparathyroidism, water and electrolyte balance, response to stress and reproductive functions) (P.332).

Objective type questions (P. 334)
Acanthosis nigricans (10): Cushing's syndrome (5): Ectopic acromegaly (6): Ectopic hormones (1): Familial hypercalcemia (7): Hypercalcemia of malignancy (2,3): MEN syndromes (8,9): SIADH (4).

• The testicular hormones; regulation; biosynthesis;in circulation and actions (P.337,F.17.1,17.2): • Sex differentiation and chromosomal disorders (P.337-341): • Pseudo-female and male hermaphroditism (P.342,F.17.5,T.17.3): • Puberty, normal and abnormal (P.343): • Assessment of testicular functions (P.343) and ovarian functions (P.344): • Prepubertal hypogonadism and delayed puberty in the male (P.345): • Differentiating constitutional delay in puberty from isolated gonadotrophic deficiency (P.346): • Differentiating hypothalamic/pituitary causes from testicular causes (P.347): • Postpubertal hypogonadism (P.347): • Gynecomastia (P.348): • The ovarian hormones (P.349): • Amenorrhea,primary and secondary (P.351-353): • Diagnosis of amenorrhea (P.353,F.17.9): • Polycystic ovarian syndrome (P.355): • Hirsutism and virilism (P.356): • Infertility (P.357): • Endocrine investigation in an infertile/sub-fertile female (P.358): • Hypospadias and cryptorchidism (P.360).

Case histories (P. 358)
CH 1. A case of female hermaphroditism: **CH 2.** A couple presenting with problem of infertility: **CH 3.** A case of delayed puberty. **CH 4.** A case of amenorrhea: **CH 5.** A case of male pseudohermaphroditism.

Objective type questions (P. 360)
Absent,rudimentary gonads (2): Androgen receptors defect (22): Constitutional delay in puberty (11): Delayed puberty (9): Estrogen formation in male (8): Gonadal function assessment (6): Gonadal dysfunction hypothalamic/pituitary (12): Gonadotropin response to GnRH (4): Hirsutism (18): Hormone estimation in the female (7): 21α-Hydroxylase deficiency (19): 17α-hydroxylase deficiency (20): Isosexual precocity/ pseudoprecocity (16,17): Kallmann syndrome (10): Klinifelter syndrome (13): Leydig cell functions (3): Male infertility (14,15), Seminiferous tubular function (5): Sex determination (1): Steroid 5α-reductase deficiency (21).

• The physiological adjustments and metabolic and hormonal changes in pregnancy (P.365): • Reference ranges of some chemistries during pregnancy (P.366): • Placental hormones and role of hCG in diagnosis of pregnancy and pregnancy related disorders (P.366): • Maternal monitoring during pregnancy (pregnancy

CHAPTER 1

Clinical Chemistry Investigations in Patient Care

Besides clinical examination, most patients need some diagnostic tests for their problems. These are imaging tests (X-ray examination and allied studies), ECG, EEG, cardiovascular, pulmonary function tests and laboratory studies (hematologic, histopathologic, microbiologic including immunologic and clinical chemistry tests). Often more than one type of tests are done to help the process of patient care. Since in a patient, different types of tests look at the same disease process from different angles, their results are mutually supportive. Often, in one diagnostic service, evidence of disease, from other diagnostic areas is helpful in interpretation of the results. Thus in all diagnostic services, those involved in interpreting results of the tests should possess adequate knowledge to make use of this supportive help.

A clinical chemistry laboratory may be involved in common biochemical tests (Table 1.1) on routine basis or it may be required to carry out emergency investigations (blood gases, urea, creatinine and electrolytes, amylase, glucose, calcium and CSF examination) or it may be undertaking specialized investigations (hormone assays, study of drugs, lipids and lipoproteins, trace elements and DNA analysis). Small laboratories, close to work place of physicians (physician office laboratories) may be required to perform some simple tests for immediate results.

Depending upon workload and budgetary considerations the laboratories may be using fully automated autoanalysis or performing their work manually. Infrequently performed investigations may be carried out by the kit methods. For special investigations procedures are more complicated and highly trained staff is needed.

Main focus of this chapter is on problems related to general biochemistry (for routine work) and emergency biochemistry laboratories.

Table 1.1. Requesting in clinical chemistry test

- Test will increase or decrease probability of diagnosis of disease. Test should not be ordered if it does not add any information. Estimation of blood glucose in a patient of glycosuria without any clinical feature of diabetes mellitus will be a very useful test. Similarly, in a jaundiced patient, study of ALT and ALP will greatly help diagnosis of cause of jaundice while study of bilirubin level will be hardly of any use from that angle.
- Result of investigation will guide management (in a patient in coma without proper history, urgent testing of blood glucose and urea is essential).
- Test will contribute to determination of prognosis (PT and serum albumin levels in a case of cirrhosis).
- Test will help to follow or manage a chronic disease. It is important to understand pathophysiology and selection of test/tests and their frequency is based on that. For example, in a patient of hypoalbuminemia serum albumin level should not be repeated before a week. In a patient of oliguria blood urea should not be repeated before 12h.
- Test/tests should only be requested after making a tentative diagnosis.

PATIENTS NEEDING BIOCHEMICAL TESTS

The clinical investigations should provide answers to specific problems in process of patient care. For example after proper history and clinical examination, a particular test may play a vital role in differential diagnosis (the probability approach is discussed later). A test may be used to screen a high risk group for a disease. A test may be required to monitor treatment of a disease. A test may be vital in deciding prognosis of the patient of a particular disease.

Tests should be requested selectively to supplement clinical sense of the clinician and not as a substitute for that. Thus a test is really required if it could change tentative diagnosis, arrived at, by clinical examination. It is useful, if it could affect treatment of the patient. In most endocrinological disorders, treatment is guided more by the laboratory results than the clinical parameters. However, investigations should not be requested, simply to fill the file or to impress the patient or fellow colleagues. An awareness on part of clinician in this regard can greatly reduce the number of tests received in a clinical chemistry laboratory and that will go a long way in improving the quality of clinical chemistry service.

The samples

Patient should be properly prepared for blood collection. Factors which affect levels of different analytes include, diet, fasting, exercise, diurnal variations, posture, smoking, alcohol and drug consumption. Drugs act by producing metabolic changes and by interfering with the method of estimation. Alcohol ingestion will increase levels of urate, lactate and triglycerides. Chronic alcohol intake increases levels of urate, HDL-cholesterol, γ-GT and mean corpuscular volume. Smokers have increased levels of carboxyhemoglobin, catecholamines and cortisol. For glucose, cholesterol, triglycerides and electrolytes, the samples should be taken in the basal state (avoiding effects of food and excessive fasting). Stress, anxiety and hyperventilation may affect hormone secretions, acid base parameters and may increase levels of lactate and free fatty acids. In general, no drug, or alcohol, no strenuous activity and no change in diet should be allowed 24h before the time of blood collection. After proper sleep, patient should get up and report for blood collection.

Levels of different proteins including albumin and immunoglobulins and protein bound substances may fall by about 15% after about an hour of recumbency due to fluid redistribution in the body. This may explain difference in levels of a number of substances between inpatient (blood collected in recumbent position) and outpatient (blood collected in sitting position) blood samples. Substances are different proteins, enzymes, calcium, bilirubin, cholesterol, triglycerides and drugs bound to proteins. Prolonged tourniquet application may also increase levels of enzymes, proteins and protein bound substances (cholesterol, calcium, triglycerides). If patient is on intravenous drip, blood should be collected from the arm other than the one used for the drip.

It is preferable to use serum or plasma for different tests. Even when the substances are freely permeable through the red cell membrane, levels in whole blood are lower than in serum or plasma since water content of red cell is less than their volume. It is obligatory to use serum or plasma if substance is unequally distributed between red cell water and serum or plasma (inorganic ions and some enzymes). Plasma and serum are equally suitable for most investigations. If the sample for analysis has to be obtained quickly, to avoid release of substances from red cells (say K$^+$ of some enzymes) or for rapid freezing (in case of unstable substances) plasma is used. Chances of hemolysis are also reduced in this case.

Anticoagulants withdraw water from red cells to dilute plasma. Those which are calcium chelators (oxalate, citrate) inhibit enzymes like amylase, lactate dehydrogenase and acid phosphatase. These plus EDTA also decrease levels of calcium by certain methods. All the three mentioned anticoagulants as sodium or potassium salts will interfere in accurate estimations of electrolytes. Heparin is quite non-interfering type of anticoagulant but it is costly. Serum or heparinized plasma are most often specimens of choice. However, sodium salt of heparin should not be used for samples for sodium estimation and its lithium salt for samples for lithium estimation. If plasma is not used within a few hours, fibrin clots will form which may interfere in automatic sampling devices.

Whole blood is useful in analysis of blood gases, pH, ammonia, pyruvate and lactate, when analytes are liable to rapid changes or when the substance of interest is mainly present in red cells, for example lead. Venous blood does not reflect acid base status of the whole body properly. It may be adequate for pH but gives incorrect values for pCO_2 and pO_2.

Ideally, the specimens should be received in the laboratory immediately after collection. One should avoid agitation of blood to avoid hemolysis. Specimens should be protected from light which causes degradation of some analytes (bilirubin). Samples for unstable analytes should be kept at 4°C immediately after collection and should be transported in ice.

Hemolysis adds red cells constituents to plasma. Thus levels of K^+, LD and acid phosphatase may increase. Because of interference in chemical reactions, hemolysis causes increase in apparent concentration of bilirubin and lowers level of alkaline phosphatase. To avoid hemolysis draw blood into the syringe slowly and remove needle before expelling blood into the vial. Centrifuge the sample at a moderate speed (at room temperature proper clotting may need 15 to 30 minutes). Excessive anticoagulant and violent mixing also promotes hemolysis.

Icteric or lactescent serum creates problems in certain estimations. In lactescent serum, reduced levels of amylase (inhibition) urate, urea, CK, bilirubin and total proteins, will be reported.

An overnight storage of a blood sample may increase levels of K^+, phosphate and certain red cell enzymes like LD.

Other samples

Venous blood samples are the commonest samples used in clinical chemistry investigations. For blood gas studies, the arterial samples are used. If these cannot be obtained capillary samples (arterialized) may be used (more details in Chapter 3). Heel is a convenient site for obtaining samples from infants.

Other samples submitted for study in clinical chemistry include urine, feces, cerebrospinal fluid, duodenal fluid, certain aspirates (pleural/ascitic fluid), biopsy specimens and calculi.

All specimens are considered potentially dangerous (because of danger of infection) but of greatest concern to the laboratory staff are those of hepatitis B and HIV patients.

SELECTION OF A TEST FOR A CLINICAL PURPOSE

Different tests differ in their sensitivity and specificity for diagnosis of a disease. For example CK-MB levels are more specific than LD-levels in diagnosis of myocardial infarction. A highly specific test gives very few false positives (Table 1.2). Thus when you want to be very sure about the presence of the disease (a disease, for example, requiring prolonged, costly or toxic treatment), a test with high specificity should be used.

Some tests are more sensitive than others for diagnosis of a disease. For example increase of ALP is more sensitive than rise of bilirubin in diagnosis of cholestasis. A highly sensitive test gives very few false negatives (Table 1.2). Thus when you do not want to miss a patient due to false

Table 1.2. Specificity, sensitivity, efficiency and predictive value of a test for a disease

Specificity:
- TN(truly negative)/(TN + FP) (false positive) x 100
- It gives %age of TN in the normal group. A person found negative in a test with high specificity for the disease, is further explored for being without disease.

Sensitivity:
- TP (truly positive)/(TP + FN) x 100
- It gives %age of truly positives in total number, tentatively, having the disease. A person found positive in a test with high sensitivity for the disease, is further explored before being declared to be suffering from the disease.

Predictive value (PV) of a positive test:
- PV = TP/(TP+FP) X 100
- It is the %age of true positive among the total positives. To have high predictive value, the test should give very few false positives.

Efficiency (overall accuracy):
- TP+TN/Total No. of tests x 100 (it is estimate of sensitivity and specificity taken together)

negativity of the test (say a patient of AIDS, lest he should spread disease to others), a test with high sensitivity should be used.

When sensitivity and specificity are equally important, a test of high efficiency should be used Table 1.2.

For confirmation of a disease the predictive value of the test should be high. Predictive value further increases if the investigated group has high frequency of the disease (screening has already been done). A test used for screening need not have a high predictive value. A screening test should be cheap, easy to perform and with high sensitivity for the disease.

If a number of tests with different predictive values are used for diagnosis of a disease, the combined predictivity becomes higher (result of the tests and their predictive values can be analyzed with the help of a computer to make diagnosis, a more objective process). The probability approach to diagnosis of disease is discussed later.

Bias, accuracy and precision of a method

Once a method, depending upon clinical requirement, is selected with adequate specificity and sensitivity, its analytical accuracy and precision should also be known. As far as possible, method should

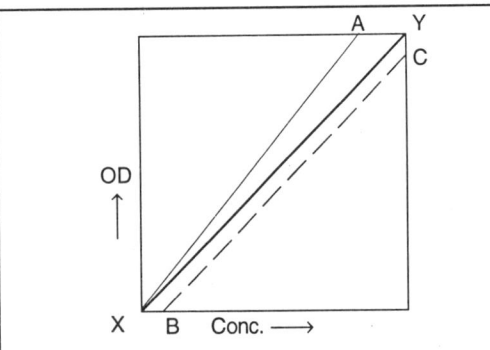

- In the operational line XY, the reported values are exactly as the actual value (unbiased reported values). Such a method would be ideal.
- In operational lines XA and BC, there are proportional, and constant biases, respectively. Those methods can also be used for which these lines are reproducible.

Fig 1.1. Proportional and constant biases in analytical methods.

be accurate without bias, although, in many cases it may not be possible. Methods with constant or proportionate or both types of biases are also used provided the operational lines for these methods are reproducible (Fig. 1.1). The bias in a method makes the analytical results correspondingly in accurate (although these may be useful and acceptable if the nature and magnitude of the bias are know). Consider, for example results of a method of glucose estimation (of constant bias) based on reducing property of glucose.

The term precision in an analytical method denotes variation between values in a replicate study (Fig. 1.2). Random analytic variations (resulting in imprecision) may be produced by a faulty automatic pipettor or weak photocells (in photometers) or by leaking electrodes. Imprecision is not uncommonly produced by errors which may arise from sample collection, mislabeling or because of a careless technician.

In a replicate study, precision is given by SD of the values. It is also denoted by co-efficient of variation (CV) which is calculated by dividing SD by the average in a replicate study and then multiplying by 100 to get percent CV. As far as allowable imprecision in a method is concerned, there is no single opinion in the matter. According to one opinion, the allowable imprecision should not be more than one fourth of the reference interval. Most people, at present, however, believe in relating method performance to biological variation of the analyte or to the need of the patient care. According to one proposal the tolerable analytical variation should be less than one half of the intrinsic biological variation.

In general, for most clinical measurements CV is not more than 5%, except that, in some enzyme estimations, CV of even 10% is acceptable.

QUALITY ASSURANCE IN BIOCHEMICAL INVESTIGATIONS

The control serum approach is widely used. The control serum is first run in replicates to workout mean and SD. Next, the control serum is run, certain times in between the clinical samples. Position of control sample values (in relation to mean ±2 SD, already worked out) is used to assess the status of quality control of the method (Fig. 1.3). In the

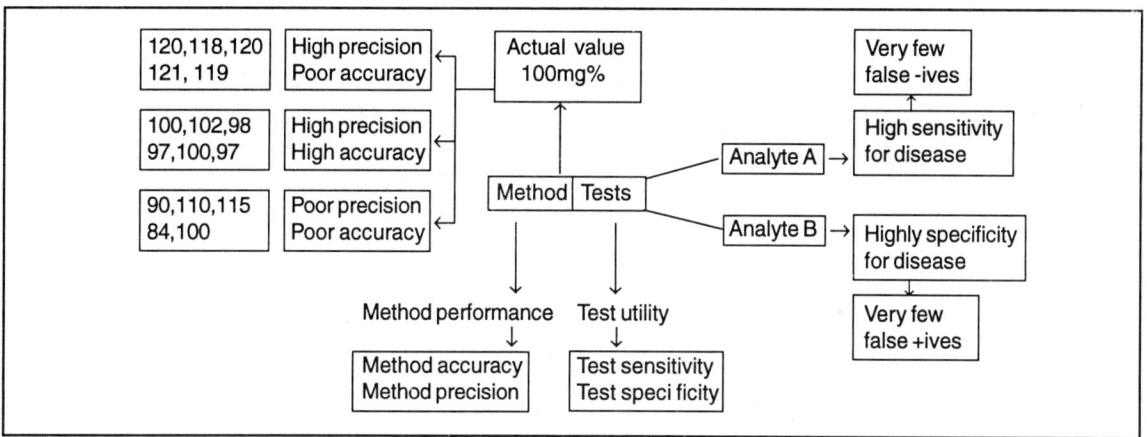

Fig. 1.2. Test suitability and method performace in clinical chemistry investigations.

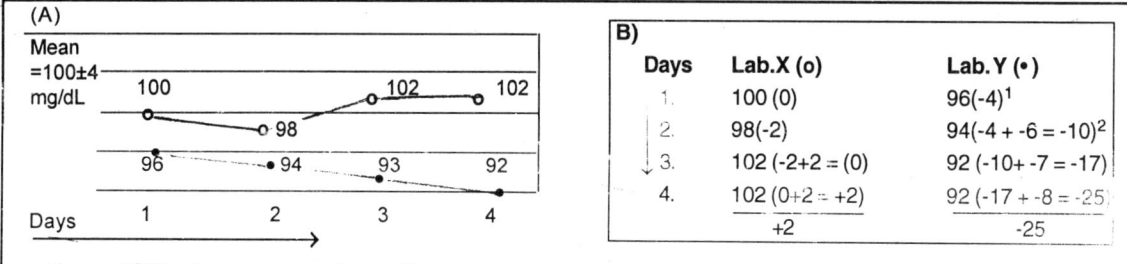

- Mean ± 2SD in the replicate analysis of the control serum was 100±4.
- Note random distribution of results (within±SD) for lab. X(o) and an increasing systemic error for lab. Y (•)
- In proper interpretation of quality control results, difference between routine conditions variance (RCV) and the optimal conditions variance (OCV) sould also be borne in mind. OCV means the variance around the actual values under ideal conditions (fresh reagents, perfectly clean glass ware and so on). RCV should not be higher than OCV by more than 3%.

Fig. 1.3. The control serum approach using Levey-Jenning control chart (A) and CUSUM control chart (B), to compare analytical errors of two laboratories X and Y for an analyte.

---

[1] CUSUM value on day 1 is the difference of the sample value from the mean value.

[2] CUSUM value on day 2 is obtained by adding the previous day's CUSUM value to the difference of the second day's actual value from the mean and so on. The CUSUM value on day 4 is - 25, indicating a significant negative systematic error.

Levey - Jenning control chart deviation from the assigned value is daily recorded in the form of a chart. Slope of the line is related to the size of the systematic error, occurring in the method. The laboratory may also participate in some regional quality control programme. In another simple approach, patient's serum is divided into two vials which are labeled like other samples but the technician is not informed about it. Difference in the two values of the sar... mple are related to the quality control status.

The total concept of quality assurance includes checks on pre-analytic, analytic and post analytic components of laboratory testing. The quality control methods mentioned above, actually test only the analytic component. And it is this component which in most laboratories is automated. It is thus equally important to take care of pre-analytic and post-analytic phases of the laboratory testing to ensure proper quality assurance. These components of laboratory work are greatly affected by excessive load of samples. Clinicians, thus can play an importa... ole in improving performance of clinical chemi... y laboratories by restricting the number of samples being submitted for analysis (Table 1.1). There is also need to increase level of awareness of the staff involved in obtaining, storing, transporting samples, about the type of errors which can make the result of analysis unacceptable. Processes like delta check and profile recognition while sending or while interpreting the reports, also help to recognize errors which might have been introduced at some stage of testing. These will be discussed under interpretation of results.

The computer based analysis is much more reliable than the manual one. However, all the medical computer programmes contain certain bugs which cannot be removed. Thus the reliability may fail at the most inconvenient time. Thus absolute faith in a single abnormal value can be disastrous even when it is computer analyzed.

INTERPRETATION OF TEST RESULTS

The reference range

In diagnosis of a disease, the results of biochemical analytes reported for the patient have to be interpreted in light of certain normal values. Because of biological variations, there are no fixed values for the levels of different analytes for the normal population. For working out the normal values,

samples from a sufficiently large number of normal individuals are analyzed. The values generally fall into a Gaussian distribution (Fig. 1.4). Two SD (Standard Deviation) above and below the mean value is described as the normal range of the analyte. It covers 95.5% of the total normal population while 4.5% of normal population will have values outside the range. If the values in normal population do not conform to a true Gaussian distribution the concept of standard deviation cannot be applied. In such cases instead of normal range the term normal reference interval is used and means the values that lie between 3rd and 97th percentiles (lowest 2% and highest 2% are not covered in the range). These days it is believed that if one actually determines analyte values in the large number of normal persons, often the values will not conform to true Gaussian distribution (since a very large group seldom remains homogeneous). Thus generally, values that lie between the 3rd and 97th percentiles (the reference interval) are used.

The reported analyte value for the patient (for diagnosis of disease) has to be interpreted in light of the reference range and the sensitivity and specificity characteristics of the analyte for diagnosis of the disease. As already pointed out the reference range does not include the lowest 2% and

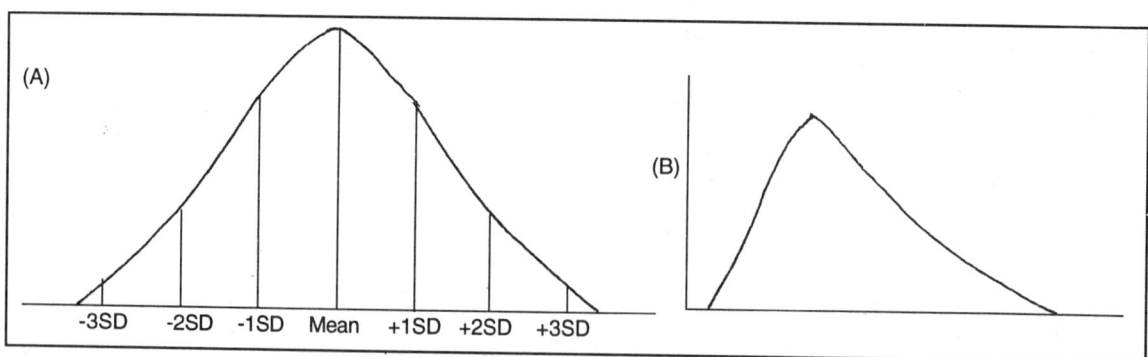

(A)

-3SD   -2SD   -1SD   Mean   +1SD   +2SD   +3SD

(B)

Fig. 1.4. Distribution of analyte values in normal population.

A)Normal Gaussian distribution of analyte values in a population. In normal population, Mean±2SD, will cover the normal range covering 95.5% of the normals. This is called normal range of the analyte for the population.

B)A skewed distribution curve (positively skewed). Positive skewing in the curve is due to mixing of a smaller group with values higher than those of the main group. The reference interval or range for the group lies between 3rd and 97th percentiles.

· These days, generally, reference range (and not the normal range) is used for interpreting the analyte results of the patients. While comparing, it should be remembered that the reference intervals are values for healthy adults not taking any drug. Further, independent effects of age, sex, diet, diurnal variations, exercise posture and pregnancy on the analyte level should be taken into account. Also effects of intravenous fluids, drugs or some diseases need to be considered.

highest 2% values for the normals. For this reason there is no sharp demarcation between the normal and the abnormal values. There is often an overlap of values between the normal population and the patients of the disease. In a test which is highly specific for the disease, in the above referred region of overlap of values, there will be very few normals beyond the cut off point. On the other hand in a test which is highly sensitive for the disease, in the overlap region, there will be very few patients, within the cut off point. See Fig. 1.5.

Other important points which need to be kept in mind while interpreting the reports are listed in Table 1.3.

Delta check and pattern recognition also help correct interpretation of the test values.

Delta check

This means comparing results of a sample with previous results (obtained for the same patient) before reporting the result. The change could be due to analytic plus physiologic variation or due to change in clinical condition of the patient. But there are limits to both type of alterations.

Pattern recognition

Change in the levels of a number of analytes provide

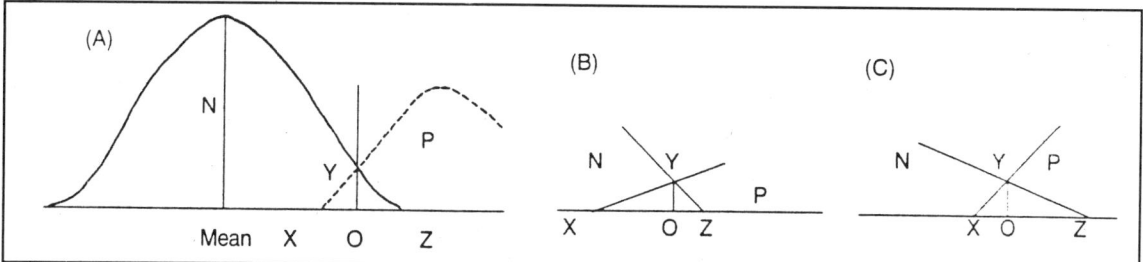

Fig. 1.5. Figures showing overlap regions between distribution curves of analyte values, for normals and the patients.

A) Showing regions XYO and ZYO. Patients included in XYO are false negatives. Normals included in ZYO are false positives.
B) Region XYO is much larger than ZYO. There are less false positives (test analyte of high specificity).
C) Region ZYO is much larger than XYO. There are very few false negatives (test analyte of high sensitivity).
Note: YO is the diagnostic cut off line (say the higher limit of the reference range) (say the higher limit of the reference range).

Table 1.3. Interpreting the reported level of an analyte

- More away a result, from the reference range, more likely that it represents the disease state; and in the probability approach (to diagnosis) more weightage of the result in changing the probability of the disease.
- Near the limit of the reference range, chances of presence of disease are more if the method is quite specific.
- Often the reference ranges are given for healthy adults. The effects of age, sex and any special physiological state of the patient are often there and must be taken into account.
- The reference range depends upon the analytic method used by the laboratory. It can vary from laboratory to laboratory. This is especially true for the ranges for enzymes. For technical reasons, different laboratories use temperatures varying from 25°C to 37°C for enzyme estimations and accordingly there will be lot of difference between their results. Differences similarly, relate to differences between the substrates and other factors (pH).
- Variations due to circadian rhythm or day to day variation may also be significant in some cases (estimation of iron and a number of hormones).
- Drug history of the patient should also be taken into account, as drugs are known to effect different analyte levels.
- Patient may also be suffering from some other disease which could effect level of test value.
- Apply delta check (useful in certain situations) and take supportive help from results of other investigations.
- In mutichannel analysis some times an unwanted abnormal value may be encountered. First its specificity to the pathological process should be known. In case of high specificity, some other confirmatory test may be required.

Table 1.4. Mutually supportive (for diagnosis of disease) tests[1]

- Liver disease (Transaminases, ALP, Albumin, Bilirubin, Ammonia): Acid base disorders (pH, Bicarbonate, pCO_2).
- Anemias (Blood film, Serum iron, Ferritin, Iron binding capacity, Haptoglobin, Bilirubin, B_{12} and Folate).
- Acute pancreatitis (Amylase, Lipase Calcium, Triglycerides, Glucose).

[1] Supportive help

mutual help in supporting diagnosis of a disease (Table 1.4). An unlikely combination in such profiles, some times can be useful in recognition of the laboratory error. The laboratory computer may be programmed to detect such unusual combinations.

In biochemical testing, there are large number of steps and each step is capable of introducing error in the laboratory results. Thus one should never rely on a single abnormal value to make diagnosis. The abnormal test must be repeated to establish the trend in values. Delta check and pattern recognition, as explained above, also help to place confidence in the abnormal values.

THE PROBABILITY APPROACH TO CLINICAL PROBLEM SOLVING

A clinician after examining a patient and after basic laboratory tests (blood counts, blood analysis and urinalysis develops a problem list for the patient. This leads to differential diagnosis and includes the most likely diagnosis which could explain patient's problems. An experienced clinician can give quantitative touch to the whole affair and give quantitative estimates of probabilities of different diseases considered in differential diagnosis (Fig. 1.6). Next, the clinician, selectively uses the laboratory tests to increase or decrease the pretest probability. This process continues till the post test probability is either high enough for the clinician to start the treatment or low enough to discard the diagnosis (Table 1.5). The level of probability, above which treatment can be started with confidence is called test-treatment threshold and the level of probability below which the diagnosis can be discarded with confidence is called test-no treatment threshold. The two thresholds referred above, differ with different

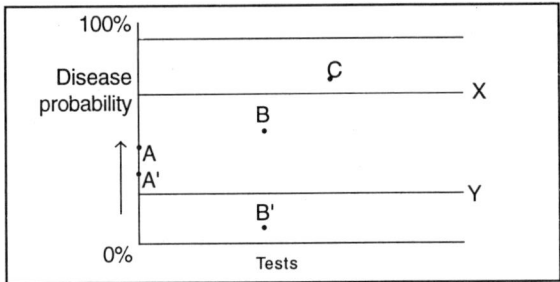

Fig.1.6. Disease probability, thresholds and test related changes in probability.

X = Treatment threshold   Y = No treatment threshold

Case 1: Position A represents disease probability at clinical evaluation; position B after the first test and position C after the second test. (disease should be treated)

Case 2: Position A' is probability at clinical evaluation; position B' after the first test (patient needs no treatment).

Table 1.5. Change in disease probability with results of a test of known sensitivity and specificity for the disease

- From clinical data of the patient the disease probability (pretest) = 20%. Test sensitivity for the disease = 90%. Test specificity for the disease = 70%

If test is positive:

Pretest odds of the disease=

  Pretest disease probability/100% - Pretest disease probability = 20/100-20

     = 1/4

[1]Likelihood ratio   = Sensitivity/1-specificity

                 = 0.90/1-0.70 = 0.90/0.30

Post test odds of the disease = 1/4 x 0.90/0.30 = 3/4

Post test disease probability = 3/7 x 100

                      = About 43%

If test is negative:

Pretest odds (as above) = 20/100-20 = 1/4

[2]Likelihood ratio = 1-Sensitivity/specificity

          = 0.10/0.7 = 1/7

Post test odds = 1/4 x 1/7 = 1/28

Post test probability = 1/29 x 100

             = About 3.5%

[1]Sensitivity = Probability of a +ive test result in a patient without the disease. (1-specificity) = Probability of a +ive test result in a patieht without the disease.

[2](1-Sensitivity) = Probability of a -ive test result in a patient with the disease. Specificity = Probability of a -ive test result in a patient without the disease.

- Disease prevalence in a group can be taken as disease probability and after a test we may find post test disease probability.

situations (the disease, the test and the test objective) and depend upon many factors like consequences of missing the diagnosis, risk of diagnostic tests, the complications of therapy and others. For example in case of liver cancer the test treatment threshold would be quite high knowing implications of diagnosis and treatment. In evaluating presence of hepatitis in a blood donar the test no-treatment threshold would be quite low as the missed diagnosis could result in great risk for the recipient.

This approach involving integration of clinical data and test results has several advantages. It presumes that neither clinical data nor the laboratory tests deserve absolute faith, but can support each other for diagnosis of disease. Pitfalls associated with accuracy of the laboratory tests have been highlighted in this chapter. Even when a laboratory is functioning under ideal conditions the value of certain test results remain ambiguous (Fig. 1.4).

This approach will also avoid unnecessary testing. The clinician will order tests, in a well planned sequence (with the objective of increasing probability of disease diagnosis at each step). For example in a patient with clinical evidence of hepatic metastases, increased bilirubin or alkaline phosphatase in serum will increase probability of disease diagnosis. On the other hand increase in bilirubin level in a jaundiced patient does not add any new information and the positive test will not increase probability of disease diagnosis.

In many recent books of Medicine such test algorithms or schemes (stepwise use of tests; each step with the objective of diagnosis in mind) for differential diagnosis of many diseases are available. Need is also realized to make available, from clinical data, well tested prediction rules. In this way a quantitative approach (using both clinical data and data from tests, each in quantitative form) to probability based patient diagnosis can be planned.

AUTOMATED ANALYZERS

These instruments help laboratories to process large number of samples quickly. Some manual steps which are automated are measuring the sample, measuring and adding reagents, incubating the sample-reagent mix, calibrating the assay, measuring and reading sample reaction and recording,

analyzing and storing sample data. The sample processing is also being automated (sorting, centrifugation, aliquotting). As per design of the pathway of analysis we have:

- Sequential testing: Multiple tests done one after another, on a given specimen.
- Batch testing: All samples are loaded at the same time and a single test is done on each sample.
- Parallel testing: More than one test done concurrently on a given sample
- Random access testing: Any test/tests performed on any sample in any sequence.

In the beginning, continuous flow chemistry analyzers were developed and the multichannel ones performed all tests on a sample, whether required or not. There was lot of wastage of reagents and confusion created by unwanted results. This lead to development of discrete systems which could analyze the sample for the test requested by the clinician. Most of the above analyzers are discrete type.

PHYSICIAN OFFICE LABORATORIES

Many analyses can be done close to the office of the physician looking after the patients. Attractive angles to the idea are, availability of the result immediately and no confusion arising from excessive load of samples, seen in the actual clinical chemistry laboratories. These laboratories however have their own problems. Generally these lack the services of properly trained persons and there is hardly any quality control of the work. Many tests will be done very infrequently. Not only quality of these will become very poor but even testing may also become uneconomical, since the kits may become out dated and wasted. In such laboratories only certain simple tests should be allowed and further these should be under control of main laboratory for training of the staff, purchase and maintenance of equipment and quality assurance.

CASE HISTORY: 1.1

A 62-year male presented with jaundice and discomfort in upper abdomen. For about previous ten days he had been passing dark urine and had anorexia. There is no prior history of hepatitis or blood transfusion or use if intravenous drugs. The attending clinician formed a problem list and the pretest probability was about 40% for malignancy and about 30% for hepatitis.

➤ How should this case be investigated further?
- In this case it can be easily persumed that bilirubin is of hepatic origin. At the first instance two investigations should be requested; ALT/AST and alkaline phosphatase.

Quite high levels of ALT/AST would have high sensitivity and specificity for hepatitis while quite high levels of alkaline phosphatase would have high sensitivity and specificity for cholestasis (and malignancy). Supposing AST was 100 U/L and alkaline phosphatase 150 U/L, probability for hepatitis would greatly increase. Subsequent attention should be focused on serology. Also, only, if Hepatitis-A IgM antibody is found negative, additional serological investigations should be undertaken. On the other hand if alkaline phosphatase level was very high (say >500 U/L) with only mild increase of AST, focus of further investigations would lie on imaging studies. Also see Table 1.5.

CASE HISTORY: 1.2

A 55-year-old man presented with abdominal pain radiating through the back. Pain started rather suddenly about 12 hours back. There was mild shock and abdomen was tender in epigastric region and there was only slight guarding.

➤ How should this case be investigated?
➤ How to avoid unnecessary investigations in general?
- The attending clinician should develop a problem list of the patient. When this list is formed probability for acute pancreatitis may be around 60%. Obviously a test with high sensitivity and specificity for acute pancreatitis should be requested. Thus estimations of serum amylase and lipase would be urgently required. A similar case could present in such a way that the problem list would point a high probability for severe hepatic damage. In that case the first investigation could be serum albumin or prothrombin time.
- In order to avoid unnecessary investigations the following points should be kept in mind: i) How high is the disease probability? ii) What is the liklihood that the diagnostic test will change the probability, sufficiently, to have an effect on either diagnosis or therapy? iii) What are costs and associated risks of the test providing new information? iv) What would be the clinical consequences if the diagnosis were missed or if the patient were misdiagnosed and treated? v) Is there scope of waiting and follow up?

OBJECTIVE TYPE QUESTIONS

Pick out the wrong statements.

1. Use of diagnostic tests in patient care

i) A test should be used if it helps diagnosis of a condition needing treatment.
ii) A test should be done to rule out a disease to save the patient from costly or harmful treatment.
iii) A test may be done to search for some new interesting fact about the disease.
iv) A test should be used if the results will be able to change the probability sufficiently to have an effect either on diagnosis or therapy.
v) Many times, it is prudent to recall the patient for observation and follow-up rather than subjecting him to a costly, potentially harmful tests of low specificity.

2. Clinical utility of a test

i) Accuracy of a test is commonly expressed in terms of its positive and negative predictive values.
ii) The predictive value depends upon the population on which the test is standardized.
iii) Once a test has high predictive value it will always have great clinical utility, for whatever purpose used.
iv) Sensitivity is probability of a positive test result in a patient with disease and 1-sensitivity indicates probability of the negative test result in a patient with the disease.
v) Specificity is probability of a negative test result in a patient without the disease, and 1-specificity is probability of a negative test result in a patient with the disease.

3. Reference range

i) It requires analysis of a sufficiently large number of normal healthy individuals.
ii) In the parametric method 95% reference interval is covered by mean±2SD.
iii) In the non-parametric method 95% reference interval is covered between 3rd and 97th percentiles.
iv) There is some overlap of values between the normal group and that of patients.
v) Because of the above referred overlap a mild increase in the analyte level above the upper limit of the reference range, leaves diagnosis of the disease uncertain.

4. Factors affecting reference values

i) Age and sex has statistically significant effect

on plasma levels of a large number of analytes.

ii) There is need for sepatate age related and sex related reference values for the population.

iii) For samples for estimations of several hormones (ACTH, cortisol, prolactin, GH), stress of venepuncture should be avoided.

iv) Mild exercise produces significant changes in plasma levels of glucose, albumin, ALT, creatinine, phosphate, urea, urate, potassium and total proteins.

v) For many analytes there are diurnal and day to day variations in the plasma levels.

5. The reference range

i) The observed intraindividual variance, in levels of repeated samples of an individual is sum of his biological variance plus the analytic variance.

ii) The group variance is larger than intra individual variance since it takes into account individual variances of a large number of persons.

iii) The reference values for the group depend upon the group variance.

iv) Reference ranges are equally sensitive to detect abnormal levels of an analyte in all individuals.

v) In some cases analytic variance is more than real biological variance.

6. Sensitivity, specificity and other terms

i) A more sensitive test shows greater percentage of true positives among the patients with disease.

ii) A more specific test shows greater percentage of true negatives in the control group.

iii) For screening a test with high specificity should be used.

iv) A test with higher predictive value shows greater percentage of true positives among total positives.

v) A test has higher overall accuracy, if it picks up greater percentage of total of true positives and true negatives among the total group.

7. Interference in clinical chemistry analysis

i) Hemolysed, lipemic or icteric serum is unsuitable for many clinical chemistry tests.

ii) Paraproteins and immunoglobulins may form complexes with certain enzymes and make their test results unreliable.

iii) Drugs/their metabolites also interfere in clinical chemistry analysis.

iv) For maintaining accuracy of the test values, the calibrating solutions should be prepared in water rather than serum as other serum constituents affect the results.

v) If there is three times increase in the number of drugs being taken by the patient, there may be 8 to 10 times increase in the number of laboratory tests being affected.

8. Sample collection

i) Bilirubin is photosensitive.

ii) Stress and anxiety may affect hormone levels.

iii) Tobacco smokers have increased plasma levels of cortisol.

iv) Addition of fluoride inhibits loss of glucose in a blood sample contaminated with bacteria or yeast.

v) Amylase activity may be inhibited by oxalate or citrate while lactate dehydrogenase and acid phosphatase are inhibited by only oxalate.

9. Hemolysis

i) It affects serum bilirubin level since Hb interferes in diazotization of bilirubin.

ii) Hb also inhibits serum lipase activity.

iii) Adenylate kinase released during hemolysis interferes in estimation of CK activity.

iv) Hemolysis will not occur if dry syringe is used for sample collection.

v) Hemolysis leads to increased serum levels of K^+, Mg^{2+} and LDH.

10. The sample

i) For estimations of glucose, triglycerides, cholesterol and electrolytes blood should be collected in basal state.

ii) Albumin and calcium levels increase if blood is collected in upright posture.

iii) Storage of serum even at 4°C leads to decrease in levels of both acid and alkaline phosphatases.

iv) Ingestion of alcohol increases plasma lactate, urate and triglyceride levels.

v) Chronic alcohol ingestion increases urate, γGT levels and leads to increase in MCV.

ANSWERS

1. No. (iii). This should not be done in clinical laboratory testing.

2. No.(iii). Not always; the test will have great utility if it is being used for the same purpose and on a similar population for which it was shown to have a high predictive value.

3. No.(v). In the probability approach of diagnosis of disease the uncertainty of the overlap region does not matter. The approach, in brief, is as under: (i) development of problem list from history, physical examination and basic laboratory

tests of the patient; (ii) development of differential diagnosis and probability; (iii) selective utilization of laboratory to rule in or rule out diagnosis.

4. No.(ii). Although statistically significant, most of these differences do not call for separate reference values (as these are a small in clinical terms) except in case of pregnant women and neonates.

5. No.(iv). If the ratio of individual variance to group variance is less than 0.6, the reference range will be insensitive to a significant change occurring in the analyte of the person; only a marked change will be detected. As the ratio increases the likelihood of small significant changes of the individual, lying outside the reference range also increase.

6. No.(iii). A cheap, sensitive and easy to perform test should be used.

7. No.(iv) To compensate for matrix bias the calibrating solution should be prepared in serum.

The matrix interference may affect performance of the instrument, reagents or it may alter properties of the analyte. It may also affect linearity of the test.

8. No.(iv). Not effective in inhibiting loss of glucose because of yeast contamination. Fluoride also decreases acid phosphatase activity, increases amylase activity and inhibits glucose oxidase activity used in estimation of glucose.

9. No.(iv). Factors which lead to hemolysis include venostasis, prolonged standing of blood, forceful ejection from syringe, violent mixing, excessive cooling and even fast centrifugation.

10. No.(iii). Level of acid phosphatase decreases (as it is very unstable) and not that of alkaline phosphatase (it may show slight increase). Level of inorganic phosphate also increases as organic phosphate is converted into inorganic phosphate.

CHAPTER 2

Fluid-Electrolyte Balance: Disorders

Water forms about 60% of body weight (Table 2.1) in men, 55% in women and 70% in infants and small children. It moves between different compartments, the movement being determined by osmotic force (interstitial fluid $\leftrightarrow$ ICF), or osmotic and hydrostatic forces (interstitial fluid $\leftrightarrow$ plasma). Water and electrolyte disturbances occur more commonly in infants and children since water constitutes a higher percent of their body weight than adults and also they have higher ECF/ICF ratio. The external exchanges of water are given in Table. 2.2.

ELECTROLYTES OF THE BODY

Important ions which determine osmotic pressure of our body fluids are Na^+ K^+, Cl^- and HCO_3^-. Concentrations of Cl^- and HCO_3^- in ECF also relate to hydrogen ion concentration (or pH) of ECF. In

Table 2.1. Water in different body comparments

Body water as percent of body weight		Distribution of water in different compartments (% of body wt.)	
Adult male	60	Intracellular fluid (ICF)	40
Adult female	50	Extracellular fluid (ECF)	20
Infants/ Small children[1]	70	Interstitial fluid	15
		Plasma	5

[1] ECF/ ICF ratio is also higher in this group than adults.

Table 2.2. The external exchanges of body water

Input (mL/d)	Output (mL/d)
As water (about 1500)	As urine (1500)(highly variable)
With food (about 1000)	Sweating (highly variable)
Metabolic water (about 300)	Feces (about 300)
	Invisible
	- Insensible perspiration (about 700)
	- In expired air (about 400)

- Invisible losses vary between 800-1200.

- Total obligatory loss is invisible loss plus obligatory urine volume (500; depends on solute load and urine concentrating ability) plus fluid loss in feces.

metabolic acidosis HCO_3^- level decreases while Cl^- may or may not increase. Reverse is true in metabolic alkalosis. Other ions like calcium, magnesium, phosphate, proteinate are much less important as electrolytes for determining osmotic pressure. Nevertheless, these are important for other functions.

Distribution of different ions in ECF and ICF is given in Table. 2.3. Na^+, Cl^- and HCO_3^- are important ions of ECF. These determine osmotic pressure and volume of the compartment. Relation of levels of Cl^- and HCO_3^- to hydrogen ion concentration of ECF was also mentioned above. K^+ is the most important cation of ICF. Other important ions are phosphate and proteinate anions. Charge on cations is balanced by charge on anions both in ECF and ICF. A large part of anion equivalence in ICF is provided by proteins, carrying about 8 negative charges per molecule.

Table 2.3. Electrolyte composition of body fluids[1]

Cations	Interstitial fluid/ plasma	ICF
Na^+	144 (142)	10
K^+	4 (4)	148
Ca^{2+}	3 (5)	2
Mg^{2+}	2 (3)	40
Anions		
Cl	114 (103)	—
HCO_3	30 (27)	10
Protein	1 (16)	40
Phosphate		
SO_4	3 (3)	150
Organic acids	5(5)	

[1]mEq/L

Sodium

Body contains about 58 mmol/kg of sodium, out of which 30% is in the bone and rest is distributed in the body fluids mainly in ECF. Na^+ of ECF along with its associated anions determines volume and osmotic pressure of ECF, which in turn, is important in determining water distribution across cell membrane.

Intake of sodium is quite variable (100 to 250 mmol/d). Kidney is highly efficient in maintaining sodium balance under highly variable intakes. Excessive intake, however, should be avoided as it

can lead to increase of blood pressure in susceptible individuals. In some population groups, low dietary K^+ has been linked with increased blood pressure. Aldosterone plays the major role in regulation of Na^+ excretion. Control of urinary excretion of Na^+ is discussed below.

Control of urinary excretion of Na^+, K^+, HCO_3^- and Cl^- in proximal tubules

In proximal tubules there is reabsorption of about 65% of filtered Na^+. The following mechanisms are involved: i) co-transport of Na^+ with solutes like glucose, amino acids and other organic acids; ii) reabsorption of Na^+ with HCO_3^- (explains about 90% of HCO_3^- reabsorption). It depends upon Na^+/H^+ exchange process at the luminal border of the tubular cells and requires involvement of carbonic anhydrase. Inhibitors of carbonic anhydrase cause bicarbonate diuresis by inhibiting the process; iii) active transport of Na^+ at no.1, above creates transepithelial potential difference (lumen negative) which promotes Cl^- reabsorption by the paracellular route; iv) reabsorption of Cl^- and some other anions also occurs by another process, probably, mediated by Na^+/H^+ exchange process; v) about 2/3rd of filtered water is reabsorbed (passively) by transepithelial osmotic gradient created by reabsorption of different types of solutes in the proximal tubules.

Control of proximal tubular sodium and water reabsorption is not well understood. An increase in ECF results in reduced reabsorption of sodium and water. It may involve change in peritubular hydrostatic pressure, or other mechanisms (arterial natriuretic peptide, angiotensin II, dopamine and others may have a role).

Thick ascending limb of loop of Henle

In this part, Na^+, K^+ and Cl^- are co-transported across the luminal border. Na^+ leaves the cell with the help of Na^+/K^+ ATPase. K^+ and Cl^- leave the cell by a cotransporter across basolateral membrane. Loop diuretics inhibit reabsorption of Na^+, K^+ and Cl^- by inhibiting the transporter.

Both in proximal tubule and the loop of Henle, total amount of Na^+ reabsorbed also depends on the filtered load crossing the sites.

Distal tubules and collecting ducts

The proximal part of distal tubules behaves like the thick ascending limb. The distal part of the distal tubules and the collecting ducts are relatively impermeable to Cl^-. Here much of Na^+ is reabsorbed in exchange for K^+ and H^+. Active Na^+ transport creates lumen negative transepithelial potential difference (TEPD). This facilitates secretions of K^+ and H^+ into the tubular fluid. Na^+ reabsorption in these segments is stimulated by aldosterone. It is also load dependent. The loop diuretics which interfere in Na^+ reabsorption in the ascending limb increase Na^+ reabsorption in the exchange segments.

Water reabsorption

About two third of filtered water is reabsorbed in proximal tubules. Water reabsorption also occurs in distal segments which is controlled by medullary interstitial concentration gradient and AVP. This facultative water reabsorption is adjusted as per body requirements, which is expressed through changes of osmotic pressure of ECF. Also see in Chapter 4.

Regulation of water balance

Water deprivation leads to increase in plasma osmolality and decrease of plasma volume. These changes bring about thirst and increased secretion of AVP. Thirst controls water intake and AVP controls loss of water in urine, to maintain water balance (Fig. 2.1). In pure water depletion, as shown in the Fig. 2.1, both increased osmolality of ECF and reduced plasma/ECF volume tend to increase AVP secretion, former being more effective than the latter. Some times however, the two mechanisms have opposing effects on AVP secretion. For example in a patient suffering from severe hypovolemia and also having reduced ECF osmolality. In such situations, volume regulating mechanism overrides the osmotic pressure regulating mechanism (read under hyponatremia).

Regulaion of ECF volume

As explained above, water in ECF is held and regulated by its osmotic effect which is provided by

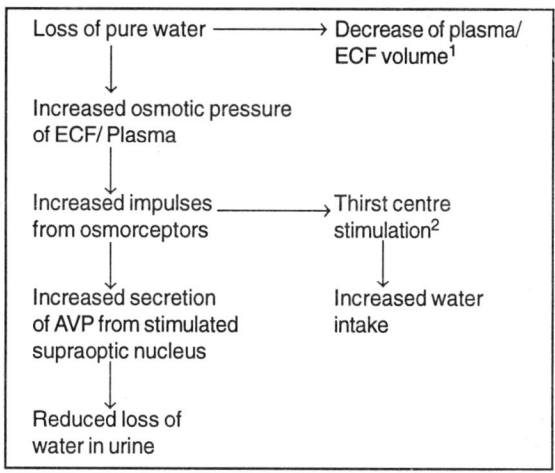

Fig. 2.1. Regulation of body water.

[1] Decreased plasma volume also stimulates AVP secretion. In pure water depletion, however, this is a much weaker stimulus than that provided by increase of ECF osmolality.

[2] In progressive dehydration increased AVP secretion occurs much earlier than stimulation of thirst centre.

Na^+ (and Cl^-). Thus with intact osmotic pressure regulating mechanism (mentioned above), the amount of Na^+ will determine ECF volume. In other words ECF volume regulation would also require ECF Na^+ regulation. Thus volume regulation is primarily done by altering Na^+ excretion (Fig. 2.2). Unlike thirst in water regulation, there is nothing like sodium thirst in sodium regulation.

Sodium and water reabsorption in some diseases

Normally, about 99% of filtered sodium is reabsorbed by renal tubules. In edematous states (congestive heart failure, nephrotic syndrome, ascites), the effective plasma volume is reduced, increasing secretion of aldosterone (by stimulating renin angiotensin system) and AVP and reducing GFR. All these lead to retention of sodium and water (more water than sodium). Failure to excrete adequate amount of free water is also a feature of hypothyroidism and Addison's disease. AVP secretion is also increased in chronic diseases, by pain and emotional and physical stress. In polycystic kidney, medullary cystic disease and tubulo interstitial disease, there is urinary wasting of sodium.

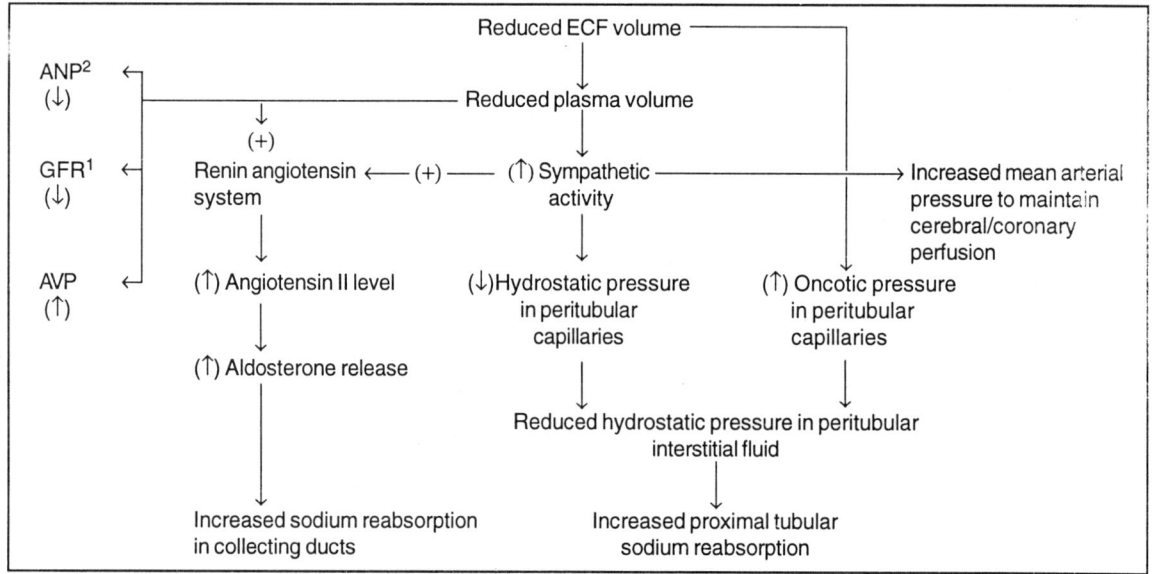

Fig. 2.2. Mechanisms involved in correction of ECF volume after its reduction.

---

[1] Reduced GFR leads to reduced urinary water and Na^+ loss.

[2] Reduced level of ANP helps actions of angiotensin II since ANP causes excretion of Na^+ and water by: i) increasing GFR; ii) inhibiting Na^+ reabsorption in proximal tubules; and iii) reducing release of renin and aldosterone.

- Local angiotensin II produced in hypothalamus (with reduced plasma volume) stimulates supraoptic nucleus (to increase ADH secretion and also the thirst centre). With increased secretions of both aldosterone and AVP, ECF volume is restored.

DISORDER OF WATER AND ELECTROLYTES

In these disorders certain changes occur in body electrolytes and water. Alterations in body sodium affect ECF volume since sodium forms backbone of ECF. Alterations in body water affect ECF osmotic pressure. Thus excessive loss of sodium from the body will reduce ECF volume and the plasma volume while excessive loss of water will increase osmotic pressure of ECF (Fig. 2.3) and also will produce hypernatremia.

Total body Na^+ determines ECF (and plasma) volume. Terms hyponatremia and hypernatremia only refer to plasma (and ECF) sodium level, without reference to total body sodium. A sodium depleted patient will have low ECF/plasma volume (condition called hypovolemia) but may be hypernatremic because of excessive loss of water. Similarly a patient with increased body sodium with increased ECF volume (hypervolemic), may be hyponatremic because of excessive water retention (as occurs in patients of edema).

In a very simple way disturbances of water and electrolytes may be classified as disorders of volume (hypovolemia and hypervolemia) related to total body sodium; concentration (hyponatremia and hypernatremia) related to body water; and composition (hypokalemia/hyperkalemia, acid base disorders and perhaps disturbances of calcium/magnesium levels). In a particular patient there may be a single problem or more than one problems presenting together. The disorders of volume and concentration may be named as under:

i) Pure water depletion (hypernatremia with near normal volume); and increased plasma and ECF osmolality.

ii) Pure water excess (hyponatremia with near normal volume); and decreased plasma osmolality.

iii) Sodium and water depletion: Patients in this group may have normal, low or high serum sodium levels. The common feature of all these patients is that they are hypovolemic and sodium depleted.

iv) Sodium and water excess (hypervolemia).

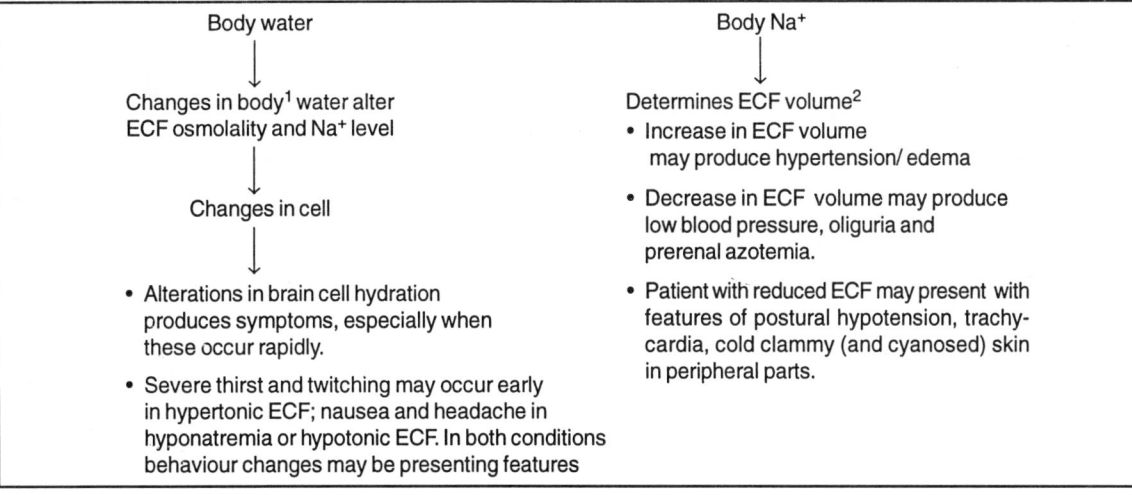

Fig. 2.3. Some fundamental relations in water and electrolyte disturbances.

[1] Monitored by plasma osmolality or by plasma Na^+.
[2] Monitored by hematocrit/ serum albumin level, and clinical parameters.

This group, mainly, includes patients of edema and ascites and may have hyponatremia. Some patients (primary aldosteronism, Cushing's syndrome, inappropriate fluid replacement) are not hyponatremic.

The above classification has etiological/pathophysiogical basis but many times the disorders are simply discussed as hyponatremia and hypernatremia. It may however be noted that a patient of hyponatremia may belong to group 2, 3 or 4. To differentiate patients of group 3 from others, these patients are said to have primary hyponatremia and others, secondary hyponatremia. Hypernatremia refers to pure water depletion, although, some patients of groups 3 and 4 can also present with hypernatremia.

Generally, there is no uniform relation between a clinical disease and the water, electrolyte disturbance it will produce. For example a patient of chronic renal failure (neither able to concentrate nor dilute urine), after excessive intake of water can present as a patient of hyponatremia and if enough water is not taken, he may present as a patient of hypernatremia. In acute secretory diarrhea or excessive vomiting, there is loss of fluid isoosmotic with plasma and often patient presents with hypovolemia with normal level of serum Na^+.

But these patients can also present with hyponatremia (read under hyponatremia). In some cases, however, the water, electrolyte disturbance can be predicted from history with greater confidence. For example a patient in coma on poor nursing care will uniformly present as a case of hypernatremia.

The point made in the above para is further emphasized in Fig. 2.4. In this figure disorders of fluid loss (hypovolemia) have been presented in three groups. In the first group of diseases, fluid loss is isoosmotic with plasma, in the second group there is more loss of Na^+ than water and in third group fluid loss is hypoosmotic with plasma.

Na^+ and K^+ are generally estimated together but their clinical significance is different and in general, altered K^+ levels carry much more clinical significance than altered Na^+ levels. Potassium metabolism is discussed separately.

Hyponatremia (Table 2.4)

It is significant fall of serum Na^+ level below the reference range (136-145 mEq/L), critical level being <120 mEq/L. It is a common water and electrolyte disturbance. It may occur as pure water excess or more commonly in conditions of water and sodium depletions. In the latter hypovolemic patients, hyponatremia occurs because of inappropriate replacement or because of natural tendency to retain more water than salt, in hypovolemia (Fig. 2.4). Hyponatremia also occurs in certain hypervolemic conditions associated with secondary aldosteronism. In these conditions body sodium is increased but paradoxically, there is hyponatremia. The sick cell syndrome also results in hyponatremia.

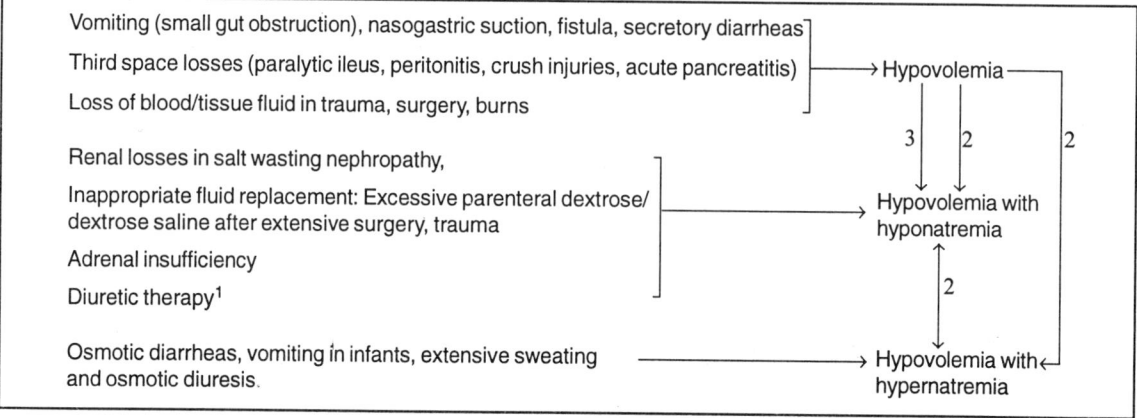

Fig. 2.4. Important causes of hypovolemia.

---

[1] Both thiazides and loop diuretics cause loss of Na$^+$ and produce hypovolemia. The AVP response (due to hypovolemia) retains more water in case of thiazides than the loop diuretics as in the latter case Na$^+$ delivery to renal interstitium is reduced, decreasing water retaining power of AVP. Thus hyponatremia is produced by thiazides and not loop diuretics.
[2] Inappropriate fluid administration.
[3] Because of overshadowing of osmotic pressure regulating mechanisms by volume regulating mechanisms in severe hypovolemia

Table 2.4. Types of hyponatremia and features

Hyponatremia and hypovolemia
- Non-renal causes include vomiting (small gut obstruction), nasogastric suction, fistulae, secretory diarrhea and third space losses (burns, crush injuries, surgery and others).
- Patients with renal losses include those with adrenal insufficiency, salt wasting nephropathies and using diuretics over prolonged periods.
- Many of these patients may be only hypovolemic to start with and develop hyponatremia, subsequently.
- Presenting features may be orthostatic hypotension, tachycardia, oliguria and prerenal azotemia.
- There is decreased plasma osmolality, decreased hematocrit/ serum albumin.
- Urine Na$^+$ is <10 mmol/L in nonrenal cases including use of diuretics in recent past (due to aldosterone response) and >20 mmol/L in renal cases or if there is lack of aldosterone response.

Hyponatremia without much alteration in ECF volume (see Table 2.5)
- Severe cases may present with features of increased brain cell hydration. Features may include nausea, headache, change in behaviour and even fits and coma (features of water intoxication).

Hyponatremia with hypervolemia
- These are patients of heart failure, hepatic cirrhosis, nephrotic syndrome and renal insuffuciency. These patients present with edema/ ascites. Not all these cases suffer from hyponatremia. Hyponatremia is due to reduced GFR which causes reduced delivery of fluid (Na$^+$ and water) to loop of Henle reducing free water excretion by kidney. In these patients (except those of chronic renal failure) secondary aldosteronism is involved in retention of Na$^+$. Na$^+$ is >20 mEq/L in acute/chronic renal failure and <10 mEq/L in other cases.

Pseudo hyponatremia in cases with high levels of plasma proteins or triglycerides (see Text).

Factitious hyponatremia in cases of high plasma osmolality due to presence of a substance which does not readily enter cells and thus causing movement of water from ICF to ECF.

Sick cell syndrome in chronic diseases like tuberculosis, carcinomatosis.

Pure water excess or hyponatremia with near normal volume

Important causes are given in Table 2.5. ECF osmolality is reduced and this causes movement of water from ECF into ICF resulting in overhydration of cells. The brain cell overhydration may cause headache, fits, confusion and coma (water intoxication). It should, however, be remembered that clinical features develop only if water accumulation and cellular hydration develop rapidly. If the process had been slow, the patient may be asymptomatic. In treatment of asymptomatic patients, only fluid restriction (say 800 mL/d) is enough. In symptomatic patients careful slow administration of 0.9% or 3.0% saline should be undertaken so that osmotic equilibrium is accomplished gradually (to avoid acute volume overload or pontine myelinosis). It is advisable to use a loop diuretic to promote excretion of isotonic urine, with use of 0.9% or 3% saline administration. During this therapy, monitoring should be done by auscultation of lung bases for crepitations and by study of jugular venous pressure.

Hyponatremia with hypovolemia (mixed sodium and water depletion)

In many patients there is excessive loss of isotonic fluids (Fig. 2.4, Table 2.4). In these patients because of reduced ECF, circulation is impaired. Initially the patient may complain of postural hypotension followed by hypotension and shock. Impaired renal circulation causes oliguria. Cell hydration is not altered. The volume and osmotic pressure regulatory mechanisms go into operation to restore plasma volume and Na^+ level. In severe cases, volume regulatory mechanisms overshadow osmotic pressure regulatory mechanisms with resultant tendency to retain water (Fig. 2.5) and perpetuate hyponatremia. If the replacement fluid is inadequate in sodium, tendency to hyponatremia is further augmented. Hypovolemia with hyponatremia is quite likely after a major surgery, if volume depleted patients are infused with normal dextrose saline. Glucose is metabolized and more water than sodium enters the system. In these patients, in the immediate postoperative period, kidney is unable to excrete dilute urine because of increased secretion of AVP. Water and electrolyte problems arise if the post operative period is prolonged due to extensive sepsis or some other complication. In such patients one should alternate dextrose saline with isotonic saline.

Adrenal insufficiency (without loss of aldosterone secretion) also leads to hypovolemia with hyponatremia. Cortisol deficiency increases secretion of AVP and also increases permeability of renal tubules to water. A similar picture may result from vigorous diuretic therapy. Diuretic treatment, in addition, alters potassium and hydrogen ion levels. There is more free water retention with thiazides than loop diuretics.

More severe hypotension results when hyponatremia complicates hypovolemia than in hypovolemia alone as in the former case ECF water enters cells further depleting ECF and plasma volumes. Regulatory reflexes also do not function well in hyponatremia with sodium depletion. Renal power to excrete dilute or concentrated urine also needs proper amount of fluid/Na^+ delivered to nephron segments involved in delivering sodium to medullary

Table 2.5. Important causes of hyponatremia with near normal ECF

- Excessive administration of 5% dextrose (surgery/trauma) or oxytocin and 5% dextrose during management of a case of delivery.
- In adrenal insufficiency and hypothyroidism there is impaired excretion of water and disordered regulation of AVP secretion ($\downarrow$GFR, $\uparrow$AVP).
- Psychogenic polydipsia: Low plasma osmolality, urine osmolality <250 mOsmol/Kg, urine Na^+ >20 mmol/L.
- Syndrome of inappropriate secretion of ADH hormone (SIADH) It is caused by disorders of central nervous system including trauma, infection and tumor, drugs, ectopic AVP (small cell lung carcinoma), and inflammatory lung diseases (tuberculosis).

- In all these cases urine sodium >20 mEq/L as there is no hypovolemia and no increased aldosterone.
- For diagnosis of SIADH, increased Na^+ excretion (>40 mEq/L), high urine osmolality (>250, often >500 mOsmol/kg), urine osmolality > serum osmolality, decreased BUN and serum uric acid are important findings. Fluid restruction causes clinical and biochemical response.

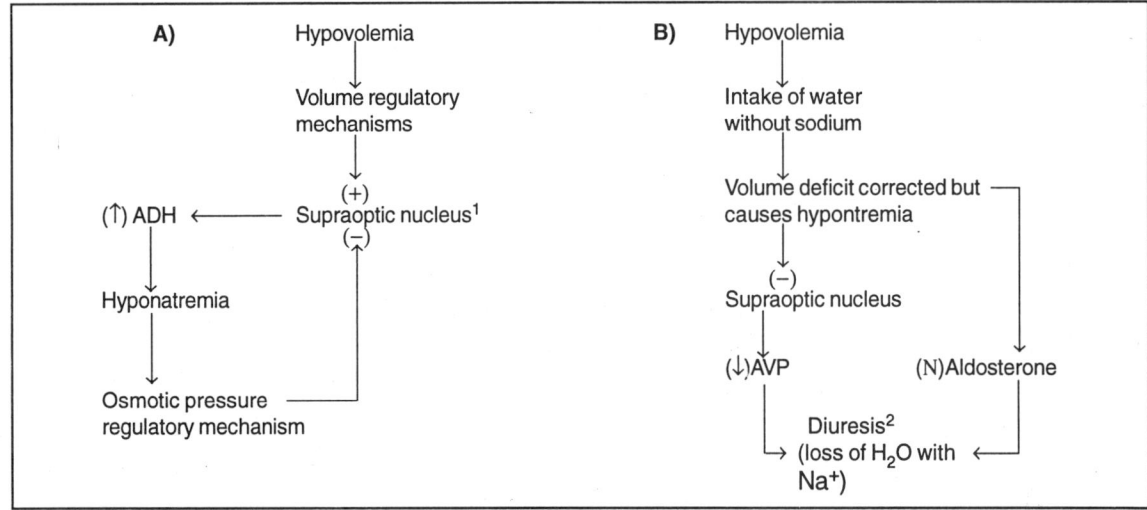

Fig. 2.5. Hypovolemia promoting urinary Na$^+$ loss and hyponatremia.

[1] The regulatory requirements of hyponatremia and hypovolemia have opposite effects on AVP secretion (the effect of the latter may overshadow the effect of the former); in severe hypovolemia, hyponatremia may result.

[2] It may be noted that correction of hypovolemia by intake of only water, not only results in hyponatremia but also promotes further loss of Na$^+$.

interstitium. This is impaired in severe sodium depletion or when GFR is reduced. Besides treating the cause, the treatment is directed towards increasing plasma volume with normal saline. In severe cases or cases with loss of protein in exudate (burns), a plasma expander may also be required along with normal saline. Patients of hyponatremia should be treated slowly and carefully. Blood pressure, JVP (CVP in critically ill patients or patients of heart disease) and urine volume are monitored during treatment. Severe acidosis if present, is treated with 1.26% sodium bicarbonate solution. Blood gases and pH monitoring will be needed in such cases.

Hyponatremia of malnutrition and chronic diseases (Table 2.4)

It is caused by movement of water from ICF to ECF because of reduced osmotic pressure of ICF, which inturn is caused by loss of cellular potassium or reduced synthesis of intracellular osmotically active particles due to disease and there is abnormal setting of hypothalamic osmoreceptors. This condition is also called sick cell syndrome and is associated with many diseases. Treatment is needed

for the primary disease and not for hyponatremia.

Hyponatremia with hypervolemia (Table 2.4)

Hypervolemia follows sodium retention. Hypervolemia with hyponatremia occurs in many conditions associated with secondary aldosteronism. It may occur in patients of edema and ascites. In these conditions of expanded ECF (due to retained Na$^+$), there may be hyponatremia because of impairment of water excretion. The renal impairment arises from increased AVP release due to reduction of effective arterial blood volume. Patients are treated with sodium and water restriction and careful use of a loop diuretic.

Diagnosis of cause of hyponatremia

Diagnosis of hyponatremia is based on history and clinical examination and by demonstrating low Na$^+$ level. History and clinical examination are also important in establishing cause of hyponatremia:

i) Rule out recent diuretic therapy and edematous states (history, clinical examination, urine Na$^+$ <10 mmol/L).

ii) Plasma osmolality is important to rule out pseudohyponatremia and psychogenic polydipsia. It is low in psychogenic polydipsia and raised in some cases of pseudohyponatremia (hyperglycemia, mannitol infusion) but remains normal in other cases (hyperproteinemia, hyperlipidemia, bladder irrigation).

iii) It is important to look for evidence of hypovolemia which may be clinical (low blood pressure, postural dizziness/hypotension, oliguria and signs of dehydration) or biochemical including increase of hematocrit/serum albumin (features of reduced plasma volume) and rise of blood urea and serum creatinine (reduced GFR resulting from reduced renal perfusion).

iv) If hypovolemia is established one may be required to differentiate between renal and extrarenal cause of excessive losses (Table 2.4). Urine Na^+ is <10 mmol/L in non-renal cases and >20 mmol/L in renal cases. The latter include acute/chronic renal failure, aldosterone ineffectivity, osmotic diuresis and during diuretic therapy.

v) In cases of pure water excess, history and clinical examination may point towards water retention as the cause for the disorder (important causes being, hypothyroidism, Addison's disease, psychogenic polydipsia and SIADH). These patients are normovolemic.

   a) Rule out sick cell syndrome as the cause, if there is pure water excess.

   b) Also rule out any stress, pain, nausea, hypotension or drugs as cause of hyponatremia. One should remember that because of these factors, mild hyponatremia is a very common finding in hospital patients.

   c) If a) and b) are ruled out, the differential diagnosis generally, lies between hypothyroidism, Addison's disease and SIADH. After ruling out Addison's disease and hypothyroidism one must establish diagnosis of SIADH (hyponatremia with appropriately low osmolality of plasma, often <280 mOsmol/kg) and find out the cause for the same (which may be curable). SIADH is often associated with hypouricemia due to mild volume expansion of the disorder.

For treatment it is important to know about presence or absence of hypovolemia. Hypovolemia is generally seen in primary hyponatremia cases. These cases, often symptomatic, require treatment.

In an otherwise healthy patient of primary hyponatremia both Na^+ and water deficiencies should be corrected simultaneously. This takes care of alkalosis due to volume contraction, also. In a patient with neurological symptoms or if hyponatremia is caused by renal salt wasting or if cardiac reserve is poor, Na^+ is first restored with an isotonic sodium containing solution. In severe cases 3% NaCl solution may also be used, initially, to be followed by slow infusion of isotonic solution.

Hypernatremia

It refers to plasma Na^+ level and not to total body Na^+. Serum Na^+ level >145 mEq/L is called hypernatremia (critical level is >160 mEq/L). Hyper natremia may occur with low, normal or high body volumes.

Hypernatremia with near normal volume (pure water depletion)

Important causes are given in Table 2.6. Water is distributed between ICF and ECF in the ratio of 2:1 and therefore in cases of pure water depletion there is two fold greater reduction of ICF than ECF water. Increased ECF osmolality leads to movement of water from ICF to ECF resulting in cellular dehydration. Brain cell dehydration results in thirst, mental confusion and other neurological features (Fig. 2.3).

Hypernatremia with hypovolemia

This occurs in infants and small children suffering from severe vomiting and/or diarrhea. At this age the intestinal fluid loss is hypoosmolar, with respect to plasma. In adults, vomiting and secretory diarrhea result in loss of iso-osmotic fluid causing only volume contraction or volume contraction with hyponatremia. (Fig. 2.4). Severe volume contraction with iso-osmotic fluid loss results in hyponatremia either due to inappropriate fluid replacement or because of the volume regulating mechanisms (Fig. 2.5).

Table 2.6. Important causes of hypernatremia with reduced or near normal volume

1. Excessive loss from lungs/skin (hot dry climate, fever, mechanical ventilation).
2. Poor nursing care in unconscious/dysphagic patients.
   - In the above two groups of cases there is excretion of minimum volume of urine which is maximally concentrated. Also ECF volume may not be much reduced.
3. Gastrointestinal fluid losses (vomiting, diarrhea). In infants the intestinal fluid is hypoosmolar with respect to plasma (it is iso-osmolar in adults). In osmotic diarrheas again fluid loss is hypoosmolar (isoosmolar in secretory diarrheas). In these patients hypernatremia may result from the fluid loss and inappropriate fluid replacement.
   - In these cases there is excretion of maximally concentrated, minimal volume of urine. ECF volume may be reduced.
4. Conditions causing diuresis with predominant loss of water (diabetes insipidus, osmotic diuretics, loop diuretics). In neurogenic diabetes insipidus 24h urine volume is more than 3L with osmolality <200 mOsmol/kg and in cases of osmotic diuresis and nephrogenic diabetes insipidus urine osmolality is >300 mOsmol/kg.

- In patients of groups 1, 2 and 3 the natural response to hypernatremia results in formation of about 500 mL of highly concentrated (osmolality >800 mOsmol/kg) per day.
- The patients of group 4 do not show urine volume and urine osmolality as mentioned above.
- Patients of group 4, with urinary osmol excretion of less than 750 mOsmol/d are likely patients of diabetes insipidus and those with higher excretion, may be patients suffering from osmotic diuresis or those with renal causes of fluid loss.
- In patients with inappropriate intake of Na^+ not shown in the Table, as there is volume expansion (with hypernatremia) there is natriuresis (sodium excretion in urine >100 mmol/L).

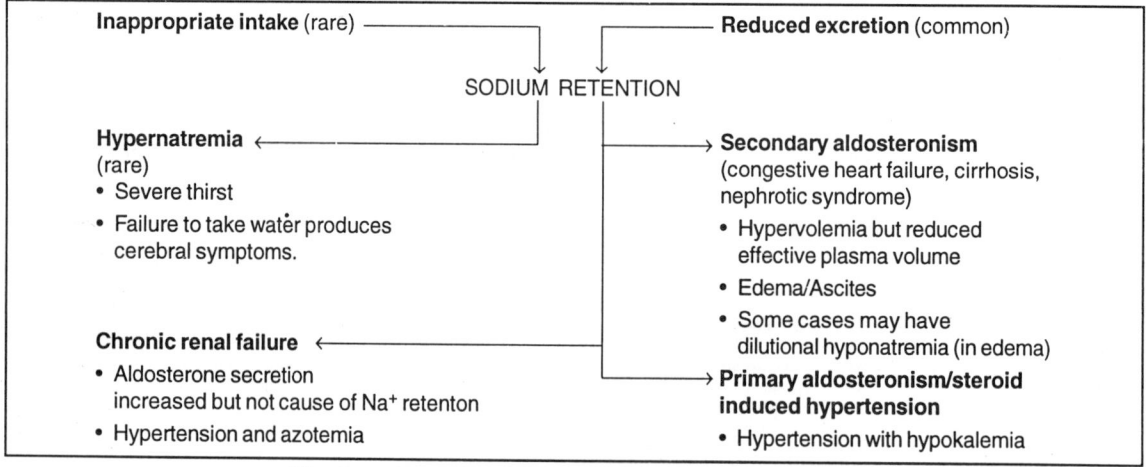

Fig. 2.6. Disorders of sodium retention (hypervolemia).

Hypernatremia with hypervolemia (Table 2.7)

This infrequent condition is often iatrogenic; produced by inappropriate administration of hypertonic NaCl or $NaHCO_3$. Other causes are administration of hypertonic tube feedings without administration of enough water and by use of high salt infant formula (sugar replaced by salt). These are cases of increased body sodium as well as hypernatremia. Other conditions with increased body sodium may not show hypernatremia (Fig. 2.6).

At this stage it is also worth referring to the terms hypoosmolality and hyperosmolality which refer to osmotic pressure of plasma. Although, Na^+ is the major determinant of osmotic pressure (and hyponatremia is almost synonymous with hypoosmolality), hyperosmolar state can also be produced by accumulation of solutes other than Na^+. However, effective hyperosmolality is produced only, when the solute does not readily enter cell (like Na^+). Some conditions of hyperosmolality, actually, produce hyponatremia (Table 2.7).

Diagnosis of hypernatremia and its cause

Clinical history and physical examination greatly help diagnosis of cause of hypernatremia which requires demonstration of high plasma Na^+ level. Features of volume contraction and presence or absence of neurological symptoms will also influence the management of the patient.

First of all, one should be able to differentiate between iatrogenic cases (administration of hypertonic NaCl or $NaHCO_3$) from others. ECF volume is increased in these patients (also urine Na^+ is high >100 mmol/L) but not in others. Supporting clinical history will be there.

After excluding the iatrogenic cases it is important to differentiate between cases with extrarenal and renal losses of hypotonic fluids. If there is extrarenal fluid loss (Table 2.6), urine volume is reduced with high osmolality (>800 mmol/kg) and low sodium (<10 mEq/L).

Once renal fluid loss has been established as the caused of hypernatremia, one should differentiate between fluid loss due to osmotic diuresis (diabetes, chronic renal disease, use of diuretics) and water diuresis (DI, neurogenic and nephrogenic). Tests related to osmolality (urine osmolality, urine osmol excretion and U/S osmol ratio) become important. In osmatic diuresis urine osmolality is generally >300 mOsmol/kg and <250 mOsmol/kg in water diuresis. For differentiating neurogenic from nephrogenic DI, see Chapter 13.

In pure water depletion without Na^+ deficit or renal dysfunction, water is given orally or intravenously, as 5% dextrose solution. In severe cases total body deficit may be calculated (see under investigations) and two third deficit corrected in first 24h and the rest in next 24 to 48h. In cases of volume deficit, as treatment of hypernatremia progresses with 5% dextrose solution, it is followed with 0.45% sodium chloride solution or with normal saline (if sodium deficit is significant).

EDEMA (Table 2.7, Fig. 2.6)

Edema is produced by accumulation of excessive fluid in the interstitial compartment. Clinical edema is produced when interstitial fluid is increased by more than 10%. Important causes of generalized

---

Table 2.7. Conditions with increased total body Na^+/other solutes

Increased body Na^+:

- Primary aldosteronism/increase of other adrenal steroids: In these cases there is increase of both ECF and plasma volumes, but plasma osmolality and Na^+ levels remain normal. Hypertension and hypokalemia are present.
- Cases of edema associated with secondary aldosteronism (heart failure, cirrhosis, nephrotic syndrome): In these cases ECF is increased while effective plasma volume is reduced. Plasma osmolality/Na^+ may be normal or reduced.
- In cases of chronic renal failure Na^+ retention is because of renal excretory failure not related to increased level aldosterone secretion. There is increase of both ECF and plasma volumes. There will be evidence of oliguric stage of chronic renal failure or that of acute renal failure.
- Inappropriate intake of Na^+: These cases present with hypernatremia and increased plasma osmolality. There is severe thirst but condition becomes serious if there if failure of water intake (in an infant, semiconscious patient or in a patient suffering from some neurological disorder).

Entry/accumulation of other solutes:

- Hyperglycemia may occur due to failure of glucose to enter cells as in diabetes or because of rapid infusion of glucose into blood.
- Mannitol infusion to reduce cerebral edema
- Fluids used for bladder irrigation during transurethral resection of prostate:
    - In all these cases there is hyponatremia produced by increased AVP secretion (and shift of water from ICF to ECF), both changes being triggered by increased ECF osmolality. Expansion of ECF will reduce, aldosterone secretion resulting in natriuresis.
- Accumulation of alcohol or urea in chronic renal failure: Urea and alcohol are rapidly equilibrated between ECF and ICF. Thus, there is neither increased secretion of ADH nor movement of water from ICF to ECF. In all cases of solute accumulation there is osmotic diuresis. Total 24h urine volume is more than 3L and urine osmolality is more than 300 mOsmol/kg.

edema are congestive heart failure, nephrotic syndrome, cirrhosis with ascites, hypoproteinemia and chronic renal disease. In these conditions, except renal failure, expansion of interstitial compartment is initiated by some primary factor followed by secondary events which actually expand the interstitial space to produce edema. The primary factor may be reduced cardiac output (in congestive heart failure), reduced plasma oncotic pressure (in hypoalbuminemia) and so on. All these result in reduced effective arterial volume, which by altering intrarenal hemodynamics, initiates the process of Na^+ and water retention. Important intrarenal changes are, reduced GFR, reduced renal interstitial hydrostatic pressure and stimulation of renin secretion from juxta glomerular cells (ultimately leading to increased secretion of aldosterone). In the presence of the primary factor (referred above) retention of Na^+ and water by the above mechanisms is not able to restore effective arterial volume and therefore Na^+ and water retention continues and edema occurs. Reduced GFR may result in more retention of water than salt and this results in hyponatremia. Arterial natriuretic peptide (ANP) is also elevated in hypervolemic states and tends to oppose vasoconstictor and Na^+ retaining actions of angiotensin II (Chapter 15). In edematous states, however there is end organ resistance to its actions and it is ineffective in counteracting the effects of angiotensin II.

Principles of treatment include, dealing with the primary factor, and increasing urinary loss of salt and water by the use of diuretics (intake of salt and water is also restricted). ACE-inhibitors may also help if kidney functions are not impaired.

INVESTIGATIONS FOR WATER AND ELECTROLYTE DISORDERS

History and clinical examination are very important in diagnosis of water and electrolyte disturbances. History will make clinician suspect a particular type of disorder. Examination of the patient should strengthen his suspicion. Features of alterations of ECF and cellular hydration are given in Fig. 2.3. The fluid balance charts help to follow the disorder during management. Certain

biochemical investigations are also useful (see below).

Serum sodium

Indications of sodium estimation are given in Table 2.8. Before attaching any significance to a serum sodium level, it should be ascertained that the level has not been influenced by high levels of serum lipids or proteins. If serum protein or lipid level is high, the aqueous phase of plasma (containing sodium and other water soluble substances) is reduced. If sodium is estimated by a flame photometer, the sample volume is not true representative of the aqueous phase of plasma containing sodium. Thus the estimated values will be lower than the true values. This is called pseudohyponatremia. Ion-selective electrodes give correct results in such cases.

Table 2.8. Some important indications of Na^+ estimation[1]

- In a disorder likely to produce hypernatremia, especially in an infant/old individual/unconscious person.
- In a patient of diabetic ketoacidosos.
- To differentiate psychogenic polydipsia from other causes of polyuria (in psychogenic polydypsia there is mild hyponatremia with low/low normal, blood urea/serum creatinine). Also see Chapter 13.
- To decide about the type of fluid to be used in a patient requiring fluid therapy.
- To monitor a patient of water and electrolyte disorder on intravenous fluid therapy.
- For urine Na^+, see Table 2.9.

[1] Effect of lipemia may be overcome by drawing sample in fasting state.
- In cases of hyperglycemia serum Na^+ level should be corrected (for each 100 mg increase in blood glucose increase the obtained value by 1.6 mmol/L.)

Urine sodium

Urine sodium is not very helpful in making initial diagnosis of the disorder but may be helpful in supporting the diagnosis once already made. For example a patient of hyponatremia with hypovolemia (or sodium depletion) should have reduced excretion of sodium in urine (due to aldosterone response to hypovolemia). If sodium excretion is not reduced the patient should be investigated for adrenal failure, or a disease at the kidney level (salt losing kidney) (Table 2.4).

During treatment of hypovolemia with extra renal fluid loss, urine sodium level may be used to judge adequacy of fluid replacement. Urine sodium level should be >30 mmol/L, once volume restoration is adequate. Urine sodium level is also used to differentiate prerenal azotemia from acute renal tubular necrosis. See Table 2.9.

Plasma and urine osmolalities

Serum sodium level is a rough guide to plasma osmolality, although, actual osmolality also depends upon other ions and molecules as shown below:

Plasma osmolality = $2[(Na^+) + (K^+)]$ + (Urea) + (Glucose) (all levels expressed as mmol/L).

Plasma osmolality can be determined with the help of an osmometer. A large discrepancy between the estimated and calculated osmolalities indicates presence of some unusual osmotically active substance (say alcohol in alcohol intoxication) in plasma.

Increased osmolality of plasma may be due to urea (renal disease), glucose (diabetes mellitus or glucose infusion), ethanol (alcohol intoxication) or some ingested drug/toxin, besides due to sodium. High plasma osmolality produces harmful effects by producing cellular dehydration. But this is only possible if the substance, accumulated in plasma does not enter cells, readily. Thus cellular dehydration does not occur in renal disease or ethanol intoxication, since both urea and ethanol, readily enter cells. As sodium is present in plasma in much higher concentration (mmol) than other substances, plasma hypoosmolality is almost always due to hyponatremia.

Ratio of urine/plasma osmolalities can be used to differentiate between different causes of polyuria (Table 2.9 and Table 4.1).

Hematocrit value

The hematocrit value, hemoglobin and serum albumin levels are important guides to the status of ECF. The values are increased with decrease of ECF volume and vice versa. Levels of these parameters also depend on nutrition of the individual. This limits their usefulness in prediction of hypo or hypervolemia, when used for the first time in a patient.

Assessment of renal circulation

Reduced renal circulation is good indicator of early stages of hypovolemic shock. It results in oliguria and increased serum levels of creatinine and urea.

Table 2.9. Use of urinary Na^+ and osmolality in diagnosis

Prerenal azotemia and azotemia due to renal disease:
- Urine Na^+ <10 mmol/L in prerenal azotemia and >20 mmol/L in azotemia due to renal disease.
- Urine osmolality >500 mOsmol/kg water in prerenal azotemia and <300 mOsmol/kg water in azotemia due to renal disease.

Diagnosis of cause of hyponatremia:
- In primary hyponatremia (Na^+ and water depletion) there is associated hypovolemia. If fluid loss is extrarenal Na^+, concentration in urine will be less than 20 mmol/L and if it is renal it will be more than 20 mmol/L.
- In SIADH urine Na^+ is >40 mmol/L (no aldosterone secretion) and urine osmolality is more than 250 mOsmol/kg.
- In primary polydipsia urine is very dilute osmolality <250 mOsmol/kg; U/S osmol ratio <1.0 which increases to >1.0 on water deprivation; urine Na^+ <20 mmol/L.

Diagnosis of cause of hypernatremia:
- In cases of volume depletion, if cause is osmotic diuresis, daily solute excretion will be >750 mmol (normal about 600 mmol on normal diet).
- In neurogenic diabetes insipidus (DI) volume depletion is minimal and urine osmolality is <250 mOsmol/kg. U/S osmol ratio is <1.0 in complete central or nephrogenic DI and does not change on water deprivation. In partial DI the ratio increases to >1.0 on water deprivation.
- If cause is lack of adequate water intake (stuporous patient), urine volume will be very small (say about 500 mL) and osmolality >800 mOsmol/kg.

Water deficit in hypernatremia

Body water is about 60% of body weight, in a well nourished lean adult. If serum sodium is 160 mEq/L, the water deficit is calculated as:

Water deficit = 0.6 × Body wt. (kg) × (160-140)/140 (where 140 mEq/L is the level of sodium prior to loss of water.) 2/3rd water deficit is corrected in first 24h and remaining in the next 24h. Water is given as 5% dextrose or as hypotonic saline.

MANAGEMENT OF WATER ELECTROLYTE DISORDERS

Fluid therapy may be in the form of simple maintenance e.g., in a patient after elective surgery. The maintenance requirement increases in a hyperthermic or hyperventilating patient. The maintenance requirement can be given in the form of any balanced salt solution (like lactated Ringer's solution). In some patients there may be fluid deficits before admission. In such a case, along with the maintenance requirement there is need to repair the existing deficit. If the amount and the type of fluid lost can be roughly assessed from history and weight loss, the existing deficit can be calculated. There are also rough methods for assessment of certain deficits. In hypovolemia cases, poor skin turgor and

dry oral mucous membrane are considered as poor markers of ECF depletion. Still in adults, a deficit of 3 to 5 litres may be present in their presence. Along with mucous membrane and skin changes the patient may also have non-specific features like weakness, muscle cramps, thirst, and postural dizziness. A more severe patient may also present with features of end organ ischemia (oliguria, cyanosis, abdominal and chest pain and a state of confusion), predicting still higher fluid deficit.

The sequestered third space losses are also included in deficits (although difficult to assess accurately). In a distal small gut obstruction there may be sequestration of 4 to 6 litres of fluid (composition similar to that of ECF).

Some patients present with existing deficits and there may also be ongoing losses (say continuous gastric suction). In such a case fluid corresponding to these losses is also included in requirement. Table 2.10 shows composition of different intestinal fluids, commonly lost from the body. The compositions can help to work out electrolyte losses when the volumes lost from the body are known with the help of fluid balance charts.

In certain cases water and Na^+ deficits can also be calculated (Table 2.11). Serum K^+ level is not a good guide to its body deficit, although, it has been used to have a rough assessment of the deficit.

Mild volume contraction can be corrected by oral route by use of some preparation based on

Table 2.10. Compositions and volumes of gastrointestinal secretions

	mEq/L				
	Na	K	Cl	HCO_3	Volume (mL/24h)
Gastric juice	60	10	120	nil	1000
Bile	145	5	75	70	400
Pancreatic juice	140	5	75	70	1500
Ileal fluid	120	5	105	20	3000
Colonic fluid	60	30[1]	40	-	250

[1] Colonic secretion of K^+ is stimulated by diarrhea.

- Roughly fluid volume lost per vomit/loose stool varies from half to one fourth of a litre.
- Secretory diarrheas (cholera, carcinoid) produce loss of fluid iso-osmotic with plasma and produce hypovolemia or hypovolemia with hyponatremia. Osmotic diarrheas (viral gastroenteritides, lactose malabsorption) produce hypovolemia with hypernatremia.

Table 2.11. Calculation of water and electrolyte deficits in patients of water and electrolyte disorders

- Water deficit in hypernatremia (see text).
- Deficits of Na^+ and Cl^- in patients of primary hyponatremia.
  - Na^+ deficit = (140-y) x (50 x 0.6) mEq Na^+
  - Where 140 mEq/L is normal plasma Na^+ level and Y is the current Na^+ level.
  - Weight of the patient is 50 kg.
  - Total body water is taken as 60% of body weight.
  - Cl^- deficit can also be calculated in the same way.
- K^+ deficit in hypokalemia.
  - K^+ deficit can not be calculated precisely from serum K^+ levels. However, serum K^+ decrease of 0.8 mEq/L, roughly represents total body deficit of 100 to 200 mEq.

WHO recommended composition. Even when patient is on intravenous fluid therapy, oral rehydration therapy (ORT) should be started concurrently if oral fluids are retained. ORT, especially with the WHO recommended fluid, is free from risk of introducing therapy induced electrolyte disturbances. For intravenous fluid therapy, in not very severe cases, one may alternate 5% dextrose with isotonic saline in the ratio of 2:1. In severe cases with hypotension and oliguria one may start with isotonic saline given rapidly (1L over half to 1h), monitoring CVP and urine flow. It may be followed by Ringer's lactate solution (this solution is more balanced than saline or dextrose and considered more useful in initial resuscitation). Once JVP and urine flow have improved, addition of K^+ to the infusion fluid can be considered under careful monitoring. In hypernatremic cases correction may require use of half normal saline or dextrose (5%) solutions. Those with significant anemia, hemorrhage or intravascular volume depletion may require blood/albumin/dextran infusion.

Monitoring needs are presented in Table 2.12. Also read under principles of management of shock in Chapter 3.

Table 2.12. Monitoring of a patient under management for a water electrolyte disorder

- Pulse, blood pressure, auscultation of lung bases (for fluid overload in old and those with compromised cardiac function) and record of urine volume (should be more than 30 mL/h, normally). (correction of tachycardia, low blood pressure and oliguria are best indications of success of fluid therapy).
- Record of body weight, signs of dehydration along with maintenance of fluid balance charts.
- Levels of Na^+, Cl^-, K^+, creatinine, urea and total plasma CO_2.
- In elderly or those with low cardiac reserve, it is important to monitor CVP and PAWP.

POTASSIUM BALANCE

Total exchangeable body K^+ is about 45 mmol/kg body weight; 98% of this is intracellular. Serum potassium level is 3.8 to 5 mmol/L. Most of the potassium loss occurs in urine, only a small amount is lost in feces. Common foods contain enough

potassium to compensate normal potassium losses from the body. Daily intake may be 50-150 mmol. Geophagy (ingestion of clay) reduces absorption of potassium and iron.

Excretion of K^+ in urine (Fig. 2.7, 4.8)

Most of potassium appearing in urine comes from K^+ secreted in the exchange process in response to reabsorption of Na^+ in distal tubular segments. This secretion depends upon the aldosterone and Na^+ load available at these segments. Thiazide and loop diuretics inhibit Na^+ reabsorption in earlier segments of the nephron and increase Na^+ load presented to the distal exchange segments. Reduced GFR, reduces this sodium load and thus K^+

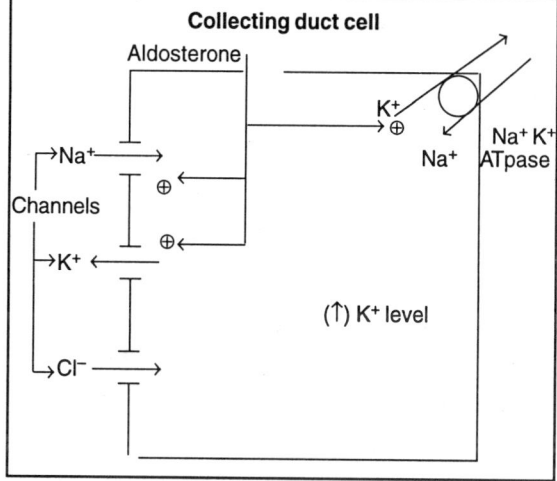

Fig. 2.7. Regulation of Na^+ reabsorption and K^+ secretion in cortical collecting duct cells, by aldosterone.

- Note effects of aldosterone on Na^+ channel, Na^+, K^+-ATPase and K^+ channel.
- Increased activity of Na^+, K^+-ATPase reduces intracellular Na^+ concentration. Low intracellular Na^+ increases activity of Na^+ channels. The Na^+, K^+-ATPase activity also increases intracellulr concentration of K^+ which in turn increases activity of K^+ channels.
- Na^+ reabsorption with Cl^- is electroneutral. Na^+ reabsorption without Cl^- is (increased presence of bicarbonate, sulphate, phosphate and acetoacetate ions) is electrogenic. It produces lumen negative transepithelial potential difference (TEPD) which promotes K^+ secretion.
- TEPD also promotes secretion of H^+. This secretion is located in intercalated cells (Na^+ reabsorption and K^+ secretion is located in principal cells of collecting ducts). However, TEPD develops in both types of cells when Na^+ is reabsorbed with out Cl^- in the principal cells.
- Control of Cl^- channel is not known.

secretion is reduced. Aldosterone increases K^+ secretion since it increases Na^+ reabsorption and has other effects (Fig. 2.7). Osmotic diuresis also increases K^+ excretion since increased rate of flow of the tubular fluid favours K^+ excretion.

K^+ excretion in urine is divided into two components: i) K^+ secretion, for which there is a driving force in the form of presence of aldosterone, increased intracellular K^+ concentration in the tubular cells, and availability of lumen negative trans epithelial potential difference (TEPD); ii) K^+ excretion increased by rate of flow of fluid in the collecting ducts (flow rate is increased by osmotic diuresis, diuretics and in Na^+ wasting nephropathies). The former component can be known by calculating transtubular K^+ concentration gradient (TTKG). This study (Table 2.13), may help in establishing etiology in certain cases of hypokalemia and hyperkalemia, produced because of inappropriate losses of K^+ in urine.

Kidney is less efficient in regulating body K^+ than Na^+. Still, K^+ excretion is reduced to <15 mmol/d in extrarenal causes of hypokalemia and increases to >200 mmol/d in extrarenal causes of hyperkalemia. These appropriate responses do not occur in the presence of factors which interfere in the normal process of K^+ secretion by the kidney.

Serum and ECF K^+ and its relation to function of excitable cells

As already pointed out most of the K^+ is inside the

Table 2.13. Calculating transtubular K^+ concentration gradient (TTKG)[1]

K^+ concentration of fluid in CCD = $[K^+_U] / (osm_U/osm_P)$

TTKG = K^+ concentration of fluid in CCD/ $[K^+_P]$.

- Factors which increase TTKG are, aldosterone, increased intracellular K^+ concentration in cells of CCD, increased lumen negative transepithelial potential difference (TEPD).
- In cases of hypokalemia and hyperkalemia due to inappropriate renal losses of K^+, this study may help to establish the etiology.

[1]These calculations are valid only if AVP is effective and urine is being concentrated.

- $[K^+_U]$ = K^+ concentration in urine; osm_U and osm_P, respectively, stand for urine and plasma osmolalities. $[K^+_P]$ = K^+ concentration in plasma. CCD = cortical collecting duct.

cells but it is ECF or serum K^+ which is important, for proper functioning of excitable cells. In many situations body K^+ may be greatly depleted but as serum K^+ is not much disturbed, there are no abnormal clinical findings. For example in diabetes mellitus (Table 2.14) cells keep on losing K^+ into ECF and from there it is excreted in urine. Thus, body may get considerably depleted in K^+ without any abnormal features related to excitable tissues. On the other hand a small change in ECF and serum K^+ by exchange at the cell level (Fig. 2.8) can be potentially dangerous. In the above example of uncontrolled diabetes mellitus when glucose and insulin are administered during treatment and K^+ enters into the cells with glucose, clinical features of hypokalemia may be produced. ECF potassium is related to resting membrane potential of cells and too low or too high level of K^+ in serum may produce serious aberrations in functioning of excitable tissues especially the heart.

Table 2.14. K^+ metabolism in diabetes mellitus

K^+ movement between ICF and ECF:
- Reduced glucose associated entry of K^+ into cells.
- Effect of reduced activity of Na^+, K^+ -ATPase. This pump is stimulated by increased intracellular Na^+. Insulin stimulates Na^+, H^+ -antiport to increase intracellular Na^+.
- Plasma hyperosmolality (due to glucose) causes movement of water from ICF to ECF and K^+ is carried along with water.
- In diabetic acidosis as H^+ moves in for intracellular buffering, K^+ moves out.

K^+ excretion in urine:
- Reduce K^+ level in tubular cells reduces K^+ secretion.
- Osmotic diuresis, if present, tends to increase K^+ secretion.

Diagnosis

There are two aspects of diagnosis of K^+ related disturbances. First, the presence of hypokalemia or hyperkalemia; the latter requiring urgent treatment. Fig. 2.8 shows the clinical conditions where one needs to be alert in this connection. Clinical features, ECG changes and plasma K^+ levels help diagnosis of hypokalemia or hyperkalemia. The second aspect is to establish the cause of hypokalemia or hyperkalemia. In most of the cases of K^+ disorders, the cause is quite apparent but in some cases it has to be established by careful history, clinical examination and investigations. This is true in patients of adrenal steroid disorders, renal tubular acidosis and certain other rare conditions. In these cases, evaluation of ECF volume, blood pressure, acid base status (Table 2.15), urinary excretion of K^+, TTKG and other investigations may be required. Table 2.16 shows important causes of hypokalemia and hyperkalemia.

Hypokalemia

It is suspected from the clinical setting (Fig. 2.8) and clinical features and confirmed from plasma K^+ level and the ECG findings. Early clinical features include muscle pain and muscle weakness which may progress to hypoventilation (respiratory muscle involvement) and paralytic ileus (involvement of smooth muscle of the intestine). There is also increased risk of rhabdomyolysis. Hypokalemia is known to produce nephrogenic diabetes insipidus

Table 2.15.　K^+ metabolism in acid base disorders

- In metabolic acidosis 60% of H^+ is buffered inside cells. As H^+ moves into cells, K^+ moves out. Movement of K^+ is more if the acid anion does not readily move into cells along with H^+ (due to limited permeability). In other acid base disorders (both acidosis and alkalosis) such transcellular migrations are less.
- Metabolic alkalosis produces K^+ depletion and reverse is also true also true (K^+ depletion produces metabolic alkalosis).
- ECF contraction causes hypokalemia and ECF expansion increases serum K^+ (effects are related to changes in Na^+ reabsorption).
- Thiazide and loop diuretics produce ECF contraction, alkalosis and hypokalemia.
- RTA type 1 and type 2 produce hypokalemia. RTA type 4 produces hyperkalemia.

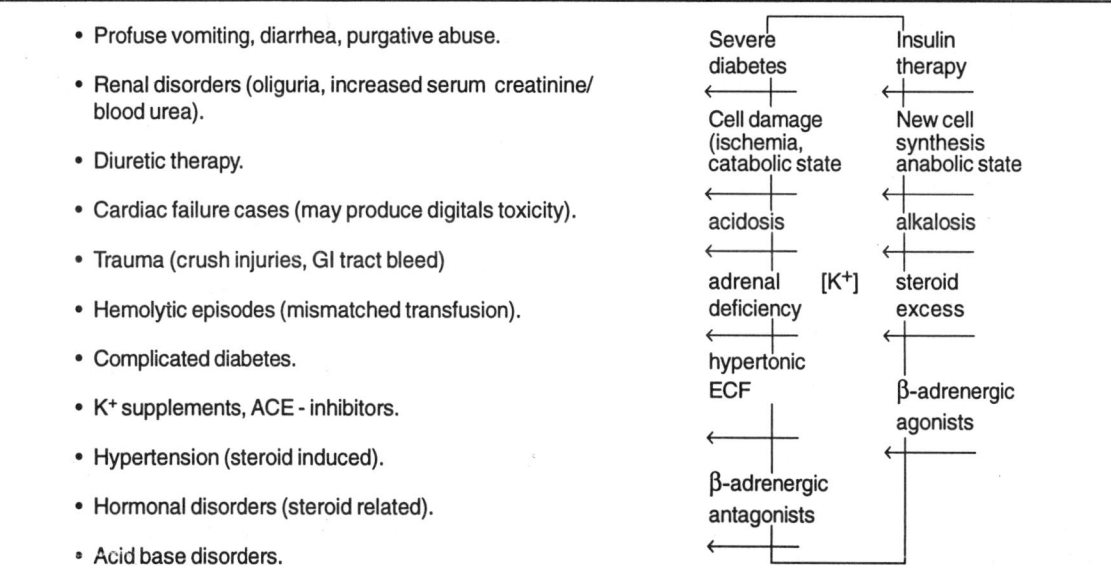

Fig. 2.8. Indications of K^+ estimation (in some cases transcellular movement of K^+ may be involved).

- Disorders of hypokalemia/hyperkalemia may result from, inappropriate intakes, inappropriate losses (renal and extrarenal) and transcellular K^+ movements. Often more than one factor is present.
- Since acidosis causes hyperkalemia (except RTA - types 1 and 2), hypokalemia associated with acidosis would mean severe K^+ depletion. Important causes of hypokalemia associated with acidosis are excessive fluid loss from gut fistulae, RTA - types 1 and 2 and transplanted ureters.
- K^+ efflux in acidosis will not occur if the corresponding acid anion readily accompanies H+ into the cell e.g. lactate.

Table 2.16. Important causes of hypokalemia and hyperkalemia

Hypokalemia	Hyperkalemia
1. Profuse vomiting (alkalosis further worsens hypokalemia by increasing K^+ excretion and migration into cells), profuse diarrhea and laxative abuse	1. Patients taking K^+ supplements.
2. Increased renal loss at distal tubular site (osmotic diuresis, diuretics, salt wasting nephropathies);	2. Oliguria of acute or chronic renal failure. Reduced K^+ secretion due to adrenal insufficiency, secondary hypoaldosteronism (hyporeninemia, drugs), resistance to aldosterone action.
3. New cell formation (parenteral nutrition, folate, B_{12} administration)	3. Due to cell damge (crush injuries, hemolysis, ischemia, malignancy)
4. Prolonged use of thiazide and loop diuretics in edema/other conditions.	4. Use of K^+ sparing diuretics/other drugs (ACE - inhibitors).
5. Alkalosis increases loss of K^+ in urine. RTA - types 1 and 2 also increase loss of K^+ in urine	5. Acidosis reduces loss of K^+ in urine: also RTA type 4.
6. Causes of transcellular movement of K^+.	6. Causes of transcellular movement of K^+.
7. During management of diabetic ketoacidosis	7. Diabetic ketoacidosis.

and glucose intolerance. In severe cases it may produce cardiac arrhythmias. Before interpreting plasma K^+ levels, pseudohypokalemia should be ruled out (Table 2.17). Hypokalemia is said to be present if plasma K^+ level is less than 3.5 mmol/L and it is said to be severe if plasma K^+ level is less than 2.0 mmol/L. Early ECG changes include prominent U-wave, flat or inverted T-wave and prolonged QU interval. Severe depletion results in prolonged PR interval, decreased voltage and widening of QRS complex. Ventricullar arrhythmias may occur.

Clinical features develop more often if hypokalemia develops rapidly. Low serum K^+ generally (although not always) indicates bodily depletion of K^+. Potassium salts can be given orally as enteric coated tablets, as these salts are irritants to gastric mucosa. Severe deficiency is corrected by intravenous infusion of K^+. It is done under ECG monitoring and fluid infused at a slow rate.

Hyperkalemia

Hyperkalemia is produced by oliguria (urine volume less than 400 mL/d.) in acute or chronic renal failure, after transfusion of stored blood and in cases of trauma with excessive tissue damage. Other causes are K^+ sparing diuretics, inappropriate K^+

administration and adrenal steroid deficiency. One should also look for some cause for transcellular shift of K^+.

It is quite common and the most serious electrolyte emergency. It is suspected from the clinical setting and established by ECG findings and plasma K^+ level. Spurious hyperkalemia should be carefully ruled out (Table 2.17). Hyperkalemia is said to be present if K^+ level is >5.5 mmol/L and it is said to be severe if plasma K^+ level is >7.5 mmol/L. ECG record can also be used to grade its severity (tall peaked T-waves → increased PR interval and QRS complex → loss of P waves → widening QRS merging with T wave → ventricular

Table 2.17. Regarding K^+ estimation

- Plasma/serum samples should be quickly separated from cells and should not be hemolysed. Plasma is better as some leakage is unavoidable in seurm after clot formation. This is especially marked if leukocyte, platelet count is high (see below).
- During muscular activity there is leakage of K^+ from muscle cells followed by uptake. Hence hand clenching should not be done during sample collection.
- Because of relationship between alkalosis and hypokalemia, K^+ and HCO_3^- levels should be estimated together.
- In leukemias there is factitious increase of K^+, due to leakage from abnormal cells after sample is withdrawn.

arrhythmia/ventricular asystole). Treatment modalities include infusion of glucose and insulin, infusion of calcium gluconate and dialysis. Preventive measures are essential and therefore clinician should be alert in clinical settings where hyperkalemia can occur.

CASE HISTORY: 2.1

A 60 year old patient with normal blood pressure and JVP reported that he had become increasingly irritable over the last few months. He had long history of persistent non-productive cough punctuated with lingering episodes of infections. X-ray revealed a mass in the lower part of right lung. There was no edema/ascites and no evidence of postural hypotension.

Some laboratory results were as under: Plasma osmolality 232 mOsmol/kg, plasma sodium 115 mEq/L, serum creatinine 1.2 mg/dL. urine volume less than 1.5 L/d, hematocrit and serum albumin in the normal range.

It is a case of hyponatremia without hypovolemia and without edema/ascites. For differential diagnosis, important conditions to be considered are, hypothyroidism, adrenal insufficiency, psychogenic polydipsia and SIADH.

As daily urine volume is less than 3 L/d, it cannot be a case of psychogenic polydipsia. There is also no history of polydipsia. In psychogenic polydipsia urine osmolality is determined by low AVP (<250 and often <100 mOsmol/kg) and urine Na^+ by low aldosterone and low AVP (>20 mEq/L).

Hypothyroidism and adrenal insufficiency were also carefully ruled out. X-ray evidence of mass in lower part of right lung is an important lead that it might be a case of SIADH. This condition is known to be present in many cases of oat cell carcinoma of lung and also in pulmonary tuberculosis. An old person presenting with a lung lesion and features like irritability or mental confusion should be investigated for hyponatremia (and water intoxication). See Table 2.5 for diagnosis.

In the present case hyponatremia requires treatment. It is, however, important to keep in mind two other types of patients which can present with mild hyponatremia but require no treatment: i) Patients with mild hyponatremia due to some stress, pain nausea, hypotension and other factors. This is quite a common finding in hospital patients; ii) patients of sick cell syndrome. For details see text.

CASE HISTORY: 2.2

A 30 year old emaciated woman presented with abdominal pain and vomiting for the last 24h. She had been feeling weak over past few months. Her blood pressure was 100/80 in supine position and 90/70 on standing. There were pigmentary patches over her buccal mucosa. On investigations: Serum Na^+ 115 mEq/L, K^+ 4.8 mEq/L and creatinine 2.5 mg/dL.

It was a case of postural hypotension and hyponatremia. Increase in creatinine level was an indication of renal circulatory impairment. Although, profuse vomiting over 24h could produce postural hypotension, urinary excretion of Na^+ was studied in view of hyponatremia. 24h urinary excretion of Na^+ was 120 mEq in 2L urine. As Na^+ excretion was unexpectedly high for a hypovolemic person, the diagnosis of adrenal deficiency was considered. The synacthen test was done which confirmed the diagnosis.

It is interesting to compare Na^+ and water excretions in adrenal failure with those in a case of thiazide diuretic abuse. In the latter case excretions of both Na^+ and water are increased, but of water more than Na^+. Thus osmotic pressure of urine is reduced. In adrenal failure excretion of only Na^+ is increased and osmotic pressure of urine is normal. Plasma and urine K^+ levels are quite different in the two conditions.

CASE HISTORY: 2.3

A 50 year female patient was on intravenous drip after an abdominal operation. On fourth day she complained of increasing muscle weakness and postural hypotension. There was no abnormal blood loss and no fever. BP was 110/80. Serum Na^+ was 120 mmol/L, serum creatinine 2.8 mg/dL. Urine Na^+ was reduced (10 mmol/L), while urine osmolality was normal.

She is a patient of hyponatremia because of inappropriate fluid therapy in the post operative period. It appears that she received inadequate Na^+ in the post operative period and became hypovolemic. This explains her raised serum creatinine (reduced renal circulation). Hypovolemia also, explains her postural hypotension. Because of hypovolemia secretions of both AVP and aldosterone increase. Likely low serum osmolality would reduce AVP. This could explain low urine Na^+ and normal osmolality.

CASE HISTORY: 2.4

A 8 month old baby had severe diarrhea of 36h duration. Child was brought in a semicomatose condition and had fever. He also had features of severe dehydration. For the previous 12h the patient had not passed any urine. Serum Na^+ was 152 mmol/L and serum creatinine 0.8 mg/dL.

It is a case of hypovolemia and hypernatremia. Oliguria is because of hypovolemia and has resulted in prerenal azotemia (increased level of serum creatinine; up to 5 years, the upper reference limit of creatinine is

5 mg/L). Hypernatremia has resulted since diarrheal fluid in infants is hypo-osmolar with respect to plasma.

In infants, severe vomiting and diarrhea produce a severer condition of dehydration than adults. This is because water constitutes a greater proportion of body water at this age than in adults. Also ECF/ICF ratio is higher in infants. It is the ECF compartment which is readily depleted with abnormal fluid loss.

Ordinarily, oral route is chosen for fluid replacement but in this case dehydration is quite severe and also because of vomiting, fluid administration should be done through the intravenous route. Total water requirement may be calculated as explained under "water deficit in hypernatremia".

CASE HISTORY: 2.5

An old beggar was picked up by a social worker from road side in semicomatose condition and was brought to hospital. He had features of severe dehydration. Skin was dry and mucous membrane of lips and tongue was dry and shrivelled. Pulse was 100/min and BP 100/70. Results of some investigations were as under:

Plasma, Na^+ 160 mEq/L, K^+ 4.0 mEq/L, creatinine 2.6 mg/dL, glucose 90.0 mg/dL, HCO_3^- 20 mEq/L., urea 110 mg/dL and Cl^- 128 mEq/L.

➤ What is the significance of HCO_3^- and Cl^- levels of the patients?

➤ What is the significance of disparity in levels of urea and creatinine?

It is a case of severe dehydration and hypernatremia leading to prerenal azotemia. All these features can be explained by lack of access of the patient to water. In hypernatremic cases, hypovolemia leading to oliguria and prerenal azotemia occurs late (compared to cases of hyponatremia) since intracellular water tends to maintain ECF volume.

• Levels of Na^+, K^+, Cl^- and HCO_3^- indicate normal anion gap. This indicates that azotemia of the patient is purely pre-renal (without renal contribution). Also; at present the patient is free from tissue hypoxia (lactic acidosis) and starvation ketoacidosis.

• Rise of urea is more than corresponding rise of creatinine (increase of urea/creatinine ratio). This is likely due to excessive protein breakdown because of starvation and reduced GFR.

CASE HISTORY: 2.6

An old woman (age about 50 years), suffered severe crush injuries in a bus accident. There were fractures of femur and pelvis. She was brought to the hospital about 8h after the accident. She was conscious. Her pulse was 106 per min. and BP was 100/60. Investigations revealed: Na^+ 140 mEq/L, K^+ 6.6 mEq/L, HCO_3^- 10 mEq/L and creatinine 2.0 mg/dL.

The patient has hypovolemic shock (increased serum creatinine), hyperkalemia, and acidosis. In a patient of trauma, first of all the vitals are checked (patency of the air way, respiration, pulse and BP). The first line of treatment is based on conditions of the vitals.

Patient needs treatment for her hypovolemic shock and also record of her urine volume should be kept. Hyperkalemia of the patient is because of release of K^+ from crushed muscles and also from hypoxic cells. hyperkalemia, will most likely improve after intravenous fluids, with improvement of kidney functions. The same is also true for her metabolic acidosis. Untreated this patient is likely to pass into acute renal failure which will worsen her hyperkalemia and metabolic acidosis.

The surgical problems of the patient would also require attention.

OBJECTIVE TYPE QUESTIONS

Pick out the wrong statement.

1. *Water and electrolytes; distribution and regulation.*

i) Charge on anions is balanced by charge on cations both in ICF and ECF.

ii) ICF and ECF are in osmotic equilibrium.

iii) A large part of anion equivalence of ICF is provided by proteins, carrying about 8 unit negative charge per molecule.

iv) Unequal distribution of K^+ across the cell membrane is because of presence of excess of negatively charged non-diffusible protein molecules in ICF.

v) Prerenal azotemia occurs earlier in hypernatremia than hyponatremia.

2. *Water and electrolytes; distribution and regulation*

i) Body water forms about 60% of body weight in adult males.

ii) Body water forms higher percent of body weight in infants.

iii) ECF/ICF ratio is also higher in infants than adults.

iv) ECF osmotic pressure regulation involves changes in aldosterone secretion.

v) ECF volume regulation involves changes in AVP and aldosterone secretions.

3. Water and electrolyte disorders

i) Biochemical and clinical evaluation should go hand in hand.

ii) Plasma volume is indicated by pulse, blood pressure, JVP and CVP.

iii) Serum Na^+ level is an indicator of ECF volume.

iv) Serum K^+ level is clinically very significant, although, not a good indicator of body K^+.

v) Hypovolemia by reducing GFR, leads to relatively greater increase in plasma urea than creatinine.

4. Fluid replacements

i) In pure water depletion there is equal volume reduction of ICF and ECF.

ii) Basal Na^+ and K^+ intakes (mmol/d) are 50-90 and 40-90, respectively.

iii) Daily maintenance needs in a surgical patient are 2L water and 80, 60 and 80 mmols of Na^+, K^+ and Cl^-, respectively.

iv) Ringer lactate is a useful maintenance fluid as it is nearer plasma in composition than normal saline, because of lactate which is converted into bicarbonate.

v) 1.26% $NaHCO_3^-$ solution is also isoosmotic with plasma.

vi) CVP is a useful means of assessing circulating blood volume and the appropriate rate of fluid replacement, except in severe hypovolemia.

5. About ECF and ICF

i) Body sodium is related to ECF volume.

ii) ECF volume is monitored by hematocrit values.

iii) Body water is related to ECF osmolality.

iv) ECF osmolality can be monitored by plasma sodium levels.

v) Plasma sodium is more often related to plasma osmolality in hypertonic states than in hypotonic states.

6. Volume depletion

i) Hematocrit and plasma albumin levels are increased.

ii) Blood urea nitrogen (BUN): creatinine ratio may be >20:1.

iii) There may be low blood pressure and increased pulse rate.

iv) Response to treatment is best indicated by increased in hematocrit.

v) Associated hypokalemia and metabolic alkalosis are present if produced by excessive use of diuretics.

vi) Associated hyperkalemia may be present in cases of adrenal insufficiency.

7. Hypernatremia

i) Important causes are extrarenal losses, loop diuretics, osmotic diuresis and diabetes insipidus.

ii) Minimal urine volume (about 500 mL) with maximum osmolality (more than 800 mOsmol/kg) means some extrarenal cause.

iii) Urine osmolality less than 200 mOsmol/kg means osmotic diuresis.

iv) In hypernatremia due to inappropate Na^+ intake urine Na^+ is >100 mmol/L

v) Often hypernatremia needs more urgent medical attention than hyponatremia.

8. About fluid and deficits

i) Osmotic diarrheas produce hypovolemia and hypernatremia.

ii) Secretory diarrheas produce simple hypovolemia or hypovolemia and hyponatremia.

iii) In intestinal obstruction, vomiting will produce hypovolemia and metabolic alkalosis.

iv) In osmotic diuresis, there is more loss of water than Na^+.

v) Reduced GFR results in retention of more water than Na^+.

9. About diuretics

i) Thiazides inhibit Na^+, Cl^- symport in early part of DCT.

ii) Loop diuretics inhibit Na^+, K^+, $2Cl^-$ symport in thick part of ascending limb of loop of Henle.

iii) Both types of diuretics increase K^+ loss and impair glucose tolerance.

iv) Both types of diuretics also produce hypocalcemia.

v) Carbonic anhydrase inhibitors lead to triggering of tubuloglomerular feed back (TGF) by increasing solute delivery to macula densa to cause afferent arteriolar constriction and decrease of GFR.

10. About diuretics

i) Thiazides and loop diuretics produce hypokalemia which may cause digitalis toxicity in a patient of congestive heart failure.

ii) In patients of ascites and edema associated with liver disease, diuretic induced hypokalemia enhances hepatic encephalopathy.

iii) Carbonic anhydrase inhibitors inhibit proximal tubular HCO_3^- reabsorption and produce acidosis.

iv) Carbonic anhydrase inhibitors increase distal tubular Na^+ and bicarbonate loads and thus produce hypokalemia.

v) Carbonic anhydrase inhibitors also produce hypophosphatemia.

vi) Loop diuretics lose effectiveness when blood volume is restored to normal levels.

11. About diuretics

i) Loop diuretics cause prostaglandin (PG) mediated increase of renal blood flow (RBF) and activation of renin angiotensinogen mechanism.

ii) Carbonic anhydrase inhibitors activate tubulo-glomerular feed back (TGF) to decrease GFR.

iii) Loop diuretics inhibit salt transport into maculdensa (thus blocking TGF) and do not produce decrease of GFR.

iv) NSAIDs interfere in diuretic response of loop diuretics by interfering in PG synthesis.

v) Osmotic diuretics produce hypovolemia and worsen pre-renal azotemia.

vi) Thiazides do not affect RBF and TGF.

ANSWERS

1. No.(v). It occurs earlier in hyponatremia since in hypernatremia intracellular water tends to maintain ECF volume.

2. No.(iv). It involves changes in AVP secretion.

3. No.(iii). Serum sodium and osmolality indicate body water.

4. No.(i). There is two fold greater reduction in ICF than ECF.

5. No.(v). Hypotonic states are commonly due to hyponatremia while hypertonic state are commonly due to increase in plasma levels of glucose, urea and other substances.

6. No.(iv). It is best indicated by clinical parameters (blood pressure, heart rate, urine volume).

7. No.(iii). In osmotic diuresis urine osmolality is >200 mOsmol/kg.

8. No.(iii). Metabolic alkalosis is not produced as there is loss of both HCO_3^- (duodenal fluid) and HCl (from gastric juice).

9. No.(iv). Loop diuretics produce hypocalcemia and hypomagnesemia; thiazides produce hypomagnesemia but hypercalcemia.

10. No.(vi). This is true for most other diuretics except the loop diuretics.

11. No.(v). Osmotic diuretics increase RBF and are useful in prerenal azotemia.

CHAPTER 3

Hydrogen Ion - Blood Gases Regulation: Disorders

In the course of metabolic reactions of the body, daily, about 20,000 mmol of CO_2 (generating equivalent amount of H_2CO_3), 40 to 60 mmol of fixed acids (H_2SO_4 and H_3PO_4) and some organic acids, are generated in the body. The special process of transporting large amount of CO_2 from tissues to lungs, without producing significant change in hydrogen ion concentration of the blood, will be discussed, separately. The fixed acids are also very efficiently handled in the body so that pH of blood is maintained between 7.38 to 7.44 (arterial) and 7.36 to 7.41 (venous).

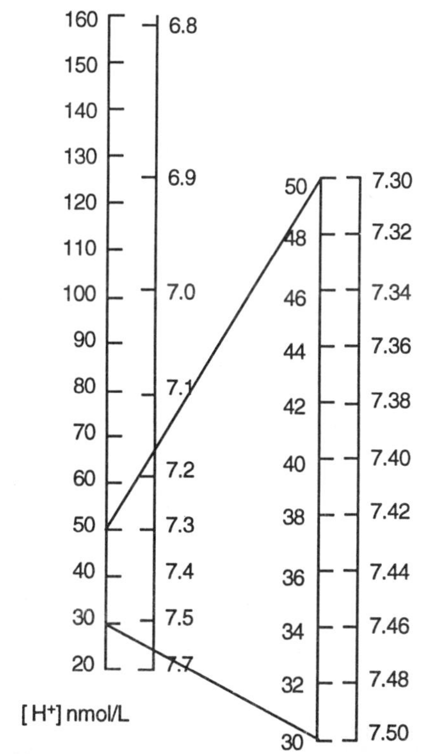

pH homeostasis is important for structural and functional integrity of proteins, nucleic acids and membranes. In this process of pH homeostasis, important roles are played by body buffers, the lung and kidney. Fig. 3.1 relates hydrogen ion concentrations to pH values.

Buffers form first line of defense against acids and alkalies, added to the body. A buffer consists of a mixture of a weak acid and its conjugate base (present in the form of a salt). When an acid is added, it reacts with conjugate base of the buffer to form the weak acid. This results in smaller change in hydrogen ion concentration (or pH), since the weak acid of the buffer dissociates less than the added acid.

In the presence of a buffer, hydrogen ion concentration of the solution is given by the ratio of the buffer components (Fig. 3.2). On addition of a strong acid to a buffer solution, there is some change in the hydrogen ion concentration of the solution indicated by change in the ratio of buffer components.

The bicarbonate buffer is the most important buffer of our body as it is an open buffer; both its components being regulated (H_2CO_3 or pCO_2 by

Fig.3.1 Relationship between pH and $[H^+]$.

pulmonary ventilation and HCO_3^- by the kidney). Conceptually, it can be considered as the central point of change produced by any acid base disturbance of the body. Acidosis is produced by two types of situations. In one type, there is increase of pCO_2 or H_2CO_3 (due to impairment of respiratory activity). This is said to produce respiratory acidosis. In the second type, the body faces excessive load of organic/inorganic acids (and their hydrogen ions). These acids might have arisen from exogenous sources (diet, drugs, poisons), endogenous metabolism or due to impaired excretion by the kidney. These react with bicarbonate component of the bicarbonate buffer and lead to its reduction. The same effect is produced by increased loss of bicarbonate from the body or by impaired H^+ secretion by the kidney. All these cases with decrease in HCO_3^- component of the bicarbonate buffer, are named as metabolic acidosis. Similarly, primary increase of HCO_3^- is termed as metabolic alkalosis and primary decrease of H_2CO_3 or pCO_2 as respiratory alkalosis.

Types of compensations available in different acid base disorders are shown in Fig. 3.3. ECF buffers act rapidly. When we talk of uncompensated cases we refer only to absence of pulmonary compensation (in metabolic acid base disorders) and absence of renal compensation (in respiratory acid base disorders).

Intracellular buffering of H^+ is rapid in respiratory disorders and provides compensation in acute cases. Intracellular buffering is more impressive in metabolic acidosis but the full effect takes time to develop.

In chronic metabolic acidosis bone salts also help H^+ buffering. It needs PTH promoted (and vitamin D supported) release of calcium salts (calcium carbonate) from the bone (acidosis $\rightarrow\uparrow$ loss of calcium in urine $\rightarrow\downarrow$ serum calcium $\rightarrow\uparrow$ PTH $\rightarrow$ bone salt mobilization for buffering H^+).

Plasma K^+ levels are altered with participation of intracellular buffers in acid base disorders. Most significant change occurs in metabolic acidosis (Fig. 3.4). Amount of calcium bound by albumin is also altered with change in anionic charge on albumin in acid base disorders.

Role of kidney in acid base disorders

Kidney compensates respiratory acidosis by decreasing excretion of HCO_3^- to normalize low arterial HCO_3^-/H_2CO_3 ratio and conversely, HCO_3^- excretion is increased in respiratory alkalosis.

In renal tubules Na^+ reabsorption with HCO_3^- (coupled to H^+ secretion) competes with Na^+ reabsorption with Cl^-. When plasma HCO_3^- is low, increased reabsorption of Cl^- from tubular fluid produces hyperchloremic acidosis. As HCO_3^- reabsorption in kidney is coupled to H^+ secretion, impairment of H^+ secretion in renal tubular acidosis also causes hyperchloremic acidosis.

Three components of renal H^+ secretion are: i) H^+ secretion with HCO_3^- reabsorption; impairment of this component increases compensatory Cl^- reabsorption; ii) H^+ secretion against tubular

---

$$H^+ = K^\dagger \frac{pCO_2^\ddagger}{[HCO_3^-]}$$

$H^+ \propto H_2CO_3/HCO_3^-$ ratio

(for $[H_2CO_3]/[HCO_3^-]$ ratio of 1/20, $H^+ = 40$ mmol/L)

• In acidosis the ratio is increased and so is H^+
• In alkalosis the ratio is reduced and so is H^+

$$pH = pK + \log \frac{[HCO_3^-]}{[H_2CO_3] \text{ or } pCO_2}$$

$pH \propto [HCO_3^-]/[H_2CO_3]$ ratio

(for $[HCO_3^-]/[H_2CO_3]$ ratio of 20/1, pH = 7.4; pK being 6.1)

• In acidosis the ratio is reduced and so is pH.
• In alkalosis the ratio is increased and so is pH.

Fig. 3.2. Relation of bicarbonate buffer component ratio to H^+ or pH.

$\dagger$ K is 178 if pCO_2 is expressed as kp$_a$; 24 if expressed as mmHg and 7.943 if expressed as mmol/L of H_2CO_3.
$\ddagger$ $pCO_2 \times 0.03 = H_2CO_3$ mmol/L (pCO_2 as mmHg).

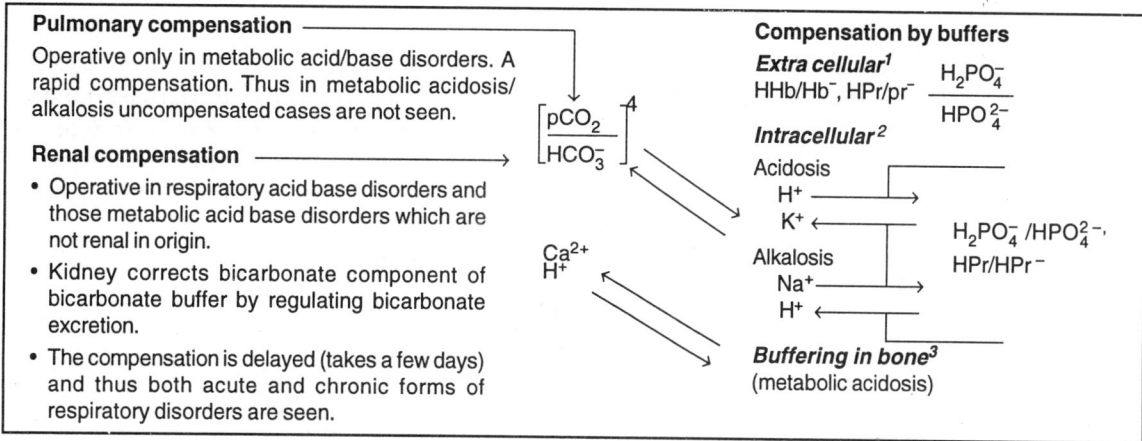

Fig. 3.3. Compensatory mechanisms in acid based disorders.

---

[1] ECF buffers act rapidly. When we talk of uncompensated cases we only refer to lack of pulmonary compensation (in metabolic acid base disorders) and lack of renal compensation (in respiratory acid base disorders).

[2] There is impressive buffering of H^+ by intracellular buffers in metabolic acidosis but full effect takes time to develop. There is less contribution of intracellular buffers in metabolic alkalosis. This compensation is rapid in respiratory acid base disorders and present in acute disorders.

[3] Buffering in bone is a prominent process in chronic metabolic acidosis. It requires parathyroid and vitamin D promoted hydroxy apatite mobilization from bone.

[4] Corresponds to Henderson equation written for $[H^+]$.

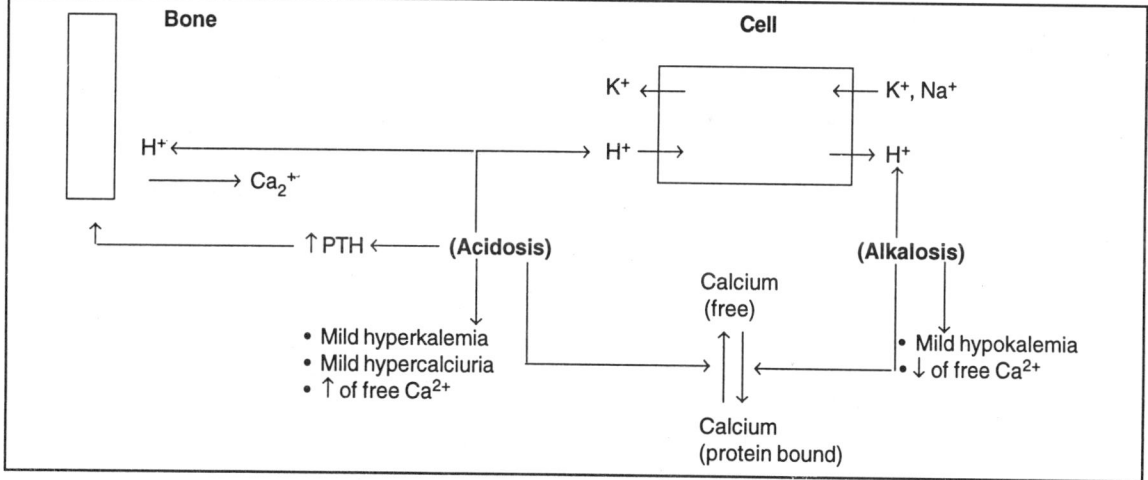

Fig. 3.4. Electrolyte changes in acidosis and alkalosis.

fluid buffers which produces titratable acidity in urine; iii) H^+ secretion with NH_3 which increases NH_4^+ in urine.

In early part of chronic renal diseases, H^+ secretion is impaired producing hyperchloremic acidosis, because of impairment of the first component of H^+ secretion. There is no increase of anion gap as excretion of fixed acid anions is adequate.

Role of lungs in acid base disorders

Lungs compensates metabolic acid base disorders by changing pCO_2/H_2CO_3 of the HCO_3^-/H_2CO_3 buffer by modifying pulmonary ventilation. Pulmonary ventilation is stimulated by increased blood pCO_2 and reduced pH and pO_2 (especially at pO_2 <60 mmHg) and depressed by reduced pCO_2 and increased pH. Both changes in pO_2 and pH affect respiration only through peripheral chemoreceptors (carotid/aortic bodies). Central chemoreceptors (lie in brain in contact with CSF and interstitial fluid of the brain) are very sensitive to changes in pCO_2 (peripheral chemoreceptor are much less responsive), but only after CO_2 enters CSF/brain interstitial fluid and alters its pH; increased H^+ being the actual stimulus. H^+ and HCO_3^- from blood also enter these compartments but slowly due to blood brain barrier to alter the pH and ventilation. For this reason, rapid normalization of blood HCO_3^- in a patient of chronic metabolic acidosis (already hyperventilating because of pulmonary compensation), exposes him to risk of respiratory alkalosis because of continuing hyperventilation due to presisting acidosis in interstitial fluid of the brain.

Mild to moderate increase in pCO_2 in arterial blood is very effective in producing increase in pulmonary ventilation but once it rises above 50 mmHg, it causes depression of both central chemoreceptors as well as the respiratory centre and in such a situation the drive for pulmonary ventilation can only come from low pO_2. Also read under chronic obstructive air way disease.

Buffering of CO_2

In tissues, large volumes of CO_2 enter capillaries. Serious problems would arise if this CO_2 was transported to lungs as CO_2 or as H_2CO_3. In the latter case, H^+ produced from dissociation of H_2CO_3 would pose a serious hazard. Blood has an effective process of CO_2 transport with only minimal changes in hydrogen ion concentration. As CO_2 enters capillaries, carbonic anhydrase, hydrates it to H_2CO_3 inside red cells. Next, H^+ generated from dissociation of H_2CO_3 protonates Hb to convert the R-form (relaxed form) to T-form (taut form). This, on one hand, serves to mop up H^+, released from dissociation of H_2CO_3 and on the other hand to release O_2, as the T-form of Hb has much reduced affinity for O_2. After H^+ has been taken up on Hb, HCO_3^- left behind crosses from red cell to plasma in exchange for Cl^- (the Cl^- shift). This HCO_3^- is transported to lungs in plasma (Fig. 3.5).

In lungs as CO_2 is exhaled, the above reactions, as occuring in tissues, are reversed. H^+ from

T-form of Hb is taken up by HCO_3^- to form H_2CO_3, which after conversion to CO_2 by carbonic anhydrase, provides more CO_2 for elimination. At the same time, R-form of Hb, formed from the T-form (with release of H^+) promotes Hb oxygenation. The reactions described are responsible for transport of most of CO_2 from tissues to lungs as HCO_3^- (Table 3.1, Fig. 3.5) without any significant change in pH of blood.

Presence of 2, 3 BPG (2, 3 biphosphoglycerate) in red cells, helps to stabilize the T-form of Hb. Thus in its presence, factors like increased H^+ and raised pCO_2 readily form T-form of Hb to release O_2 in tissues. Excessive 2, 3 BPG (in hypoxic conditions, as hypoxia stimulates synthesis of 2, 3 BPG), interferes in formation of R-form of Hb, reducing uptake of O_2 by Hb in lungs.

Table 3.1. Measured and calculated HCO_3^- in blood

- Total blood CO_2 (measured) in mmol/L is 23-30 for venous and 19-25 for arterial blood (about 2 mmol/L ($0.03 \times pCO_2$) is present as carbamino plus dissolved CO_2 and rest as HCO_3^-).
- Arterial blood HCO_3^- (calculated from arterial pCO_2) is 21-27 mmol/L.

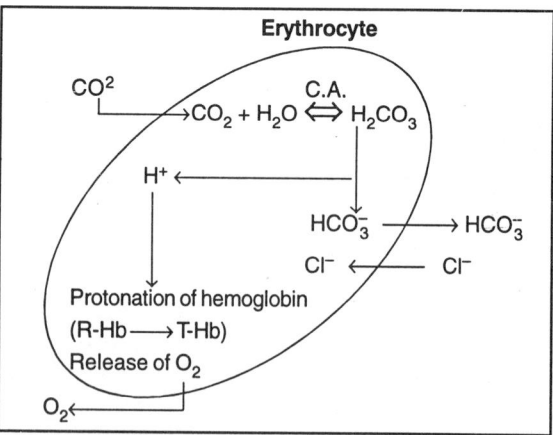

Fig. 3.5. Formation of plasma HCO_3^- from CO_2 in tissues.

- The above relations are reversed in the lung resulting in release of CO_2 and oxygenation of hemoglobin.
- To CO_2 of arterial blood (about 48 mL/dL), is added about 3.7 mL CO_2 in tissues (2.5 as HCO_3^-, 0.8 as carbamino compounds and 0.4 in soluble form) to increase venous blood CO_2 to about 51.7 mL/dL.
- CA = carbonic hydratase

The blood gases and other parameters, including pCO_2, pH, HCO_3^- and pO_2 are studied in arterial samples. In venous blood, the levels of these are affected by variable amounts of CO_2 produced and O_2 released in tissues. Arterial blood pCO_2 and pO_2 should actually reflect the pulmonary efficiency.

ACID BASE DISORDERS

Acid base disorders are classified according to changes in components of bicarbonate-carbonic acid buffer, since these are easily evaluated. The three components of this buffer are related as follows (the Henderson-Hasselbalch equation) (Fig. 3.2).

$$pH = pK + \log [HCO_3^-]/[H_2CO_3] \text{ or } pH = pK + \log [HCO_3^-]/pCO_2$$

In defining acid base disorders, primary decrease of $[HCO_3^-]$ is called metabolic acidosis and its primary increase, metabolic alkalosis. Primary increase in pCO_2 is called respiratory acidosis and its primary decrease, respiratory alkalosis (Figs. 3.6, 3.7).

Metabolic acidosis

Four important causes of metabolic acidosis with increased anion gap (explained below) are, diabetic ketoacidosis, renal disease, lactic acidosis, and drug/toxin poisoning. Acidosis with normal anion gap is caused by chronic diarrhea, intestinal fistular fluid loss and renal tubular acidosis (Table 3.2).

Clinical features arise from stimulation of respiratory centre (Kussmaul's respiration), depression of central nervous system function (confusion,

Metabolic acidosis	Normal	Metabolic alkalosis
Increased generation of acids(hydrogen ions).	$\dfrac{HCO_3^{-\dagger}}{H_2CO_3}$	Increased loss of H$^+$(gastric juice).
Reduced renal loss of H$^+$.		Use of diuretics.
Increased loss of HCO_3^-.		Hypokalemia, volume depletion.
	Normal ratio = 20/1	
$\dfrac{HCO_3^-}{H_2CO_3}$ ratio < 20/1 pH < 7.4 H$^+$ > 40 nmol/L	pH = 7.4 H$^+$ = 40 nmol/L	$\dfrac{HCO_3^-}{H_2CO_3}$ ratio > 20/1 pH > 7.4 H$^+$ < 40 nmol/L

Fig. 3.6. Primary decrease of HCO_3^- causes metabolic acidosis and primary increase of the same parameter causes metabolic alkalosis.

[†] Corresponds to Henderson equation written for pH.

Table 3.2. Important causes of metabolic acidosis

With high anion gap[1]	With normal anion gap (hyperchloremic acidosis)
• Lactic acidosis • Ketoacidosis (diabetic, alcoholic, starvation) • Formation of acids during metabolism of drugs and toxins (methanol, salicylates) • Acute renal failure and advanced chronic renal failure	• Gastrointestinal HCO_3^- loss (diarrhea, fistular fluid loss, ureterosigmoidostomy) • Renal tubular acidosis types 1 and 2 • Renal tubular acidosis type 4 (mineralocorticoid deficiency or resistance, tubulointerstitial renal disease, ammonium excretion defect) • Early renal insufficiency • Drugs (K$^+$ sparing diuretics) • Expansion acidosis (rapid saline infusion)

[1] Anion gap = $[Na^+]-([HCO_3^-]+[Cl^-])$ (normal value is 10 to 12 mmol/L). In calculating the anion gap, some authorities include concentration of K^+ along with that of Na^+).

lethargy, stupor even coma) and effects on cardio-vascular system. There may be peripheral arterial vasodilatation along with central venoconstriction. The situation predisposes to pulmonary edema, even with small fluid overload. Acidosis per se depresses cardiac contractility but simultaneous release of catecholamines keeps up the inotropic function. Acidosis may produce glucose intolerance.

In metabolic acidosis, pulmonary compensation is rapid and biochemical features (Fig. 3.6) include, reduced pH, reduced HCO_3^- and reduced pCO_2 (pulmonary compensation). In acidosis produced by HCO_3^- wasting there is no change in the anion gap (decrease of HCO_3^- causes increase of Cl^-). Increase of anion gap is present in other cases (Table 3.2).

Management includes, removal of the cause, and meeting water and electrolyte needs of the patient. Kidney, gradually, corrects the acidosis. If response is poor or pH is less than 7.2, bicarbonate administration is considered. Correction is applied slowly and not to exact normal value, under check of repeated investigations.

Anion gap

Normally, positive charge of Na^+ is balanced by negative charges of Cl^-, HCO_3^- and certain unmeasured anions (phosphate, sulfate, anionic proteins, organic anions) which constitute the anion gap. Normal anion gap is 10 to 12 mmol/L. In acidosis of certain etiologies decrease of HCO_3^- is accompanied with corresponding increase of Cl^- and thus the anion gap is not altered, while in acidosis of other etiologies (Table 3.2), plasma Cl^- level is not increased and loss of negative charge of HCO_3^- is compensated by the negative charge of certain anions of weak acids. This results in increase of anion gap. Presence of high anion gap may help to identify an acidosis (in a mixed disorder) when a superimposed metabolic alkalosis has normalized pH, pCO_2 and HCO_3^-. In such mixed disorders the increased anion gap of metabolic acidosis does not disappear, when other parameters get normalized.

Information on anion gap and about the nature of the accumulated anions may also be useful to decide about HCO_3^- administration, during management. Administration of HCO_3^- in patients of high anion gap produced by accumulation of anions of metabolizable organic acids is controversial since these anions (acetoacetate, β-hydroxy butyrate, lactate) will generate HCO_3^- in plasma. In other cases HCO_3^- administration is recommended, to slowly increase HCO_3^- to about 21 mmol/L.

For proper use of information provided by change in the anion gap, the following points should be borne in mind: i) anion gap can also be changed by change in plasma levels of endogenous cations like K^+, Ca^{2+}, Mg^{2+} or by presence of exogenous cations (Li^+); ii) it can also be changed by change in level of albumin or by change in its anionic charge, which increases in alkalosis and decreases in acidosis; iii) it is also affected by presence of certain paraproteins; iv) the calculated value of anion gap will be imprecise if levels of Na^+ and Cl^- are not accurately determined (in case of plasma with high osmolaity or in the presence of lipidemia.

Lactic acidosis

It is produced by tissue hypoxia either due to hypoxemia or due to poor tissue perfusion. It is often present in a severly ill patient. Important causes are shock, acute septicemia, cardiac decompensation, acute pancreatitis, respiratory failure and, CO poisoning. In these conditions mitochondrial oxidative reactions are affected. ATP deficiency and increased $NADH/NAD^+$ ratio stimulates glycolytic reactions with increased formation of lactate.

Lactic acidosis produced as above is called type 1 lactic acidosis. Type 2 lactic acidosis is produced in liver and kidney diseases (poor lactate disposal), in leukemia, extensively disseminated cancer (high glycolytic rates of malignant cells), in alcoholism, and by intake of certain drugs (phenformin used in diabetes promotes glucose disposal by glycolytic reactions) and poisons (methanol, ethylene glycol).

In lactic acidosis, there is marked hyperventilation and CNS depression (mental confusion, stupor and coma). There are biochemical features of severe acidosis (low pH, low HCO_3^-). There is increased anion gap due to lactate accumulation.

For diagnosis of lactic acidosis: i) rule out chronic

renal failure (estimate serum creatinine); ii) rule out diabetic ketoacidosis; iii) rule out drug intake (history, osmolar gap). Confirmation requires demonstration of serum lactate level of >5 mEq/L (upper normal limit is 1.6 mEq/L).

For lactate estimation blood should be collected without hand clinching and deproteinized immediately, by adding it to a tube, containing perchloric acid. At room temperature (unchilled sample), in presence of red cells, 20% increase in the sample lactate, occurs in about 3 min.

Condition is difficult to treat. Best is to treat the cause. Once treated, lactate will be converted into bicarbonate with production of metabolic alkalosis. Hypotension or shock is treated with fluids. HCO_3^- administration is controversial. It may improve cardiac function when given carefully in severe acidosis. Excessive administration, besides producing fluid overload, may stimualte phosphofructokinase to further increase lactate formation. Never raise pH to more than 7.2. Dialysis may be better than large doses of HCO_3^-.

Renal failure

With decrease of renal mass the available nephron number is not adequate to deal with net acid, produced, daily. When GFR falls to about 30 mL/min, there is development of hyperchloremic acidosis. With further decrease of GFR, uremic type acidosis develops with increase of anion gap, especially, in tubulointerstitial type of disease. HCO_3^- level generally, does not fall below 15 mmol/L. At this stage the daily generated H^+, is buffered by the salt released from the bone.

Metabolic alkalosis

It may be caused by excessive loss of gastric juice (pyloric stenosis and nasogastric aspiration), excessive use of diuretics, following treatment of ketoacidosis or lactic acidosis and rapid correction of chronic hypercapnia. In all these cases there is ECF contraction and urinary chloride is low (<10 mEq/L). Metabolic alkalosis may also be caused by corticosteroid excess (in these patients there is ECF expansion and urinary chloride is >20 mEq/L). Hypokalemia causes modest alkalosis which res-

ponds to K^+ administration. Hypoalbuminemia may worsen metabolic alkalosis (decreased albumin of 1 gm/dL increases HCO_3^- by about 3.4 mEq/L).

There may not be any clinical features in alkalosis, although, severe cases may show features of reduced level of free Ca^{2+} (muscle cramps, paresthesia or even tetany). Some features may result from K^+ and phosphate depletions which may accompany alkalosis.

Pulmonary compensation occurs and biochemical features (Fig. 3.6) include elevated pH, raised HCO_3^- and raised PCO_2 (pulmonary compensation).

Two important aspects of management are the removal of the cause and treating the factors that maintain alkalosis (hypovolemia, hypochloremia and K^+ depletion). Isotonic normal saline should be administered and serum K^+ corrected. The chloride depleted patients readily respond to chloride replacement (adequate replacement is indicated by increase of urinary chloride to >40 mEq/L). Excretion of HCO_3^- may be enhanced by use of acetazolamide, if renal functions are normal. It may, however, worsen hypokalemia.

Respiratory acidosis (Fig. 3.7)

Both acute and chronic forms occur. Acute respiratory acidosis may be produced by respiratory centre depression (drugs, stroke, infection), respiratory muscle dysfunction (poliomyelitis), airway block (aspiration, asthma), and lung diseases (bronchopneumonia, respiratory distress syndrome). With sudden hypoventilation there is increase of pCO_2 and reduced pH and pO_2. The triad of biochemical changes leads to early coma and death. No renal compensation is possible (which takes 48 to 72h). In these cases, although compensation is provided by cellular buffers, acidosis is severe (pH of about 7.1) but HCO_3^- is only 29-30 mEq/L.

In management, cause should be removed (since it is often removable). In these cases fall of pO_2 is more damaging than rise of pCO_2 and H^+. Oxygen should be given and can be given safely without adverse effect on respiratory centre stimulation (see below).

Long standing chronic obstructive air way

Respiratory acidosis	Normal	Respiratory alkalosis
Hypoventilation due to respiratory centre failure, neuromuscular disorders of respiratory muscles, air way obst. and pulmonary diseases.	$\dfrac{HCO_3^{-\dagger}}{H_2CO_3}$	Mechanical ventilation, hypoxemia, hypotension, cerebral causes, gram negative sepsis, anxiety, hysterical.
	Normal ratio = 20/1	
$\dfrac{HCO_3^-}{H_2CO_3}$ ratio < 20/1	pH = 7.4 H^+ = 40 nmol/L	$\dfrac{HCO_3^-}{H_2CO_3}$ ratio > 20/1
pH < 7.4		pH > 7.4
H^+ > 40 nmol/L		H^+ < 40 nmol/L

Fig. 3.7. Primary increase of pCO_2 causes respiratory acidosis and primary decrease in the same parameter causes respiratory alkalosis.

---

† Corresponds to Henderson equation written for pH.

disease (chronic bronchitis, emphysema) is the common cause of chronic respiratory acidosis. In these cases also, like the acute cases, poor alveolar ventilation results in increased pCO_2 and reduced pH and pO_2, but there is well developed renal compensation (reduced HCO_3^- excretion). Increased HCO_3^- results in near normal pH despite high pCO_2. In these patients respiratory centre becomes insensitive to high pCO_2 and hypoxemia is the major stimulus to respiratory centre.

In management, the cause cannot be removed. However, the acute exacerbation (see under chronic obstructive airway disease) should be treated with antibiotics, bronchodilators to improved alveolar ventilation.

Both hypoxemia and hypercapnia need careful corrections. As respiratory acidosis is compensated both pCO_2 and HCO_3^- are high. Rapid correction of pCO_2 will leave HCO_3^- inappropriately high (as its renal loss takes time), leading to metabolic alkalosis. For danger of rapid correction of low pO_2 read under chronic obstructive airway disease.

Respiratory alkalosis (Fig. 3.7)

It may be produced by excessive ventilation on a mechanical ventilator or by overbreathing by a hysterical patient. Hypoxia (high altitude, severe anemia) and increased intracranial pressure and encephalitis also cause overbreathing. Respiration is also stimulated by gram negative sepsis, (toxins stimulate respiratory centre), fever and hypotension.

Hepatic failure (accumulation of respiratory centre stimulating metabolites) and drugs (salicylate overdose) are other causes.

It is the most common acid base disorder in critically ill patients and its presence predicts poor prognosis. Rapid decrease of pCO_2 may produce cerebral features (dizziness, mental confusion, convulsions) due to reduced cerebral blood flow. The cardiovascular effect of sudden hypocapnia may produce arrhythmias in a patient of cardiac disease and may create problems during mechanical ventilation or in an anesthetized patient. Intracellular shifts of Na^+, K^+ and phosphate and reduced free calcium may create their specific problems.

Chronic respiratory alkalosis, common in pregnancy often remains without significant clinical features.

Patients of hyperventilation syndrome (paresthesia, chest wall tightness, dizziness, problems in breathing and some times tetany) need reassurance and rebreathing from a paper bag to increase pCO_2 of the inspired air. The cause of the disorder should be treated.

Mixed acid base disorders

In salicylate overdose, respiratory centre stimulation causes respiratory alkalosis and the metabolic effects (ketogenesis and accumulation of lactic acid due to inhibition of citric acid cycle) produce metabolic acidosis. Next, consider a patient of chronic airway disease, having respiratory acidosis. Because of prolonged use of diuretics for his corpulmonale he may develop hypokalemia and metabolic alkalosis. In this way a mixed disorder of respiratory acidosis and metabolic alkalosis can result. In critically ill patients a number of pathophysiological mechanisms may be operative to produce mixed acid base disorders.

Significance of data in acid base disorders

In interpretation of biochemical results in acid base disorders, history and clinical features are important in deciding about the type of disorder. Biochemical findings confirm the suspicion and reveal its severity.

Blood gas and pH analyzers are commonly used in providing the biochemical data in acid base disorders. pCO_2 and pH are measured in arterial blood with specific electrodes and the data is used to calculate HCO_3^-. Commonly used instruments also contain an electrode for measurement of pO_2, since this parameter is often disturbed in acid base disorders.

In some laboratories venous blood is used to measure plasma total CO_2 (venous blood is centrifuged in such a way that there is minimal loss of CO_2 of the sample) alongwith other estimations in an autoanalyzer (not in a blood gas and pH analyzer). Method may be based on colour change of an indicator in a carbonate, bicarbonate buffer, following release of CO_2 on acidification of sample. Normal range of total CO_2 in venous blood is 23 to 30 mmol/L (19 to 25 mmol/L in arterial blood). These values approximate the HCO_3^- values very closely since 89 to 90% of total serum CO_2 comes from HCO_3^- (Fig. 3.5, Table 3.1). In a large number of cases (in the presence of clinical history and clinical findings), this parameter alone is enough for diagnosis of the acid base disorders (Table 3.3). The detailed analysis of arterial blood sample for pH, pCO_2 and HCO_3^- should be undertaken if interpretation of abnormal total pCO_2 of the patient does not lead to a logical diagnosis. Even in these cases the calculated HCO_3^- should be compared with measured total pCO_2 which is also a measure of HCO_3^- as explained above.

In simple disorders, diagrams giving limits of compensatory response may be used to plot the data (Fig. 3.8). This helps to monitor a patient under treatment. Alternatively, limits of compensation may

Table 3.3. Diagnosis of acid base disorders based on total venous CO_2

High total CO_2[†]
- It could be respiratory acidosis or metabolic alkalosis. Clinical history and features will easily differentiate the two conditions. If diuretic administration is the cause of metabolic alkalosis, estimation of serum K+ will also be helpful.

Low total CO_2[‡]
- In this case it should be first ensured that only fresh and properly centrifuged sample (no undue leakage of CO_2) has been analysed. Then clinical history and clinical exaination will easily decide between metabolic acidosis and respiratory alkalosis.

[†] In this case one should carefully look for obstructive air way disease. Once respiratory acidosis has been ruled out, search should be made for metabolic cause of alkalosis. The patient might be taking some K+ losing diuretic (confirm by serum K+ level). Patient might be having dyspepsia and ingesting HCO_3^- for his dyspepsia.

[‡] Once clinical examination reveals normal respiration, the patient is likely to be suffering from mtabolic acidosis. One should carefully look for some cause of metabolic acidosis. It could be diabetes, tissue hypoxia (hypotension, hypovolemia), renal impairment (confirm by estimating serum creatinine), excessive loss of bicarbonate (diarrhoea, fistula) or some drug toxicity.

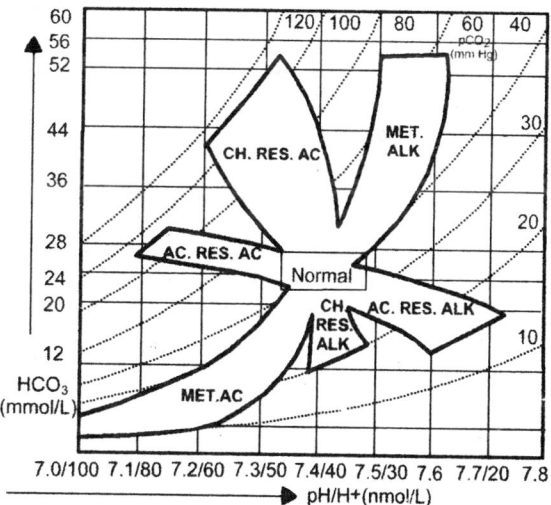

Fig. 3.8. Acid base nomogram, showing 90% confidence limits of normal compensations for primary acid base disorders.

- The diagram gives 90% probability range of values for pure acid base disorders as specially demarcated bands. Generally, the values lying in the bands indicate pure disorders (although in some cases it may not be so) and those lying in between the bands, a mixed disorder of at least two acid base disorders.

Table 3.4. Expected compensatory response in simple acid base disorders

Metabolic disorders (change in pCO_2 (mmHg) per mmol/L change in HCO_3^-) • Acidosis: 1.25 (↓) for (↓) in HCO_3^- • Alkalosis: 0.75 (↑) for (↑) in HCO_3^-	Respiratory disorders (change in HCO_3^- (mmol/L) per 10 mmHg change in pCO_2) • Acute acidosis: 1.0 (↑) ⎤ • Chronic acidosis: 4.0 (↑) ⎦ for (↑) in pCO_2 • Acute alkalosis: 2.0 (↓) ⎤ • Chronic alkalosis: 4.0 (↓) ⎦ for (↓) in pCO_2

Table 3.5. Some examples of parameters in acid base disorders

Disorder	pCO_2	HCO_3^-	pH
Respiratory acidosis acute (mild)	50	24	7.3
Respiratory acidosis acute (severe)	90	30	7.1
Respiratory acidosis chronic(mild)	50	28	7.35
Respiratory acidosis chronic(severe)	90	48	7.35
Respiratory alkalosis acute (mild)	30	24	7.45
Respiratory alkalosis acute (severe)	20	22	7.55
Respiratory alkalosis chronic (mild)	30	18	7.40
Respiratory alkalosis chronic (severe)	20	14	7.45
Metabolic acidosis (mild)	38	20	7.35
Metabolic acidosis (severe)	20	9	7.3
Metabolic alkalosis (mild)	40	30	7.5
Metabolic alkalosis (severe)	50	42	7.55

Table 3.6. Interpreting data in diagnosis of acid base disorders

- Is it acidosis or alkalosis? (consider pH)
- Is it respiratory or metabolic acid base disorder? (this will be decided by the dominant change; in pCO_2 or HCO_3^-; history will also help)
- Is the disorder compensated? (consider the parameter other than that responsible for the primary disorder)
- If it is a single disorder, pH should be appropriate for the primary disorder either compensated or uncompensated. If not consider possibility of a superimposed second disorder. Consider clinical state of the patient.

be calculated (Table 3.4). Table 3.5 indicates magnitudes of changes seen in compensated and uncompensated, both mild as well as severe cases.

Difficulties in interpretation can arise in mixed cases. Some times decision has to be made about the change in the compensatory parameter (Table 3.6). Is it simple compensation to the primary disorder or an indication of superimposed second acid base disorder? In the first case pH should be appropriate to the primary (first) disorder. History and

clinical examination and sound knowledge of patho-physiological mechanisms of the disorders, are helpful to use the acid base data for the benefit of the patient. *Unless the detailed knowledge of acid base parameters is going to influence treatment of the patient, arterial blood sampling should not be undertaken.* Arterial samples are preferable over the capillary samples. If, however, the capillary sample has to be used (often in infants) the sample collection should be done carefully (Table 3.7).

Table 3.7. Precautions in collecting capillary sample for blood gas estimation

- The area from which capillary blood has to be collected should be made pink by warming. In a cyanotic patient the capillary sample should not be used.
- It should be free flowing blood taken in a heparinized capillary. No squeezing should be required.
- The capillary tube shold be completely filled with blood without presence of any air bubble, and should be immediately sealed at both ends.
- The arterial sample is collected in a heparinized syringe, excluding air from the syringe both before and after collection of blood. Analysis should be performed immediately or else the syringe is capped and transported in a plastic bag surrounded by ice water.

THE BLOOD GASES

CO_2 transport in the blood and its relation to acid base disorders has already been discussed.

Transport and utilization of O_2

In pulmonary circulation, gaseous exchanges occur between blood and the alveoli (Fig. 3.9). CO_2 diffuses from the blood into alveolar air and O_2 in the reverse direction. In tissues oxy Hb is deoxygenated as the blood takes up CO_2 as HCO_3^- (Fig. 3.5). The oxygenated blood at a pO_2 of about 100 mmHg, leaves the lung. At pO_2 of 100 mmHg, blood carries about 20 mL of oxygen per dL, of which only about 0.3 mL/dL is in solution and rest bound to Hb as oxyHb.

There are two ways of indicating the amount of oxygen present in blood (ignoring effects of Hb amount and type). It may be indicated as pO_2 of blood which is measured with the help of an oxygen electrode. Alternatively, oxygen in blood may be estimated as its oxygen saturation (it is % of total Hb present as oxyHb.). Oxygen saturation of blood is studied with the help of a pulse oximeter. It is a non-invasive method using a probe clipped over patient's finger and gives continuous estimation of oxygen saturation of Hb. The device measures absorption of two wavelengths by oxygenated and deoxygenated Hbs. Based on differential absorption of the two wavelengths, the percentage of oxygen saturated Hb is calculated. Accuracy is affected in the presence of abnormal or modified Hbs. (Table 3.8). Smokers may carry about 10% carboxy-Hb in their Hb.

Table 3.8. Problems in use of pulse oximetry

- Oximetry is sensitive upto 90% oxygen saturation of Hb (pO_2 of 60%).
- Oxygen available in tissues will depend upon shape of O_2 dissociation curve, about which the oximetry values contain no information.
- Oximeter readings are less reliable if cutaneous perfusion is reduced because of low cardiac output or during use of vasoconstrictors.
- There is interference from presence of other forms of Hb. like carboxy Hb., met Hb. Thus reports of oximeter are not reliable when such Hbs. are present in significant amounts. In this respect co-oximeter (needs arterial blood) is better.

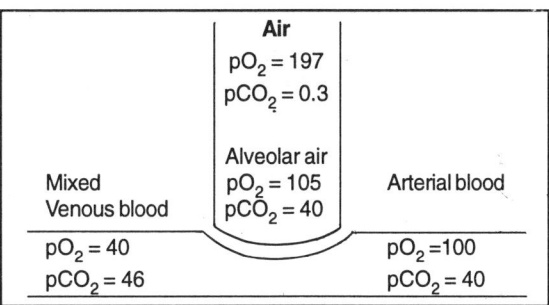

Fig. 3.9. Gas exchanges at pulmonary alveolar-capillary junction (values in mmHg).

- CO_2 diffuses 20 times faster than O_2, because of higher solubility coefficient of CO_2.
- Normally the exchange are complete in 1/3rd of the transit time of erythrocytes through the pulmonary capillary bed.
- Resistance to diffusion of O_2 due to altered alveolar-capillary junction, alone, does not result in hypoxemia.
- Hypoxemia may be caused by reduced alveolar pO_2 due to hypoventilation/low pO_2 in inspired air, ventilation-perfusion mismatch or if desaturated blood bypasses oxygenation at alveolar-capillary level (shunting).

Delivery and utilization of O_2 in tissues

Blood carries O_2 for delivery to tissues for their oxidative reactions. Failure to use adequate amount of O_2 in tissues is called tissue hypoxia. Hypoxia may occur if blood is not carrying enough O_2 to tissues. In some instances blood may be carrying enough O_2 (normal level of normal Hb, normal pO_2/oxygen saturation) but hypoxia is caused due to reduced release of O_2 from oxyHb. In diabetic ketoacidosis, there is erythrocyte depletion of 2, 3 BPG because of phosphate depletion. If acidosis is corrected rapidly, metabolic alkalosis may occur since hyperventilation may continue (inspite of HCO_3^- infusion and correction of acidosis in the blood) because of persisting acidosis of the brain interstitial compartment due to slow entry of infused HCO_3^- into that compartment. It is further augmented by HCO_3^- formation from metabolism of accumulated ketones, as circulation improves). All this would lead to reduced release of O_2 in tissues (by left shift of oxygen dissociation curve: Fig. 3.10).

It is important to understand about O_2 carried by oxyHb at different pO_2 values. Hb is almost fully saturated with O_2 at pO_2 of >75 mmHg; even at pO_2 of 60 mmHg it is about 90% saturated (see

- The upper, almost horizontal, part of the curve ensures high % saturation of Hb even at moderately reduced pO_2.

- The next vertical part determines release of oxygen in tissues depending upon the slope in this part (right or left shift of the curve).

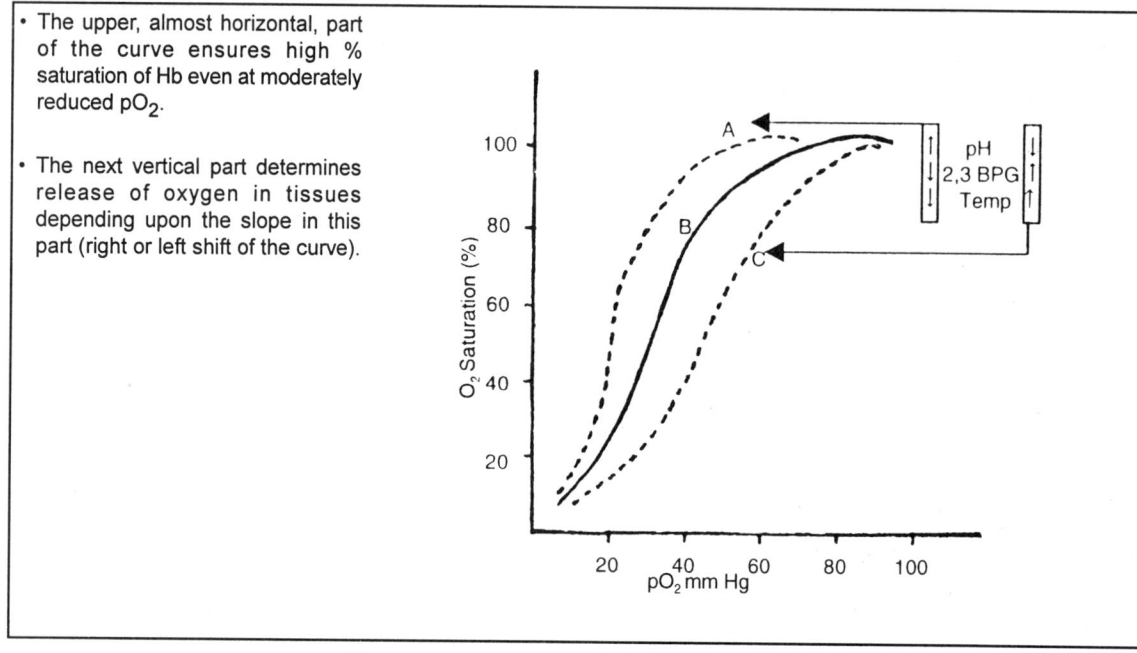

Fig. 3.10. Oxyhemoglobin dissociation curve.

- Normally, arterial blood with pO_2 of 100 mmHg (oxygen saturation of 100%) reaches tissues which have pO_2 of about 40 mmHg. pO_2 of blood falls to about 40 mmHg (and saturation to about 70%) with release of about 5-6 mL of O_2/100 mL of blood.
- Above pO_2 of 75 mmHg oxygen saturation of blood is almost 100%. Percent saturation is about 90% even at pO_2 of 60 mmHg. Because of steep descent of the oxygen dissociation curve at this level, any decrease of pO_2 below 60 mmHg of arterial blood causes substantial desaturation of blood, resulting in tissue hypoxia.
- A person is said to be in respiratory failure, if breathing at rest his arterial pO_2 is less than 50 mmHg.
- Increased H^+ concentration, tissue temperature and level of 2,3 BPG (in erythrocytes), shift oxygen dissociation curve to the right.(curve C). This leads to decrease in oxygen binding power of Hb. Shifted to left (curve A) leads to less release of O_2 in tissues. Curve B is normal.

oxygen dissociation curve of Hb_2O). Thus at pO_2 of 60 mmHg or more, blood is carrying enough O_2 for tissue needs. However, if pO_2 falls below 60 mmHg, substantial desaturation of Hb is present (see, steep descent of oxygen dissociation curve) and O_2 released in tissues is also greatly reduced, resulting in tissue hypoxia. Thus, to fulfil tissue O_2 needs, blood must carry enough oxygen (adequate normal Hb, pO_2/oxygen saturation) and oxygen must be properly delivered in tissues. Tissue hypoxia may also occur if tissues are not properly perfused with blood (as in shock). Also see Table 3.9.

In tissue hypoxia cells switch over to anaerobic metabolism with excessive formation of lactic acid. Respiratory centre is stimulated by H^+ (acidosis) and low pO_2 (especially when pO_2 is <60 mmHg; ordinarily pCO_2 is the most important stimulus for

Table 3.9. Different types of hypoxia

Respiratory hypoxia

- Three important causes are V̇/Q̇ mismatching, hypoventilation and shunting. First two are correct-able by 100% O_2 inhalation (third one is not).

Anemic hypoxia

- In anemia, pO_2 remains normal, oxygen saturation is also normal but O_2 carried by blood is reduced. It is also produced in the presence of altered Hbs e.g., methemoglobin, carboxy hemoglobin. CarboxyHb. cannot carry O_2; it also shifts oxygen dissociation curve to left. Thus tissue hypoxia is much more than in simple anemia.

Stagnant hypoxia (circulating hypoxia)

- Arterial pO_2 is normal but tissue pO_2 is reduced due to reduced tissue perfusion (shock, heart failure)

Histotoxic hypoxia

- It is produced by interference in mitochondrial oxidation process as produced by cyanide.

respiratory centre). Hyperventilation and lactic acid accumulation may produce a mixed acid base disorder. Cellular deficiency of ATP will lead to complex disturbance of cellular functions. Other effects of hypoxia are shown in Table 3.10.

Table 3.10. Some important effects of hypoxia

- Anaerobic metabloism (lactic acidosis).
- Complex cellular dysfunctions due to reduced ATP formation.[1]
- Reduced cerebrovascular resistance (increased cerebral blood flow). If pCO_2 is also reduced cerebrovascular resistance will increase worsening cerebral hypoxia.
- Pulmonary vascular constriction, increasing pulmonary vascular resistance (increased right ventricular load).
- Reduced pO_2 in tissues causes vasodilatation increasing cardiac output and work of heart.
- Prolonged severe hypoxia impairs hepatic/renal functions.
- Chronic hypoxia causes polycythemia.

[1]Cerebral functions are affected (clinical picture like that of acute alcoholism). In severe hypoxia brain stem centres are affected.

- Protein synthesis is inhibited and enzymes/proteins leak out from cells.

Importance of monitoring of oxygen delivery and consumption in patients of shock.

Different hemodynamics develop in different types of shock. In hypovolemic shock the intravascular volume is reduced. This causes decrease of ventricle preload demonstrated by markedly reduced central venous pressure (CVP) and pulmonary artery wedge pressure (PAWP). Because of reduced ventricular preload, cardiac output (CO) is secondarily reduced. In cardiogenic shock, there is cardiac dysfunction (ischemia, infarction, arrhythmia, valvular disease or cardiomyopathy) leading to reduced CO, causing increased CVP and PAWP. In both conditions because of reduced CO, reflex systemic vasconstriction and increased heart rate (HR) occur. Systemic vascular resistance (SVR) increases. In septic and neurogenic shocks there is dilatation of peripheral vascular beds. Other features are shown in Fig. 3.11.

In patients of shock or other critically ill patients it has been found that oxygen delivery to tissues and oxygen consumption by tissues (Fig. 3.12) are

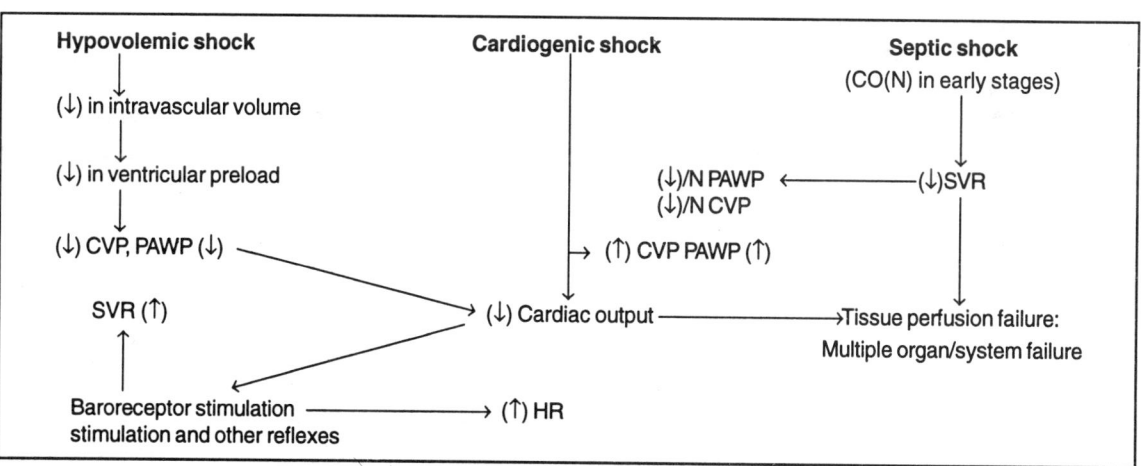

Fig. 3.11. Hemodynamics during different types of shock.

CO = cardiac out put, CVP = central venous pressure, PAWP = pulmonary artery wedge pressure, SVR = systemic vascular resistance

- A baloon tipped catheter is passed via left subclavian and advanced through right heart into pulmonary artery and made to wedge in a branch of the artery to record PAWP which provides indirect measure of left atrial pressure. Catheter tip in superior vena cava (or even right atrium) records CVP.
- Noninvasively inspection of right internal jugular vein in the neck is commonly used to have idea of CVP.

important parameters for guiding management and for predicting outcome. For studying these parameters, there is need to determine pO_2 of arterial blood and pO_2 of mixed venous blood collected through the arterial catheter used to measure CVP.

In hypovolemic or cardiogenic shock there is marked decrease in oxygen delivery to tissues while oxygen consumption remains unaffected. Ratio of oxygen delivery to oxygen consumption becomes much reduced. In normal conditions oxygen delivery exceeds oxygen consumption by about five fold, and because of that, oxygen consumption is quite independent of oxygen delivery. On the other hand in hypovolemic and cardiogenic shocks oxygen consumption gets limited by oxygen delivery. In septic shock total body oxygen requirement increases dramatically but a parallel increase in oxygen delivery does not occur. Thus tissue oxygen needs may not be met with.

Fig. 3.12 shows calculation of parameters of oxygen delivery and oxygen consumption. In critically ill patients, management aims at increasing the reduced gap between oxygen consumption and oxygen delivery. Oxygen delivery may be improved by correcting hemodynamics, by increasing hemoglobin level and by improving cardiac functioning (this may require treatment of arrhythmia, increasing coronary blood flow and by the careful use of inotropic agents for the heart). High oxygen consumption may be reduced by treating the cause. It may require treatment of fever, treatment of sepsis and other measures.

Principles of management

In hypovolemic shock hemodynamics are corrected mainly, by fluid administration. PAWP is monitored to ensure adequate preload of left ventricle to maintain proper CO. Mean BP is maintained atleast above 60 mmHg. to ensure proper tissue perfusion.

Management of cardiogenic shock greatly depends upon the cause. In general, myocardial ischemia, if present, is urgently attended to (oxygen administration). If systolic BP permits, SVR is reduced to reduce afterload and therefore, the work of heart. Improved myocardial functioning will increase CO to increase coronary artery perfusion without increasing cardiac work. Tachycardia is treated as it increases cardiac work and its oxygen demand.

In septic shock, treatment aims at increasing SVR. Dopamine is used which raises BP while maintaining or enhancing blood flow to renal and splanchnic areas. After correcting hypotension a cardioinotropic may be used to improve cardiac out put. Sepsis and the septic focus, of course, also need management.

Oxygen delivery[1] (mL oxygen/min)

Cardiac output (mL/min) x Arterial O_2 conc.[2]/mL of blood.

When arterial O_2 conc./mL of blood

=Hb (g/mL) x percent oxygen saturation of blood/100 x 1.34

(at 100% arterial oxygen saturation, lg Hb carries 1.34 mL of oxygen)

• Normal oxygen delivery to tissues is 700 to 1400 mL oxygen/min.

Oxygen consumption (mL oxygen/min)

= Cardiac output (mL/min) x Arterial, venous oxygen conc. difference/mL of blood.

When Arterial, venous oxygen difference/mL blood

= Hb (g/mL) x arterial, venous percent oxygen saturation differnce/100 x 1.34

(in normal mixed venous blood oxygen percent saturation is around 79% and normal oxygen consumption is around 200 mL oxygen/min)

Fig. 3.12. Calculating oxygen delivery and oxygen consumption in critically ill patients.

---

[1] Under normal conditions oxygen delivery exceeds oxygen consumption by about five fold, making oxygen consumption almost independent of oxygen delivery.

[2] mL of O_2.

Monitoring

Patient needs to be monitored for hemodynamics (pulse, BP, JVP, CVP, PAWP) as well as for adequacy of tissue of O_2 delivery and O_2 consumption. During fluid administration, to avoid overhydration, auscultation of lung bases for rales is useful. For monitoring adequacy of tissue perfusion urine output and serum creatinine and blood urea levels should be studied. Other investigations are serum bilirubin and lactate levels.

The gas exchanges in the lung

In the lung O_2 and CO_2 diffuse down their respective concentration gradients, through the alveolar wall and pulmonary capillary endothelium (Fig. 3.9). Hypoxemia is a common condition resulting from different diseases affecting lungs or other parts of respiratory system. Different mechanism resulting in hypoxemia are as under (Table 3.11):

i) Decrease in inspired air pO_2: This can occur if concentration of O_2 is less than 21% in the inspired air. It may happen in a patient on ventilatory support or during smoke inhalation. In these patients arterial pO_2 is reduced but pCO_2 remains normal.

ii) Hypoventilation as a cause of hypoxemia: Hypoventilation may be due to decrease of ventilatory drive or because of neuromuscular disease. Similar effect is produced if there is increase of pulmonary dead space as in cases with $\dot{V}/\dot{Q}$ mismatching (see below). In hypoventilation cases arterial pO_2 is reduced and pCO_2 may be increased.

In the two above mentioned causes of hypoxemia, gas exchanges at the capillary - alveolar level occur normally and alveolar - arterial pO_2 difference (A-a gradient) remains normal. Further, administration of 100% oxygen improves arterial pO_2.

iii) Hypoxemia due to shunting and $\dot{V}/\dot{Q}$ mismatching: In alveolar collapse and intralveolar block (pneumonia, pulmonary edema) deoxygenated blood bypasses oxygenation at alveolar-capillary membrane (Fig. 3.13). This is called shunting.

Examples of $\dot{V}/\dot{Q}$ mismatching are chronic obstructive pulmonary disease (COPD), asthma,

Table 3.11. Evaluation of hypoxemia/reduced tissue O_2 utilization

pO_2 in arterial blood ⎤ Oxygen saturation by pulse oximetry ⎦ (along with level and type of Hb)	• These are two basic parameters. Ear/pulse oximeters give continuous, noninvasive estimation of arterial oxygen saturation.
Alveolar-arterial pO_2 difference (A-a gradient)[1] ⟶ pCO_2 (hypercapnia is mostly caused by hypoventilation; also see the text)	• Normal in low inspired pO_2 and hypoventilation. (corrected by oxygen) • Increased A-a gradient in $\dot{V}\dot{Q}$ mismatching (corrected by oxygen) • Increased A-a gradient in pulmonary shunting[2] (not corrected by oxygen) • Shunting cardiac (R →L) (not corrected by oxygen) • Hypercapnia is mostly caused by hypoventilation (also see the text).
Blood lactate ⟶	• Reduced tissue perfusion in shock.
Diffusing capacity ⟶	• In itself rarely responsible for hypoxemia, but may have contributory role in certain pulmonary diseases (interstitial lung disease). Important indicator of functional integrity of alveolar-capillary membrane.

[1] To caluclate alveolar-arterial O_2 gradient (A-a O_2 gradient)
[2] Shunting is $\dot{V}/\dot{Q}$ mismatching in which $\dot{v}$ is zero and $\dot{\varrho}$ is normal.
- Measure arterial pO_2 by oxygen electrode.
- Calculate alveolar pO_2 as follows:
- pO_2 (alveolar) = pO_2 (inspired air) - pCO_2 (arterial)/RQ,   RQ = Respiratory quotient
- A-a O_2 gradient=normal value is 10 to 15 mmHg.
- (A-a O_2 gradient is increased in hypoxemia due to shunting or $\dot{V}/\dot{Q}$ mismatching but not in hypoventilation or with decreased pO_2 in inspired air).

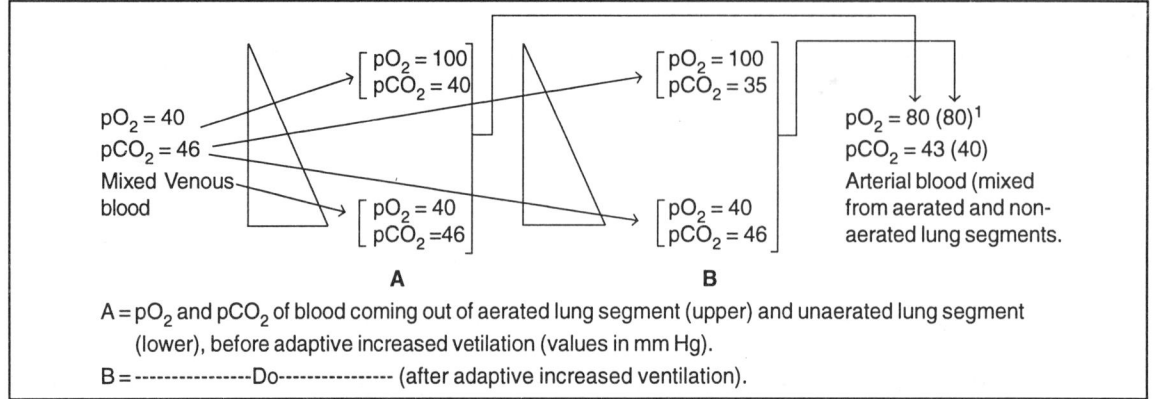

Fig. 3.13. Mechanism of hypoxemia in shunting.

[1] Values in brackets are obtained after adaptive increase in ventilation which reduces pCO_2 (in blood from the ventilated segment) below 40 but cannot increase pO_2 above 100.

- In lobar pneumonia/partial lung collapse, blood coming out of unaerated segment does not exchange gases with alveolar air. Immediately after the development of the lung pathology, slight adaptive increase in ventilation occurs (due to $\uparrow pCO_2$).

interstitial lung disease and pulmonary vascular disease. In some regions of affected lung, alveolar ventilation ($\dot{v}$) is normal but perfusion ($\dot{Q}$) is reduced (high $\dot{v}/\dot{Q}$ratio). These regions add to the volume of pulmonary dead space (see above). In some other regions of the affected lung $\dot{v}/\dot{Q}$ ratio may be low (the region is perfused but not ventilated).

In both shunting and $\dot{v}/\dot{Q}$mismatching, A-a gradient is increased. Administration of 100% oxygen administration corrects hypoxemia in $\dot{v}/\dot{Q}$mismatching but not in shunting.

iv) In some diseases, diffusing capacity of oxygen across alveolar-capillary membrane may be reduced. But this defect alone is not expected to produce hypoxemia, although it may add to hypoxemia producing effect of other mechanisms (see above) operative in a pulmonary disease.

Hypoxemia with hypercapnia

Hypercapnia (increased arterial pCO_2) is mostly because of hypoventilation. In cardiac shunt patients (R→L shunt); as blood bypasses pulmonary circulation there is both hypoxemia and hypercapnia. Presence of low pO_2 (<50 mmHg) and high pCO_2 (>49.5 mmHg) is called respiratory failure type 2. It occurs, as explained above in cases of hypoventilation (respiratory centre failure, and neuromuscular diseases involving thoracic cage) and the

cardiac shunt patients. Impaired ventilation may also be present in patients having hypoxemia due to $\dot{v}/\dot{Q}$ mismatch or because of shunting. In patients of $\dot{v}/\dot{Q}$ mismatch, increased pulmonary dead space becomes cause of ineffective ventilation. Loss of normal elasticity of the lung tissue or thoracic cage may be the cause of impaired ventilation in some cases. In COPD increased airway resistance may impair ventilation. Thus respiratory failure type 2 also occurs in COPD, bronchial pneumonia and others. Many of these patients start with respiratory failure type 1 with low levels of pO_2 and normal pCO_2 but with advance of disease respiratory failure type 2 supervenes.

Chronic obstructive airway disease

In this group there are three important conditions. First is persistent chronic bronchitis, generally related to smoking and worsening with time. Second is emphysema (permanent, abnormal distension of air spaces distal to terminal bronchioles with destruction of alveolar septa). Thirdly, some cases of asthma, especially those not managed properly become indistinguishable from those of chronic bronchitis. In all these disorders there is impaired ability of expiration, either due to spasm of bronchioles or due to loss of elasticity of alveolar walls. If main damage lies in alveolar walls (emphysema), there is loss of both alveolar capillaries and the alveolar elastic tissue. Thus there is loss of both perfusion (capillary damage) and ventilation (loss of alveolar tissue). There may be hypoxemia but no hypercapnia, for quite a long time. Hypoxemia stimulates respiratory centre and there may be alkalosis due to hyperventilation. There is less marked increase in pulmonary vascular resistance and its consequences. Eventually, however, CO_2 retention and respiratory acidosis also occur.

In cases with chronic bronchitis, mainly alveolar walls are damaged and not capillary walls. Thus alveoli are perfused but not ventilated. There is large ventilation/perfusion imbalance and there is not only hypoxemia but also hypercapnia. In these patients chemoreceptors lack sensitivity to both pO_2 and pCO_2 and hyperventilation may not be marked. Further, there is marked increase in pulmonary vascular resistance and early right ventricular failure. Unlike the emphysematous patients, these patients

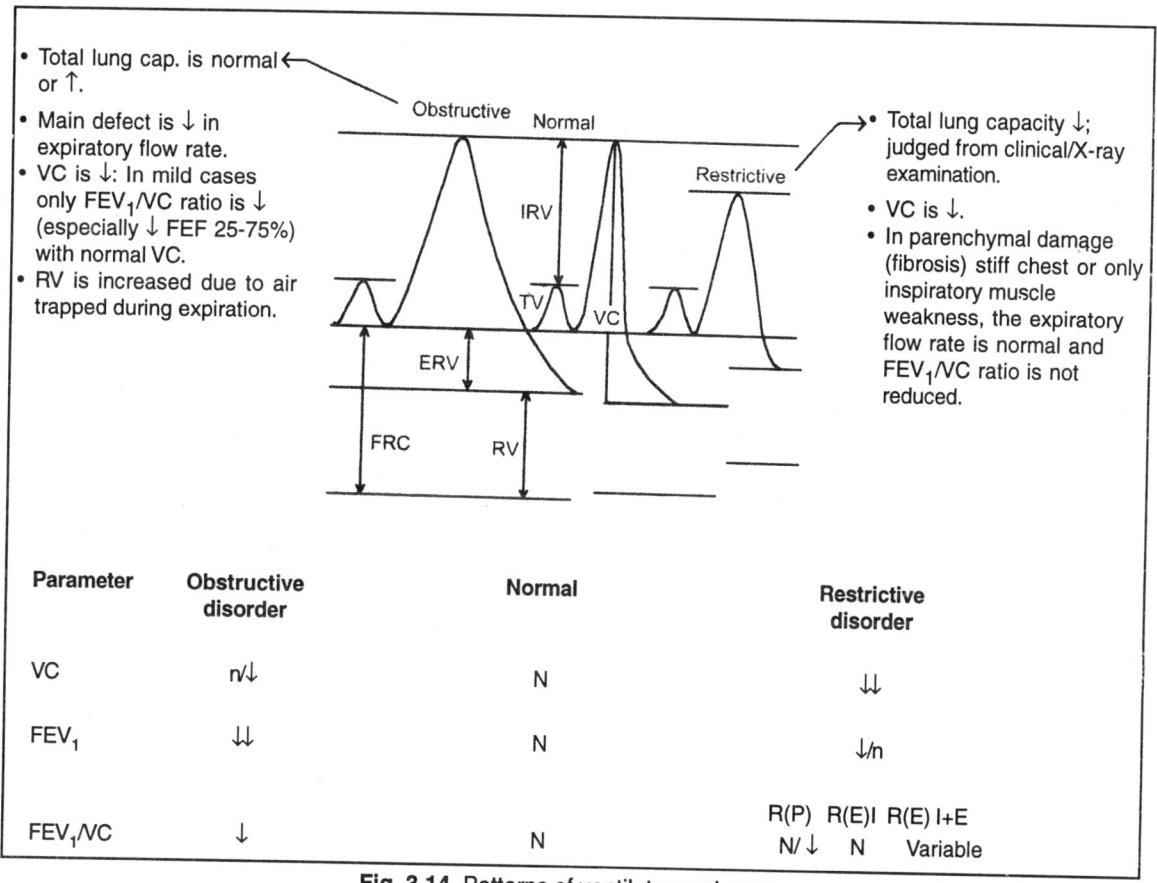

- Total lung cap. is normal or ↑.
- Main defect is ↓ in expiratory flow rate.
- VC is ↓: In mild cases only FEV$_1$/VC ratio is ↓ (especially ↓ FEF 25-75%) with normal VC.
- RV is increased due to air trapped during expiration.

- Total lung capacity ↓; judged from clinical/X-ray examination.
- VC is ↓.
- In parenchymal damage (fibrosis) stiff chest or only inspiratory muscle weakness, the expiratory flow rate is normal and FEV$_1$/VC ratio is not reduced.

Parameter	Obstructive disorder	Normal	Restrictive disorder
VC	n/↓	N	↓↓
FEV$_1$	↓↓	N	↓/n
FEV$_1$/VC	↓	N	R(P) N/↓ R(E)I N R(E) I+E Variable

Fig. 3.14. Patterns of ventilatory volumes.

Note: In obstructive disease both FEV$_1$ and VC are reduced (the former more than the latter). In restrictive disease (especially the pulmonary restrictive disease VC is reduced more than FEV$_1$.

R(P) = Restrictive (pulmonary) disease: R(E)I = Restrictive (extrapulmonary) inspiratory

R(E)I+E = Restrictive (extrapulmonary) inspiratory + expiratory

VC = Maximum volume of air expired after a maximum inspiration (both recorded on a spirometer)

FEV$_1$ = Volume of air expired in 1 sec. by maximum effort, after maxium inspiration. It also represents peak expiratory flow rate (PEFR) in a flow meter: FEF 25-75% = Forced expiratory flow between 25-75% of VC, also called max. midexpiratory flow rate.

TV = Tidal volume, VC = Vital capacity, FRC = Functional residual capacity, RV = Residual volume and IRV = Inspiratory reserve volume. Normal: VC = 3-6L; varies with age, sex and height: FEV$_1$/VC = 0.75-0.80.

suffer from both hypoxemia and hypercapnia and respiratory acidosis.

In advanced cases of all above disorders, a uniform sort of picture is produced. There is hypoxemia and respiratory acidosis. Because of renal compensation, there is near normal pH despite high pCO_2. Disease may show acute exacerbation because of factors like infection, dusty environment and excessive smoking. There will be worsening of hypoxemia and hypercapnia with appreciable decrease of pH as the changes may be produced rather rapidly without much renal compensation. The patient is likely to go into respiratory failure type 2 unless treated vigorously with antibiotics, bronchodilators, and expectorants alongwith postural drainage of secretions. With all this treatment, controlled O_2 administration can be done to produce a small increase in pO_2 at which tissues can obtain adequate release of O_2, resulting in improved tissue oxygenation. Excessive increase of pO_2 can be dangerous as in these patients, hypoxemia is the only stimulus for respiratory centre. Thus careless increase in pO_2 may cause dangerous increase in pCO_2 by inhibiting respiratory centre. If this cannot be avoided, it is better to put the patient on mechanical ventilation.

Patients of COPD may suffer from acute respiratory acidosis superimposed on chronic respiratory acidosis (as mentioned above) or metabolic alkalosis complicating their respiratory disorders because of vomiting or use of diuretics.

Dyspnea is unpleasant awareness of act of breathing. It is a common finding in respiratory and cardiac diseases. A number of factors are involved in mechanism of dyspnea. In COPD increased sense of effort, hypoxia, hypercapnia and dynamic airway compression may be responsible for dyspnea.

Fig. 3.14 compares obstructive and restrictive types of ventilatory volumes.

CASE HISTORY: 3.1

A patient with long previous history of dyspepsia started with persistent vomiting 4 days back and presented with marked muscle weakness. Arterial blood gas findings are: pCO_2 48.0 mmHg, H^+ 25 nmol/L (pH 7.6), HCO_3^- 40 mmol/L, pO_2 76 mmHg, K^+ 2.3 mmol/L.

Gastric vomiting produces metabolic alkalosis because of loss of H^+ of gastric juice. For secretion of one hydrogen ion in gastric juice, one HCO_3^- ion is added to blood. With loss of hydrogen ion in gastric juice, the corresponding HCO_3^- ion permanently stays in blood (normally, when gastric juice is reabsorbed, and hydrogen ions diffuse back, these rejoin HCO_3^- ions to form H_2CO_3). Increase of HCO_3^- in the present case is the primary change in the bicarbonate buffer, producing metabolic alkalosis.

➤ What are other effects of vomiting on parameters of water and electrolyte metabolism in this case?

➤ What is relation between water, electrolyte disturbances produced by vomiting in this case to alkalosis?

➤ How are effects of vomiting without pyloric stenosis (acute intestinal obstruction) different from those with pyloric stenosis (duodenal ulcer)?

➤ Is there any evidence of K^+ depletion in clinical picture of this case? How to correct K^+ depletion?

➤ Will tissue oxygenation be appropriate in this case with arterial pO_2 of 76 mmHg?

• Besides alkalosis due to loss of hydrogen ions, there will be hypochloremia because of excessive loss of chloride ions, hypovolemia, because of loss of Na^+ and water and hypokalemia because of loss of K^+ in gastric juice. Volume depletion could reduce renal circulation resulting in azotemia. Thus blood urea and serum creatinine levels should be studied in this case.

• Hypovolemia, hypochloremia and hypokalemia of this case will tend to worsen metabolic alkalosis. Na^+ depletion enhances Na^+ reabsorption from the tubular fluid both in proximal and distal segments of kidney. In proximal tubules, Na^+ is reabsorbed with HCO_3^- because of reduced level of Cl^- in the tubular fluid. This tends to maintain alkalosis. In distal segments Na^+ is reabsorbed in exchange for K^+ and H^+. Because of hypokalemia, less K^+ is available for exchange and therefore more H^+ is secreted and a paradoxic finding of increased H^+ excretion in urine, in a person suffering from metabolic alkalosis. K^+ excretion will also be more than appropriate. Thus there will be worsening of both alkalosis and hypokalemia.

• In the absence of pyloric stenosis, persistent vomiting would lead to loss of gastric juice from stomach and of duodenal juice (rich in HCO_3^-). This will produce loss of Na^+, H_2O, K^+, HCO_3^-, Cl^- and H^+. There will be hypovolemia, hypokalemia but no alkalosis.

• Severe muscle weakness is most likely because

of K^+ deficiency in the present case. The most important part of management is infusion of isotonic saline to remove volume (and Na^+) deficit. However, as K^+ is very low, some K^+ should be given in the intravenous fluids. Intravenous K^+ should be given slowly (not more than 20 mmol/h) and under ECG check.

- Ordinarily, at pO_2 of 76 mmHg, there should be no problem of tissue oxygenation. However, in the presence of alkalosis, the shape of oxygen dissociation curve is changed (shift to left) and there is impaired release of oxygen at the prevailing pO_2 in tissues. It will tend to make metabolism anaerobic in tissues.

CASE HISTORY: 3.2

In a patient of chest injury in a road accident, blood gas analysis results were:

H^+=66 nmol/L (pH 7.18), pCO_2=62 mmHg, HCO_3^-=26 mmol/L

Explain the results.

H^+=66 mmol/L means severe acidosis. pCO_2 is raised, implying that it is respiratory acidosis. In such cases renal compensation increases HCO_3^-. In the present case HCO_3^- is not much increased and it is a case of uncompensated respiratory acidosis.

CASE HISTORY: 3.3

A patient of COPD arterial blood gas analysis revealed:

pCO_2=80.2 mmHg, HCO_3^-=36 mmol/L and H^+=60 nmol/L (pH 7.2).

He was put on artificial respiration and a few hours after, his arterial blood gas analysis showed:

pCO_2=42.0 mmHg, HCO_3^-=36 mmol/L, and H^+=28 nmol/L (pH 7.52).

Explain the results.

Initial high pCO_2 and pH of 7.2 means respiratory acidosis. Bicarbonate is increased, indicating renal compensation. The patient has chronic partially compensated respiratory acidosis.

After a few hours on ventilator, pCO_2 was normalized but not HCO_3^-. This is because excess CO_2 is rapidly washed off on a ventilator but HCO_3^- which was raised due to renal response, changes only very slowly. The patient has blood gas parameters of metabolic alkalosis. At H^+ of 28 nmol/L he is likely to show features of tetany. The inference is that such patients need slow, careful artificial ventilation.

CASE HISTORY: 3.4

During exacerbation of COPD the arterial blood gas analysis results were:

pCO_2=71.0 mmHg, H^+=63 nmol/L, HCO_3^-=28 mmol/L

and pO_2=48 mmHg. His condition persisted for about 10 days when a repeat blood gas analysis showed:

pCO_2=64.0 mmHg, H^+=40 nmol/L (pH 7.4), HCO_3^-=37 mmol/L, pO_2=60 mmHg.

- In the first group of results, increased H^+ is due to high pCO_2; the patient has respiratory acidosis. As HCO_3^- is almost in the normal range, there is no renal compensation. So it is an acute case of respiratory acidosis.
- In the second group of results, pCO_2 has been reduced to 64.0 mmHg and pO_2 increased to 60 mmHg, showing some improvement in pulmonary functions. Further renal compensation has raised HCO_3^- to normalize H^+. A period of 10 days is sufficient for adequate compensation.

CASE HISTORY: 3.5

A 30 year old patient (female) had severe vomiting of about a week and then she was admitted to the hospital.

Explain the following findings of the patient:

➤ Serum Na^+ 150 mEq/L and urine Na^+ 15 mmol/L

➤ Arterial blood H^+ of 26 nmol/L (pH 7.6) and HCO_3^- of 41 mmol/L) and urine pH 5.2.

➤ Blood urea 120 mg/dL and serum creatinine 2.1 mg/dL.

➤ Serum K^+ 2.6 mmol/L.

➤ Arterial blood HCO_3^- 42 mmol/L and pCO_2 52 mmHg.

- There is conservation of Na^+. Excretion in urine is reduced inspite of mild hypernatremia. This is because of increased aldosterone secretion in hypovolemia.
- It is a case of metabolic alkalosis produced by severe prolonged vomiting. Formation of acid urine means paradoxic aciduria. In severe, prolonged gastric vomiting, HCO_3^- is being added to blood (alkalosis) and there is ECF contraction. The latter change reduce GFR and increases renal reabsorption of Na^+ (with HCO_3^-). During the active stage of HCl loss, plasma HCO_3^- rises above its the proximal tubular threshold leading to increased HCO_3^- load of distal nephron segments. In these exchange segments there is increased TEPD (lumen negative transepithelial potential difference) because of increased load of $NaHCO_3$ in the presence of elevated aldosterone due to ECF contraction. Increased TEPD promotes loss of both K^+ and H^+. In this way the events in both proximal and distal segments explain hypokalemia and formation of acid urine. After the acute stage of HCl loss is over, metabolic alkalosis still continues because of increased threshold for HCO_3^- (produced by ECF contraction, low K^+ and increased aldosterone secretion).
- Hypovolemia is produced by loss of Na^+ and

water in vomits. Hypovolemia leads to pre renal azotemia. With reduced GFR there is greater reabsorption of urea than creatinine in proximal tubules.

- There is hypokalemia due to loss of K^+ in vomits and in urine because of alkalosis.
- The results indicate compensation of metabolic alkalosis.

CASE HISTORY: 3.6

Arterial blood gas analysis results in two cases of acute aspirin poisoning are given below:

- pCO_2=12 mmHg, H^+=26 nmol/L (pH 7.6), pO_2=96 mmHg.
- pCO_2=26 mmHg, H^+=62 nmol/L (pH 7.2), pO_2=94 mmHg.

Explain the two results

- There is hyperventilation (due to stimulation of respiratory centre), in early phase of aspirin poisoning. In an acute case, with pCO_2 of 12 mmHg, and without any renal compensation, one would expect H^+ lower than 26 nmol/L. It could be metabolic acidosis superadded on respiratory alkalosis. Aspirin produces metabolic acidosis by promoting lipolysis (and ketogenesis) and by inhibiting citric acid cycle reactions.
- The data means metabolic acidosis with compensatory hyperventilation. In aspirin poisoning metabolic acidosis occurs following early respiratory alkalosis. Metabolic acidosis following respiratory alkalosis is generally more severe since during respiratory alkalosis renal response leads to HCO_3^- depletion and subsequent metabolic acidosis is poorly buffered. Arterial blood HCO_3^- should be quite low in this patient, although, the actual figure has not been mentioned.

CASE HISTORY: 3.7

A baby had cyanotic attack 8h after birth and had grunting respiration. His birth weight was 1.8 kg and gestational age was 36 weeks. Apgar score was poor. At the time of examination pulse was 136/min and respiratory rate 65/min. X-ray chest showed ground glass appearance of lungs. Results of blood gas analysis were: pO_2 50 mmHg, pCO_2 50 mmHg, HCO_3^- 15 mEq/L and pH 7.14 (H^+ 70 nmol/L).

It is most likely a case of respiratory distress syndrome (RDS). One must, however, rule out certain congenital anomalies and complications commonly, seen in low birth weight babies. Diaphragmatic hernia is ruled out because of delayed onset of respiratory distress. From X-ray findings of the present case, possibility of inhalation of regurgitated stomach contents is ruled out.

Congenital heart disease can be differentiated with the help of the hyperoxia test. In this test administration of high level of O_2 improves pO_2, dramatically, in RDS but not in congenital heart disease.

CASE HISTORY: 3.8

A 26 year old man presented with chest tightness, coughing and wheezing for the last 6h. In the past few months he had many such attacks. Attacks were often induced by exercise or emotional situations. In the present attack the clinical examination showed that the patient was dyspneic. In chest there were rhonchi and coarse crepitations. Results of blood gas analysis were:

pO_2 66 mmHg, pCO_2 32 mmHg and pH 7.5 (H^+ 30 nmol/L).

➤ Does this patient need assisted ventilation?
➤ What is role of pulmonary function tests in diagnosis and management of asthmatics?

- Hypoxemia, mild hypocapnia and mild alkalosis (As seen in this case) is not uncommon in an attack of asthma and is not an indication of assisted ventilation. Need for assisted ventilation is apparent in a severe attack of asthma when progressive type 2 failure develops; pO_2 starts falling below 50 mmHg, pCO_2 starts rising above 50 mmHg and pH starts dipping below 7.3. Clinically patient gets exhausted, and starts becoming confused and drowsy.
- In asthmatics, FEV_1, VC and PEF (peak expiratory flow) are used to evaluate degree of air flow obstruction. These parameters also help to identify the triggering factor in an asthmatic attack. For example, a bout of exercise or exposure to a particular environment may lead to sudden drop in above parameters. Serial estimations of PEF show morning decrease in patients of asthma. This finding helps to differentiate asthma from chronic bronchitis and emphysema (morning decrease of PEF is not seen). Another way to differentiate these conditions from asthma is to find out bronchial reactivity (as decrease in PEF) after inhalation of increasing amounts of methacholine which stimulates the bronchiolar muscle. Decrease of PEF occurs at much lower level in asthma than the other conditions. The same test is also used to monitor benefit of a proposed drug therapy.

CASE HISTORY: 3.9

A 60 year old man had urinary tract symptoms of enlarged prostate. His BP was 136/92. Transurethral resection was done and was uneventful. About 30 hours after the operation he developed severe chill and his temperature was 40°C. BP came down to 95/60. There was no evidence of excessive bleeding from the resected area. ECG ruled out myocardial infarction, and any arrhythmia. X-ray chest was normal. The patient had developed endotoxic shock. This condition may develop gradually, after surgery on infected urinary tract or after a difficult intestinal surgery. It is confirmed by blood culture. In endotoxic shock patient develops shivering and high fever. There may also be respiratory distress and hyperventilation. Bacterial endotoxemia causes peripheral vasodilation. Peripheral parts feel warm. In early stages of the disorder, cardiac output is normal. As the condition progresses both systolic and diastolic blood pressures fall. Because of hypotension and peripheral stagnation of blood, there is fall in pO_2 and reduced oxygen delivery to tissues.

➤ What acid base disorders such a patient is likely to suffer, during the course of illness?

➤ How should such a patient be monitored?

• Because of fever, hypoxemia and endotoxins there is hyperventilation which may produce respiratory alkalosis. Further due to reduced pO_2 and poor O_2 delivery in tissues (pooling of blood due to vasodilatation), metabolic acidosis will be produced.

• The patient needs to be monitored for central venous pressure, blood gases and H^+. Patients of endotoxic shock are at risk of developing DIC. This tendency should be monitored by suitable investigations. Management of the patient includes steps to control infection and to improve hemodynamics.

CASE HISTORY: 3.10

In a case of septic shock blood pressure was 80/50 mmHg, and the patient was cold to touch. His arterial blood gas analysis results were as under:

pCO_2 43.5 mmHg, H^+ 80 nmol/L (pH 7.1), HCO_3^- 14 mmol/L, pO_2 60.0 mmHg.

Give comments on the results

• It is a case of acidosis since H^+ is 80 nmol/L.

• pCO_2 is in the normal reference range while HCO_3^- is appreciably reduced. It is a case of metabolic acidosis. It is also in agreement with the clinical condition of the patient. In septic shock there is lactic acidosis (poor tissue perfusion), and azotemia (poor renal circulation).

• After compensation pCO_2 (expected) would be <30 mmHg. Actual pCO_2 of 43.5, indicates super added respiratory acidosis. This is also suggested from H^+ concentration. H^+ concentration of 80 nmol/L is too high for HCO_3^- level of 14 mmol/L.

• In this patient there is super added respiratory distress syndrome which explains inappropriately

high H^+ concentration for HCO_3^- of 14 mmol/L and also accounts for pO_2 of 60 mmHg.

OBJECTIVE TYPE QUESTIONS

Pick out the wrong statement.

1. H^+, pH and buffers

i) It is easier to think of acid base disorders in terms of H^+ than pH.

ii) Between pH of 6.0 to 8.0 for each increase of 0.01 pH, there is decrease of 1 nmol of H^+.

iii) Buffer base represents sum of the blood buffers and its value varies from 46 to 52 mmol/L.

iv) Hb forms a good buffer because of histidine residues it contains.

v) Phosphate buffer is more important in ICF and tubular fluid than in ECF.

2. About acid base disorders

i) The commonest cause of metabolic alkalosis is gastric vomiting or prolonged gastric suction.

ii) The commonest causes of metabolic acidosis are diabetes mellitus, lactic acidosis and renal disease.

iii) Respiratory alkalosis is the most common disorder of critically ill patients.

iv) The initial acid base disturbance of salicylate poisoning in children is generally respiratory alkalosis.

v) Patients of with pneumonia, sepsis or cardiac failure frequently present with respiratory alkalosis.

3. Anion gap

i) The anion gap results form presence of certain unmeasured anions in plasma.

ii) Study of anion gap may be helpful in diagnosing the cause of metabolic acidosis.

iii) The unmeasured anionic charge is also provided by albumin.

iv) The anionic charge of albumin is reduced in acidosis.

v) All case of renal failure acidosis, present with increased anion gap.

vi) Anion gap remains unchanged in hyperchloremic acidosis.

4. Hypertension with hypokalemia and alkalosis

i) There is ECF expansion.

ii) It may be caused by primary aldosteronism.

iii) It may be caused by renal artery stenosis.

iv) It may be caused by licorice or tobacco chewing.

v) In licorice and tobacco chewing there is increased renin activity.

vi) Renin activity is also increased in renal artery stenosis.

5. Metabolic alkalosis with hypokalemia and ECF contraction

i) Most common cause is loss of gastric fluid.

ii) It could be caused by prolonged use of diuretics.

iii) Renal compensation for metabolic alkalosis fails in the presence of hypokalemia, ECF contraction and chloride depletion.

iv) Generally, in management, saline infusion is enough, along with correction of the causative factor.

v) In cases of kidney damage, however, acetazolamide may help.

6. RTA type 2

i) In RTA type 2 there may be general proximal tubular dysfunction with increased fractional excretion of bicarbonate.

ii) RTA type 2 may be primary or secondary.

iii) Hypokalemia results from increased bicarbonate load on distal segments.

iv) Reduced citrate reabsorption in proximal tubules causes citruria which prevents formation of renal stones inspite of hypercalciuria.

v) In RTA type 1 (but not in RTA type 2) urine pH can be lowered to below 5.0 with a load of ammonium chloride.

vi) RTA type 1 requires smaller amounts of HCO_3^- for treatment compared to RTA type 2.

7. RTA type 1

i) One or both of the active proton pumps (H^+ - ATPase, and H^+, K^+ - ATPase) are defective.

ii) Patient is not able to lower urine pH below 5.5.

iii) There is increased reabsorption of Cl^-.

iv) Because of defect in NH_3 formation, its excretion is reduced.

v) Patient suffers from hyperchloremic acidosis, hypokalemia and low ammonium excretion.

8. RTA

i) Hyperchloremic acidosis may occur in RTA, in the presence of profuse diarrhea, or in some cases of parenteral hyperalimentation with use of chloride salts of basic amino acids.

ii) Urinary ammonium level is increased in extrarenal causes of hyperchloremic acidosis, compared to renal causes.

iii) In urine there is equivalence of charge between cations (Na^+, K^+, NH_4^+) and anions (Cl^-, HCO_3^-).

iv) Hyperchloremic metabolic acidosis and hyperkalemia found in chronic renal disease is called RTA type 4.

v) In both RTA types 1 and 2, rickets/osteomalacia may be present.

9. Respiratory acid base disorders

i) Acute cases are compensated by cellular buffers.

ii) In chronic cases renal compensation starts within 12 to 24h but takes a few days to develop fully.

iii) Respiratory alkalosis is the most common acid base disorder in critically ill patients.

iv) In respiratory alkalosis tissue oxygenation improves as ventilatory process is increased.

v) In severe hypercapnia a patient may present with features like that of a cerebral tumor.

10. Hypoxemia

i) In pulmonary edema $\dot{V}/\dot{Q}$ mismatch produces hypoxemia.

ii) In alveolar collapse shunting is the cause of hypoxemia.

iii) In $\dot{V}/\dot{Q}$ mismatch and shunting, alveolar - arterial pO_2 difference is increased.

iv) Both in $\dot{V}/\dot{Q}$ mismatch and shunting, oxygen administration improves alveolar-arterial pO_2 difference.

v) Hypoventilation or low inspired pO_2, may produce hypoxemia.

11. Respiratory acid base disorders

i) In respiratory alkalosis of sepsis there may be later superimposed metabolic acidosis; in such a case both pH and HCO_3^- may be normal.

ii) Pink puffers (COPD) present with mild hypoxemia, normal pH and normal pCO_2.

iii) Blue bloaters present with hypoxemia, elevated pCO_2 and low pH.

iv) In asthmatics, without bronchitis or emphysema, during an attack, along with hypoxemia, presence of normal pCO_2 (>40 mmHg) indicates need for ventilatory assistance.

v) In pulmonary edema (acute) hypoxemia without increase of pCO_2 is the common finding.

vi) In pulmonary embolism hypoxemia (related to size of embolus) with mild to moderate alkalosis is the common finding.

ANSWERS

1. No.(ii). This relationship holds between pH values 7.3 and 7.5.

2. No.(iv). It is true in adults (metabolic acidosis follows initial respiratory alkalosis), not in children who generally present with metabolic acidosis right from the beginning. Respiratory alkalosis preceding metabolic acidosis depletes the bicarbonate buffer and results in increased severity of the subsequent disorder.

3. No.(v). Early cases of chronic renal failure may present with normal anion gap.

4. No.(v). Some metabolites of licorice/tobacco act like mineralocorticoids.

5. No.(v). Acetazolamide is effective only in the absence of renal insufficiency.

6. No.(v). In RTA type 2 pH of urine can be lowered to <5.0 with an ammonium chloride load.

7. No.(iv). There is failure of H^+ secretion and as ammonia can not be trapped in urine, in the absence of H^+, excretion of NH_4^+ in urine is reduced.

8. No.(iv). Although some degree of renal failure is associated with RTA type 4, it is a different entity (see in the Chapter 4).

9. No.(iv). Tissue oxygenation is reduced because of 'shift to left' of the oxygen dissociation curve of oxygen.

10. No.(iv). In cases of shunting, oxygen administration does not improve alveolar - arterial pO_2 difference.

11. No.(iii). pH may be low (decompensated state) or normal (compensated state).

CHAPTER 4

Renal Functions and Disorders

There are two kidneys, each having about a million nephrons which are the functional units. Renal functions include: i) excretion of waste products like urea, creatinine, uric acid, sulphate and phosphate, derived from metabolism of proteins and nucleic acids; ii) maintenance of ECF volume and composition (electrolytes, pH, calcium and phosphate). These functions are achieved by the actions of hormones like AVP, aldosterone and PTH; iii) kidney is also site of formation of renin, erythropoietin and calcitriol.

From about 700 mL of plasma passing through the two kidneys, about 125 mL of glomerular filtrate (protein and cell free fluid) is formed per minute. The filtration membrane is composed of three layers; the endothelial layer of glomerular capillaries, the middle basement layer and the outer epithelial layer. The ultrafiltrate character of glomerular fluid is determined by the health of the three layers especially the middle one. The glomerular filtration rate (GFR) depends upon: i) rate of circulation through kidneys; ii) hydrostatic pressure in glomerular capillaries; iii) hydrostatic pressure of the tubular fluid (this pressure increases in case of obstruction in the urinary tract); iv) oncotic pressure of plasma; v) patency of glomerular capillaries.

Systemic hypotension is an important cause of reduced GFR. Reduced plasma volume, in congestive heart failure, also tends to reduce GFR, although release of certain vasodilatory prostaglandins in renal circulation help to maintain GFR. GFR is greatly reduced in nephritic disorders, as the proliferative changes in glomeruli interfere in their patency. In nephrotic disorders the pathological changes mainly occur in the filtration membrane and glomerular patency is maintained and GFR is not reduced.

From GFR of about 125 mL/min, about 1 mL urine is formed per minute. As the glomerular filtrate passes through the tubules, not only its volume is greatly reduced but also, it undergoes extensive qualitative changes. There is extensive removal (reabsorption) of the useful materials like glucose, amino acids, sodium and others (along with passive reabsorption of water), while the waste materials are not reabsorbed or only poorly reabsorbed. Infact, these may be further added to the tubular fluid by the secretory activity of the tubules.

Substances whose concentrations in ECF are regulated by the kidney, are handled in a facultative manner by the tubules. This facultative property is the outcome of the morphological and biochemical characters of the tubular cells as well as their interactions with different hormones. These functions are carried out by the part of the nephron distal to the proximal tubule. The proximal tubule has the main function of reabsorbing useful substances and retaining the waste substances in the tubular fluid while reducing the volume of filtrate and reducing the amounts of substances to be regulated, to desired limits, so that the distal segments can perform their facultative actions, effectively.

There is a large reserve of renal functions. Further, from what has been said above, it can be inferred that moderate decrease of GFR may not much impair the renal ability to perform its functions. The following points, however, should be kept in mind:

1. The first evident change that occurs with decrease of GFR, in a renal or prerenal disease, is increase in plasma levels of urea and creatinine (waste substances). When GFR is reduced to less than 50% of the normal, the normal plasma ranges of urea and creatinine concentrations are exceeded.

2. Fall in GFR does not lead to oliguria (unless GFR falls to quite a low level). On the other hand, the accumulated waste substances (see above) cause osmotic diuresis, to increase urine volume.

3. In severe hypotention, GFR is reduced but the tubular functions are normal in the beginning, also there is increased secretion of aldosterone and AVP and urine of high osmolarity and low Na^+ is produced (see later).

4. Although specific tubular mechanisms are involved in excretions of H^+, K^+, urate and phosphate, reduced GFR reduces the required load on the tubules for adequate excretion of these substances. Normal plasma ranges of these substances exceed when GFR falls below 25% of the normal value.

The important facultative functions of the tubules are as under:

1. Water reabsorption and urine concentration

Specific gravity of urine in a normal person may vary from about 1.003 (50 mosmol/L) to about 1.030 (1400 mosmol/L). Renal concentrating power of urine can be taken as normal if specific gravity of a random urine sample is 1.023 or more. Three important requirements of urine diluting and concentrating mechanism are: i) functionally normal loops and distal segments; ii) adequate delivery of salts and urea to distal segments; iii) slow rate of flow of fluid in the loops and distal segments. All these help to establish renal medullary interstitial

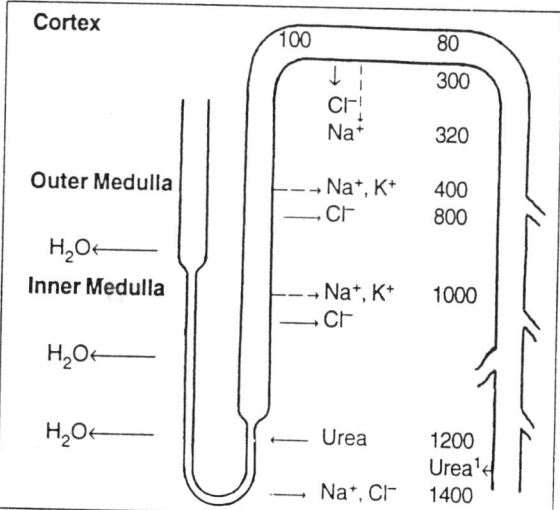

Fig. 4.1. Generation of renal medullary interstitial concentration gradient.

---

[1] In the presence of AVP, the collecting ducts in inner medulla become permeable to urea. In this way urea has a major role in producing high interstitial concentration in deeper parts of medulla.

Condition for generation of suitable concentration gradient:
- Healthy loops.
- Proper salt and protein intake for normal levels of urea, Na^+, Cl^- in plasma.
- Slow flow of fluid in distal segments.
- Normal levels of serum Ca^{2+} and K^+ (hypercalcemia and hypokalemia impair the process).
- AVP for permeability of urea.

concentration gradient; iv) appropriate availability of AVP for the process of urine concentration (Fig. 4.1).

The ascending limb of the loop has the main role in establishing the medullary interstitial concentration gradient by reabsorbing Na^+, K^+ and Cl^- without reabsorption of water and producing dilute fluid. The process continues in the proximal part of the distal convoluted tubule. Urine is said to have been diluted when the above dilute fluid is passed, as such, as urine (more precisely this fluid is further diluted by reabsorption of Na^+ in onward segments).

For urine concentration, water from the above fluid (while flowing down the collecting ducts) is reabsorbed because of increasing medullary concentration gradient. AVP makes the collecting duct cells permeable to water. Thus any damage to the collecting ducts, any impairment of AVP secretion or action or defective medullary interstitial gradient will interfere in urine concentration process, while damage to the loop of Henle will impair both diluting as well as concentrating powers of the kidney.

2. Exchange of reabsorbed Na^+ for H^+ and K^+ secretions

Na^+ is reabsorbed in different ways in different parts of the nephron. In proximal tubular cells there is Na^+ - solute symport, (the transporter carries Na^+ alongwith some solute like glucose, amino acid etc.), and the transepithelial potential gradient generated helps reabsorption of chloride through the leaky junctions between the cells. In the same region there is Na^+ - H^+ antiport which may be linked with bicarbonate reabsorption or chloride (cellular route) reabsorption. In thick part of the ascending limb, there is Na^+, K^+ - $2Cl^-$ symport and Na^+ - Cl^- symport in proximal part of distal tubule, without water reabsorption. In distal part of distal tubule and the collecting duct there is active Na^+ reabsorption. In all these Na^+ reabsorptive processes, Na^+ reabsorption is active except perhaps in the thick part of the ascending limb where chloride reabsorption may be active and Na^+/K^+ reabsorption linked to that.

In the collecting ducts and distal part of distal convoluted tubules, Na^+ is reabsorbed through the

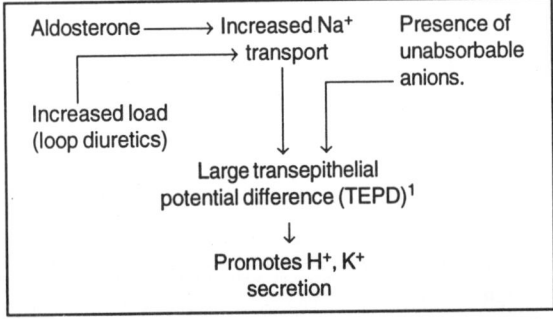

Fig.4.2. Factors affecting sodium reabsorption and K^+, H^+ secretions in exchange segments.

---

[1] TEPD is created by electrogenic Na^+ reabsorption (Na^+ reabsorption in excess of any accompanying anion).

sodium conducting channels which creates a high transepithelial potential difference (if Na^+ is accompanied by anions other than Cl^- with low permeability) which helps secretions of H^+ and K^+. This is what is called Na^+ reabsorption through the exchange process. Na^+ reabsorption with Cl^- is non-electrogenic. All this sodium reabsorption is under control of aldosterone. Other factors influencing this reabsorption are shown in Fig.4.2. Increased Na^+ reabsorption through this exchange process increases secretions of H^+ and K^+. There is reciprocity in secretions of the two ions depending upon their relative levels in distal tubular cells.

Renal disorders and renal function tests

GFR is very commonly affected in renal diseases or systemic disorders influencing functioning of kidneys. A number of immune complex and auto-immune diseases produce pathological lesions in glomeruli. If blood flow through glomeruli is reduced, GFR will be reduced. If the filtration membrane is damaged, proteins and blood cells will start appearing in the filtrate and urine. Effect of systemic hypotention on GFR has already been mentioned. In all these disorders, it is important to evaluate GFR and integrity of the filtration membrane (see Appendix B).

Tubular damage without involvement of glomeruli is less common. In pyelonephritis, however, involvement of tubular system occurs earlier than glomeruli. Tubular damage is evaluated by studying the renal ability to concentrate and dilute urine and to secrete H^+. Renal ability to concentrate urine, is also affected in a systemic disease that generates excessive solute load to be cleared by the kidney (also see Table 4.1). Many diseases start with involvement of glomeruli but ultimately lead to loss of the whole nephrons, since the lesion at the glomerular level may affect the vascular supply to the tubular system of the nephron. Some vascular diseases also lead to gradual nephron loss. In all such diseases a stage comes when surviving nephrons experience excessive solute load per nephron and osmotic diuresis results, along with decrease in GFR. Tubular cells express different transport proteins for different reabsorptive processes. A

Table 4.1. Conditions in which urine concentrating ability of kidney is impaired

---

Reduced ADH formation[1]:
- Excessive water intake (eg; primary polydipsia)
- Central diabetes insipidus
- Drug induced inhibition of ADH release

Renal tubular unresponsiveness:
- Nephrogenic diabetes insipidus familial (congenital)
- Nephrogenic diabetes insipidus acquired
  - after obstructive uropathy
  - after acute tubular necrosis
  - many chronic renal diseases (pyelonephritis, interstitial nephritis) and congenital renal diseases (polycystic, medullary cystic disease).
  - chronic hypercalcemia, potassium depletion
    drugs like lithium, ethanol, demeclocycline, systemic diseases like multiple myeloma, sickle cell disease, amyloidosis.

Osmotic diuresis:
- Diabetes mellitus
- Diuretics

Poor intake of salt/protein

- Urine output >3L/d is called polyuria.
[1] Polyuria is due to water diuresis, if urine osmolality is <250 mOsmol/kg and total mOsmol excretion is normal (600-800 mOsmol/d).
- Polyuria is due to solute or osmotic diuresis if urine osmolality is >300 mOsmol/kg (group 3 and most cases of group 2).

number of inborn errors are known with defective transport proteins. In this category we have Fanconi syndrome, phosphate diabetes (vitamin D resistant rickets) and renal tubular acidosis. Certain hormones regulate the tubular transport processes. Assessment of tubular functions have also been used in evaluating the status of these hormones.

Glomerulonephritis or glomerulopathy

Glomerular injury can be produced by various factors which may be immunogenic, metabolic, hemodynamic, genetic or infections. The disease process may be renal limited (primary disorder) or part of a systemic disease (secondary disorder or secondary glomerulopathy). Quite commonly, the glomerular injury is immunogenic. The antigen involved may be exogenous (bacterial, viral, other proteins) or endogenous (immune complexes resulting from some systemic autoimmune disorder) or local.

The glomerular injury may be with evidence of glomerular inflammation and increased cellularity of glomeruli. Increased cellularity is because of proliferation of glomerular cells or because of infiltration of leukocytes. Such a lesion is called proliferative glomerulonephritis or proliferative glomerulopathy. Some people use the term glomerulopathy for any type of glomerular injury and the term glomerulonephritis when glomerular injury is accompanied with an inflammatory reaction. The proliferative injury produces nephritic type of clinical disease (see below).

The term membranous, used with a glomerulopathy, indicates that the damage involves the filtration membrane (without proliferative changes). Such a pathological change produces nephrotic type of clinical presentation. Same is true about glomerulopathies in which there is increased formation of material whose structure resembles that of basement membrane (the process is termed glomerulosclerosis).

Besides the two common clinical forms, the nephritic and nephrotic syndromes, other less common clinical presentations are, recurrent hematuria, chronic renal failure, hypertension and persistent proteinuria and rapidly progressive renal failure (Table 4.2).

A glomerulopathy should be first defined from its clinical presentation. Next, its pathological pattern should be known. Finally, primary or secondary nature of the glomerulopathy should be explored.

Nephritic syndrome

The proliferative inflammatory reaction obstructs glomerular capillary lumen leading to fall in GFR. GFR is further reduced by intrarenal vasoconstriction and mesangial cell contraction because of imbalance between local vasoconstrictors (leukotrienes, PAF, thromboxanes, endothelins) and vasodilator substances (NO, PGI_2) in renal microcirculation. Fall in GFR may cause oliguria (urine volume <400 mL/d). There is ECF expansion, edema, and hypertension due to reduced GFR and increased tubular reabsorption of salt and water. Because of injury to glomerular capillary wall, urine shows red

Table 4.2. About glomerulopathies

Immunologic injury mediated by Igs, T-cells, cytokines, complement activation	Metabolic (hyperglycemia in diabetes)	Hemodynamic (systemic hypertension, intraglomerular hypertension)

Causes of glomerular Injury ←
- Toxic (drugs)
- Induced by deposits (amyloid/light chains)
- Thrombotic microangiopathy
- In born

Acute nephritic syndrome (acute proliferative GN)	Post streptococcal and other immune complex primary cases/ secondary cases (SLE/SBE/HSP)	Acute renal failure for days/weeks. Azotemia, oliguria, hypertension, edema. Nephritic type active urine sediment (red cells, red cell casts, WBC, cellular casts). Subnephrotic proteinuria.
Rapidly progressive GN (crescentic GN)	Immune complex (as above) Pauci-immune GN primary/ secondary Anti - GBM disease	Subacute renal failure for weeks to months. Azotemia, oliguria, hypertension, edema. Active urine sediment. Subnephrotic proteinuria.
Milder form of GN (focal proliferative GN, mesangial proliferative GN)	Immune complex cases (milder forms), IgA nephropathy, HSP	In focal proliferative cases, mild to moderate decrease in GFR, active urine sediment. In mesangial proliferative cases (more chronic) effect on GFR variable, hypertension, proteinuria, hematuria.
Nephrotic syndrome (minimal change GN, membranous GN)	Idiopathic/drug induced/ Hodgkin's, lymphomas/ hepatitis, malaria, leprosy/ autoimmune disorders	Proteinuria>3g/d, hypoalbuminemia, edema, lipidemia, lipiduria, thrombotic tendency. Slow decline in GFR in 10 to 30% cases.
Variable nephritic/ nephrotic mixed picture (membranoproliferative GN) and others (see next column)	Immune complex (see above), thrombotic microangiopathic cases (malignant hypertension), disposition disease (myeloma, amyloid)	Proteinuria in nephrotic range. Active urine sediment, acute or subacute decline in GFR.
Proteinuria and chronic renal failure (nodular/global sclerosis)	Diabetic nephropathy/may occur with long term changes in most glomerulopathies.	Proteinuria and chronic renal failure.

cells casts, dysmorphic red cells, leukocytes and subnephrotic proteinuria (<3 g/d). Hematuria is often microscopic.

Most patients of acute glomerulonephritis are having immune complex glomerulonephritis in which an immune inflammatory reaction plays an important role, in development of the pathological lesion. Most commonly, it occurs as a post infectious disorder and poststreptococcal glomerulonephritis is the commonest acute immune complex glomerulonephritis. This is a primary glomerulonephritis.

The immune complex glomerulonephritis can also occur in other bacterial, viral, fungal and parasitic infections. Secondary glomerular injury can be produced in many multisystem diseases. The mechanism of injury may be immunogenic or non-immunogenic. The resulting disorders may have different pathological forms and different clinical presentations (Table 4.2). Two most important multisystem diseases which involve glomeruli are hypertension and diabetes mellitus. In both cases glomerular injury occurs by non-immune mechanisms. In malignant hypertension, thrombotic microangiopathy (microthrombi in glomerular capillaries, along with endothelial damage) results in acute renal failure and nephritic type of urinary sediment. In diabetes, there occurs, nodular or global sclerosis and clinical form of nephrotic syndrome. SLE,

Henoch - Schonlein purpura (HSP), microscopic polyartheritis nodosa, Wegner's granulomatosis and Churg - Strauss syndrome, all produce immunogenic glomerular injury.

Nephrotic syndrome

This condition is produced when damage is confined to filtration membrane and inflammatory changes are much less marked. There is heavy proteinuria (more selective than in nephritic disorders), but GFR is not reduced (no oliguria) and also urine is free from cellular elements (there are no red cells and cellular casts). The central feature of nephrotic syndrome is urinary protein excretion of 3 to 3.5 g/d and hypoalbuminemia. Many other features are related to this loss of protein in urine. These features are edema, hyperlipidemia, lipiduria, and hypercoagulability.

Hypoalbuminemia is caused by urinary loss, reduced hepatic synthesis and increased catabolism of albumin in kidney. Hypoalbuminemia causes reduced plasma oncotic pressure leading to reduced plasma volume, which in turn, stimulates renin-angiotensin-aldosterone axis and sympathetic system and also increases secretion of AVP. Reduced plasma volume also reduces release of ANP (atrial natriuretic peptide). All these changes contribute to edema of nephrotic syndrome (Chapter 2). Urinary losses of transferrin, thyroxine binding globulin, vitamin D_3 binding globulin, metal binding proteins and other proteins, produce metabolic abnormalities. IgG deficiency may produce compromised immune status. Increased urinary loss of antithrombin, increased hepatic synthesis of fibrinogen, increased platelet aggregation, reduced fibrinolysis and other changes result in hypercoagulability of blood.

Urinary loss of certain regulatory proteins and low plasma oncotic pressure, stimulate hepatic lipoprotein and α_2 – macroglobulin synthesis. The latter tends to maintain plasma oncotic pressure (in the presence of hypoalbuminemia).

Diagnosis of glomerulopathies

A glomerulopathy may present as acute nephritic syndrome, rapidly progressive glomerulonephritis

Table 4.3. Protein selectivity in proteinuria

Highly selective proteinuria
- Urine contains albumin and other low mol. wt. proteins like antithrombin, prealbumin, α_1 antitrypsin, α_1 acid glycoprotein and transferrin.
- Occurs in nephrotic syndrome in children, especially with minimal change disease.

Low selective proteinuria
- Besides low mol. wt. proteins urine also contains high mol. wt. proteins like IgG, α_2-macroglobulin and β-lipoprotein.
- Occurs in membranous nephropathy and proliferative glomerulonephritis.

Calculating selectivity index (SI)
- SI = IgG clearance/Albumin clearance x 100: Protein clearance = Conc. in urine/Conc. in plasma (SI <15% means high selectivity and SI>30 means low selectivity)

- Low selectivity indicates injury to podocytes and loss of -ive charge of filtration membrane.

(RPGN), nephrotic syndrome, asymptomatic abnormalities of urinary sediment (isolated proteinuria, isolated hematuria) or chronic glomerulonephritis. To define the clinical form, urine examination for different types of cells and casts and also for study of protein excretion in 24h, is required (Appendix B). There will also be need to study plasma levels of urea, creatinine, albumin and lipids. Study of excretion of protein in urine and selectivity of urinary protein (Table 4.3) should be done.

The histopathological pattern of the glomerulopathy is known from the kidney biopsy as well as certain serological features. Three important serological markers are serum C_3 levels, titres of anti-GMB antibody (glomerular membrane antibody) and anti-neutrophil cytoplasmic antibody (ANCA). The histological forms, crescentic glomerulonephritis and pauci-immune glomerulonephritis, commonly, present as RPGN. These studies will define prognosis of the disorder and also form basis for treatment. Age of the patient, in many instances, is also related to prognosis.

In poststreptococcal glomerulonephritis, antibiotics are used to eliminate the infection. The patient is also given supportive treatment till the glomerular inflammation resolves. Salt and water restriction depends upon oliguria, circulatory overload and edema. There is need to monitor serum K^+ level. For diet, liberal intake of carbohydrate is advised to reduce endogenous protein break down. Protein intake depends upon degree of oliguria and plasma urea level.

Acute renal failure (ARF)

It is sudden failure of kidney functions (occurring within hours to weeks) with decrease in GFR resulting in increased plasma levels of creatinine and urea, metabolic acidosis (reduced secretion of H^+) and hyperkalemia. Frequently, urine volume is reduced to less than 400 mL/d (oliguria). The last finding is encountered in about 50% cases. ARF is generally asymptomatic and diagnosed with biochemical investigations.

Depending upon the causative disorder, it may be prerenal ARF (prerenal azotemia) or renal ARF (renal azotemia) or postrenal ARF (postrenal azotemia) (Table 4.4). In most cases, ARF is recoverable, but when occurring as complication of a serious disease, it may get associated with morbidity or mortality of the patient.

Prerenal azotemia

It results from poor renal perfusion. It may result from any condition producing systemic hypotension (hypovolemic/cardiogenic/septic shock). Fig. 4.3. shows mechanisms which tend to maintain renal perfusion in such situations. The importance of these mechanisms in maintaining proper renal perfusion is clear from the fact that some drugs (ACE-inhibitors, cyclooxygenase inhibitors) which impair these responses produce prerenal azotemia without already existing hypotension. These intrarenal responses maintain a sort of systemic, renal vascular resistance gradient. This gradient is also impaired in the presence of severe systemic vasodilatation (sepsis, anti-hypertensives, anaesthesia), drugs producing renal vasconstriction (hypercalcemia, cyclosporine, catecholamines, amphotericin) and in many cases of cirrhosis with ascites (hepatorenal syndrome). All these conditions also produce prerenal azotemia.

In conditions resulting in severe systemic hypotension, the above referred mechanism tend to maintain renal perfusion. Although renal perfusion is below normal (and there is prerenal azotemia), no hypoxic damage to renal parenchyma occurs. This damage occurs to produce *ischemic ARF* only when the above mentioned mechanisms are overwhelmed (see below). To avoid development of

Table 4.4. Causes of different types of acute renal failure (ARF)

Prerenal ARF (prerenal azotemia):	**Intrinsic renal ARF** (intrinsic renal azotemia):
• Water electrolyte losses producing severe hypovolemia.	• Acute tubular necrosis.
• Hemorrhage, burns.	- Ischemic renal ARF: severe continuing prerenal azotemia.
• In septic shock, crush injuries (rhabdomyolysis) and intravascular hemolysis, (acute tubular necrosis can develop with element of prerenal ARF).	- Nephrotoxic renal ARF: It may be caused by exogenous toxins (radiocontrast compounds, drugs like cyclosporine, aminoglycosides and ethylene glycol) or endogenous toxins (rhabdomyolysis, hemolysis, uric acid, oxalate, L-chains in myeloma).
• Cardiogenic shock	• Diseases of glomeruli/microcirculation
• Relative increase of renal vascular resistance (compared to systemic vascular resistance)	- Glomerulonephritis and vasculitis
- Systemic vasodilatation (septic shock)	- Malignant hypertension, HUS, TTP, DIC, toxemia of pregnancy, SLE.
- Renal vasoconstriction (hypercalcemia, catechol amines, cyclosporine, amphotericin-β). It also occurs in hepato renal syndrome.	• Interstitial nephritis
Post renal ARF (postrenal azotemia):	• Tubular obstruction Myeloma L-chains, uric acid, oxalate
• Bladder neck obstruction, neurogenic bladder, cancer, blood clot)	• Renovascular obstruction
• Urethra (stricture, congenital valve)	- Renal artery thrombosis, atheroma, embolism, renal vein thrombosis
• Ureteric (retroperitoneal fibrosis).	

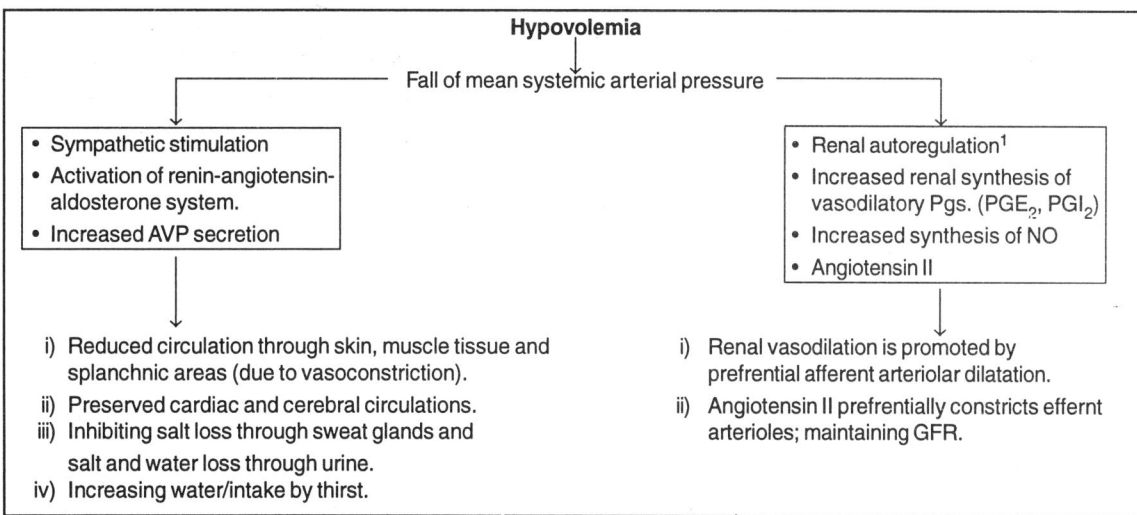

Fig. 4.3. Important hemodynamic alterations with hypovolemia and fall in mean systemic arterial pressure.

---

[1] Breakdown of these mechanisms results in ischemic ARF. Damage starts in tubular cells and there is decrease in GFR due to reduced blood flow through glomeruli, obstruction in tubules and leakage of fluid from tubules. This state of affair continues even when systemic blood pressure has been corrected (for a period of 1 to 2 weeks). Factors released from damaged tubular cells (less of NO and more of endothelin) and from leucocytes play important role in this phenomenon.

prerenal azotemia into ischemic ARF such patients should be vigorously treated. Further, in hypovolemic patients, use of drugs producing renal vasoconstriction or inhibiting renal vasodilatory responses should be avoided.

Intrinsic renal azotemia (intrinsic renal ARF)

Two most common causes are ischemia following prerenal azotemia (ischemic ARF) and nephrotoxins (nephrotoxic ARF). In both conditions there is typical acute tubular necrosis (ATN). Thus intrinsic renal ARF produced by these two causes may also be called as ATN. In ATN, two important pathophysiological changes are ischemia of glomeruli (no pathological damage) causing low GFR and patchy and focal necrosis in tubular cells (most commonly in pars recta of proximal tubules and medullary portion of thick ascending limb of loop of Henle). These tubular changes (which precede the glomerular changes) cause, tubular obstruction and leakage, thereby, decreasing effective GFR. Tubular functions are also impaired. Damaged cells appear in urine as muddy brown granular or epithelial casts.

Ischemic ARF is produced by severe/prolonged renal hypoperfusion (milder hypoperfusion produces prerenal azotemia). Severe hypoperfusion produces damage to tubular cells (see above). The damaged tubular cells, by dysregulated release of different mediators (less of NO and more of endothelin) and/or by other less well defined mechanisms, keep up renal hypoperfusion even when systemic hypotension has been corrected. This explains the oliguric phase (1 to 2 weeks) till tubular cell regeneration starts. In nephrotoxic ARF, the drug/toxin causes damage to the tubular cells which in turn produce renal hypoperfusion as explained above. In some cases (radiocontrast dyes, cyclosporine) the toxic agent besides causing tubular damage also, directly, causes renal hypoperfusion.

Besides ischemic ARF and nephrotoxic ARF, intrinsic renal ARF (much less commonly) is induced in acute tubulointerstitial diseases, renal microcirculation diseases (glomerulonephritis, malignant hypertension hemolytic uremic syndrome) and diseases of large renal vessels (thrombosis, atheroembolism).

After the oliguric phase, kidney functions

gradually return to normal. Between the oliguric phase and the recovery phase, often, there is a short diuretic phase, due to excretion of accumulated salt, water and other solutes and also because full reabsorptive functions have not yet developed in recently formed tubular epithelial cells. Poor urine concentration may also be due to loss of medullary interstitial concentration gradient during oliguric phase. During the recovery phase GFR and the tubular functions gradually return to normal.

Prevention has a very important role in management of ATN. In the high risk patient (after major surgery, severe trauma, burns, cholera), volume depletion should be vigorously treated. Plasma volume should be carefully monitored in patients receiving chemotherapy or nephrotoxic drugs. Forced alkaline diuresis may help patients suffering from rhabdomyolysis or those receiving chemotherapy.

Important diagnostic aspects

In a patient of azotemia, one should enquire whether condition is acute or chronic. Important indicators of chronic renal failure are, anemia, neuropathy, and radiological evidence of small kidneys or osteodystrophic changes in bone (Table 4.5).

Table 4.5. Biochemical differences between acute and chronic renal failure

- There is more uniformity in biochemical parameters in acute renal failure than chronic renal failure. In the latter disorder, these parameters will depend upon GFR (or stage of the disease).
- Hyperkalemia (often associated with acidosis) is more common in ARF than CRF. In CRF it may occur only at advanced stage of the disease when GFR is greatly reduced.
- Hyperphosphatemia and hypocalcemia are features of CRF.
- Anemia is quite a constant feature of CRF when GFR is less than 20 mL/min.
- Urine in CRF may often show a few red cells and a few broad casts. In ARF these microscopic findings are related to the etiology of the disorder.

- CRF may come to notice by accidental urine examination (broad casts due to dilated tubules), abdominal imaging (bilateral small kidneys) or blood examination (high creatinine, urea).
- Some times ARF is superadded on CRF.

Table 4.6. Investigations used to differentiate prerenal azotemia from intrinsic renal azotemia

Parameter	Prerenal azotemia	Intrinsic renal azotemia
Fractional sodium excretion (%) $\dfrac{U_{Na} \times P_{Cr}}{P_{Na} \times U_{Cr}} \times 100$	<1	>1 (often > 2.0)
Renal failure index $\dfrac{U_{Na}}{U_{Cr}/P_{Cr}}$	<1	>1
Urine creatinine to plasma creatinine ratio	>40	>20
Urine urea-N to plasma urea-N ratio	>8	<3
Plasma urea-N to plasma creatinine ratio	>20	<10-15

- In prerenal azotemia and intrinsic renal azotemia, urine osmolaties (mosmol/kg) and sodium concentrations (mmol/L) are >500 and <300 and <10 and >20, respectively.
- Urine contains hyaline casts in pre-renal azotemia and muddy brown granular casts in intrinsic renal azotemia.

In a patient of shock presenting with azotemia, one should find out if ischemic ARF has set in. In prerenal azotemia urinary sediment consists of hyaline casts, only, while in ischemic ARF sediment consists of muddy brown granular and epithelial casts. There may also be microscopic hematuria and mild tubular proteinuria (<1g/d). Similar features are present in nephrotoxic ARF. Fractional excretion of Na^+ is another useful test (Table 4.6). Rapid recovery after correction of hemodynamics indicates prerenal azotemia and persistance of azotemia increases likelihood of ischemic ARF.

A attempt should be made to find cause of intrinsic renal ARF. 90% of cases of intrinsic renal ARF are due to ischemic and nephrotoxic causes. In most of the cases there is quite apparent evidence of hypovolemia, hypotension or history of some drug intake. In other cases some indirect evidence may be available to arrive at the diagnosis. Myoglobinuria, hemoglobinuria, excessive urate excretion and L-chain excretion in myeloma, can all produce nephrotoxic renal ARF. Besides crush injuries, rhabdomyolysis and myoglobinuria may also occur during seizures, or in coma. Besides history of mismatched transfusion, severe anemia in the absence of hemorrhage may indicate possibility of hemolysis (also of myeloma or thrombotic micro-angiopathy). Tumor lysis and hyperuricosuria may occur after cancer chemotherapy. In cases of rhabdomyolysis and hemolysis, urine will show presence of heme (tested by reagent strips based on pseudoperoxidase activity of heme) and there will be alterations in plasma levels of K^+ ($\uparrow$), Ca^{+2} ($\downarrow$), PO_4^{-3}($\uparrow$) and uric acid ($\uparrow$). Further increased level of CPK-MM and myoglobin may be demonstrated in rhabdomyolysis and increased plasma level of hemoglobin in cases of hemolysis. In tumor lysis cases again hyperuricemia, hyperkalemia and hyperphosphatemia will be present (Chapter 16). Clue to myeloma may come from bone pains or anemia (see above). Urine may show presence of Bence-Jones protein. A monoclonal band may be demonstrated by electrophoresis.

In case of an acute glomerulopathy there may be history of a recent acute infection followed by (after a suitable interval) oliguria and presence of red cell casts, red cells and proteinuria. In a case of allergic interstitial nephritis there may be history of some drug intake, fever, rash and urine examination showing proteinuria, presence of eosinophils, red cells and white cell casts. There may also be systemic eosinophilia. Table 4.7 records some features of tubointerstitial diseases. The above urinary findings are also present in atheroembolic disease which may also produce ischemic renal ARF in old age (above 50 years).

In non-ischemic and non-nephrotoxic ARF cases, renal biopsy may be required for confirmation of diagnosis, proper treatment and knowing prognosis.

Metabolic disturbances and management of ARF

In the oliguric phase there is failure of excretion of nitrogenous and other waste products and patient may develop uremic syndrome. More catabolic the patient more rapidly this complication develops. Because of loss of homeostatic functions of the kidney, patient may develop volume overload, hyponatremia, hyperkalemia, hyperphosphatemia, hypocalcemia, hypermagnesemia and metabolic acidosis.

Volume overload occurs because of reduced renal loss of salt and water. It may lead to weight gain, increased JVP, rales at lung bases, dependent edema and pulmonary edema in severe cases. Excessive intake of free water may cause hyponatremia, which may lead to cerebral edema. For management both salt (1 to 2 g/d) and water (1L/d) are restricted.

In severe oliguric patients serum K^+ may rise by 0.5 mmol/L per day. Mild hyperphosphatemia is also an almost invariable finding. Both hypermagnesemia and hyperphosphatemia are severe in presence of rhabdomyolysis, hemolysis and tumor lysis syndrome. Metastatic calcification (in the presence of hyperphosphtemia) may produce hypocalcemia. Other factors contributing for hypocalcemia are

Table 4.7. Dysfunctions produced in tubulointerstitial diseases of kidney

- Loss of microvasculature and obstruction of tubules produces reduced GFR.
- Hyperchloremic acidosis is produced by HCO_3^- wasting (proximal tubular damage), impaired ammonia production and inability to generate titratable acid.
- Tubular proteinuria (α_1-microglobulin, β_2-microglobulin, lysozyme, L-chains).
- Damage to medullary structures impairs powers of the urine dilution and concentration.
- Impaired K^+ secretion, partly by aldosterone resistance.
- Hyperkalemia is produced by impaired K^+ secretion.
- There is salt wasting due to distal tubular defect.
- In some cases the proximal tubular damage may result in Fanconi syndrome.

- Tubulointerstitial disease may be caused by toxins (lead, analgesics, metals), metabolic disorders (hyperuricemia, hypercalcemia, hypokalemia), infections (acute/chronic pyelonephritis), neoplasia (multiple myeloma, lymphoma), immune disorders (hypersensitivity nephropathy, Sjogren's syndrome), vascular disorders (sickle cell nephropathy) and hereditary factors (Alport's syndrome, medullary cystic disease, polycystic kidney disease).

reduced formation of calcitriol and resistance to actions of PTH. For management, dietary intake of K^+ and phosphate is restricted. Other active measures (see under hyperkalemia (Chapter 2) and chronic renal failure) may also be required in certain cases.

Patients of ARF also suffer from metabolic acidosis. Acidosis may become severe in the presence of diabetes, prolonged fasting, tissue hypoperfusion, sepsis or liver disease. Acidosis is treated with sodium bicarbonate to keep HCO_3^- >15 mmol/L (or pH >7.2).

Dialysis is indicated in the presence of signs and symptoms of uremia, and when fluid overload, hyperkalemia or acidosis are not being controlled by conservative measures. Prophylactic dialysis is controversial.

Aim of dietary management is to provide sufficient calories to avoid ketoacidosis and protein catabolism of starvation while minimizing formation of nitrogenous waste to be eliminated by the kidney. Protein intake is restricted to 0.6 g/kg/d (protein of high biological value). Calories are provided as carbohydrate; about 100 g/d.

Severe diuresis during early part of recovery phase may produce volume depletion and hypernatremia (as fluid loss is hypoosmolar). Thus secondary prerenal azotemia may develop and delay recovery of patient.

Post renal ARF

Post renal ARF is uncommon (5% of cases of ARF). The most common cause is bladder neck obstruction due to prostatic disease (producing acute obstruction) and may require some radiological investigation for confirmation. Other causes are urethral stricture, neurogenic bladder dysfunction (diabetic neuropathy, multiple sclerosis) or obstruction of both ureters (infiltrating neoplasm, retroperitoneal fibrosis etc). Decrease of GFR is due to increase in intraluminal pressure due to accumulated fluid in the tubules as well as due to arteriolar vasoconstriction produced. There is tubular damage and impaired medullary osmolality. Urine concentrating ability is reduced. In partial obstruction urine volume may be normal or increased (due to reduced urine concentrating ability). After removal

of the obstruction there is rapid improvement in renal function. In long standing complete obstruction (>4 months), functional recovery of the kidney will not occur.

Chronic post renal obstruction is more common and produces gradual damage. Hydronephrosis may occur.

CHRONIC RENAL FAILURE (CRF)

The syndrome of chronic renal failure results from reduction in the number of functional nephrons. It may result from glomerulonephritis, pyelonephritis, malignant hypertension, diabetic nephropathy, a collagen disease or a congenital anomaly (like polycystic kidney). With progressive loss of nephrons the remaining nephrons hypertrophy, there is increase in glomerular capillary hydrostatic pressure and increased formation of filtrate per surviving nephron. Although, this helps to slow down process of reduction of GFR, it tends to produce proteinuria and promotes focal and segmental glomerulosclerosis Fig. 4.4.

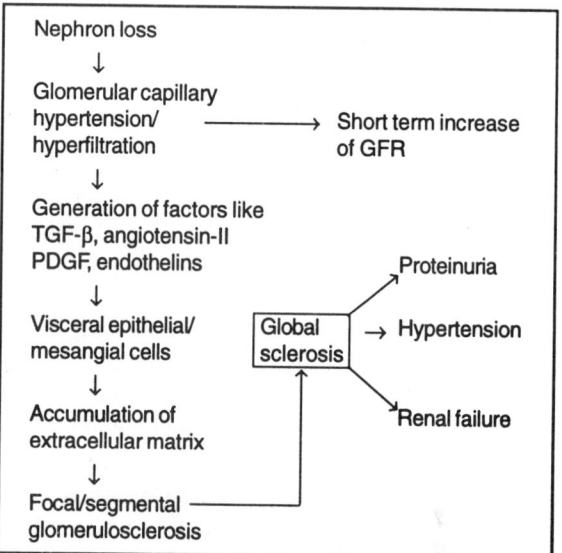

Fig. 4.4. Long term damage of surviving hyperfunctioning nephrons in chronic renal failure.

- If glomerular capillary blood pressure can be kept reduced (by use of ACE-inhibitors and by reducing dietary protein intake) the progression of renal disease can be slowed down.

There is a large reserve of renal functions. Thus even easily affected functions (those which depend only upon GFR; eg; excretion of creatinine/urea) are quite well maintained with GFR falling by about 50%. With 50% reduction in GFR, plasma creatinine level remains within the normal range. For many other functions (in which tubules also participate) there is extensive adaptation and adequate functions are maintained even when GFR is greatly, reduced. When GFR is reduced, because of increased fractional excretions, there is no retention of Na^+ and water, at normal daily intakes (explained below). However, in view of increased fraction excretions, it may become difficult to achieve balance at low intakes. In general, too high intakes or too low intakes of water and electrolytes are poorly tolerated in CRF. Normal intakes are quite will tolerated even when GFR is greatly reduced.

Sodium chloride excretion

With normal salt intake, plasma Na^+ is maintained in normal range even when GFR is reduced down to about 5 mL/min by increasing fractional excretion of Na^+ from 0.5% to about 30%. A large number of factors may be involved in this process. There is reduced proximal tubular reabsorption of NaCl and water due to increased peritubular interstitial hydrostatic pressure, produced by increased peritubular capillary hydrostatic pressure (caused by systemic hypertension, commonly associated with CRF) and low oncotic pressure (caused by hypoalbuminemia and reduced filtration fraction). ANP is increased in CRF which causes afferent arteriolar dilatation to increase peritubular capillary hydrostatic pressure and also increase in single nephron GRF (hence increase in filtered Na^+). ANP is also inhibitor of Na^+ transport process. Same is true about vasodilatory prostaglandins, increased in CRF. Osmotic diuresis also increases urinary loss of Na^+ and Cl^-. Aldosterone level however, is not reduced in CRF.

In tubulointerstitial diseases (pyelonephritis), polycystic disease and medullary cystic disease (salt wasting nephropathies) there is greater medullary

and interstitial damage and tendency to increased sodium chloride excretion is still more.

Water excretion

Just as for sodium chloride, fractional excretion of water also increases with reduction of GFR. Thus with certain restrictions water excretion can be maintained even when GFR is reduced to about 5 mL/min. This results from failure of kidney to concentrate urine (osmolality varies between 250 to 350 mOsmol/kg water). The causative factors are, osmotic diuresis, non-responsiveness to AVP, changes in medullary blood flow, defective reabsorption of Na^+ and Cl^- in the ascending limb and disease induced change in morphology of medulla. It is again stressed that in CRF both urine concentrating and diluting abilities are impaired.

H+/pH balance

Arterial pH and plasma HCO_3^- remain in the normal range when GFR falls to about 30% of normal. With reduced GFR, it is not possible to increase H^+ secretion (per nephron) against the tubular fluid buffers as pH of tubular fluid cannot be reduced below 4.5. The required increased H^+ secretion (and new HCO_3^- formation) is achieved by increased ammonia genesis in tubular cells. In proximal tubular cells, increased metabolism of glutamine not only generates NH_4^+ for exchange for Na^+ (Na^+, NH_4 antiport at luminal broder) but also forms increased amount of HCO_3^-, reabsorbed as new HCO_3^-. In collecting ducts increased formation of NH_3 helps secretion of H^+ to form NH_4^+ in the tubular fluid. As GFR is further reduced even this increased formation of NH_3 per nephron is not enough to excrete the load of fixed acids added to the body, daily. Thus metabolic acidosis results.

In the initial phase of renal acidosis, the functional tubular mass is not enough to secrete enough H^+ but GFR is still adequate for excretion of anions like phosphate and sulphate. Thus hyperchloremic acidosis results. With further decline in GFR retention of these anions also occurs and acidosis with increased anion gap is produced. In any case, in acidosis of chronic renal failure plasma HCO_3^-

does not fall below 14 mmol/L as bone salts are used for buffering H^+.

K^+ balance

Kidney is also able to maintain plasm K^+ level in the normal range, in chronic renal failure, until GFR falls to quite a low level (although, renal K^+ regulation is much less efficient than Na^+ regulation). Factors causing increased fractional loss of K^+ are, increased aldosterone level, osmotic diuresis and increased lumen negative transepithelial potential difference (TEPD) due to increased concentration of phosphate/sulphate in tubular fluid accompanying Na^+.

Water and electrolytes

Renal efficiency in excreting water and electrolytes, in chronic renal failure, has already been discussed. Generally, patients with stable CRF show moderate increase of total body Na^+ and water. Increased salt intake contributes to congestive heart failure, hypertension and edema. Patients with edema (those not on dialysis) are treated with diuretics and moderate restriction of salt. Extrarenal loss of salt and water (vomiting, diarrhea, sweating) can cause ECF and plasma volume depletion leading to further deterioration of renal functions.

Hyperkalemia occurs in CRF when GFR is greatly reduced (about 10 mL/min.) or when some other factor producing hyperkalemia operates (trauma, infection. drugs, hemolysis, administration of stored blood). Acidosis also promotes hyperkalemia. Hyperkalemia may produce rhythm disturbances.

Phosphate, calcium and bone abnormalities

In chronic renal failure retention of phosphate and secondary hyperparathyroidism have important roles in development of bone disorder (Fig. 4.5). Before dialysis has been started, radiological examination may reveal; bone changes as seen in rickets (widened osteoid seams at growth margins of bones), bone changes of secondary hyperparathyroidism (bone resorption especially in terminal phalanges) and osteosclerosis (at upper and lower

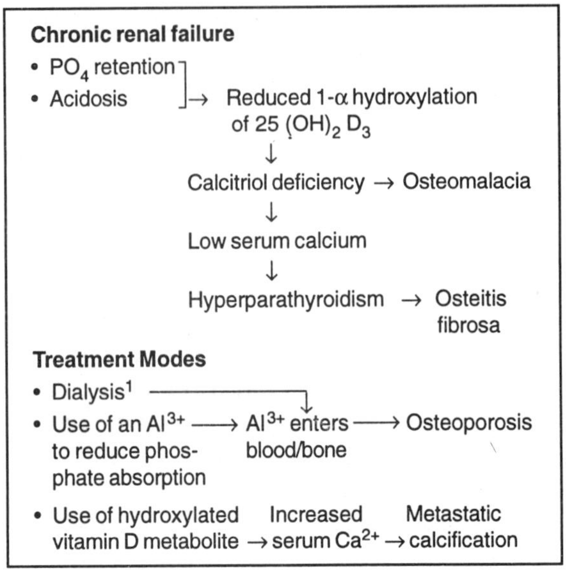

Fig. 4.5. Osteodystrophic changes in chronic renal disease and following dialysis.

---

[1] If tap water is used in prepration of dialysis fluid, Al^{3+} level in blood and bone biopsy material is used to follow toxicity. Al^{3++} toxicity also causes dementia.

- Bony changes of osteomalacia and osteitis fibrosa with progression of chronic renal failure.

- Osteoporosis and metastatic calcification with the management modes of renal osteodystrophy.

margins of vertebrae). In children bone growth is reduced. After the dialysis treatment is started two other bone abnormalities develop. Aluminium induced osteoporosis and adynamic bone disease. These abnormalities are not often detected in radiological examination and need bone biopsy study. All above bone disorders are included in the term metabolic bone disease or renal osteodystrophy.

The central issue in management of bone disorder is to suppress parathyroid hypertrophy and for that, levels of PO_4^- and Ca^{2+} are kept in the normal range (product <70). This is achieved by reducing dietary phosphate, using phosphate binders orally and administration of some vitamin D metabolite to increase calcium absorption. Use of aluminium salts is avoided (for phosphate binding) to avoid aluminium induced bone disorder. Adynamic bone disease is believed to result from over suppression of PTH.

Abnormalities related to carbohydrate, lipid and protein metabolism

There is glucose intolerance due to resistance to peripheral glucose utilization. Acidosis, cellular K^+ deficit and increased levels of hormones like glucagon, catecholamines, prolactin and GH, along with accumulated uremic toxins may account for this insulin resistance. Hypoglycemia may occur in advanced renal disease due to reduced renal gluconeogenesis and reduced degradation of insulin. Important changes in lipid metabolism are hypertriglyceridemia, increased level of Lp(a) and reduced level of HDL-C (total C level, often remains normal). These lipid abnormalities do not improve by dialysis. Also see Chapter 9.

Two important metabolic features of uremia are hypercatabolism and reduced elimination of end products of protein catabolism. There is accumulation of urea, uric acid, creatinine, guanidine compounds, aliphatic amines, derivatives of aromatic amino acids and a host of other compounds. Precise role of these compounds in uremic toxicity is unclear. There is also accumulation of so called middle molecules along with cytokines and growth factors because of reduced excretion and impaired catabolism in kidney. Plasma levels of a number of peptide hormones also rise in uremia. These include PTH, insulin, glucagon, LH and prolactin. PTH may produce toxic effects by increasing cytosolic calcium in many tissues.

Uremic toxins may inhibit different ion fluxes across cell membranes, partly by inhibiting Na^+, K^+ - stimulated ATPase. Calcium flux is also inhibited in uremia. The resulting cellular disturbances include, change in resting membrane potential, increased intracellular Na^+, leading to osmotically induced overhydration of cells and cellular depletion of K^+. Inhibition of Na^+ pump may also produce hypothermia. The basic cellular dysfunctions may produce a variety of bodily disturbances, including metabolic and endocrine abnormalities, neuromuscular, cardiovascular, pulmonary and gastrointestinal disturbances and abnormalities of hematologic and immune systems. The catabolic state produced in uremia is completely normalized by kidney transplant but not by dialysis.

Anemia

It is a regular feature of CRF. Reduced level of erythropoietin appears to be the most important factor responsible for anemia of CRF since administration of recombinant human erythropoietin causes rapid increase in hematocrit. Bone marrow inhibition by toxins and the hemolytic component are less important. The erythropoietin therapy may increase severity of hypertension probably by increasing production of endothelin. Iron deficiency or PTH induced marrow fibrosis may cause resistance to erythropoitin therapy. Repeated transfusions for treatment of anemia have their own complications.

Investigations

Long history, increased urine formation, raised blood urea/serum creatinine, anemia, hypertension and small kidneys on x-ray examination, make diagnosis of chronic renal failure an easy affair. Table 4.5 mentions some differences between acute and chronic renal failures.

It is also important to investigate and identify, remediable factors which tend to worsen chronic renal failure (by promoting further nephron damage). These include hypertension, heart failure, urinary tract infection, urinary tract obstruction and water and electrolyte disturbances.

Serum creatinine level is more useful in following a case of chronic renal failure (Fig. 4.6), as it is not influenced by dietary protein intake or endogenous protein catabolism (fever, sepsis, internal hemorrhage). Creatinine clearance tends to overestimate GFR and urea clearance tends to underestimate GFR. Of the isotopic methods ^{125}I-iothalamate clearance involving collection of the urine sample over a period of 2 to 4h, is more accurate.

Initially, the patient is managed on conservative treatment. This includes, restricting his dietary protein intake, maintaining his water and electrolyte balance (appropriate intakes and use of diuretics), maintaining serum calcium (oral calcium supplements and vitamin D), reducing serum phosphate by use of calcium carbonate (to reduce phosphate absorption), treating acidosis with sodium carbonate and lowering serum uric acid with allopurinol.

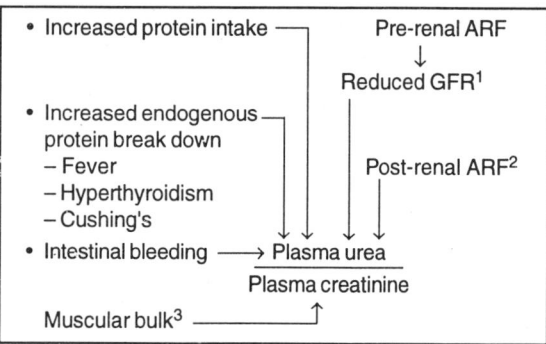

Fig. 4.6. Factors affecting plasma levels of urea and creatinine.

---

[1] When GFR is reduced, urea reabsorption from tubules is increased while creatinine reabsorption is not much affected.

[2] From the tubular fluid above the obstruction, there is greater reabsorption of urea than creatinine.

[3] Only muscular bulk of a person affects plasma creatinine level.

- Normally blood urea nitrogen/plasma creatinine ratio, remains between 12: 1 to 16: 1; diagnostic significance is only attached to ratios <10:1 and >20:1.

Diuretics are used to increase urine flow and patient is given sufficient salt so that he does not become sodium depleted but not too much to worsen his hypertension or produce edema.

Reduced protein intake (not >0.6 g/kg) improves anorexia and nausea and also causes modest decrease in progression of the disease. However, if serum albumin is <3.0 g/dL with some other evidence of malnutrition, the above said protein restriction may prove harmful. In advanced cases hypertriglyceridemia, hypermagnesemia, hyperamylasemia and mild carbohydrate intolerance are generally resistant to treatment.

Indications of dialysis include, clinical evidence of uremia, conservative treatment resistant volume overload, hyperkalemia and acidosis and if creatinine level is >10 mg/dL. In a patient of chronic renal failure, it is often possible to predict, as to when the patient will need dialysis. This is because once serum creatinine level of about 4.0 mg/dL has reached, further deterioration of renal functions and increase of serum creatinine occur at a predictable constant rate.

In a patient on dialysis, the clinical condition improves; the water, electrolyte and acid base disturbances are also corrected. Other metabolic, hematological or endocrine abnormalities, however, are not reversed. Patient still needs treatment for his anemia and osteodystrophy. Blood urea and serum creatinine are also not normalized.

Renal transplant gives better quality of life (than dialysis) since no dietary restrictions are required. These patients, however, require life long immunosuppressive therapy with cyclosporine (or azathioprine). Cyclosporine A, is nephrotoxic, when used in high doses. Thus proper monitoring of levels of serum creatinine and cyclosporine has to be done.

Renal tubular acidosis (RTA)

In this group of disorders, there is defect in renal mechanism of H^+ secretion, and as a result, hyperchloremic acidosis may be produced. In RTA type 1, there is defect in one or both distal tubular proton pumps (H^+-ATPase, H^+, K^+-ATPase). Both inherited and acquired/secondary cases occur (Table 4.8), the latter being more common. Conditions producing nephrocalcinosis and the nephrotoxic drugs may also produce RTA type 1.

In RTA type 1, distal tubular H^+ secretion is defective and pH of urine remains above 5.5 even in the presence of acidosis. Because of impaired H^+ secretion, levels of urinary NH_4^+ and titratable acid are low and K^+ excretion is increased, resulting in hypokalemia. The retained H^+ is buffered by bone salts and there is hypercalciuria (Fig. 4.7), nephrocalcinosis and renal stones. Stone formation is promoted by low citrate level in alkaline urine. Low urinary citrate excretion is due to increased proximal tubular citrate reabsorption caused by acidosis and hypokalemia. Rickets in children and osteomalacia in adults result from chronic acidosis induced hypophosphatemia, resistance to actions of vitamin D and reduced tubular reabsorption of calcium, producing hypercalciuria.

RTA type 2 also occurs as a primary (familial and sporadic) and as a secondary disorder (Table 4.8). Primary RTA type 2 may occur as part of Fanconi syndrome (impaired proximal tubular reabsorption of bicarbonate, amino acids, phosphate,

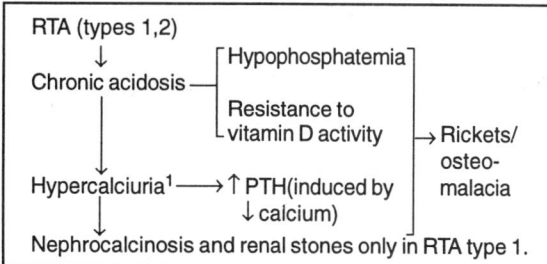

Fig. 4.7. Effects of chronic acidosis of RTA types 1 and 2.

---

[1]Hypercalciuria predisposes to nephrocalcinosis and renal stones. But these are not seen RTA type 2 because of hypercitruria.

- Nephrocalcinosis produces tubulointerstitial renal disease (Table 4.7).

citrate and urate) or as an isolated proximal tubular reabsorption defect for bicarbonate. At normal plasma bicarbonate level, there is bicarbonaturia (and urine pH >5.6) and at a lower bicarbonate level (metabolic acidosis), the distal nephron segments lower pH of urine (urine pH <5.5) in a normal fashion (the distal H^+ secretion is not defective) (Fig. 4.8). There is hypercalciuria but renal stone formation does not occur as citrate level of urine is high. Rickets/osteomalacia occurs because of hypophosphatemia and low calcitriol levels.

RTA type 4 is an acquired disorder producing hyperchloremic acidosis with hyperkalemia (both RTA type 1 and type 2 are associated with hypokalemia). It appears to be a generalized dysfunction of distal tubules in many cases bearing relation to low aldosterone activity. Secretions of both H^+ and K^+ are reduced. Ammonia production is also low. However, RTA type 4 differs from type 1, since, in the former pH of urine is <5.5 during acidosis. The reason for acidosis inspite of acid urine is reduced ammonia production. Unlike RTA type 2, fractional excretion of HCO_3^- is normal in RTA type 4.

In majority of cases of RTA type 4 there is moderate degree of renal insufficiency. In earlier stages of chronic renal failure also, hyperchloremic acidosis is a common finding. However, renal insufficiency accompanying RTA type 4 is often so mild that of its own, it will not produce acidosis.

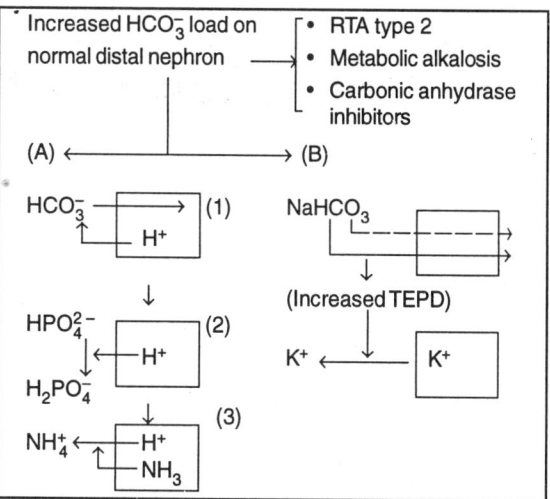

Fig. 4.8. Effect of HCO_3^- load on distal segments and on pH of urine.

- Total capacity of H^+ secretion of distal segments as mechanisms (1), (2) and (3) (mechanisms occur in the same order as shown) is fixed. If HCO_3^- load is quite high, all the capcity is used as (1); pH of urine remains high and no NH_4^+ is excreted.

- If HCO_3^- load is low mechanism (1) utilizes only insignificant part of H^+ secretion capacity and urine pH is reduced and NH_4^+ exretion is also increased.

- As HCO_3^- is not easily reabsorbed with Na^+, it leads to development of lumen negative transepithelial potential difference (TEPD), which in turn, promotes K^+ secretion. This is shown in column (B).

Diagnostic issues

If the patient has metabolic acidosis (hyperchloremic, with normal plasma anion gap) and hypokalemia, it may not be difficult to differentiate RTA type 1 from type 2. pH of urine should be >5.5 in RTA type 1 and <5.5 in RTA type 2. Other differences are low titratable acidity of urine in type 1 (and normal in type 2). If there is no acidosis, in incomplete form of disease, the patient is given an acid load (NH_4Cl 0.1 g/kg body weight in a gelatine capsules to avoid irritation to gastric mucosa). Urine samples, between 4 to 8h of NH_4Cl administration, are collected for analysis. All the samples, should have pH >5.5 (type 1). Also during this period plasma HCO_3^- should be 22 mEq/L or less (to indicate NH_4Cl produced acidosis).

For confirmation of RTA type 2, 7.5% $NaHCO_3$

solution is infused at a rate of 2 mL/min. When pH of urine rises to 6.1, plasma HCO_3^- is measured. This is HCO_3^- threshold level at which HCO_3^- reabsorption is saturated and it starts appearing in urine. Normally, it occurs at HCO_3^- level of 24 to 26 mEq/L. In RTA type 2 the threshold is much reduced.

Presence of RTA type 4 may explain hyper-chloremic acidosis and/or hyperkalemia (or worsening of these parameters) in disorders, with which it may be associated. For example it may explain unexplained severity of hyperkalemia in diabetes or chronic pyelonephritis (Table 4.8). It may also explain unexpectedly severe acidosis in a patient having only moderate degree of renal insufficiency.

Table 4.8. Causes and important features of renal tubular acidoses

RTA TYPE 1

Inherited:

- Familial, commonly autosomal dominant; X-linked; autosomal recessive; sporadic cases
- *Associated with other inherited diseases:* Wilson's disease, galactosemia, Ehler-Danlos syndrome, Fabry's disease, medullary sponge kidney.

Acquired (*Associated with systemic diseases:* Sjogren's syndrome, hypergammaglobinemia, chronic active hepatitis, SLE):

– Urine pH>5.5 in presence of acidosis .
– Hypokalemia
– Presence of nephrocalcinosis, renal stones.
– No proximal tubular reabsorptive defects.
– In acidosis, daily HCO_3^- need is small.

RTA TYPE 2

Inherited:

(It may occur as an isolated proximal tubular bicarbonate reabsorptive defect but commonly as Fanconi syndrome.)

- Familial autosomal dominant; autosomal recessive; X-liked: sporadic cases.
- *Associated with other inherited diseases*[1]: Wilson's disease, galactomsemia, cystinosis, tyrosinemia, fructose intolerance.

Acquired[2]

- *Associated with systemic diseases:* Multiple myeloma, amyloidosis, heavy metal poisoning.

– Urine pH < 5.5 in presence of acidosis.
– Hypokalemia.
– No nephrocalcinosis.
– No renal stones.
– Other proximal tubular reabsorptive defects, may be there.
– In acidosis, daily HCO_3^- need is large.
– Proteinuria (<2 g/d)

RTA TYPE 4

(it is an acquired, generalized dysfunction of distal tubules and in many cases may bear relation to aldosterone inactivity)

- *Inadequate aldosterone production:* Diabetic nephropathy, tubulointerstitial nephropathies. (renin aldosterone levels are low even with low ECF volume).
- *Adrenal disease producing aldosterone deficiency:* Aldosterone deficiency in isolation or along with deficiency of other corticosteroids.
- *Tubular resistance to aldosterone:* Obstructive uropathy, tubulointerstitial nephropathies)
- *Drug related:* Non-steroid anti-inflammatory drugs, ACE-inhibitors.
- *Chloride Shunt:* Increased distal electroneutral Na^+ reabsorption. Patients are volume expanded with suppressed renin and aldosterone levels. GFR is normal.

– Urine pH < 5.5 in presence of acidosis.
– No proximal tubular reabsorptive defect.
– Hyperkalemia.
– No nephrocalcinosis, no stones.
– In acidosis, daily HCO_3^- need is small.

[1] These patients and those associated with systemic diseases (secondary RTA) mostly present as Fanconi syndrome. Cystinosis is a disorder with intralysomal accumulation of cystine crystals in different tissues and leading to their damage. The infantile form and the juvenile form produce renal damage (Fanconi syndrome ⟶ renal failure); the adult form is benign (cystine crystals in cornea only). Diagnosed by demonstrating cystine crystals in cornea, leukocytes or cultured fibroblasts.
[2] Acquired forms of both RTA types 1 and 2 are more common than inherited ones.

Table 4.9. Plasma and urinary anion gaps in the three types of acidosis

Cause of metabolic acidosis	Anion gap	
	Plasma	Urine[1]
Increased generation of some acid (diabetic ketoacidosis)	Increased	Non-informative
Increased loss of bicarbonate	Normal[2]	Negative
Renal tubular acidosis	Normal	Positive

[1]It is calculated as follows: $[Na^+] + [K^+] - [Cl^-]$ (it is, infact, a measure of NH_4^+ excretion). In patients with increased loss of HCO_3^- (as NH_4^+ excretion is increased) Cl^- is balanced by $Na^+ + K^+ + NH_4^+$ and $[Na^+] + [K^+] - [Cl^-]$ will have a negative value. In RTA, there is very little excretion of NH_4^+, moreover urine contains appreciable amount of HCO_3^- besides Cl^- and equation between anions and cations, in urine, will be: $[Na^+] + [K^+] = [Cl^-] + [HCO_3^-]$ and $[Na^+] + [K^+] - [Cl^-]$ will have positive value.
[2]Acidosis with normal plasma anion gap is called hyperchloremic acidosis.

Hyperchloremic acidosis with hypokalemia may be produced in RTA type 1 and type 2, as well as in patients with excessive loss of HCO_3^- rich fluid from the intestine. Urinary excretion of NH_4^+ may be studied in such a situation for arriving at the correct diagnosis (Table 4.9).

Renal hypertension

It may be due to renovascular disease (renal artery stenosis, pre-eclampsia) or renal parenchymal disease. In renal parenchymal disease (like renovascular hypertension), activation of renin angiotensin system might have a role in causation of hypertension but the most favoured explanation is, ineffective disposal of Na^+ playing a key role in causing increase of blood pressure. This is because, removal of salt by dialysis or by the use of diuretics is quite effective in lowering blood pressure, in most of the cases of chronic renal failure. Further in patients of chronic renal failure having salt wasting kidneys, hypertension is not found.

Renovascular hypertension

It is produced by renal vessel narrowing which activates renin angiotensin system increasing formation of angiotensin II. Angiotensin II produces hypertension by direct vasoconstrictor action, by increasing aldosterone secretion (causing Na^+ retention) and by stimulating adrenergic nervous system. Renal vessel narrowing may be produced by atherosclerosis (hypertension appearing after 50 years of age) or by fibromuscular hyperplasia (hypertension appearing before 25 years of age in females: rare). Raised blood pressure suppresses renin secretion from the healthy side. Thus renin level in peripheral blood may not be very high.

This condition is suspected if hypertension starts before 20 years or after 50 years; if hypertension is accelerated or severe; if there is accompanying hypokalemia; if an abdominal bruit is present. There is no family history in this condition. Common laboratory findings are, hypokalemia, poorly concentrated alkaline urine, mild proteinuria, low urine sodium, mild elevation of serum creatinine and difference in kidney size on the two sides. For screening, the captopril test may be done. In this test plasma renin level is measured before and after (1h) captopril administration. Captopril (a converting enzyme inhibitor) blocks angiotensin II formation, removing inhibition (feed back) from renin secreting cells leading to hypereninemia and also rapid fall of blood pressure. Effect is much less pronounced in essential hypertension. Angiography will also demonstrate stenosed vessel on the affected side. Other screening tests include intravenous pyelography (delayed excretion and appearance of contrast medium on the affected side), captopril induced renogram (drug causes reduced uptake and delayed excretion on the affected side) by accentuating the excretory deficiency, and renal duplex ultrasound which gives both anatomic and functional assessment but is technically difficult to perform and interpret, properly.

Before surgery, renal vein samples of the two sides are studied for renin activity. Surgery is expected to give benefit, if renin activity on the stenosed side is ≥ 1.5 times that on the other side. This study should be done carefully. Patient is not given any

Table 4.10. Factors affecting plasma renin levels

- Sodium content of diet.
- Age, sex and race.
- Position of the body and physical activity.
- Use of drugs.
- Severity of hypertension.
- Presence of some other disease.

- There are lot of variations in assay procedures used in different laboratories.

renin suppressor for previous ten days and is given low salt diet for four days or ACE inhibitor before undertaking the test.

Before surgery, biopsy of the contralateral kidney should also be studied. If it shows severe form of arteriolonephrosclerosis (and therefore, likely to perpetuate hypertension), it should be removed along with repair of the stenosed vessel, during surgery.

Other biochemical tests for diagnosis of renal vessel stenosis involve study of urine samples collected separately from the two ureters. On the affected side, urine volume is reduced, osmolality is increased (reduced tubular functions) and Na^+ concentration is reduced (increased Na^+ reabsorption from slowly moving fluid). These tests, however, are not easy to do and not very popular.

Other renal disorders may also cause hypertension. These include polycystic kidney, hydronephrosis and pyelonephritis. It is also associated with nephritic type of glomerulopathies. In SLE and polyarteritis nodasa, hypertension occurs due to renal vasculitic changes. Hypertension also occurs in end stage kidney (mentioned above). Hypertension during transplant rejection is due to renal ischemia.

Renin secreting tumor of J.G. cells is very rare but can be mistaken for primary aldosteronism as it causes increased plasma level of aldosterone, marked hypokalemia and hypertension. Plasma renin is elevated (unlike primary aldosteronism). Tumor is located by renal vein catheterization. Wilms' tumor also secretes renin.

Renin and essential hypertension

The renin angiotensin system is not easy to assess. A large number of factors influence plasma renin activity (Table 4.10). There is a definite correlation between plasma renin level and sodium content of the diet (as judged from sodium excretion in 24h urine) in normal individuals. Higher the sodium content lower the plasma renin level. When this study was conducted in patients of essential hypertension, around 15% of patient showed significantly higher plasma renin levels (at all salt contents of the diet) compared to others. Similarly around 30% patients showed significantly lower plasma renin levels (at all salt intakes) compared to the rest. This study could have practical significance, because of the general observation that patient of the hypertension with low renin level, respond better to channel blockers and diuretics and those with higher renin levels respond better to converting enzyme inhibitors and ß-adrenergic blockers. However, even patients with normal plasma renin level, show considerable variation of this type when the two regimens are used on them. Thus the concept is not very popular (Fig. 4.9).

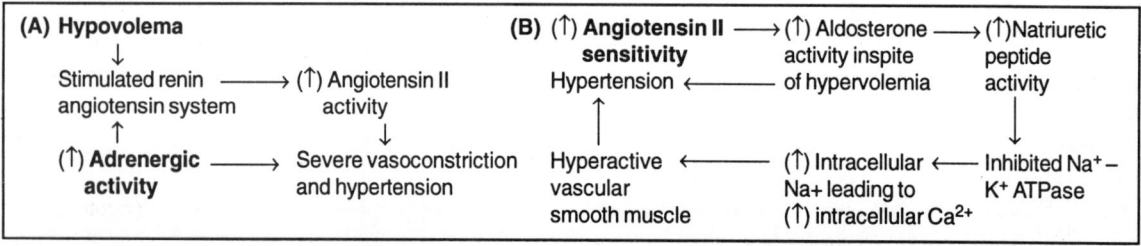

Fig. 4.9. The concept of low renin (B) and high renin (A) essential hypertension.

A) These are considered hypovolemic, intensely vasoconstrictive and more prone to myocardial ischemic injury (have added risk of myocardial infarction. These patients of "dry hypertension" are better responsive to β-blockers and converting enzyme inhibitors.

B) These are considered hypervolemic and show exaggerated response of aldosterone secretion in response to angiotensin II. These patients of "wet hypertension" are better responsive to diuretics and calcium channel blockers.

CASE HISTORY: 4.1

An adult male presented with massive proteinuria (more than 3 g/d). There was no hypertension and serum creatinine was in the normal range.

➢ Discuss two, possible, widely different, courses the disorder can follow.

➢ Suppose, after a period of ten years, the patient, gets acute flank pain and gross hematuria. What could be the reason?

• It may be a case of persistent proteinuria (Appendix B). This condition needs only follow up (every 6 months) and no treatment. Second possibility is membranous glomerulopathy which can also present with only proteinuria. Microscopic hematuria is present in 50% of cases. Hypertension occurs in about 20% of the cases, at the first presentation. Hypertension, however, commonly appears subsequently, in patients who develop progressive renal failure.

Majority of cases of membranous glomerulopathy are idiopathic. However, it may occur secondary to infections (hepatitis types B and C, malaria, leprosy), autoimmune diseases (SLE, rheumatoid arthritis), neoplasia and drugs (penicillamine, captopril).

• It could be due to renal vein thrombosis. Renal vein thrombosis may occur in a patient of nephrotic syndrome due to membranous glomerulopathy and amyloidosis (other associations are pregnancy, trauma, use of oral contraceptives). In an acute case there is sudden onset of flank or abdominal pain, gross hematuria, left sided varicocele and acute reduction in GFR. Proteinuria also increases. Chronic renal vein thrombosis is asymptomatic. It may however, ultimately lead to Fanconi syndrome type features.

CASE HISTORY: 4.2

A 5 year old boy presents with anasarca, developing over the previous week. Serum albumin level is 2.1 g/L. There is heavy proteinuria which is highly selective. There is no oliguria and serum creatinine level is 0.5 mg/dL. Blood pressure is not raised.

Rapidly developing anasarca (with rapid weight gain), heavy proteinuria and hypoalbuminemia suggest an acute nephrotic type glomerulopathy. As proteinuria is highly selective, the pathological diagnosis, is most likely minimal change glomerulonephritis. A patient of nephrotic syndrome carries better prognosis, if he is a child, the pathology of disease is minimal change glomerulonephritis and proteinuria is high selective. This condition readily responds to prednisolone as well as cyclophosphamide.

CASE HISTORY: 4.3

An 18 year old boy presents with fever, oliguria, and mild generalized edema about two weeks after an upper respiratory tract infection. His blood pressure is 160/100 (previously he was not hypertensive). He has proteinuria and microscopic hematuria. Urine also shows presence of hyaline and erythrocyte casts. Serum creatinine is 2.1 mg/dL.

Patient is suffering from a nephritic disorder. Treatment is conservative. He should be given bed rest till hematuria, edema and hypertension disappear. Protein intake is restricted and guided by his blood urea level. Fluid intake is also restricted and guided by his urine out put. A loop diuretic may be given to treat his edema.

➢ How to predict the prognosis of the case?

➢ Suppose this boy had developed hematuria and mild proteinuria (without oliguria and increase of serum creatinine level) only three days after his respiratory tract infection, what would have been the diagnosis?

• Prognosis depends upon both clinical presentation as well as the histological form of the disease. The two most benign clinical forms are nephrotic syndrome with highly selective proteinuria and persistant proteinuria and the two most benign histological forms are the minimum change nephropathy and focal proliferative glomerulonephritis. Clinical presentation of renal failure (acute or chronic) carries the poorest prognosis and same is true for the crescentic glomerulonephritis. Pauciimmune glomerulonephritis also carries poor prognosis. The prognosis of other forms (diffuse proliferative glomerulonephritis, membranous glomerulonephritis and mesangiocapillary glomerulonephritis) lie between the two extremes. Age of the patient may also determine prognosis. Younger the patient, better the prognosis.

• The clinical presentation of recurrent hematuria can occur in some forms of glomerulonephritis (focal proliferative glomerulonephritis and others) but glomerulonephritis (post streptococcal) would develop only 10 to 14 days after an upper respiratory tract infection. Recurrent hematuria can also occur in Henoch-Schonlein purpura (skin lesions, gastrointestinal or joint symptoms) or in septic endocarditis (presence of cardiac murmurs). Benign recurrent hematuria also occurs in a milder and common glomerulopathy called IgA nephropathy with mesangial deposits of IgA. Exacerbation may occur in upper respiratory disease. It requires no treatment.

CASE HISTORY: 4.4

A 40 year old man complained of pelvic and back pain. X-ray examination of spine showed presence of cod fish vertebrae. X-ray examination of abdomen showed evidence of nephrocalcinosis in medullary area. pH of urine varied between 6.5 to 7.0. Arterial pH was 7.3. Levels of serum calcium and phosphate were in the normal range.

The patient has RTA type 1 (in a patient with osteomalacia/nephrocalcinosis, presence of acidosis with neutral or mildly acidic urine is strongly suggestive of RTA type 1).

The patient has complete form of the disease.

➤ How is incomplete form of RTA type 1 investigated?

➤ What is the cause of bone pains in this case?

• In the incomplete form of the disease urine pH is near about 7.0, but there is no acidemia. Patient may present with bone pains, nephrocalcinosis or renal stones. There is hypercalciuria, caused by calcium mobilized from bones. Hypokalemia can also occur, as in distal exchange segments more Na^+ is exchanged for K^+. The patient is diagnosed by the acid load test (see the text).

2. Acidemia of distal tubular acidosis is buffered by $CaCO_3$ of bone (Fig.4.7); resulting osteoporosis produces bone pain.

CASE HISTORY: 4.5

A 22 year old female underwent D and C after a septic abortion, for the retained septic material. She had fever with rigors and was passing dark coloured urine. Her blood pressure was 90/60. Urine volume/24h was only 350 mL. Urine osmolality was 350 mosmol/kg and urine Na^+ 60 mmol/L. Serum urea level was 140 mg/dL and serum creatinine 2.0 mg/dL.

In view of her presenting features and the results of biochemical investigations, she was most likely a case of acute renal failure with acute tubular necrosis.

➤ What is probable cause of acute tubular necrosis?

➤ How should the case be investigated for DIC?

➤ How do you explain serum urea and creatinine levels in this case?

• In septic abortion cases, Clostridium welchii is known to produce shock with dark coloured urine. The enzyme lecithinase produced by the organism causes red cell hemolysis. Although, unlike myoglobin (and certain nephrotoxic substances released in crush injuries), hemoglobin is not considered nephrotoxic, it can produce nephrotoxicity during gram negative septicemia, especially in pregnancy.

• DIC is suspected in obstetrical cases (abruptio placenta, retained placenta after septic abortion, pre-eclampsia, amniotic fluid embolism), certain infections and certain cancers. Once DIC is suspected, it can be varified by certain laboratory tests. There is drop in platelet count, and PTT, PT and TT are prolonged. TT (thrombin time) is commonly used both for diagnosis and to monitor heparin therapy during DIC. Fibrin degradation products (FDP) are elevated because of stimulated secondary fibrinolysis. Often cross linked fibrin derivatives are measured (D-dimer immunoassay). Two other useful tests are antithrombin III and protamine sulfate levels. Generally, a number of repeated tests are required for firm diagnosis. Plasma fibrinogen level is measured to know chances of further bleeding.

• Excessive rise of urea compared to creatinine was due to fever and hypercatabolic state of the patient (due to septicemia).

CASE HISTORY: 4.6

A 50 year old man presented with history of progressive weakness, weight loss and anorexia of about four months duration. He had also been passing excessive urine compared to his urine volume about 6 months back. On examination he was found anemic and his blood pressure was 190/110. X-ray examination showed presence of small kidneys.

In the clinical presentation there is indication that the patient had been suffering from progressive renal failure. It was confirmed by finding high levels of blood urea and serum creatinine. HCO_3^- level was 17 mEq/L.

➤ In what other ways a patient of chronic renal failure may present?

➤ What is the role of investigations in a case of chronic renal failure?

➤ How to decide about salt intake in patients of chronic renal failure?

➤ How are osteodystrophic changes produced in chronic renal failure?

• Patient may present with severe hypertension, resulting in retinal damage, encephalopathy, or cardiac failure. He may present with some hemorrhagic episode (cerebral, gastrointestinal or nasal). He may present with bone pains and osteodystrophic features. A child may present with growth retardation.

• Blood urea and serum creatinine levels are used to have an idea of kidney functions; serum calcium, phosphate and alkaline phosphate to know about osteodystrophic changes. Bone radiology and biopsy may be done to know about bone changes, in detail. Patient should be investigated for urinary tract infection or urinary tract obstruction and other remediable causes leading to renal damage. Blood urea and serum K^+ and HCO_3^- estimations help to plan protein intake and salt intake of the patient.

• Sodium loss in a patient of chronic renal failure varies with stage of the disease and also depends upon the renal disease which has lead to renal failure (in some diseases there is increased wastage of salt and water). Excessive intake would cause edema and worsen hypertension while reduced intake would reduce GFR and urine flow and worsen azotemia. Depending upon presence and severeity of acidosis, part of sodium should be taken as sodium bicarbonate (instead of sodium chloride). Undue salt restriction affects nephron function while some excess of salt can be covered up with the use of a diuretic. In advanced stage of the disease (GFR falling to about 10 mL/min.), serum K^+ level needs to be monitored carefully. It is advisable to avoid foods rich in K^+ (banana, tomato, coffee and others).

Adequate fluid intake (about 3 L) is allowed. Fluid restriction becomes reasonable only when GFR falls to about 5 mL/min.

• Phosphate retention plays an important role in bone related problems in chronic renal failure (Fig. 4.5). Oral intake of calcium or magnesium carbonate is required to reduce phosphate absorption from the intestine. Calcium from these salts binds phosphate in the gut and reduces its absorption. In addition, some hydroxylated vitamin D metabolite is used to increase serum calcium and reduce formation of PTH. This will prevent bone changes. Increase of calcium may, however, cause metastatic calcification.

OBJECTIVE TYPE QUESTIONS

Pick out the wrong statement

1) Hematuria

i) Hematuria is defined as 2 to 5 red cells/high power field.

ii) Persistent or significant hematuria (>100 red cells/high power field), always needs to be investigated.

iii) Gross hematuria with presence of blood clots is almost diagnostic of glomerulonephritis.

iv) Hematuria with pus cells or WBC casts indicates renal infection.

v) In hyperuricosuria and hypercalciuria patients may have hematuria without pus cells and significant proteinuria.

2) Proteinuria

i) Normally urine contains <200 mg of protein/d, out of which about 30 mg is albumin.

ii) Proteins excreted in normal urine are Tamm-Horsfall, IgA, urokinase besides albumin.

iii) Barrier to protein filtration is mostly, constituted by basement membrane (size restriction) and negatively charged slits of epithelial cells.

iv) In multiple myeloma or other lymphoproliferative malignancies, there is tubular proteinuria.

v) In multiple myeloma or other lymphoproliferative malignancies there is discrepancy between sulfosalicylic acid precipitation method and dipstick method estimates of urinary protein.

3) Proteinuria

i) Dipstick method, mostly measures albumin.

ii) Microalbuminuria is not detected by dipsticks.

iii) Urinary protein excretion of >3.5 g/d is often an indication of nephrotic syndrome.

iv) Urinary protein excretion of >3.5 g/d can also occur in multiple myeloma.

v) Urinary protein excretion of <1 g/d is common in acute tubular necrosis.

4) Hematuria

i) Hematuria with dysmorphic red cells, red cell casts and proteinuria >500 mg/d is virtually diagnostic of glomerulonephritis.

ii) Asymptomatic isolated microscopic hematuria may also be a presenting feature in inactive phase of most primary and secondary proliferative glomerulopathies.

iii) Most common causes of isolated asymptomatic hematuria are IgA nephropathy (Berger's disease) and thin basement membrane disease.

iv) In a patient of IgA nephropathy, common presentation is gross hematuria, 24 to 48h after some infection (pharyngeal) or vaccination or severe physical exertion.

v) A rare hereditary cause of benign isolated hematuria is Alport's syndrome.

vi) Henoch-Schonlein purpura has glomerular lesions quite identical to those of Berger's disease.

5) Renal circulation and glomerular perfusion

i) Fall of mean systemic arterial blood pressure triggers certain renal responses to maintain GFR.

ii) In systemic hypotension, mediators of local renal responses maintaining GFR, are prostaglandins and Angiotensin II.

iii) Prostaglandins cause afferent arteriolar relaxation.

iv) Angiotensin II causes constriction of efferent arterioles.

v) Severe renal vasconstriction is cause of low GFR in congestive heart failure and renal artery stenosis.

vi) ACE inhibitors reduce renal vasoconstriction and benefit cases of renal artery stenosis.

vii) Renal local vasoregulatory responses fail when systemic blood falls below 70 mmHg, thus producing dramatic fall in GFR.

6) Azotemia (diagnosis of cause)

i) It is important to rule out hydronephrosis.

ii) Cause is chronic renal failure if kidneys are small and there is cortical thinning.

iii) It could be prerenal azotemia, if kidneys are of normal size and urine analysis shows normal results.

iv) In acute tubular necrosis, often, protein and casts are present.

v) If red cell casts are present, it is an indication for kidney biopsy.

vi) The biopsy study will be of academic interest as it will establish specific cause of intrinsic renal azotemia which is non-ischemic and non-nephrotoxic.

7) Tubointerstitial nephritis

i) It is caused by drugs, infections, systemic and infiltrative diseases.

ii) There is mild to moderate proteinuria, hematuria (pyuria in certain cases) and presence of white cell casts.

iii) Presence of eosinophils in urine will indicate allergic interstitial nephritis or atheroembolic vascular occlusion.

iv) Renal artery thrombosis causes heavy proteinuria and hematuria.

v) Renal vein/artery disorders often require angiography for confirmation.

8) Azotemia with kidney of normal size/ parenchyma

i) Presence of protein and red cell casts indicates glomerulonephritis or vasculitis.

ii) Presence of WBC, casts and bacteria make diagnosis of pyelonephritis, likely.

iii) Presence of WBC, casts and eosinophils make diagnosis of interstitial nephritis, likely.

iv) Presence of only red cells may indicate large vessel occlusion.

v) Glomerulonephritis or vasculitis are the commonest causes of acute intrinsic renal failure.

9) Acute renal failure

i) Urine protein <1g/d is a common finding in acute tubular necrosis (ATN).

ii) Urine protein concentration >1g/d suggests presence of glomerular lesion or excretion of myeloma proteins.

iii) The dipstick method does not detect myeloma proteins.

iv) Dipstick detection of urinary protein is not affected by bacterial contamination of urine.

v) Urine strongly positive for heme dipstick indicates presence of hemoglobinuria or myoglobinuria.

vi) In hemoglobinuria urine contains only a few red cells.

vii) In hepatorenal syndrome urine will be positive for bilirubin.

10) Diagnosis of acute renal failure

i) Exclude prerenal causes.

ii) Exclude postrenal causes.

iii) Find out if ARF has been superadded on already existing CRF.

iv) Some times diagnosis of intrinsic renal azotemia is established while treating a patient for prerenal azotemia.

v) There is no place for kidney biopsy in diagnosis of ARF.

11) Diabetic nephropathy

i) It occurs both in IDDM and NIDDM.

ii) Glomerular hyperfiltration may be followed by microalbuminuria after a period of about 5 years.

iii) Microalbuminuria develops into frank proteinuria in about 5 to 10 years.

iv) Patients may also present features of tubulointerstitial renal disease like hyperkalemia and RTA type 4.

v) Diagnosis often requires renal biopsy.

12) Hypertension in CRF

i) Hypertension is the most common complication of the end stage renal disease.

ii) A patient of CRF may not have hypertension if he is suffering from salt wasting type of renal disease.

iii) A patient of CRF may not have hypertension if is volume depleted.

iv) Because of hyperreninemia most patients remain

hypertensive even after strict salt and water restriction or dialysis.

v) A patient of CRF may suffer from pulmonary congestion even without any fluid overload.

13) Hematologic/immune disturbance in uremia

i) There is normochromic normocytic anemia.

ii) Gastrointestinal bleeds occur due to CRF produced lesions and by abnormal platelet function.

iii) There is dramatic response to administration of recombinant human erythropoietin.

iv) There is also increased tendency to hemolysis in CRF due to defect in red cell membrane.

v) Anemia of uremia does not respond to hematinics.

vi) Hb level in CRF should not be raised above 8.5 g/dL as it may worsen plasma flow and uremia.

14) Hemodialysis in CRF

i) Increase in level of urea in uremia may contribute to features like headache, anorexia, malaise and vomiting.

ii) Accumulated guanidinosuccinic acid interferes with activation of platelet factor III by ADP.

iii) Uremia results in a catabolic state which may lead to protein energy malnutrition.

iv) Impaired growth and development in a child readily improves after patient is put on regular dialysis.

v) A patient on regular dialysis may develop aluminium induced osteomalacia.

ANSWERS

1. No.(iii). Frank bleeding almost never occurs in glomerulonephritis.

2. No.(iv). It is an overflow type of proteinuria. A large concentration of L-chains present in the glomerular fluid, exceed the reabsorptive capacity of proximal tubules.

3. No.(ii). Originally microalbuminuria was defined as proteinuria not detected by dipstick method. But now dipsticks are available which can detect microalbuminuria. However, sulfosalicylic acid precipitation method is more accurate for study of microalbuminuria.

4. No.(v). Alport's syndrome (most common form of herediatry nephritis) is not a benign disorder. It is associated with progressive renal insufficiency. The thin basement membrane disease (in cases of isolated hematuria) is the most benign disease.

5. No.(vi). In renal artery stenosis GFR is maintained by efferent arteriolar constriction. ACE inhibitors will reduced formation of angiotensin II and reduce the efferent arteriolar constriction leading to decrease of GFR. In conditions where prostaglandins (by producing afferent arteriolar vasodilatation) are involved in maintaining renal perfusion (eg; CHF) use of non-steroidal anti-inflammatory drugs (NSAID) which inhibit prostaglandin synthesis, will result in profound renal vasoconstriction and fall in GFR.

6. No.(vi). The pathological nature of the disorder is important for treatment as well as knowing prognosis of such diseases.

7. No.(iv). Heavy proteinuria and hematuria occur in renal vein thrombosis. In renal artery thrombosis there is only mild proteinuria and hematuria.

8. No.(v). Ischemic and nephrotoxic ARF account for more than 90% cases of intrinsic renal azotemia.

9. No.(iv). False positives occur if urine is alkaline, contaminated with bacteria, highly concentrated or contaminated with blood.

10. No.(v). It is important in diagnosis of a non-ischemic, non-nephrotoxic cause.

11. No.(v). It is commonly diagnosed without biopsy. Diagnostic features are microalbuminuria (or frank proteinuria), kidneys of normal size or enlarged, urinary sediment containing only hyaline casts (without cells), presence of hypertension and proliferative retinopathy.

12. No.(iv). Only some patients remain hypertensive even after strict salt and water restriction.

13. No.(iv). There is no defect of red cell membrane.

14. No.(iv). Impaired growth and development persists despite regular dialysis.

CHAPTER 5

Plasma Enzymes and Proteins including Immunoglobulins and Tumor Markers

Plasma contains a large number of enzymes and proteins with different functions. Evaluation of plasma for activities of different enzymes, total protein, certain groups of proteins or individual proteins, has become quite important in diagnosis and management of a large number of diseases. Enzymes may be measured in terms of their activities or by immunochemical methods. Ordinary chemical methods are used for estimation of total protein and its albumin fraction. Different electrophoretic techniques are used to separate different plasma/serum proteins. Immunochemical and immuno-nephlometric methods are now available for almost any specific plasma protein, including hormones and also for enzymes.

ENZYMES

Enzyme activities or concentrations in serum may be elevated by a number of factors. It may be increased production. Level of alkaline phosphatase (ALP) increases when production of this enzyme (in liver or by osteoblasts in bone) increases. It may be leakage of an enzyme from certain damaged cells. In hepatic damage ALT, AST and LDH, which normally, remain inside cells, are released into circulation because of increased permeability of the damaged cells. Similarly certain enzymes leak out of myocardial cells, when these cells are damaged in myocardial infarction (MI). In acute pancreatitis there is necrosis of pancreatic tissue.

This leads to activation and leakage of pancreatic enzymes into circulation. Certain enzymes catalyze reactions in plasma itself. These are produced in some tissues but enter circulation for their actions. Lecithin cholesterol acyl transferase (LCAT) for example, is synthesized in liver and functions in blood. In liver disease, as its synthesis is reduced, its level in blood decreases.

To determine activity of an enzyme present in serum, most commonly, serum is added to the specific substrate at a concentration, much higher than Km, and incubation started. Enzyme activity is calculated from the initial rate of reaction in kinetic assays. In end point assays, the incubation is completed for a fixed period and enzyme activity is calculated from either decrease in concentration of the substrate or from increase in concentration of the reaction product. Problems in enzyme assays include, rapid inactivation at room temperature and need for transport/storage at a suitable temperature, need to avoid hemolysis of the sample (the leaked red cell enzymes may make results inaccurate), non-availability of control material and need for meticulous control of conditions of reaction. Also see Chapter 1.

Immunochemical assays

Immunoassays are used for determination of enzyme protein levels. These assays are primarily used to determine the levels of specific isoenzymes of an enzyme and take advantage of difference in amino acid sequence between different isoenzymes. Isoenzymes of CK have been studied by these methods.

Aminotransferases

These are aspartate aminotransferase (AST) and alanine aminotransferase (ALT). Muscle tissue (skeletal, cardiac) does not contain ALT which comes mainly, from liver. AST is found in muscle, liver and red cells (hemolysis, however, significantly increases only LD and acid phosphatase). AST along with CK increases in muscle disorders. AST is increased (along with reticulocytosis and low levels of haptoglobin) in hemolytic disorders. 25% of cases of pulmonary embolism (important in differential diagnosis of myocardial infarction) have raised levels of AST. LD increase (total) is associated with all above referred disorders and is thus nonspecific. In liver ALT is a cytoplasmic enzyme while AST is both cytoplasmic and mitochondrial. In viral hepatitis there is greater rise of ALT than AST. Reverse happens in most other diseases of hepatocellular damage. Delay in analysis of sample can increase level of AST.

In congestive heart failure (due to hepatic cell necrosis secondary to hepatic congestion), LD and AST increase along with ALP and with slight increase of bilirubin. In pulmonary embolism/infarction, there is increase of LD, bilirubin (in about 20% patients) and occasionally of AST.

Lactate dehydrogenase (LDH/LD)

Total LD lacks specificity. LD isoenzymes offer greater specificity and have greater clinical importance. In myocardial infarction levels of LD_1 and LD_2 are important. These can be estimated electrophoretically. One may estimate total LD and the heat stable LD_1 (65°C for 30 min). LD_1 can also be estimated as α-hydroxy butyrate dehydrogenase (HBD) activity (using α-hydroxy butyrate as the substrate instead of lactate). Normal LD/HBD ratio is 1.2 to 1.6. In myocardial infarction, it is 0.8 to 1.2. LD_1 can also be determined by an immuno chemical (more expensive) method.

In hepatic diseases LD_5 is increased (also see under liver disease). Quite high levels of LD (LD_1 and LD_2) are seen in megaloblastic anemias. In hemolytic anemias LD levels increase proportional to extent of hemolysis. LD levels are impressively increased in metastasizing tumors (not in localized, small ones) and these can be used to indicate prognosis or response to treatment.

While interpreting the significance of raised levels of LD it should be kept in mind that both hypoxia and shock cause rise in LD levels. The samples, also, should not be delayed.

Creatine phosphokinase (CPK) or creatine kinase (CK)

CK has three isoenzymes, BB (CK_3), MM (CK_1) and MB (CK_2). In brain 90% of CK is BB, in skeletal muscle 99% is MM and in cardiac muscle 80% is MM and about 20% is MB type.

For diagnosis of acute MI, CK or CK-MB may be analyzed. As CK-MB is mostly present in cardiac muscle, increase in levels of this isoenzyme has higher specificity for diagnosis of MI. However, in conditions of rhabdomyolysis, along with rise of CK-MM, there is sufficient rise of CK-MB to give a false positive for MI. Significant rhabdomyolysis occurs in hypothermia, hyperthermia, uremia, diabetic ketoacidosis and septic shock. Thus for proper diagnosis of MI one should know the level of CK-MB and also the fraction it forms of total CK. CK isoenzymes are assayed immunochemically. For use of CK and CK-MB in diagnosis of MI the samples should be obtained between 4 to 72h of the acute episode. Ratio of CK-MB activity: CK activity > 6% is highly suggestive of MI.

In about 5% of acute MI patients, especially old individuals, presence of peak (increase followed by decrease) of CK-MB is the only abnormality found as total CK and CK-MB levels vary only in the normal range. Thus it is best to take multiple samples at 8 to 12h intervals and study CK-MB in all these samples. If source of CK or CK-MB is skeletal muscle a plateau pattern is seen (no peaking occurs). Besides, above mentioned disorders with associated rhabdomyolysis, CK is also increased in muscular diseases (muscular dystrophies, myopathies, polymyositis), hypothyroidism, cardiac catheterization, electric cardioversion, stroke, trauma, convulsions and prolonged immobilization.

Alkaline phosphatase (ALP)

Liver and bone are two major tissues which produce ALP and the enzyme helps diagnosis of many diseases related to these tissues (Table. 5.1). Other tissues which produce ALP are intestinal epithelial cells and placenta (some tumors also produce ALP). Because of placental origin, the fetal ALP level is increased in pregnancy (third trimester). The high level, at birth, comes down rapidly, still remaining 2 to 3 times the adult level and this is maintained till a moderate rise, coinciding with pubertal growth spurt, occurs. The higher levels of these age groups are because of more rapid bone turnover at these ages, compared to adults. Osteoblasts are the source of ALP and the amounts produced relate to their activity.

All above referred tissues (liver, bone, intestinal epithelium, placenta, tumors) produce different isoenzymes. These isoenzymes can be separated by electrophoresis or by the use of heat inactivation. The placental isoenzyme and one tumor related isoenzyme (Reagen isoenzyme) are more stable at

Table 5.1. Pathological conditions with increased levels of ALP in serum

Quite high levels (often 5 to 6 times higher than upper normal limit)**:**
- Paget's disease of bone.
- Rickets/osteomalacia.
- Extrahepatic cholestatic liver disease.
- Primary biliary cirrhosis, post necrotic cirrhosis.
- Drug induced cholestasis.

Levels are high but less than in the first group:
- Bone disorders in which osteoblastic activity is increased (healing fractures, bone tumors, renal osteodystrophy, osteomyelitis, hyperparathyroidism with bone involvement).
- Liver disorders (acute hepatitis, cirrhosis, acute fatty liver).
- Primary and metastatic liver cancer; infiltrative liver disease
- Shock, congestive heart faiilure and drug hepatitis.

- There is no rise of ALP in a bone disease if bone formation is not stimulated (multiple myeloma and osteoporosis without a fracture).
- Serial estimations of ALP help monitoring of healing of osteomalacia, renal osteodystrophy and paget's disease.
- ALP estimation also helps to differentiate cholestatic liver disease from other types of liver disorders.

Table 5.2. Biochemical findings which increase specificity of ALP of hepatic origin

If there is increased activity of 5´-Nucleotidase

If there is increased level of serum bilirubin (cholestasis stimulates synthesis of ALP by bile ductules and amphipathic nature of bile salts facilitates release of ALP from membrane bound sites).
- In hepatic malignancy or hepatic infiltrative disease, high levels of ALP may occur without much increase in bilirubin.

If there is also increased level of γ-GT
- γ-GT is very sensitive to detect cholestatic liver disease. Both, in intrahepatic (viral, drug induced) and extrahepatic cholestatic liver diseases, levels increase 2-5 times (increase is more in extrahepatic cholestasis) the upper normal limit.
- γ-GT increase is from moderate to high in chronic alcoholics.
- Other conditions with less marked increase include pancreatic, prostatic and renal diseases; slight increase may also occur in obesity and diabetes mellitus.

65°C than other isoenzymes. Another way of confirming hepatic origin of ALP is to, simultaneously study some other liver specific enzyme (Table. 5.2).

Indications of estimations of ALP are (Table 5.1): i) diagnosis of bone disease; ii) differential diagnosis of jaundice; iii) serial measurements to monitor healing of fractures or progress of certain diseases (Paget's disease). ALP level is also increased in inflammatory bowel disease. Levels are reduced in arrested bone growth, cretinism and achondroplasia. Genetic deficiency of ALP, in hypophosphatasia, causes rickets or osteomalacia.

Acid phosphatase (ACP)

50 to 75% of patients of cancer prostate, in which tumor is extending beyond the capsule, show high levels of ACP. This enzyme helps to detect metastatic carcinoma of prostate but has no role in diagnosis of resectable tumor, confined within the capsule. Other sources of ACP are red cells and platelets and hemolysed sample of blood is not assayed for ACP. ACP from prostate (and platelets) is inhibited by tartrate but not that from red cells. In diagnosis of cancer prostate, tartrate inhibited ACP is more useful than the total ACP. After collection

of the sample, assay of ACP should not be delayed as its activity in the sample declines rapidly. Any pressure on prostate during rectal digital examination can cause release of ACP into circulation. The sample for assay of ACP should be drawn before such an examination or instrumentation.

A prostate specific protease also called prostate specific antigen (PSA) and located in acinar and ductal cells and present in seminal fluid, is also present in serum and can be estimated using ELISA technology. Its level is raised in prostatic disorders (both hypertrophy and cancer). If level of this marker is raised, search should be made for prostatic malignancy.

In two other conditions ACP estimation has been used to help diagnosis. In hairy cell leukemia there is rise in serum level of ACP (tartrate resistant). Rape can be confirmed by demonstrating high level of ACP in vaginal secretions (seminal fluid is rich in ACP). In Paget's disease and many cancers metastasizing in bone, increased osteoclastic activity, increases ACP level (ACP released from osteoclasts).

Gamma glutamyl transferase (γ-GT)

It is one of the most sensitive indicators of the liver disease. It is a microsomal enzyme, widely distributed in tissues including liver. There is enzyme induction in liver disease. Alcohol also induces γ-GT. Its level is increased in alcoholics even when there is no involvement of liver. In acute hepatic damage levels of γ-GT and aminotransferases run in a parallel fashion. Rise of γ-GT alongwith that of ALP suggests that ALP has arisen from the biliary tract.

Amylase

Normally this enzyme is mostly derived from salivary glands and pancreas. Because of its low mol. wt. it is readily excreted in urine. In normals, amylase - creatinine clearance ratio is 1-5% and rises to 8% in acute pancreatitis. The main use of estimation of serum amylase lies in diagnosis of acute pancreatitis as a cause of acute abdomen. In this condition rise in serum level of the enzyme may be five to ten times the upper limit of the reference range. In a few other conditions, some times, a similar high rise may occur and these conditions, should be borne in mind. These conditions are, chronic renal failure (due to reduced GFR), severe diabetic ketoacidosis, and perforated peptic ulcer. Same can also occur in macroamylasemia in which amylase is bound to a high mol. wt. protein leading to reduced clearance.

Salivary amylase activity is strongly inhibited by a wheat germ protein. This inhibition forms basis of a method used to study, specifically, pancreatic type of amylase raised in acute pancreatitis and chronic renal failure. For study of amylase, a fresh sample should be used or the sample should be immediately refrigerated.

Angiotensin converting enzyme (ACE)

The main sources of this enzyme are endothelial cells of pulmonary artery, testes and brain. Serum levels are increased in leprosy and sarcoidosis especially pulmonary sarcoidosis, when disease is active. ACE may be used in diagnosis of sarcoidosis but 5% of the positive cases turnout to be false positives because of elevated levels occuring in granulomatous conditions of the lung (tuberculosis, mycotic infections and berylliosis) and other disorders. Enzyme levels are also elevated in Gaucher's disease, amyloidosis, primary biliary cirrhosis and hyperthyroidism. CSF studies of this enzyme have indicated neuronal dysfunctions of Alzheimer disease. Radioimmunoassay and automated methods are available for the enzyme assay.

Cholinesterase (CHS)

This enzyme (CHS) is also called pseudo-CHS and is derived from liver. It is different from acetyl-CHS or true CHS which is an intracellular enzyme present in erythrocytes and nerve cells. There is difference in substrate preference between the two enzymes, and that is the basis of their differential analysis. Serum CHS (or pseudo-CHS) levels are reduced in different hepatic diseases but the enzyme is not used for diagnosis of these disorders. Serum CHS is also depressed in poisoning by organophosphorous compounds (insecticides) and is used for diagnosis of this condition.

Succinyl choline (scoline) is a muscle relaxant

often used during anaesthesia. The enzyme CHS inactivates succinyl choline to limit its duration of action during anaesthesia. An individual may have CHS in one of the three forms given below. The three forms have different activities towards succinyl choline as mentioned below.

Normal CHS	78% activity inhibited by dibucaine (dibucaine number 78).	Inactivates scoline rapidly
Atypical heterozygous	Dibucaine number 60.	Inactivates scoline less rapidly
Atypical homozygous	Dibucaine number 16.	Poor inactivation activity

If scoline is used in a patient who is homozygous for the atypical enzyme the action of scoline is prolonged and he may develop prolonged apnea. Thus before using this muscle relaxant the enzyme form of the patient should be properly defined.

Table 5.3. Levels of different enzymes after myocardial infarction

	Behaviour of enzyme after chest pain		
	Appears	Peaks	Disappears
CK-MB	4-8h	12-24h	72h
CK(total)	4-8h	18-36h	4-5d
AST	Follows CK	48h	5d
LD	Follows AST	72h	>10d

- CK-MB rises early, rises sharply (mean rise more than 5 times the upper normal limit (UNL); declines sharply. Often estimation of this isoenzyme is enough.
- For CK, the peak level is more than 4 times UNL and for AST peak level is less than 3 times UNL. Both the enzymes decline sharply.
- For LD peak level is less than 3 times UNL. Decline is very gradual.

Diagnosis of myocardial infarction (MI)

In majority of cases of MI, study of serum enzymes is not required for diagnosis of the condition (clinical features and the ECG changes are enough for the purpose). In less than 30% of cases when clinical features are not typical (in elderly patients there may be no pain) or when ECG changes are not helpful (intramural, posterior or lateral infarct; ECG changes masked by bundle branch block or residual changes from a previous infarct), the enzyme studies become essential.

As already mentioned myocardial tissue contains about 80% of CK as CK-MM and about 20% as CK-MB. Following MI both isoenzymes rise in serum. CK-MB appears within 4 to 8h, peaks at 12 to 24h and comes down within 3 days. CK-MM remains elevated for 4 to 5 days. CK-MM alone has poor specificity for MI since exercise, trauma, surgery or even intramuscular injection can cause rise of CK-MM (originating from muscle tissue). Time courses of different enzymes, for appearing, peaking and disappearing from serum are given in Table. 5.3.

Protocols using CK-MB, CK and CK-MB together and CK-MB in serial samples were mentioned earlier. Another protocol is shown in Table 5.4. Generally, however, LD (total and isoenzymes) and AST are only, occasionally, useful in samples which are available late.

Pulmonary embolism may simulate an attack of MI. ECG may however, show right axis deviation and there will be a source of embolus. It may be followed by pulmonary infarction with findings in the chest. Commonly, 24h after chest pain there is elevated LD; AST may or may not be increased; CK-MB is not elevated.

Table 5.4. Use of CK-MB, LD_1 and LD_2 in diagnosis of myocardial infarction (MI)

Sample on admission (earlier than 12h after chest pain)	Sample at 24h	Sample at 48h
Absence of CK-MB is 100% predictive of absence of MI	CK-MB present; $LD_2 > LD_1$ (MI or some other cause)	CK-MB present and $LD_1 > LD_2$ (100% predictive of MI)

- In MI both LD_1 and LD_2 enter blood from cardiac tissue but more of LD_1 than LD_2. Thus there is more of LD_1 than LD_2 (flipped LD). This pattern appears within 12 to 24h and within 48h is present in sera of 80% cases of MI. This a highly specific finding in diagnosis of MI.

MI may get complicated with shock or congestive heart failure. In the latter condition both LD and aminotransferases may be elevated. Shock can also lead to increase in levels of AST.

The enzyme estimations are also useful in diagnosis of extension or recurrence of infarction during convalescence. Other uses are to judge prognosis and to select patients for thrombolytic therapy and also to monitor success of this therapy. Marked elevation of serum enzymes with increased incidence of ventricular arrhythmia, shock and heart failure indicate poor prognosis. Thrombolytic therapy should be given within 4-6h of the acute episode. Thus there was search for some test which could indicate cardiac damage rather early.

CK-MB from cardiac muscle (CK-MB$_2$) and not that from skeletal muscle is cleaved by lysine carboxy peptidase to produce CK-MB$_1$. CK-MB$_2$: CK-MB$_1$ ratio of >1.5 at 6h after the episode, has sensitivity of 97% and specificity of 94% for diagnosis of MI. Total CK-MB at 6h has sensitivity of only 48%.

Myoglobin has also been found useful in diagnosis of MI. Myoglobin can be estimated in serum by an ELISA assay and has been shown to rise in serum very early after MI since it is released from the heart muscle within two hours after the episode (and its level normalizes in 24h). It could help as a screening test and could also be helpful in selecting the patient for thrombolytic therapy. It should however, be realized that specificity of myoglobin estimation in diagnosis of MI is quite low since it is present in all types of muscles and any myolytic condition would increase its level in serum.

Cardiac-specific-troponins T and I are different from skeletal muscle troponins. These are new serum cardiac markers when differentiation is required between skeletal muscle damage and MI and are considered superior to CK-MB or CK. These markers increase in serum as early as CK-MB but their peaks are much sharper and thus have much greater sensitivity than CK-MB. Further troponin I may remain elevated for 7-10 days and troponin T for 10-14 days. These markers are also useful in selecting patients for thrombolytic therapy and predicting prognosis of patients of unstable angina. In these patients, the levels of these troponins may increase (indicating probable microinfarction) while levels of CK or CK-MB do not increase.

Once thrombolytic therapy is given its success is monitored by levels of CK-MB or myoglobin (as reperfusion is established there is rapid rise in levels of these markers).

Diagnosis of liver disease

Important enzymes used in diagnosis of liver disease are, AST, ALT, ALP and γ-GT. Ornithine transcarbamoylase is most specific to liver but is not much used since its method of assay is complex. Both AST and ALT levels rise in liver cell damage but AST is more sensitive indicator of liver damage. Advantage of ALT is that it is more specific for liver involvement. For liver cell damage γ-GT is as good as AST. In infective hepatitis rise in levels of these enzymes occurs before rise of bilirubin.

In cholestatic liver disease there is greater rise in level of ALP than in hepatitis. 5′-Nucleotidase is a sort of hepatic isoenzyme of ALP, but it is more difficult to estimate. γ-GT is more sensitive than ALP in diagnosis of biliary obstruction. It is not altered in bone disease.

Significant, isolated elevations of ALP and LD suggest presence of space occupying lesion in liver. Studies of serum enzymes greatly help: i) to differentiate liver disease from myocardial infarction or other conditions accompanied with pain in upper abdomen/chest; ii) to differentiate between hepatic cell damage and cholestasis; iii) to follow course of chronic hepatitis.

Serum enzymes in muscle disorders (Table 5.5)

In the dystrophic group there are a number of inherited diseases with difference in age of onset and the muscles involved. The commonest is Duchenne muscular dystrophy. In these disorders (especially Duchenne dystrophy) muscle tissue associated enzymes, CK, aldolase, LD and AST are raised. CK-MM isoenzyme is most specific for these disorders. Electromyography is helpful to differentiate these myopathies from neurotropic muscle disorders.

Table 5.5. Diagnostic features of certain skeletal muscle disorders

HEREDITARY MYOPATHIES

Muscular dystrophies (These disorders are progressive in nature. Individual diseases differ in age of onset and the muscle groups involved. The commonest condition is Duchenne dystrophy.):

- CK levels are 20 to 100 times the normal at birth and decline with age due to loss of muscle tissue.
- EMG (differentiates between dystrophic, atrophic and disorders due to receptor or channel defects).
- Muscle biopsy (differentiates atrophic, dystrophic and muscles affected in connective tissue disorders).
- For definitive diagnosis of Duchenne dystrophy, dystrophin deficiency is demonstrated in muscle biopsy by Western blot analysis.
- Mutant DNA analysis can also be done on peripheral leucocytes for definitive diagnosis. This procedure can also be used for carrier detection and for prenatal diagnosis.

Congenital myopathies (It is a non-progressive group of hereditary myopathies with early appearance of clinical features. One disorder in this group predisposes the patient to malignant hyperthermia).

- EMG and muscle biopsy are used for diagnosis of these disorders:
- CK levels are usually normal.

METABOLIC MYOPATHIES

Glycogen storage diseases (producing exercise intolerance): It includes glycogenesis type V (most common, muscle phosphorylase deficiency), type VII (phosphofructokinase deficiency), type IX (phosphoglycerate kinase deficiency), type X (phosphoglycerate mutase deficiency) and type XI (lactate dehydrogenase deficiency).

- All these disorders have autosomal recessive inheritance except type IX, which is X-linked recessive.
- Manifestations of these disorders generally start in adolescence.
- After a short severe bout of exercise muscles become stiff and painful. There is myoglobinuria and increase of CK.
- There is associated hemolytic anemia in type VII (mild) and type IX (severe).
- Type IX, more commonly, presents with mental retardation and seizures than with exercise intolerance.
- In the forearm exercise test, there is impaired increase in venous blood pyruvate and lactate (in type XI there is increase of pyruvate but not lactate)
- For confirmation, enzyme levels are studied in the muscle biopsy samples.

Carnitine palmitoyl transferase deficiency[1]: This also produces a myopathy which starts in teenage and is the most common cause of recurrent myoglobinuria (more common than glycogen storage disorders).

- Muscle pain and myoglobinuria occurs after prolonged severe exercise (fasting predisposes to the trouble).
- CK level increases only during the episode of myoglobinuria.
- In the forearm exercise test there is normal increase in venous lactate level.
- For confirmation, enzyme level is studied in the muscle biopsy sample.

Myoadenylate deaminase deficiency

- This enzyme regulates ATP level in skeletal muscle.
- Deficiency may cause exertional faigue, myalgia and myoglobinuria in some cases; but often there are no symptoms.

MYASTHENIA GRAVIS AND CHANNEL RELATED DISORDERS

Myasthenia gravis: Diagnosis is based on special groups of muscles involved and demonstration of improved muscle strength with edrophonium chloride (the anticholinesterase test). One should look for other disorders which may aggravate the disease (thyroid disorders, occult infection, certain drugs) or which interfere in treatment of disease with anticholinesterase drugs or immunosuppressives (tuberculosis, diabetes, peptic ulcer, renal disease, hypertension, asthma, osteoporosis).

- The anticholinesterase test is commonly used for diagnosis; other tests are:
- The repetitive nerve stimulation test.
- Acetyl choline receptor assay.
- Single fiber EMG.

Familial periodic paralysis and related disorders: In these disorders episodic (for less than an hour to several hours duration) muscle weakness or flaccid paralysis occurs but not during vigorous activity. The disorders manifest in the first two decades of life.   *Contd.....*

- Serum K^+ is often high (hyperkalemic periodic paralysis) or low (hypokalemic periodic paralysis) at the time of attack.
- Attacks can be provoked by lowering of serum K^+ (glucose and insulin administration; a heavy carbohydrate meal) or by loading with K^+.

Polymositis-dermatomyositis, scleroderma:
- These may require differentiation from peripheral neuropathy with the help of EMG.
- Biopsy may help to confirm diagnosis.

Myopathies associated with endocrinal disorders: Both increased and reduced levels of thyroid, parathyroid, and adrenal hormones may be associated with muscle weakness. Primary hyperaldosteronism produces hypokalemia which can produce muscle weakness. Muscle weakness is also associted with diabetes and vitamin D deficiency.
- CK levels are normal or reduced.
- Establish the hormone status of the patient.

Post-infective/toxic myopathies:
- CK level is increased in acute state and reduced in chronic state.

Muscular atrophies (secondary to lower motor neuron damage)**:**
- CK level is reduced.

Crush injuries:
- CK level is increased.

---

[1] A similar but less common myopathy is "Myopathic Carnitine deficiency", with overlapping features of muscular dystrophy and polymyositis. Carnitine is deficient in muscle but not in blood. CK is increased. Muscle biopsy shows lipid accumulation.

- For muscle disorders useful enzymes are CK, CK(MM) and aldolase. CK(MM) and aldolase are equally sensitive but aldolase is less specific. Less commonly used enzymes are LD (LD_3 and LD_4) and AST. Muscle tissue does not contain ALT.

- Liver glycogenoses are grouped as: i) with hepatomegaly and hypoglycemia (type Ia, defective glucose-6-phosphatase, Ib, glucose-6-pO_4 translocase defect; IIIa, liver and muscle debrancher defects, IIIb, liver debrancher defect only; type VI, liver phosphorylase defect and the liver phosphorylase kinase defect (formerly called type VIa or type IX)) and ii) with cirrhosis and hepatomegaly (type IIIa and IIIb; type IV brancher defect).

- Muscle glycogenoses are grouped as: i) with muscle energy impairment (type V, type VIII, phosphofructokinase/ phosphoglycerate kinase/phosphoglycerate mutase/lactate dehydrogenase/muscle phosphorylase kinase defects) and ii) with progressive skeletal muscle weakness, atrophy and/or cardiomyopathy (type II, lysosomal acid α-glucosidase defect; type IIIa and type IV, brancher and cardiac specific phosphorylase kinase defects).

In the group of endocrine myopathy, diagnosis needs evaluation of thyroid, adrenal, parathyroid and vitamin D status of the patient. Also serum levels of K^+; Ca^{2+} and Mg^{2+}. In elderly, often hypokalemia, hypomagnesemia, vitamin D and other deficiencies develop over time and may cause muscle weakness. In case of toxic myopathy history of drug intake is important. Alcohol, steroids and thiazide diuretics may produce this type of muscle weakness. Diabetes and renal, hepatic, pulmonary and cardiac diseases can also produce muscular weakness.

Some myopathies can be recognized from their special features. Myasthenia gravis is a disorder of neuromuscular junction. There is weakness of muscles of lids (causing ptosis), ocular muscles (causing diplopia), and muscles of chewing, swallowing and speech. There is improved muscle strength with endrophonium (a short acting anti-cholinesterase inhibitor). Familial periodic paralysis is a rare disorder in which attacks of severe muscle weakness are associated with low serum K^+ level. A high carbohydrate diet may induce an attack by promoting K^+ entry into cells.

Some myopathies arise in diffuse connective tissue disorders with muscle weakness and inflammatory changes in muscle and skin (polymyositis - dermatomyositis, scleroderma). Test for rheumatoid factor is positive and there are antibodies to certain nuclear antigens. EMG helps to differentiate from peripheral neuropathy. Levels of aminotransferases, LD and aldolase indicate disease activity. MRI can also reveal active myositis noninvasively. These connective tissue disorders may be secondary to some malignancy. Search for that is important.

Glycogen storage disease may also produce myopathy. In these cases confirmation of disorder requires study of certain enzymes in muscle biopsy. The investigated enzymes are phosphorylase, phosphofructokinase, lactate dehydrogenase and others. Myopathies with mitochondrial enzyme defects (and mitochondrial inheritance) are also known (objective type question 25, Chapter 18).

Post viral/bacterial myopathy may also occur. In acute stage, CK is raised but is reduced in chronic stage.

Progressive muscular atrophies (motor neuron disease) are due to progressive damage to lower motor neurons. These are more common, late in life (dystrophies occur in childhood), and commonly affect distal muscle groups. Muscles in process of atrophy show fasciculations (not seen in dystrophic muscles). EMG differentiates dystrophic from atrophic muscles. It can also demonstrate abnormality at neuromuscular junction. Muscle biopsy can differentiate atrophic, dystrophic and muscles involved in connective tissue disorders. The tissue can also be studied for activities of certain enzymes of some other substances. Features of important myopathic groups are summarized in Table 5.5.

Crush injuries

Such injuries result in leakage of CK, myoglobin and K^+ from muscle cells into the blood. Generally, there is simultaneous loss of blood and sequestration of fluid in damaged tissue. Hypovolemia and myoglobinuria can result in acute renal failure (acute tubular necrosis). Also read under acute renal failure in Chapter 4.

Leakage of cellular contents (see above) from damaged muscle cells is called rhabdomyolysis. Besides trauma significant rhabdomyolysis occurs in hypothermia, hyperthermia, uremia, diabetic ketoacidosis and septic shock. Quite high serum levels of CK-MM are seen in these disorders. Also read under 'haptoglobin'.

PLASMA PROTEINS (Table 5.6)

Low level of total protein in plasma provides information about status of nutrition or about some severe organ disease (protein losing state, liver disease). It may also indicate overhydration if it develops, rather rapidly. Raised level indicates presence of some paraprotein and patient should

Table 5.6. Feature of certain plasma proteins[§]

†1. Prealbumin (62,000), (0.15-0.36)
 2. Albumin (66,000), (39-51)
 3. α_1-Antitrypsin (54,000), (2.0-4.0)
 4. α_2-Macroglobulin (725,000), (1.5-3.5)
 5. Haptoglobulin (1,000,000), (0.4-2.9)
 6. Transferrin (80,000), (2.0-4.0)
 7. C3 — (185,000), (0.6-1.4)
 8. Fibrinogen (340,000), (1.0 -4.0)
††9. Ceruloplasmin (132,000), (20-30)
 10. Hemopexin (70,000), (50-120)
 11. Gc-Globulin (51,000), (20-55)
‡12. C-reactive protein (118,000-144,000), (470-1340)

[†]Nos 1 to 8: (Mol. wt.), (Conc. in g/L).
[††]Nos 9 to 11: (Mol. wt.), (Conc. in mg/dL).
[‡]No.12: (Mol. wt.), (Conc. in ng/mL in adults), conc. in children 170 ng/mL.
[§]Nos. 3,5,8,9,10 are acute inflammatory reactants. Others are α_1-acid glycoprotein and ferritin as well as ESR and neutrophils.

be further investigated. It may also indicate dehydration if develops rapidly. Albumin levels are more useful as indicators of nutritional status. This investigation is also important in a chronic liver disease and nephrotic syndrome. In septicemia and general inflammatory disorders, hypoalbuminemia can occur due to leakage of albumin into interstitial compartment. Albumin level alongwith total protein level gives indication of the globulin level.

Protein electrophoresis is carried out on serum, since plasma contains fibrinogen which migrates in β region and its band could be mistaken for a myeloma band. For electrophoresis cellulose acetate and agarose produce better separations than paper. Bands of albumin, and α_1, α_2, β and γ globulins are seen. Occasionally, discrete bands of C-reactive protein and α-fetoprotein may be seen if these proteins are present in excess. The prealbumin band may be seen depending on the method used. Paraproteins (or M-proteins), if present, are often seen as discrete bands (called M-bands).

The most important use of electrophoresis is in study of paraproteins. It can also easily display deficiency of IgG by reduced density of the γ-globulin band. IgA and IgM changes are not revealed since the amounts of these immunoglobulins are rather small and these proteins might migrate with other globulins. The electrophoretic studies are also important in long term follow up of cases of myeloma, cirrhosis, nephrotic syndrome and extensive burns.

Some specific protein studies are also important in certain clinical disorders. α_1-Antitrypsin (genetic deficiency causes emphysema in childhood and neonatal hepatitis progressing to cirrhosis), transferrin (important in diagnosis of hematological disorders), C3 (to monitor rheumatic disease activity), fibrinogen (in cases of hemorrhagic diathesis and intravascular coagulation), ceruloplasmin (in diagnosis of Wilson's disease), the C-reactive protein (to monitor the active phase of certain autoimmune disorders), haptoglobulin (in hemolytic disorders) and α-fetoprotein (for diagnosis of hepatoma and neural tube defects), are the important examples (discussed later). For most of these nephlometric methods (Fig. 5.1) are used in automated immunochemistry analyzers instead of previous radial immunodiffusion measurements.

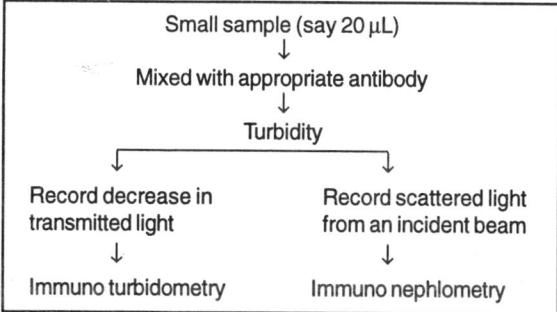

Fig. 5.1. Immune nephlometry/immune turbidometry.

- The major advantage of these methods is that these are easily automated but there is interference from lipemic or turbid sample (due to repeated freezing and thawing).

Albumin

It is synthesized in liver. Fetal liver synthesizes α-fetoprotein which has regions of homology with albumin. The two are synthesized from the same ancestral gene. In an inborn error, modified albumin is synthesized and in heterozygotes for the modified albumin, two albumin bands are seen, because of difference in rates of migration of normal and mutant albumin. Another mutant albumin has much higher affinity for thyroid hormones.

Albumin is main determinant of plasma oncotic

pressure. However, in congenital absence of albumin (analbuminemia), there is no peripheral edema, unlike other causes of low albumin (malnutrition, malabsorption, chronic liver disease, ascites, protein losing enteropathy and nephrotic syndrome).

Albumin has multiple binding sites to bind thyroxine, bilirubin, cortisol, estrogen, FFA, Ca^{2+}, Mg^{2+}, heme and certain drugs. Albumin acts as a carrier of amino acids from liver to peripheral tissues.

Normally, 8% of albumin is glycosylated while in diabetes upto 25% may be glycosylated. As half life of albumin is 17 days, glycosylated albumin can be used to monitor diabetics over a shorter period compared with glycosylated Hb.

An immunologic measurement is used to study microalbuminuria of diabetes for early detection of diabetic complications. Table. 5.7 presents clinical situation in which study of serm albumin/albuminuria may be helpful.

Table 5.7. Clinical significance of altered serum albumin levels and albuminuria

- Low levels indicate malnutrition/malabsorption. It is a good parameter to indicate protein nutritional status in chronic malnutrition, chronic illness and chronic malabsorption but not a good parameter to monitor nutritional intervention.
- Low levels occur in nephrotic syndrome (increased α_2-macroglobulin level partly compensates for the reduced plasma oncotic pressure).
- Low level in septicemia is due to leakage of albumin into interstitial compartment.
- In liver diseases serum albumin levels may determine prognosis of the disease.
- In Rh incompatibility cases, low albumin increases risk of kernicterus.
- Low serum albumin levels may interfere in proper interpretation of levels of those hormones which bind to albumin.
- Low serum albumin levels are produced by enteropathies, burns, hemorrhage and catabolic states like fever/septicemia/trauma/wide spread cancer.
- Rapidly produced changes in serum albumin level may indicate changes in plasma volume. Same is also true of rapidly produced changes in hematocrit, Hb and total protein levels.
- Glycosylated albumin level (normal about 8%) has been used to monitor diabetic control.
- Microalbuminuria is studied to monitor progression of chronic complications of diabetes (with time micro albuminuria of diabetes changes into albuminuria).

Pre-albumin

It migrates faster than albumin in electrophoresis. It binds to retinol binding protein and prevents its loss in urine. It is a marker for nutritional state of an individual. Its half life is only about two days. In nutritional intervention, it is considered better than albumin and transferrin which have longer half lives and are also affected by certain factors other than nutrition. It also binds thyroxine. When CSF protein electrophoresis is done to detect a monoclonal band, absence of band of pre-albumin is used to confirm that the sample is that of CSF. It is best quantitated by immunologic assay (nephlometric).

α_1-Antitrypsin (ATT)

In electrophoretic separation, it migrates in α_1-globulin fraction. ATT acts as a natural defence against protease action. In an inflammatory reaction or on exposure to irritants, leukocytes release proteases, which could cause tissue damage (in lungs emphysema and in liver, cirrhosis can be produced), and ATT gives protection against this damage.

There are at least 75 different alleles for ATT. Normal genotype is MM. The most common abnormal allele is called Z and some others are F and S. Individuals with genotype ZZ are at great risk of developing the above referred diseases. Individuals with genotype MZ (heterozygous) have about 60% of normal ATT activity and have no risk of developing the disorders. Similarly individuals with genotypes, MS, SS, MF or FF are not at increased risk.However, those with genotype SZ have some risk.

Risk of developing emphysema is greatly increased by smoking. Smoke oxidizes thiol group at active site of ATT and makes it ineffective.

Screening of family members and the antenatal diagnosis is possible. Isoelectric focussing is used for study of different phenotypes of ATT. Antenatal screening based on DNA analysis, is also available. DNA obtained from chorionic villus sampling is first amplified using PCR, before analysis.

Fibrinogen

It is most abundant of the coagulation factors. It is an acute phase protein and its level is directly related to elevation of ESR. Level also rises in pregnancy and with use of oral contraceptives. Low level of fibrinogen along with increased level of fibrinogen split products is an index of intravascular coagulation. There are many inherited variants of fibrinogen (dysfibrinogenemia) in which clotting is excessive (thrombotic tendency) or impaired (hemorragic diathesis). In electrophoresis of plasma, it appears as a distinct band between β and γ regions and looks like a monoclonal band).

Transferrin

It is the major β-globulin protein which transports iron from stored ferritin of mucosal and other cells, to bone marrow. In normal serum transferrin protein level is 240-480 mg/dL (App. B). It is also measured as total iron binding capacity of serum. A more useful allied parameter is percent saturation of transferrin. In iron deficiency anemia, transferrin synthesis is increased and serum iron is reduced. Thus percent saturation is greatly reduced. In idiopathic hemochromatosis and transfusional siderosis percent saturation of transferrin is very high (Chapter 6). There is deposition of iron (same is also true in congenital deficiency of transferrin) in tissues.

In iron deficiency, increased level of transferrin leads to a sharp band on electrophoresis simulating a monoclonal band.

Ceruloplasmin

It is also an acute phase protein but unlike fibrinogen, its level does not, directly, influence ESR. It may be involved in transferring iron from ferritin to transferrin since it can oxidize ferrous iron to ferric. In Wilson's disease, ceruloplasmin level is reduced and there is impaired excretion of Cu in bile (and Cu is deposited in tissues). Wilson's disease is discussed in Chapter 6. A simple colorimetric assay using p-phenylenediamine as the substrate (which is oxidized) is available besides the immunochemical method, for ceruloplasmin estimation.

Complement

C3 is a sub fraction of β-globulin. C3 and C4 (not seen in electrophoresis), are easily measured by

Table 5.8. Some primary immune deficiency diseases and AIDS

Congenital X-linked agammaglobulinemia:

- Increased susceptibility to pyogenic infection in second year of life (staphylococcal skin abscesses, pneumonia, meningitis) but not to viral infection.
    - Deficiency of B-cells and IgG, IgA and IgM.
    - Peripheral lymphocyte count is normal.
    - Skin tests are normal.

Selective IgA deficiency

- It is common in Caucasians (1 in 500) and is associated with inheritance of certain class III histocompatibility antigens. Increased susceptibility to respiratory tract or gastrointestinal tract infections, is produced. Selective IgM deficiency makes patient more susceptible to blood borne infections (septicemia). In another pattern, there is reduced/absent IgM and IgA but normal to increased IgG.

Common variable immunodeficiency:

- Patient is prone to secondary immune deficiency and he may present in this way or he may present as a case of late onset (adult form) of primary hypogammaglobulinemia. There is high incidence of autoimmune diseases (pernicious anemia/hemolytic anemia). He may also have malabsorption due to giardia infection. There may be reduced level of any class of Ig (generally, IgA).

Hypogammaglobulinemia of infancy (transient):

- In these cases there is increased incidence of bacterial infections, for a limited period, after birth. Prophylactic IgG treatment helps.

X-linked immunodeficiency with increased IgM:

- Patient suffers from pneumocystis pneumonia and often has associated cyclic neutropenia. Normal to elevated levels of IgM and absent IgA and IgG.

Severe combined immunodeficiency[1]:

- It is caused by IL-2 receptor defect (X-linked inheritance) and a number of other inherited defects including the one caused by adenosine deaminase deficiency. There is stem cell defect which leads to impairment of both T-cell and B-cell functions. About 50% of infants with autosomal recessive form of the disease have deficiency of adenosine deaminase. The detection of this deficiency helps prenatal diagnosis of these cases. The affected infants suffer from both bacterial and severe viral infections. If the infants are given small pox or BCG vaccines they may develop severe forms of the respective diseases.

Hyper IgE syndrome (Job - Buckley syndrome)[1]:

- T-cells defect is poorly defined. There are severe staphylococcal abscesses of skin.

Thymic hypoplasia (DiGeorge's syndrome)[2]:

- It is a primary T-cell deficiency. There is characteristic facies, heart lesions and hypoparathyroidism. There is increased susceptibility to viral, fungal and bacterial infections
    - Peripheral lymphocyte count is low, and there are no T-cells in peripheral blood.
    - Response to skin tests is poor.
    - Igs may be normal or low depending on degree of T-cells deficiency.

Nezelof syndrome[2]:

- Congenital fault in thymic embryogenesis.
    - Specific antibody response is poor.

Wiskott-Aldrich syndrome[1]:

- It is an X-linked combined T and B-cell functional deficit. The condition is associated with eczema and thrombocytopenia. There is high incidence of lymphoreticular malignancy.
    - IgM level is low. IgA and IgE levels are often elevated.
    - Skin tests are impaired to fungal antigens..
    - Decrease, in vitro, response to phytohemagglutinin stimulation

Ataxia-telangiectasia associated immunodeficiency (A chromosomal repair defect)[1]:

- It is an autosomal recessive disorder. There is ataxia and choreoathetoid movements in infancy and telangiectasia (face, conjunctiva etc.) seen a few years afterwards.

  - IgE and IgA deficiencies are seen commonly along with T-cell deficit.

Acquired immune deficiency syndrome (AIDS):

- Hallmark of HIV infection is progressive deficiency of Helper or inducer - T-cells (HIV, a retrovirus passes through lysogenic pathway inside these cells). When the number of these (CD4 + T-cells) declines below a certain level, the patient suffers from AIDS - related disorders including opportunistic diseases particularly infections and neoplasms. All these diseases cannot be explained completely by immunosuppressive effects of HIV infection. This is especially true for disorders like Kaposi's sarcoma and neurologic abnormalities. Thus multiple pathogenic mechanisms (which may vary with phase of the disease) are involved in the disease process.

- After HIV infection the course of the disease is divided into acute HIV syndrome with widespread virus dissemination and seeding (9 to 12 months), the clinically latent period (about 8 years), constitutional symptoms (low fever, diarrhea), opportunistic diseases and death.

- The tests used in diagnosis of HIV infection include: i) antibody detection by ELISA, the test is highly sensitive but less specific (false positive test is caused by antibodies to class II antigens, autoantibodies, hepatic disease and recent influenza vaccination); ii) Western blot test (WB), in which viral antigens are separated and transferred to a filter paper and reacted with test serum followed by addition of enzyme-linked antihuman globulin antibody to reveal the separated antigens (this test is highly specific and the commercial kits contain viral antigens both from HIV-1 and HIV-2); iii) polymerase chain reaction (PCR) is used to study viral RNA and proviral DNA. RNA PCR is more commonly used to detect HIV infection at an early stage before antibodies become detectable; iv) detection of p24 antigen by an ELISA type assay. This test is positive in about 50% of patients before development of antibodies and the test is quite simple.

- The following sequence of testing may be followed in HIV infection: i) do ELISA; if positive, on two separate occasions, confirmation is done by WB (if negative, there is no infection); ii) if WB is negative but there is strong suspicion of HIV infection, do PCR to take final decision from the results.

---

[1] Combined T-cell, B-cell deficiency syndromes (primary).

[2] Primary T-cell deficiency syndromes: Rest are primary B-cell deficiency syndromes.

- Besides the above conditions, T-cell functional deficiency can be produced by inosine phosphorylase deficiency, by non-expression of CD_3 on T-cells and other causes. Primary immune deficiency may also be produced by C_3 deficiency (mimics antibody deficiency syndromes), leukocytic defects, and other causes.

nephlometry to monitor rheumatic disease activity (both C3 and C4 are reduced in autoimmune disorders, SLE and rheumatoid arthritis). Increased levels of C3 and C4 have very little clinical significance except as indicators of acute phase response.

Haptoglobin

One of the major proteins migrating in α_2-region, in electrophoresis. Blood may contain different molecular forms. In one major form the structure resembles that of immunoglobulins. Because of presence of different forms, haptoglobin, estimation (immunologic method or method based on Hb binding capacity) presents difficulty. Thus its study is most useful when required in serial estimations, otherwise, only those levels are helpful which are quite away from the normal range.

It is an acute phase protein and level increases in stress, infection, inflammation or tissue necrosis. Its level is reduced in cases of hemolysis as hapto-globin - Hb complexes are cleared from circulation. Change may be sharp after a massive hemolytic episode. It may also be useful to follow cases with slow but steady hemolysis (mechanical heart valves). Haptoglobin - Hb complex migrates differently from haptoglobin and may simulate a M-band.

A red coloured fluid from hemolysis will show test for pseduo-peroxidase (the reagent strip urine test for heme), low level of haptoglobin and presence of LD_1. On the other hand a red solution from rhabdomyolysis will be pseudoperoxidase positive, with no change in level of haptoglobin and presence of LD_5. Level of haptoglobin can also be low in hepatic disease (reduced synthesis) and in cases of hereditary deficiency.

Hemopexin also binds Hb when level of free Hb exceeds binding capacity of haptoglobin. Reduced level of this protein also helps diagnosis of intravascular hemolysis. This protein migrates in β-globulin region and is quantitated by immunologic methods.

α₂ - Macroglobulin

One of the largest serum non-immunoglobulin. It is an endogenous protease inhibitor like AAT but its low level is not related to any disease. Level of this protein greatly increases in nephrotic syndrome (its synthesis is increased), and it assumes role of maintaining oncotic pressure.

Some other proteins are, Gc-globulin (a transport protein for vitamin D which is lost in urine in nephrotic syndrome alongwith vitamin D), α_1-acid glycoprotein which is very rich in carbohydrate content, and is excreted in urine and binds progesterone, may be for its transport (level increases in pregnancy) and C-reactive protein (CRP). The last mentioned protein increases in serum in conditions of tissue necrosis. It is a γ-region migrating protein (it may form a monoclonal type band, when its level is high). It is used to monitor the active phase of certain autoimmune disorders. It can also be used to distinguish between bacterial (rise occurs) and viral (no rise) infections. It can bind many substances like different lipids, polysaccharides, DNA and nucleotides. It appears to be a general scavenger molecule.

Quantitative analysis of CRP is better than ESR, as non-specific indicator of intensity of inflammatory reactions. Generally changes in CRP parallel those in ESR except that unlike ESR, CRP does not change in anemia, congestive heart failure and hypergammaglobulinemia. CRP is most useful in monitoring a rheumatic disease.

PROTEINS CONCERNING THE IMMUNE SYSTEM

Proper assessment of immune system requires, evaluation of cell mediated immunity, humoral immunity, the complement system and the granulocyte functions. Table 5.8 gives important primary immune deficiency disorders. Acquired immune deficiency syndrome, although not a primary disorder has been included in the Table. Table 5.9 mentions important causes of secondary immune deficiency.

Table 5.9. Some factors which may cause secondary immuno deficiency

- Viral infections (especially Epstein-Barr virus and HIV) may occur in utero and produce immune deficiency state in fetus.
- Nutritional deficiencies of calories, protein and micronutrients (especially biotin, zinc and selenium).
- After irradiation or use of immunosuppressive drugs.
- Certain malignant disorders (chronic lymphoid leukemia, multiple myeloma and Hodgkin's disease).
- In old age impaired immune system functioning leads to increased chances of autoimmune diseases besides reduced T-cell functions.
- Patients remain in relative immune deficiency for several days in the post operative period.

Proper evaluation of immune system requires a careful history and physical examination. This may suggest the immune system component needing further exploration. Table 5.10 lists some points which should be borne in mind while examining the patient.

Investigations start with total and differential counts. An absolute lymphocyte deficiency represents T-cell deficiency, since only 12% of total lymphocytes are B-lymphocytes. More specifically, number of small lymphocytes (T-cells) should be normally, more than 1200/cmm. The skin tests are done to qualitatively, assess cell mediated immunity.

Table 5.10. Some features suggestive of primary immune deficiency disorders

- Frequent infections with extracellular pyogens (B-cell defect).
- An ordinary benign virus causing a severe infection (T-cell defect).
- Infections caused by opportunistic organisms (T-cell defect).
- Live virus/attenuated bacterial vaccine produces systemic illness or severe untoward effect.
- Chronic/recurrent osteomyelitis or abscesses of skin, liver or lymph nodes.
- X-ray changes in ribs, scapulae and vertabrae.
- Neonatal tetany and uncommon face.
- Eczema and thrombocytopenia.
- Telangiectasia of sclerae and ears.
- Short limb dwarfism.
- Family history of recurrent infections.

Skin sensitivity is noted after intradermal injection of certain antigens against which humans are frequently sensitized. However, skin tests are reliable only after 3 to 5 years of life (after the infant has sufficient previous exposure to the employed antigens). The reliability is in doubt when need for testing T-cell immunity is maximum.

Humoral immunity is assessed by determination of serum immunoglobulins. For the first few months of life IgG (placental transfer from mother) is the major immunoglobulin Ig. Thus for diagnosing panhypoglobulinemia presence of IgM and IgA is a good evidence against the condition. Panhypogamma globulinemia is the usual presenting form of X-linked or autosomal primary hypogammaglobulinemias. As immunoglobulin levels increase with age the levels in patients should be reported with age related controls.

Besides panhypoglobulinemia, a careful note should be taken of: i) absent IgA with normal or high IgM; ii) a marked increase of IgE; iii) low IgM with marked elevation of IgA. IgG subclass deficiencies also occur but may go undetected (total IgG may remain normal).

More useful than simple immunoglobulin levels, is measurement of specific antibody response to previously administered or ubiquitous naturally occurring antigens. Thus isohemagglutinin titres and febrile titres should be assessed. If the child has received usual immunizations, their titres should be assessed. If not, immunization response after vaccine administration should be measured. However, no live virus vaccine should be given, if immune status of the child is under doubt.

See Table 5.8 for diagnosis of acquired immune deficiency syndrome (AIDS).

A note on techniques for studying immunoglobulins will be presented in the next section.

Polyclonal gammopathy and paraproteins in disease

In a number of diseases there is polyclonal increase of immunoglobulins (Igs), seen as diffuse increase in the γ-globulin band on ordinary electrophoresis. It may be related to antigenic stimulation or loss of immunoglobulin regulation. The finding, however is, generally, of very little help in diagnosis. Polyclonal increase is seen in chronic liver disease, chronic infections (leprosy, all Igs, helminthic infections, IgE or all Igs, chronic granulomatous disease of childhood, all Igs, infectious mononucleosis, IgM or all Igs and others), certain immune deficiency diseases, autoimmune diseases, sarcoidosis (all Igs), amyloidosis (all Igs), down's syndrome (all Igs), narcotic addictions (IgM) and others.

Increase of monoclonal immunoglobulins or fragments of immunoglobulins (called paraproteins or M-proteins) are also associated with a number of diseases (multiple myeloma, Waldestroms macroglobinemia, B-cell neoplasm, chronic lymphatic leukemia, lymphomas and monoclonal gammopathy of undetermined significance (MGUS). Patients of chronic liver disease and those of autoimmune disorders may also have monoclonal immunoglobulin (paraprotein) increase. Monoclonal immunoglobulins appear as sharp discrete bands in electrophoresis (Tables. 5.11 & 5.12).

Laboratory evaluation of Ig deficiencies or for presence of paraprotein

Generally, simple electrophoresis is first performed. The agarose medium results in better separations than paper or cellulose acetate. Based on results of this investigation other investigations are undertaken. Some times the specialized investigations

Table 5.11. About estimation of serum proteins and electrophoresis

- Assumption of upright posture and application of tourniquet before venepuncture lead to increased diffusion of fluid from vascular compartment into interstitial compartment and increase in serum protein concentration.

- In electrophoresis, serum (and not plasma) is used since fibrinogen, migrating in β–γ region, may produce a sharp band which may be mistaken as a paraprotein.

- Presence of acute phase proteins, haptoglobin and ATT increase the size of α_1/α_2 band, and reduce albumin.

- Presence of bilirubin or drugs binding with albumin, modify migration of albumin band. Thus one may see two albumin bands in such conditions.

- Hb when present free in serum (after saturating haptoglobin) migrates in β or α_2 region. Hapto-globulin Hb complex travels separate from free Hb.

Table 5.12. Proteins which may appear as an M-band in serum electrophoresis

- Paraproteins (from abnormal plasma cells)
- Haptoglobin-hemoglobin complexes
- C3
- β-Lipoprotein
- Transferrin
- Fibrinogen (when plasma is used as the sample)
- Immune complexes
- α_1-Macroglobulin
- C-reactive protein (CRP)

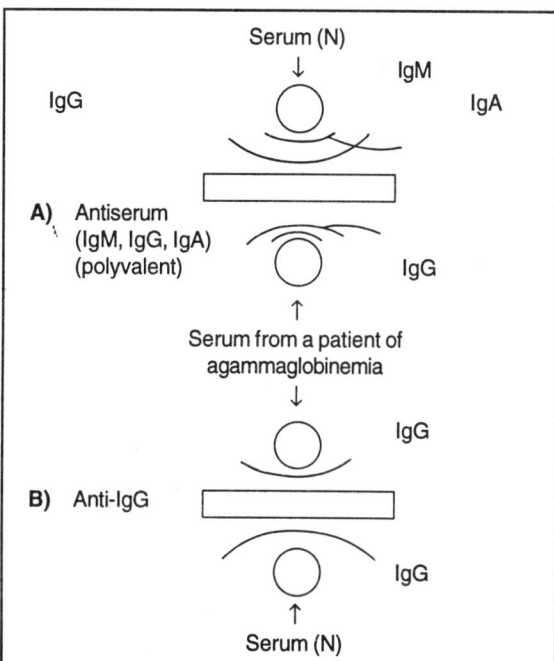

Fig. 5.2. Serum immune protein analysis by immuno-electrophoresis.

- In the round wells cut in the gel are added normal/test sera, as shown. In the elongated gutters antisera, polyvalent or against a particular Ig (anti-IgG, anti-IgM, anti-IgA, anti-K, anti-γ) are added. The test serum of this patient contains reduced amount of only IgG.

may be directly performed depending upon clinical symptoms and signs of the patients.

Immunoelectrophoresis is the most useful screening method for evaluation (semiquantitative) of IgG, IgA or IgM and for identifying abnormal immunoglobulin molecules such as myeloma proteins (Fig. 5.2). Immunologic nephlometry (Fig. 5.1) and radial

immunodiffusion techniques are used to quantitate individual Igs and other proteins. In radial immunodiffusion method, circular wells are cut in a gel plate impregnated with specific antiserum directed against a single immunoglobulin class (or Ig component). A circular precipitin ring will form after the sample protein placed in the well diffuses through the gel. The radius of the precipitin ring is proportional to the concentration of the serum immunoglobulin. In the immunofixation technique, test serum replicates are subjected to electrophoresis on agarose gel (the number of replicates depends upon the number of antisera to be used). Six replicates will be required if five antisera have to be used. After electrophoresis, five gels are reacted with five antisera (anti-IgG, anti-IgA, anti-IgM, anti-K and anti-γ) one for each gel. Next, the gels are washed and then stained for proteins. The sixth gel, after electrophoresis, is neither reacted with any antiserum nor washed. It is directly stained for proteins. In this gel the position of the monoclonal band is revealed by comparison with other gels.

In autoimmune diseases antigen is known and serum is tested for autoantibodies by methods like, tanned red cell hemagglutination, radioimmune precipitation, immunofluorescence microscopy and complement fixation.

Different autoantibodies and other investigative parameters used in detection and follow up of chronic rheumatic diseases/collagen diseases are ANA (antibody, nuclear antigen), Anti-DNA, ANCA (antibody, neutrophil cytoplasmic antigen), C3, C4, C-reactive protein and ESR.

Multiple myeloma

It is a malignant disorder of plasma cells with peak incidence after 60 years. The malignant cells produce the same immunoglobulin, meaning thereby, that the tumor represents clone of a single B-cell. The immunoglobulin produced, thereby, is monoclonal. The paraprotein belongs to one of immunoglobulin type (with one or other of the two light chains). The light chains may be produced in excess and because of small size, pass in urine. These Ig light chains in urine are called Bence Jones protein. This protein is present in urine in about 50% of myeloma cases and in about 20%, only light chains are synthesized and Bence-Jones proteinuria occurs without the myeloma band in simple serum electrophoresis.

With malignant proliferation of plasma cells (single clone), in bone marrow, there is increased synthesis of abnormal Ig, reduced synthesis of normal Igs, and reduced formation of red cells, white cells and platelets. There is often anemia and increased susceptibility to infections.

The presymptomatic phase of multiple myeloma (may last many years) may show: unexplained proteinuria, elevated ESR, the myeloma protein in serum and/or urine, increased incidence of infections and amyloidosis.

Table 5.13 indicates the systems involved and the basis of investigations, in multiple myeloma. Some cases of B-cell lymphoma and chronic lymphatic leukemia also produce paraproteins. In some old individuals a benign paraprotein band may be seen, in electrophoresis. It however, does not increase in size with passage of time and is not accompanied with Bence Jones protein in urine. Further there is no decrease in normal Igs (Table 5.14). Also read Case history 5.1.

The factors determining the tumor mass or stage of the disease, with values indicated for stage III (high tumor mass) are as follows: i) Hb (<8.5 g/dL); ii) corrected serum calcium (>12 g/dL); Bence-

Table 5.13. Systems involved with relevant investigations in multiple myeloma

Growth of malignant cells in bone marrow:
- Marrow biopsy shows a large number of malignant plasma cells.
- Osteolytic lesions in X-ray.
- Increased serum calcium and alkaline phosphatase levels.

Immune system:
- Reduced levels of normal serum immunoglobulins.
- M-Band in electrophoresis.
- Bence Jones protein in urine.

Kidney:
- Increased serum levels of urea, uric and creatinine.

- Plasma cell neoplasms are often associated with primary or secondary amyloidosis. Amyloid material arises from abnormal immunoglobulin products. Renal involvement may cause glomerular damage (nephrotic syndrome), renal tubular acidosis, or diabetese insipidus. Chronic renal failure occurs in about half of the patients with renal involvement.

Table 5.14. Monoclonal gammapathies of uncertain significance (MGUS)

- More common than myeloma (in 1% of population above 50 years of age; upto 10% above the age of 70 years).
- Features compared to those of myeloma;
  - Bone marrow plasma cells <10% (>10% in myeloma).
  - M-component level <30g/L.
  - No Bence Jones protein.
  - No lytic bone lesions, no anemia, no renal failure.
  - In bone marrow cells, labeling index <1% (cells exposed to radioactive thymidine).
  - Low plasma cell acid phosphatase and β-glucuronidase.
  - Salmon calcitonin stimulation test negative.

- In long term follow up about 25% of patients with MGUS develop myeloma or some other B-cell malignancy.

Jones proteinuria (>12 g/d); serum IgG and IgA (>7 g/dL and >5 g/dL) and bone involvement (generalized lytic lesions in bones).

Myeloma needs treatment (with cytotoxic drugs) when paraprotein level rises above 5 g/dL or progressive bone lesions develop.

Waldenstroms macroglobinemia

The condition is less common than multiple myeloma. It is a varient of chronic lymphatic leukemia with greater number of plasma cells. It is characterized by presence of monoclonal IgM detected by immunoelectrophoresis. Vascular blockage due to high viscosity of serum may result in retinal hemorrhages, visual impairment and transient neurological problems. The macroglobulin binds with red cells to produce hemolytic anemia and with coagulation factors to produce hemorrhages. The macroglobulins may show features of cryoglobulins (precipitation on cooling to 4°C) and may be associated with Raynaud's phenomenon (episodic vasoconstriction of small arteries and arterioles of fingers/toes, causing pallor and/or cyanosis). Cryoglobulin formation is more common in this condition than in multiple myeloma. Cryoglobulinemia also occurs in other conditions associated with abnormal globulins (SLE). In Waldenstroms macroglobinemia, unlike multiple myeloma, there are no bone pains and no osteolytic lesions in bones, on X-ray.

Heavy chain disease

It is a rare disorder in which abnormal serum and urine protein is homogeneous α, γ or μ chain. Presentation in γ-chain disease is more like lymphoma (lymph adenopathy, hepato-splenomegaly, fever and propensity to infection) than multiple myeloma. In the α-chain disease, there is abnormal plasma cell infiltration of lamina propria of small gut resulting in severe diarrhea and malabsorption. Immuno-electrophoresis is needed for correct diagnosis, as ordinary electrophoresis may only show hypogammaglobulinemia.

Amyloidosis

Primary amyloidosis is a paraprotein disorder with monoclonal L-chain deposits in tissues and there is associated Bence-Jones proteinuria. Secondary amyloidosis (deposition of amyloid A protein) with Bence-Jones proteinuria, occurs in chronic infections (tuberculosis, leprosy), chronic inflammation (including rheumatic disorders), neoplasms or as a familial disorder. Amyloid deposits in the heart produce congestive heart failure, in kidney, proteinuria and azotemia, in intestinal tract, malabsorption and in nerves, peripheral neuropathy and other functional impairments.

Diagnosis is established by demonstration of amyloid in tissues. In primary amyloidosis monoclonal proteins can be demonstrated in serum and urine.

TUMOR MARKERS

Mitogenesis is a multistep process, starting with activation of a growth factor receptor. This in turn leads to activation of other membrane and cytosolic proteins and second messenger molecules, that transduce the mitogenic signal to the nucleus. Defects in the components of this intracellular cascade result in loss of cellular control on the mitogenic pathway. Generally, lesions in a number of components of this pathway are required for malignant change in the cell; defects in one or two components may not be enough. The normal components of the cascade are encoded by proto-oncogenes and oncogenes formed from these proto-oncogenes encode abnormal protein components (oncoproteins). With loss of control over mitogenesis, there is rapid cell proliferation, in tumor cells. Besides mitogenesis, the process of differentiation is equally important in the process of growth. Control of this process is less well understood but lesions in the components of the control process of differentiation (leading to de-differentiation) are very important in malignant transformation of tumors. The third fundamental property of malignant tissue is related to its capability to metastasize. Mechanism by which this property is acquired is not well understood. *In formation of malignant tissue, as explained above, new proteins are produced corresponding to the changes of the transformation process.*

The molecules involved in the above mentioned process of malignant transformation may act as tumor markers. The transformed cells may also produce certain substances which are unusual for the normal tissue. These will also out as tumor markers. Thus tumor markers are produced related to the process of malignant transformation, cell de-differentiation, rapid cell proliferation and other tumor associated events. Related to malignant transformation, c-erbB-2 protein (p185) and its cleaved product have been studied. Serum level of cleaved product of p185 correlates with change in concentration of many other major tumor markers in serum.

Proteins encoded by mutated suppressor genes (for suppressing cell growth) may become tumor markers for certain tumors. Mutant p53 proteins belong to this group. Other suppressor genes of interest are BRCA-1 and BRCA-2. Their mutations are of interest in cancer breast. However, their encoded proteins cannot be studied at present.

Carcinoembryonic proteins are produced in the dedifferentiation process. Substances like hCG, LD, AP, HVA and 5-HIAA may be produced in increased amounts in relation to rapid cell proliferation process. In relation to metastases, tumor cells produce certain proteolytic enzymes. Activities of various tissue specific glycosyltransferases are also altered in tumor cells. This would lead to alteration in structures of certain glycoproteins, mucins, blood group substances and AFP.

Most human cancers are monoclonal in origin. But as the clone develops, further mutations occur and this gives rise to cell heterogeneity in tumors. For the same reason the antigenic profile of tumor cells and epitope profile of tumor antigens goes on changing with time.

Some tumor markers are discussed below.

Human chorionic gonadotropin

It is glycoprotein hormone, made up of noncovalently linked α and β subunits. Both malignant and non-neoplastic trophoblast cells produce intact hCG as well as free α and β subunits. Assay of hCG is specific for β subunit. Further the free α and β subunits can also be assayed separately.

Hydatidiform mole is a potentially malignant proliferation of trophoblastic tissue which is treated by uterine curettage. If some tissue is left behind there is risk of developing chriocarcinoma (it is malignant proliferation of trophoblastic tissue). hCG is an excellent tumor marker for this tumor. Free β -subunit is more useful in detection of recurrence, as intact hCG level may remain normal. It is useful in monitoring response to treatment as well.

α-hCG (free) is a tumor marker for pituitary endocrine tumors. Use of hCG, as a tumor marker, for germ cell tumors, is discussed separately.

Prostatic specific antigen (PSA)

It is perhaps the best tumor marker discovered so far. It is synthesized by epithelial cells of prostate gland and its usefulness is because of high tissue specificity, although, there is lack of cancer specificity. PSA levels are increased in both prostatic hypertrophy and prostatic cancer. Together with rectal digital examination or transrectal ultra-sound, it may be used for screening of clinically significant prostatic cancer. Major amount of PSA, in serum is present as PSA-antichymotrypsin complex. Further the complexed fraction increase is higher in cancer cases than those of prostatic hypertrophy. Thus assay of complexed form has higher specificity for detection of cancer prostate. PSA assay is particularly useful in monitoring surgical prostatectomy. Measurable PSA level after the operation means residual prostatic tissue or metastases.

Table 5.15. Superiority of monoclonal assays over polyclonal assays

- Give better reproducibility.
- Give better specificity as there is reduced non-specific cross reactivity.
- Give wider linear concentration range in assay.
- Better agreement between results of different kits.

- The tumor markers CA 19-9, CA 125 and CA 15-3 detected by monoclonal antibodies are more specific and sensitive than CEA detected by using polyclonal assay.

Carbohydrate antigens (CA) markers

CA 19-9, CA 125 and CA 15-3 (detected by monoclonal antibodies) are much more sensitive and specific (Table 5.15) than CEA (using polyclonal assay) for pancreatic, ovarian and breast carcinomas. These markers have been used with CEA and other tumor markers to increase both sensitivity and specificity for tumor diagnosis (Table 5.16). CA 125 is expressed by more than 80% of non-mucinous epithelial ovarian carcinomas. CA 125 is found in most serous, endometriod and clear cell carcinomas of ovary. Ovarian tumors also have a strong familial incidence. Thus CA 125 estimation along with ultrasound examination and clinical examination can be used to screen relatives of a patient of an ovarian tumor.

Alpha-fetoprotein (AFP)

It is a major fetal serum protein and also one of the major carcinoembryonic proteins. It resembles serum albumin in many physiochemical properties. It is the most useful marker for diagnosis and management of hepatocellular carcinoma (HCC). But its level is also increased in pregnancy and many benign hepatic diseases. AFP has been used for screening population for hepatoma in China and certain nearby countries (also Eskimos). There is high incidence of this tumor in these parts of the World. Increased fucosylation of AFP in primary HCC (determined by lentil lectin reactivity of serum AFP) is used to differentiate the condition from benign liver disorders and also to indicate beginning of hepatoma in cirrhosis. Use of AFP in screening for neural tube disorders is discussed elsewhere (Chapter 18).

Table 5.16. Use of some tumor markers in different malignancies

hCG	Choriocarcinoma Gonadal germ cell tumours (D,P,MT,R)	ACP, PSA	Cancer prostate (D,MT,R)
		Paraprotein	Myeloma (D.MT,R)
AFP	Hepatoma, Gonadal germ cell tumor (D,P,MT,R)	Calcitonin	Medullary carcinoma thyroid(S.D,MT,R)
CEA	Colorectal carcinoma (MT,R)	CA-125	Ovarian carcinoma (D,MT,R)

Some other important tumor markers are catecholamines for pheochromocytoma, CD-30 for Hodgkins disease and anaplastic large cell lymphoma, CD-25 for hairy cell leukemia, neuron specific enolase for neuroblastoma and small cell cancer lung.

- Some substances act as nonspecific but sensitive markers of activity of many tumors (lactic dehydrogenase, lipid associated sialic acid, β2M, tennessee antigen, tissue polypeptide antigen). These can be used in monitoring efficacy of tumor therapy.
- Some tumor makers are produced when tumor becomes highly de-differentiated and highly malignant. Some examples are AFP (gastrointestinal, renal, bladder, breast and ovarian carcinomas), free α-hCG (colorectal and pancreatic endocrine tumors) and chromogranin A (medullary thyroid carcinoma and certain other endocrine tumors).

S = screening, D = diagnosis, P = prognosis (higher the levels more disseminated the tumor) MT = monitoring treatment (successful treatment lowers the levels), R = recurrence, after levels were once normalized.

For abbreviation of tumor marker, see the text.

Table 5.17. The screening procedures for certain malignancies

Cervical cancer	• Pappanicolaou smear, every 1 to 3 years between 18 to 65 years.
Ovarian Cancer	• Abdominal examination, transvaginal ultrasound and CA-125 level in plasma in high risk groups.
Breast cancer	• Clinical examination of breast, every year, over 50 years in females. • Mammography between 50 to 75 years, every 1 to 2 years. • Some clinicians recommend breast self examination every month.
Cancer prostate	• Evaluation of PSA level every year in men over 50 years of age.
Cancer colon	• Fecal occult blood, periodically, in people over 50 years. • Periodic sigmoidoscopy.

- It should be clear from this table that tumor markers are not recommended for population screening of malignancies except probably for cancer prostate which is also controversial. Screening, however, is recommended in high risk groups (CA-125 for ovarian cancer, AFP for hepatoma in certain regions of China. Also see Table 5.16.

Use of AFP, as a tumor marker for germ cell tumors is discussed separately.

Carcinoembryonic antigen (CEA)

It is the first carcinoembryonic protein and still most widely used tumor marker. Its levels are increased in cases of colorectal cancer, especially when hepatic metastases are present. Table 5.16 indicates its utility in cases of colorectal cancer.

Population screening or screening of high risk groups is recommended for certain malignancies (Table 5.17).

Tumor markers for germ cell tumors

These tumors arise from gonads or from extragonadal sites (retroperitoneum, mediastinum, pineal gland and others). About 50% of the germ cell tumors of testis are non-seminomatous type (pure embryonal type without much differentiatioin, endodermal sinus tumors arising from yolk sac elements, choriocarcinoma and teratomas including different cell types) and commonly present in the third decade and are associated with elevated levels of hCG and AFP. The rest 50% of the testicular germ cell tumors are seminomatous type (more differentiated and less malignant) and are associated with elevated levels of only hCG.

In female the germ cell tumors constitute 75% of all ovarian tumors in women under 30 years of age. The ovarian germ cell tumors are: i) the benign tumors (usually it is dermoid cyst lined by epidermis bearing hair. It may contain teeth or calcified bone which may be seen in pelvic X-ray); ii) malignant tumors arising from dermoid cysts; iii) primitive malignant germ cell tumors (dysgerminoma, yolk sac tumors, immatue teratomas, embryonal carcinoma and choriocarcinoma).

AFP and hCG are useful in diagnosis, knowing prognosis and management of the germ cell testicular tumor and the malignant ovarian germ cell tumors. Chemotherapy is very effective against these gonadal tumors.

CEREBROSPINAL FLUID

Cerebrospinal fluid (CSF) is produced at a rate of about 500 mL/d. 70% of this fluid is derived by ultrafiltration and secretion from the choroid plexuses, and the rest from ependymal lining of the ventricles and cerebral subarachnoid space. It leaves the ventricular system through the medial and lateral formina of the fourth ventricle, into the subarachnoid space. Resorption of CSF occurs at the arachnoid villi. It circulates nutrients and collects wastes from central nervous system. It has also functions of lubricating and cushioning the brain.

Subarachnoid space contains CSF around the brain and spinal cord. This space extends as perivascular space around blood vessels entering and leaving the brain. In meningeal inflammatory diseases, proteins and cells enter CSF via these perivascular spaces. Resorption of CSF occurs at the arachnoid villi into venous sinuses and other veins. In the region of spinal cord, it is also resorbed into venous plexuses surrounding the duramater. Spinal tumors may press on this drainage system leading to increase in pressure of CSF below the tumor site and also leakage of proteins from congested vessels. The spinal cord ends near the first lumbar vertebra and the spinal subarachnoid space is punctured between the third and fourth lumbar vertebrae to obtain a sample of CSF.

Any space occupying lesion of the brain will press the surface of brain against the vault and interfere in resorption of CSF leading to increase in CSF pressure. In this case collection of CSF may cause herniation of brain tissue through foramen magnum and should be avoided. A dramatic drop in CSF pressure after removal of 1 to 2 mL of CSF, suggests herniation or spinal block above the puncture site and no further fluid should be withdrawn in such a case.

CSF should be submitted separately, for different studies: i) chemistry and immunology studies; ii) microbiological examination; iii) total and differential cell counts (for this purpose do not use glass tubes to avoid cell adherence and process quickly to avoid cell degradation); iv) cytology, if malignancy is suspected. The four major categories of diseases in which CSF examination is generally required are; meningeal infection, subarachnoid hemorrhage, CNS malignancy and demyelinating diseases. (Table 5.18)

In meningeal infections there is increase in cell count. In pyogenic cases, there is granulocytic cell reaction; in viral cases, there is lymphocytic cell reaction and in tubercular cases there is mixed cell reaction. In areas of inflammation, there is leakage of proteins (mostly albumin) form the vessels and the infecting organisms may consume CSF glucose. Changes in these two biochemical parameters, are often, not seen in viral cases. In postinfective polyneuritis, there is disproportionate increase in CSF protein, compared to cellular reaction because of hypersensitivity reaction.

Blood in CSF may indicate subarachnoid or intracranial hemorrhage. In such cases, xanthochromia (yellow colour of supernatant after centrifugation of sample of CSF) may also occur. No xanthochromia will be seen if hemorrhage is fresh due to puncture of some vein by the lumbar puncture needle. A commercially available, latex agglutination immunoassay for cross-linked fibrin derivative D-dimer is specific for fibrin degradation and is negative in traumatic taps. False positive, however, can be expected in DIC, fibrinolysis or trauma from repeated lumbar punctures.

In case of meningeal tumors, the drainage of

CSF is blocked and leakage occurs from distended veins. There is greatly increased CSF pressure, not affected by jugular vein compression. There is also a large increase in CSF protein. There is only slight increase in mononuclear cells while CSF glucose is reduced by metabolic activity of the tumor cells. Some times carcinoma elsewhere causes diffuse involvement of meninges (carcinomatosis meningitis). The clinical condition runs a chronic course with mild mixed cell reaction, increase of CSF protein and decrease of CSF glucose.

In degenerative states like multiple sclerosis and neurosyphilis, there is mild hypersensitivity reaction to the damaged tissue components, leading to mononuclear cell pleocytosis, an elevation of total immunoglobulin and presence of oligoclonal IgG. There is selective production of IgG in CNS. Thus CSF IgG is increased while total protein level is normal. The CSF IgG index is used to distinguish locally synthesized IgG from serum IgG, that may have entered CSF across a disruptive blood brain barrier. It is calculated by dividing CSF/serum IgG index (CSF IgG/serum IgG) by CSF/serum albumin index (CSF albumin/serum albumin). If the levels of IgG and albumin are expressed in mg/dL in CSF and g/dL in serum, 0.8 may be taken as upper normal limit. IgG index is abnormal multiple sclerosis, neurosyphilis, brain tumors and after cerebrovascular accidents.

One or more oligoclonal bands of CSF IgG may be demonstrated by agarose gel electrophoresis in multiple sclerosis. Simultaneous serum study will exclude a systemic origin of the bands. These oligoclonal bands are absent at onset of the disease and their number goes on increasing with time.

TRANSUDATES AND EXUDATES

Excess of fluid present in the pleural space is called pleural effusion and in the peritoneal space, ascites. The fluid, if derived by filtration across the capillary endothelium by altered systemic factors, is called a transudate and if formed in response to some local factors like infection or malignant involvement, is called an exudate. Exudates are distinguished from transudates by higher protein concentration of the former.

Table 5.18. Some CSF findings in normals and in certain disorders

Parameter (normal values)	Meningitis			Multiple sclerosis	Subarachnoid hemorrhage
	Pyogenic	Tubercular	Viral		
Pressure (50-180 mm water)	↑	↑/↓ with spinal block	N	N	↑
Cells (0-4 lymphocytes/mL)	(1000-10,000) (PMNs)	(100-5000) (Lymphos.)	10-2000 (Lymphos.)	0-100 (Lymphos.)	Large no. (Red Cells)
Glucose (40-70 mg/dL) (2/3rd of blood glucose level)	↓	↓	N	N	N
Protein (20-50 mg/dL)	↑	↑	N/↑	N/↑	↑
IgG (0.9-5.7 mg/dL)/total protein)% (<13%)	-	-	-	↑	-
IgG index (0.29-0.59)	-	-	-	↑	-

- A CSF to blood glucose conc. ratio <0.23, CSF protein >2.2g/L and >1180 × 10^6 neutrophils/L favour diagnosis of pyogenic than any other form of meningitis.
- Gram staining and CSF culture should also be done in pyogenic cases.
- Low neutrophil count in pyogenic meningitis carries poor prognosis.
- Certain other tests used in diagnosis of bacterial meningitis include levels of C-reactive protein, and TNF (both levels ↑), certain bacterial antigens and bacterial DNA after amplification by PCR.
- In certain viral infections viral DNA/RNA is studied (after PCR) for proper diagnosis.
- Newer tests for tuberculous meningitis include studies of adenosine deaminase, Mycobacterium tuberculosis antigens/antibodies and bacterium DNA after amplification. The last mentioned test holds maximum promise and is likely to become most useful test in paucibacillary forms of pulmonary tuberculosis and extrapulmonary disease, in near future.

Pleural effusion

The exudative effusion should have at least one of the following three characteristics: i) pleural fluid protein/serum protein ratio >0.5; ii) pleural fluid LDH/serum LDH ratio >0.6; iii) pleural fluid LDH more than two-thirds of normal upper limit for serum. The pleural effusion is a transudate if none of the three characteristics is there. Three important causes of transudative pleural effusion are, congestive heart failure, hepatic cirrhosis and hypoproteinemia (fourth cause is pulmonary embolism and infarction).

Important causes of exudative pleural effusions are tuberculosis and other infections (pulmonary), malignancy (metastatic and pulmonary), pleural involvement in SLE and rheumatoid disease, pancreatitis and ruptured esophagus. Important tests to arrive at the cause are as under; pleural fluid (PF) pH, and levels of glucose and amylase; gram staining, cytology and culture of PF. Needle biopsy of pleura may be needed.

Any of the following is an indication for tube thoracostomy (for drainage of fluid): presence of gross pus; organisms revealed by Gram staining; glucose level <50 mg/dL and pH<7.0 or 0.15 units lower than arterial pH.

Ascites

Important causes of ascites include, cirrhosis, congestive heart failure, nephrosis, tuberculosis and disseminated carcinomatosis. It is important that the cause of ascites is firmly established before treatment is started. For example ascites due to cirrhosis may get worsened by superadded tuberculous infection and in that case simple treatment with salt restriction and diuretic may appear ineffective.

It is best to characterize ascites on basis of serum-ascites albumin gradient. In exudative type it is <1.1 (pyogenic, tuberculous, neoplasm and pancreatitis). In transudative type it is >1.1 (cirrhosis, congestive heart failure). In nephrosis although the ascites is transudative type the gradient is <1.1 because of low serum albumin level. Also see Table 5.19.

Table 5.19. Ascitic fluid characteristics in certain diseases

Condition	Protein (g/L)	Cells(per μL)	Other tests
Cirrhosis	<25	Predominantly mesothelial cells(<250)	
CHF	15-50	Mesothelial, mononuclear (<1000)	
Nephrosis	<25	Mesothelial, mononuclear (<250)	May be chylous
Pyogenic	>25 (if purulent)	Predominantly polymorphonuclear	Gram stain: Culture
Tuberculous	>25	Lymphocytes (>1000) Also red cells	Stain for acid fast bacilli: Peritoneal biopsy
Malignancy	>25	Variable cell types (>1000) Also red cells	Cytology: Peritoneal biopsy
Pancreatitis	Often >25 (variable)	Variable May be blood stained	Increased amylase level in peritoneal fluid/blood: Chylous

- Serum - ascites albumin difference or gradient >1.1 in cirrhosis, CHF and <1.1 in the rest.
- Blood stained fluid with protein level >25 g/L often in malignancy, tuberculosis. In pancreatitis it may be chylous/blood stained.

CASE HISTORY: 5.1

A 62 year old patient presented with complaints of bone pains, loss of weight and increased frequency of intercurrent infections. Patient had proteinuria, better demonstrated by sulfosalicylic precipitation method than by the dipstick method. There was suspicion of multiple myeloma.

➤ How to confirm the diagnosis?
➤ What is the cause of increased frequency of infections?
• Three important investigations used in diagnosis of multiple myeloma are: i) demonstration of Bence Jones protein in urine and/or a paraprotein band (M-band) in serum electrophoresis.

Bence Jones protein is found in urine in about 50% of the patients and in about 20%, this finding occurs without presence of the M-band; ii) excess of plasma cells in bone marrow biopsy; iii) X-ray evidence of typical bone lesions. Two of the three findings are considered sufficient for diagnosis. Many patients have the initial finding of increased serum globulin level. Subsequently, M-band would be demonstrated on electrophoresis.

- As bone marrow is dominated by plasma cells synthesizing abnormal immunoglobulin, synthesis of normal immunoglobulins is reduced. This explains increased frequency of infections.

CASE HISTORY: 5.2

A 54 year old employee of a hospital developed breathlessness soon after his lunch. He also complained of dizziness. His blood pressure was 110/70 (previously recorded level was 170/100). ECG record indicated a recent myocardial infarction. Within 2h of the episode he was admitted to ICCU.

➤ Comment on clinical presentation of the patient.

➤ What is role of enzyme studies at the time of admission?

➤ What supportive meausres and drugs are used to limit the infarct size?

➤ What are biochemical indiations of multple organ failure in case of severe shock following AMI?

- Clinical presentation indicates early left ventricular failure due to myocardial infarction. Lowering of blood pressure and dizziness are pointers to the episode. Many times especially, in old individuals there is no chest pain.

- The earliest enzyme change is increase of CK-MB in serum, occurring at 4 to 8h and peaking at 12 to 24h. Thus no enzymes changes can be expected at this stage. However, it may be useful to establish baseline values for enzymes at this stage. About the protocols for use of serum enzymes in diagnosis of MI, it may be said: i) CK-MB is better than CK; ii) CK-MB and CK together (to express CK-MB as % of CK) are better than CK-MB alone; iii) CK or CK-MB estimatioins in multiple samples (to look for peak levels) are better than single sample studies; iv) AST/LDH are occasionally useful in late samples.

- It is done by protecting ischemic myocardium by proper O_2 administration, pain control, minimizing tachycardia, controlling hypertension and treating congestive heart failure. Drugs used for thrombolysis, anti-thrombotic agents, β-blockers and ACE inhibitors are employed for restricting the size of infarct.

- Prolonged severe hypotension produced by cardiogenic shock, (hypovolemic shock is much less damaging) can produce multi-organ failure syndrome and is associated with high mortality. The shock stage is followed by a period of hypermetabolism of 7-10 days showing hyperglycemia; lactic acidemia and polyuria with excessive nitrogen excretion in urine (>15 g/d). During this period evidence of lung injury and hepatic failure appear. After a progressive increase of bilirubin for about a week evidence of renal failure appears (progressive increase of serum creatinine). This is followed by encephalopathy, consumption coagulopathy, gastrointestinal bleeding and failure of immune system.

With progressive increase of blood glucose, serum lactate and urinary N-excretion, there is decrease in levels of serum albumin and other liver proteins.

Poor prognostic features are initial mean arterial pO_2/FIO_2 ratio of <250 (normal = 400) and blood lactate of ≥3.4 mg/dL (normal <1.5 mg/dL) on day 2. Subsequently rapidly developing hepatic and renal failures confirm a bad prognosis.

CASE HISTORY: 5.3

A 58 year old patient was admitted with complaints of pain in upper abdomen, loss of weight and mailase. There was long history of excessive alcohol intake. Examination showed dullness on both the lung bases. There was no jaundice. There was only modest increase of ALT and AST. Levels of ALP and γ-GT were 2080 U/L and 940 U/L, respectively.

In this case there is no parallel increase in bilirubin and ALP levels and at the same time there is only a small increase in levels of ALT and AST. This combination of findings strongly suggests presence of primary or secondary hepatic malignancy. This combination of findings can also occur in infiltrative conditions of liver (amyloidosis). In case of secondary liver malignancy, one should look for the primary tumor. Also the enlarged liver is hard and irregular. Hepatocellular carcinoma may develop in a patient of cirrhosis or chronic hepatitis following HBV infection and following hepatic injury produced by various carcinogens including aflatoxins. High level of γ-GT in the present case indicates that the hepatic damage could be because of chronic alcoholism, which in turn could be a factor in development of hepatocellular carcinoma.

α-Fetoprotein is a good marker for hepatocellular carcinoma. Liver biopsy and fetoprotein level are two investigations which will help confirmation of diagnosis.

OBJECTIVE TYPE QUESTIONS

Pick out the incorrect statement

1. Myocardial infarction

i) CK-MB is more specific for diagnosis of myocardial infarction than total CK.

ii) In pulmonary embolism, levels of both AST and LDH may increase.

iii) In a hemolysed sample level of CK will increase due to its release from red cells.

iv) γ-Glutamyl transpeptidase (γ-GT) levels increase in chronic alcoholics.

v) In a patient without jaundice, high level of ALP may indicate hepatocellular carcinoma.

2. Myocardial infarction

i) A silent episode of MI may subsequently be detected by ECG.

ii) Three commonly used enzymes for diagnosis of MI are CK, LDH and AST.

iii) CK rises most rapidly of the three and peaks at 24h.

iv) Raised CK levels can be demonstrated even 1h after an attack of MI.

v) Increase of serum enzymes in MI, in isolation, cannot be used to indicate size of infarct.

3. Transaminases

i) Serum ALT, primarily, arises from liver.

ii) Serum AST can arise from different tissues like heart, muscle, kidney, brain, besides liver.

iii) ALT is cytosolic enzyme.

iv) AST is present in cytosol as well as mitochondria.

v) In viral hepatitis AST/ALT ratio is generally, more than 1.0.

4. Plasma proteins

i) Increase of serum proteins is usually due to increase of globulins.

ii) A serum with high globulin level may show a paraprotein band.

iii) All patients of multiple myeloma show presence of Bence-Jones protein in urine.

iv) In multiple myeloma there may be evidence of bone lesions in X-ray examination.

v) Multiple myeloma may show presence of large number of plasma cells in bone marrow biopsy.

5. Diagnostic use of certain specific proteins

i) Reduced ceruloplasmin levels occur in patients of Wilson's disease.

ii) α_2-Macroglobulin level, in plasma, increases, in nephrotic syndrome.

iii) C-reactive protein increases in acute infections.

iv) Haptoglobin levels are reduced in hemolytic disorders.

v) Transferrin level gives an idea of iron stores.

vi) Antitrypsin deficiency may cause pulmonary disease.

6. Electrophoresis

i) The most important use of electrophoresis is to study the presence of M-band.

ii) If plasma is used for electrophoresis, fibrinogen may appear as a separate band which may be mistaken as a M-band.

iii) In the presence of bilirubin or drugs binding with albumin, one may see two bands for albumin.

iv) The M-band and Bence Jones protein in urine are also features of MGUS.

v) Haptoglobin-hemoglobin complexes may also appear as a M-band.

7. Electrophoresis

i) In hemolytic condition, hemoglobin appears as a sepatate band in electrophoresis, only after haptoglobin has been depleted.

ii) In acute phase response, electrophoresis shows increased level of haptoglobin and reduced level of albumin.

iii) In chronic response to stress, there is increase of haptoglobin, greater decrease of albumin (than acute phase response) and increase in size of γ-globulin band due to polyclonal increase of immunoglobulins.

iv) Once a myeloma band is seen in electrophoresis, in a patient of myeloma, there is no need to quantitate immunoglobulins.

v) In cirrhosis, besides decrease of albumin, there is polyclonal increase of all immunoglobulins causing increase of γ–globulin and β-globulin, causing β–γ bridging.

vi) In adults hypogammaglobulinemia (poor γ–globulin band on electrophoresis) is commonly seen in lymphorticular disorders and also after chemotherapy for malignancies.

8. Immunodeficiency (primary)

i) Absolute lymphocyte count is primarily related to T cell function and not B cell function.

ii) Presence of IgG in first few months of life rules out X-linked or autosomal primary panhypoglobulinemia.

iii) Congenital X-linked agammaglobulinemia is

familial and is caused by mutation in Bruton tyrosine kinase gene.

iv) Common variable immunodeficiency and IgA deficiency may be two different clinical forms of the same underlying gene defect in a large number of patients.

v) In some primary B cell deficiency states levels of some immunoglobulins may be reduced while of others increased.

vi) Severe T cell abnormalities with or without hypogammaglobulinemia are often treated with bone marrow transplantation.

vii) Human immunoglobulin replacement therapy should be used only in IgG deficient patients with recurrent bacterial infections.

9. Immunodeficiency

i) In DiGeorge syndrome there is primary T cell deficiency with heart lesions and hypoparathyroidism.

ii) In DiGeorge syndrome, the immune defect usually, spontaneously, improves.

iii) In ataxia-telangiectasia there is DNA repair defect and cells are highly susceptible to radiation induced chromosomal damage.

iv) In ataxia-telangiectasia there is high incidence of lymphoreticular malignancy.

v) In primary T cell deficiency states immunoglobulin levels are not affected.

10. Myeloma (bone lesions)

i) Myeloma cells produce osteoclastic activity factor (OAF) which stimulates osteoclasts to produce bone lesions.

ii) Myeloma bone osteolytic lesions are not followed by osteoblastic (bone formation) activity.

iii) Bone lesions are not used in staging myeloma.

iv) In patients of MGUS, there are no bone lesions.

v) The salmon calcitonin simulation test is positive in myeloma but not in MGUS.

11. Myeloma (renal involvement)

i) Over half the patients of myeloma suffer from some renal pathology.

ii) Renal failure occurs in about 25% of myeloma patients.

iii) Myeloma associated hypercalcemia and hyperuricemia contribute to renal failure.

iv) Glomerular deposits of amyloid also contribute to renal failure.

v) L-chains passing through filtration membrane, produce glomerular injury.

vi) Kidney infection may also occur as there is general increased tendency to infections.

12. Multiple myeloma

i) The M-component is cationic leading to decreased anion gap.

ii) Increased plasma protein level may produce pseudohyponatremia.

iii) Interaction between M-component and the clotting factors may produce clotting abnormalities.

iv) The M-component may form cryoglobulins producing Raynaud's phenomenon and hyperviscosity syndrome.

v) Besides change in bone marrow, plasma cell expansion often leads to enlargement of spleen and lymph nodes.

13. Tumor markers

i) AFP and hCG are tumor markers for testicular teratoma.

ii) Very high serum level of AFP in teratoma, means poor prognosis.

iii) Management of teratoma may require surgical excision followed by chemotherapy.

iv) Steady increase in post treatment low level of AFP means recurrence.

v) Tumor markers are not used for screening purpose.

14. Tumor markers

i) Tumor markers may be hormones/proteins/enzymes secreted by the tumor cells.

ii) Tumor markers may be certain tumor antigens.

iii) A positive pregnancy test in a male is always a false positive.

iv) Prostatic specific antigen (PSA) has high tissue specificity but lacks cancer specificity.

v) CEA is used for monitoring success of treatment in colorectal carcinoma.

15. CSF examination

i) Early diagnosis of meningeal disorders is important to reduce mortality/morbidity.

ii) In bacterial meningitis, the rapid bacterial antigen tests have become quite popular because of high sensitivity and ease of use.

iii) Early diagnosis of tubercular meningitis from CSF examination, at present, is quite difficult.

iv) Increased IgG index and presence of oligoclonal bands are highly diagnostic of multiple sclerosis.

v) Diagnosis of viral meningitis is mostly a matter of exclusion.

ANSWERS

1. No.(iii). Hemolysis increases serum LD and acid phosphatase but does not affect levels of serum amylase, ALP and ALT. Hemolysis is visible in serum at Hb level of >20 mg/dL.
2. No.(iv). Increases at 4 to 8h.
3. No.(v). In viral hepatitis AST/ALT ratio is generally less than 1.0. In most other types of hepatic damage this ratio is generally more than 1.0.
4. No.(iii). Only 50% of the myeloma patients show this abnormality.
5. No.(v). Ferritin level gives an idea of iron stores.
6. No.(iv). There is no Bence-Jones proteinuria.
7. No.(iv). It is required to provide a baseline to monitor response to treatment during management of the patient.
8. No.(ii). It is presence of IgM and IgA which rules out primary panhypoglobulinemia. IgG may be there because of transfer from mother.
9. No.(v). T-cells help β-cell function.
10. No.(iii). Staging of myeloma to predict prognosis is based on hemoglobin, calcium and paraprotein levels, degree of skeletal involvement, and total body tumor burden.
11. No.(v). The L-chains present in tubular fluid are reabsorbed and catabolized by the tubular cells. The process leads to damage to these cells. This process produces Fanconi type syndrome and not renal failure.
12. No.(v). Plasma cells mostly remain in bone marrow. In solitary bone plasmacytoma there is a single bone lesion. In extramedullary plasmacytoma there is involvement of lymphoid tissue in regions of nasopharynx or paranasal sinuses.
13. No.(v). In certain familial malignancies these may be used to screen rest of the family members.
14. No.(iii). It may indicate a testicular tumor.
15. No.(iv). Positive predictive value of the test is largely dependant upon degree of clinical suspicion. Thus the tests have a complementary value only.

CHAPTER 6

Gastrointestinal Tract
Including Liver and Pancreas

THE LIVER

Liver cells are arranged in columns radiating from portal tracts. In these radiating columns, the liver cells either face each other (canalicular side) or the sinusoids which run between the columns. The sinusoids are lined by endothelial cells and Kupffer cells (phagocytes) and receive blood from branches of hepatic artery and portal vein running in the portal tracts. The blood drains into the central veins (of the conventional liver lobules) to ultimately reach hepatic vein. Between the liver cells and the lining cells of sinusoids lies the space of Disse which forms the interstitial space of liver. Large molecules secreted into space of Disse, easily enter sinusoids because these lack basement membrane. Stellate cells in the space of Disse store vitamin A. Between the liver cells, away from sinusoid, lie bile canaliculi, from which bile drains into terminal bile ductules. Microvilli (and secretory functions) exist on liver cells towards sinusoids as well as bile canaliculi. Liver cell damage in hepatitis leads to obstruction of bile canaliculi (or secretory failure of liver cells toward canaliculi) while liver cell necrosis followed by fibrosis (cirrhosis) distorts both bile canaliculi and hepatic sinusoids. Thus in cirrhosis, in addition to cholestasis, portal hypertension also occurs. There is also loss of Kupffer cells. This leads to entry of a number of unwanted antigens from intestine (normally destroyed by the Kupffer cells), into systemic circulation with formation of unwanted immunoglobulins (non-functional) causing increase of γ-globulin fraction of plasma.

Functions of liver are, excretory (bile pigments, bile salts, cholesterol, lipid soluble drugs and toxic metabolites), biosynthetic (albumin, coagulation proteins, glycogen), metabolic (gluconeogenesis, formation of glucose from galactose, metabolism of lipoproteins), storage (vitamins A, B_{12} and glycogen) and phagocytic.

The liver function tests (LFTs) may be grouped according to hepatic functions listed above. It is, however, of clinical advantage to group them according to certain pathophysiological mechanisms. Thus there are tests which indicate excessive hemolysis, cholestasis, liver cell damage, reduced number of liver cells, greatly reduced number of liver cells and loss of phagocytic functions of the liver (Fig. 6.1).

Formation and fate of bilirubin

Reticuloendothelial cells of liver and spleen form bilirubin from heme of Hb and other similar compounds (myoglobin, cytochromes). It is transported to liver bound to albumin. This is called unconjugated bilirubin and being bound to albumin, it does not appear in urine. In small infants it can cross blood brain barrier to produce kernicterus. From serum albumin, bilirubin is taken up in liver by a specific binding protein called ligandin to be actively transported to smooth endoplasmic reticulum where

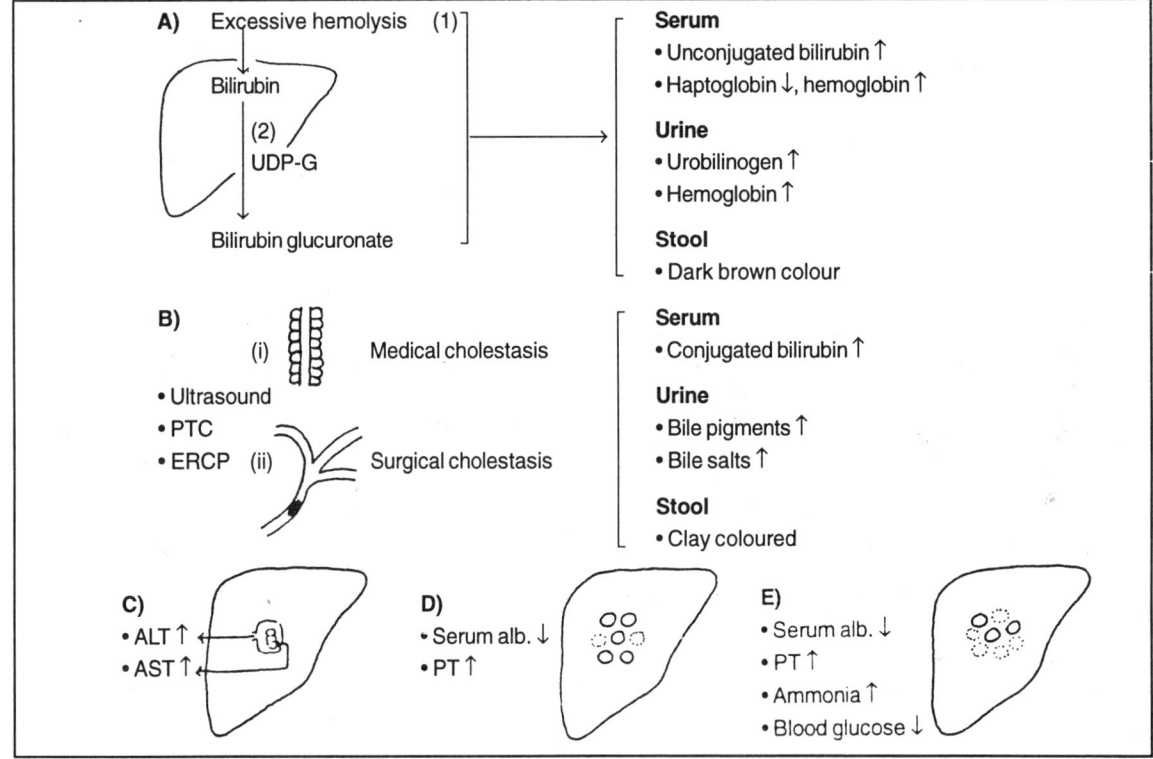

Fig. 6.1. Pathophysiology of liver function tests.

A) Hemolytic jaundice (1), bilirubin conjugation failure (2).

B) Cholestatic jaundice; (Ultrasound, Percutaneous transabdominal cholangiography (PTC) and Endoscopic retrograde cholangio pancreatography (ERCP), differentiate intrahepatic (i) from extrahepatic (ii) cholestasis.

C) In mild hepatocyte damage (permeability changes) in ordinary infective hepatitis, ALT> AST while in presence of mitochondrial damage (cirrhosis, severe hepatitis), AST>ALT and more cell necrosis in the latter case.

D) Reduced number of functional liver cells (cirrhosis).

E) Number of functional liver cells greatly reduced (hepatic failure).

it is conjugated with glucuronate by glucuronyl transferase. Bilirubin monoglucuronate passes to canalicular side of hepatocytes and from here after addition of second glucuronate molecule conjugated bilirubin is actively secreted into bile canaliculi. This active secretion is affected in functionally impaired liver cells (hepatitis, hypoxia, septicemia) and also when there is increased pressure in biliary tract. Many anions (salicylates, FFA, sulfonamides) which bind to ligandin, impair bilirubin uptake by liver cells, its conjugation and excretion. Fig. 6.2 shows certain inborn errors related to defective handling of bilirubin by liver cells.

After entering the intestine, bilirubin is freed from

glucuronate and next, a number of products are formed, collectively called urobilinogen, by reducing activities of bacterial enzymes. Some of urobilinogen is absorbed into portal blood, and rest is lost in feces. In feces urobilinogen is oxidized to urobilin (brown coloured pigment) by atmospheric oxygen. A small part of urobilinogen from portal circulation appears in urine to be oxidized to coloured urobilin in urine. Rest of urobilinogen from portal circulation is re-excreted in bile, as conjugated bilirubin.

In excessive hemolysis, increased amount of bilirubin (unconjugated) is taken up into liver cells and passed as conjugated bilirubin into the gut.

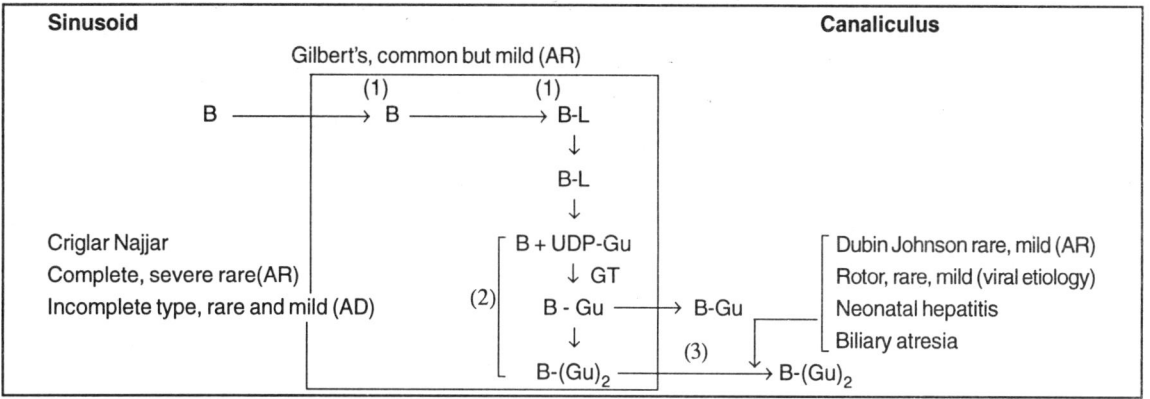

Fig. 6.2. Inborn errors of transport (also neonatal hepatitis) and secretion of bilirubin by hepatocytes.

- Defects in steps (1) (transport defect in the sinusoidal membrane) and step (2) (Glucuronyl transferase activity) result in accumulation of unconjugated bilirubin in serum. Gilbert's is a mild and harmless condition. As it is common, it needs to be kept in mind in differential diagnosis, in any age group of patients. Criglar Najjar complete type can cause kernicterus in neonates. Criglar Najjar incomplete type benefits from administration of phenobarbitone.
- Note the four disorders due to canalicular secretory defects (3). In all these there is accumulation of conjugated bilirubin. Differentiation between Dubin Jonson and Rotor disorders is possible only by liver biopsy.
- B=Bilirubin, B-L = Bilirubin ligand complex, GT=Glucuronyl transferase, B-Gu = Bilirubin mono glucuronide, B-$(GU)_2$ = Bilirubin diglucuronide.

This leads to increased loss of urobilinogen in feces and urine and colour of stool changes from normal yellow to dark brown. The Watson-Schwartz test (Chapter 8) gives semi-quantitative estimate of urobilinogen in urine. A commercial strip is also available. For these tests, fresh urine should be used. To summarize, in hemolytic jaundice, level of unconjugated bilirubin increases in serum, stool becomes dark in colour, urine is free from bilirubin (bile pigment) and shows increased excretion of urobilinogen but normal amounts of bile salts (Hay's test is negative). In post hepatic jaundice, level of conjugated bilirubin increases in serum, and excretion of bile pigment (bilirubin) in urine. Bile salt excretion in urine also increases. Since very little bilirubin enters the intestine, stool becomes clay coloured and urine is also free from urobilinogen. Bile pigment excretion profile in hepatic jaundice resembles that of post hepatic jaundice, since functionally impaired liver cells can still take up unconjugated bilirubin, quite well, but processes of conjugation and especially secretion into canaliculi is impaired. In this condition, re-excretion of urobilinogen into bile by liver is also impaired. Some times increased excretion of urobilinogen in urine is an important indication of the early stage of hepatitis.

Aminotransferases

ALT is present in cytoplasm and occurs in much higher concentration in liver than other tissues. AST is present both in cytoplasm and mitochondria. ALT is more specific for liver damage. Levels of these enzymes can rise with loss of plasma membrane integrity, even when cellular functions are not much disturbed (especially ALT) and there is no necrosis. Thus the increased levels indicate liver cell insult but do not relate to the severity of damage and therefore to prognosis of the disease.

In acute viral hepatitis the AST/ALT ratio is 1.0 or less. In more severe hepatocellular injury, with mitochondrial damage, the above ratio is increased. In alcoholic liver disease the ratio lies between 3 to 4. This is because alcohol is a mitochondrial toxin and also alcoholics are deficient in pyridoxine, which is more limiting in analysis of ALT than AST. AST is used to monitor therapy with potentially, hepatotoxic drugs. Donor blood is screened for elevated ALT levels; to exclude patients (donors) with viral hepatitis.

Chronic elevation of aminotransferases in an asymptomatic patient may be because of alcohol abuse, use of some drugs, chronic viral hepatitis, non-alcoholic fatty liver and overweight individuals.

In viral hepatitis, maximal aminotransferase levels (>200 U/L, often 500 to 1000 U/L) occur when jaundice, just, starts appearing. Similar levels may occur due to drugs (especially paracetamol), in exacerbation of chronic active hepatitis and in acute circulatory failure. In obstructive jaundice rise is only mild but increases with development of cholangitis.

Alkaline phosphatase

The hepatic alkaline phosphatase is mostly located, in the canalicular and sinusoidal membranes of the liver cells. In cholestasis there is increased synthesis of this enzyme which is passed into circulation. There is also reduced biliary secretion of the enzyme. This leads to increase of ALP more than 2 to 3 times the upper normal limit in cholestasis. In case of complete obstruction the rates of rise of bilirubin and ALP run parallel but in case of incomplete obstruction rise of bilirubin is relatively much less. After cholestasis is relieved fall of serum ALP is much slower than that of bilirubin. In jaundice of hepatic cell injury there is only moderate increase of ALP. The same is also true in passive liver congestion. In the latter condition rise of ALP is more than that of bilirubin.

Some times rise of serum ALP is found as the sole biochemical finding. It may be due to hepatobiliary disease but one should be able to demonstrate presence of some other marker of liver disease, say, increase in level of γ-GT.

γ-Glutamyl transferase

This enzyme helps transport of amino acids across the cell membrane and also increases formation of glutathione required for drug detoxication. This enzyme increases in serum in three types of disorders associated with liver. Firstly, certain drugs induce proliferation of endoplasmic reticulum (location of γ-GT) which increases formation of the enzyme. The drugs inducing the enzyme include, alcohol, phenobarbitone, phenytoin and others. The enzyme may be used to detect and follow alcohol abuse (provided other drugs that induce the enzyme are not being used). The second liver related disorder in which γ-GT level is increased, is cholestatic jaundice. Elevations of γ-GT and ALP commonly, run parallel except in pregnancy since in cholestatic jaundice of pregnancy, γ-GT does not increase. The third hepatic disorder associated with increase of γ-GT is hepatocellular damage. But in this condition levels of transaminases are more sensitive indicators of the damage.

Prothrombin time

Liver synthesizes all coagulation factors (except factor VIII) and brings about activation of factors II, VII, IX and X with the help of vitamin K. In liver disease prothrombin time is prolonged because of impairment of the above referred functions of liver. Prothrombin time (PT) depends upon factors I, II, V, VII and X. PT is prolonged in severe liver damage and prolonged biliary obstruction. The latter condition produces vitamin K deficiency. If, after administration of vitamin K, PT is still prolonged, it implies liver cell damage. Because of very short half life of coagulation factors (upto 72h), PT changes can be used to assess liver cell damage of both acute and chronic liver disease. In cases of hepatic failure increasing PT carries bad prognosis.

Disseminated intravascular coagulation (DIC) may accompany cirrhosis and acute fulminant hepatic failure. This has been attributed to reduced synthesis of clotting inhibitory factors, decreased clearance of activated clotting factors or release of tissue thromboplastin from hepatocytes.

Patients of liver disease may also present platelet deficiency or dysfunction.

Plasma albumin

Liver is the only site for synthesis of this protein. Reduced level of serum albumin indicates reduced mass of functioning liver cells, as occurs in chronic diseases especially cirrhosis. Other factors, which can reduce serum albumin level are malnutrition, fever and increased plasma volume. Falling level of serum albumin carries bad prognosis, in a chronic liver disease.

Globulins

In cirrhosis while serum albumin level falls, that of

Table 6.1. Some more specifically used tests

Ceruloplasmin:
- Serum level is reduced in Wilson's disease. Increased urinary excretion of copper may be used for screening of Wilson's disease.

Percent transferrin saturation (serum iron/TIBC x 100 : normal 20-55%)**:**
- It is the most sensitive test for screening of hemochromatosis; serum ferritin level is also used.

α_1**-Antitrypsin:**
- This deficiency may produce neonatal hepatitis or cirrhosis in children/young adults. In ordinary serum electrophoresis the α-band is much reduced, in α_1-antitrypsin deficiency.

α**-Fetoprotein:**
- Increased levels are encountered in hepatoma but also in other liver diseases because of regenerating liver cells (eg; chronic active hepatitis). High levels which specifically indicate hepatocellular carcinoma often occur at a late stage of the disease. α-Fetoprotein estimation has been used in screening populations with high incidence of hepatoma. It may also be used for the same purpose in liver diseases associated with high degree of development of hepatoma (cirrhosis, chronic hepatitis with B virus and hemochromatosis). Also read under tumor markers in chapter 5.

Procollagen Type III propetide[1] and PGA index:
- The first one is studied by immunoassay and is used to follow active cirrhosis. PGA index (computed from serum levels of γ-GT, prothrombin time and apo A-1 levels (apo A-1 level decreases with disease severity) is also used for the same purpose.

[1] Increased level of propeptide in chronic hepatitis and cirrhosis is related to increased connective tissue biosynthesis in hepatocellular disease.

globulin increases. Thus there is reversing of albumin/globulin ratio (there is also β-γ bridging in cirrhosis during electrophoretic separation). Increase of globulin, without change in albumin may occur in chronic active hepatitis or prolonged viral hepatitis.

One important function of hepatic macrophages is to prevent entry of a number of antigens from portal circulation into systemic circulation to prevent undesirable immunological response. Loss of this hepatic function may partly explain increase of serum globulins in liver diseases. The patients of cirrhosis are however, generally, immunosuppressed and this pattern of serum proteins (fall of albumin and increase of globulin) is also seen in some other immunosuppressed states, like AIDS and some times in diabetes. A common finding in each of the above conditions is reduced number of CD4-positive T-cell function.

Marked elevation of γ-globulin (IgG) occurs in autoimmune chronic hepatitis and primary biliary cirrhosis (IgM). Mild elevation also occur in biliary cirrhosis (IgA), chronic viral hepatitis (IgG) and chronic alcoholic liver disease (IgG, IgA).

Some other tests used in certain hepatic diseases are given in Table 6.1.

HEMOLYSIS AND HEMOLYTIC JAUNDICE

Hemolysis may be intravascular or extravascular. Intravascular hemolysis may be non-immune (G6PD deficiency, sickle crisis, toxins as those produced by Clostridium welchii) or immune (use of ABO - incompatible blood) and generally occurs as an acute process (Fig. 6.3). In case of ABO-incompatible blood, anti-A or anti-B, which can fix complement, cause hemolysis. There is fever, hypotension, chest pain, shock, hemoglobinuria, renal failure and in severe cases even generalized bleeding (from DIC). DIC is produced by early, excessive formation of certain cytokines, the most important of which is TNF. The laboratory findings in intravascular hemolysis include decrease in levels of haptoglobin and hemopexin, increase in lactate dehydrogenase and presence of hemoglobinuria and hemosiderinuria along with free hemoglobin in plasma. In the immune cases, direct anti-immunoglobulin test (DAT) or direct coomb's test is positive.

Examples of immune extravascular hemolysis are Rh blood group incompatibility in a new born, drug induced hemolytic anemia and cold agglutinin disease. Acute extravascular hemolysis can also occur in incompatible transfusion due to non-ABO

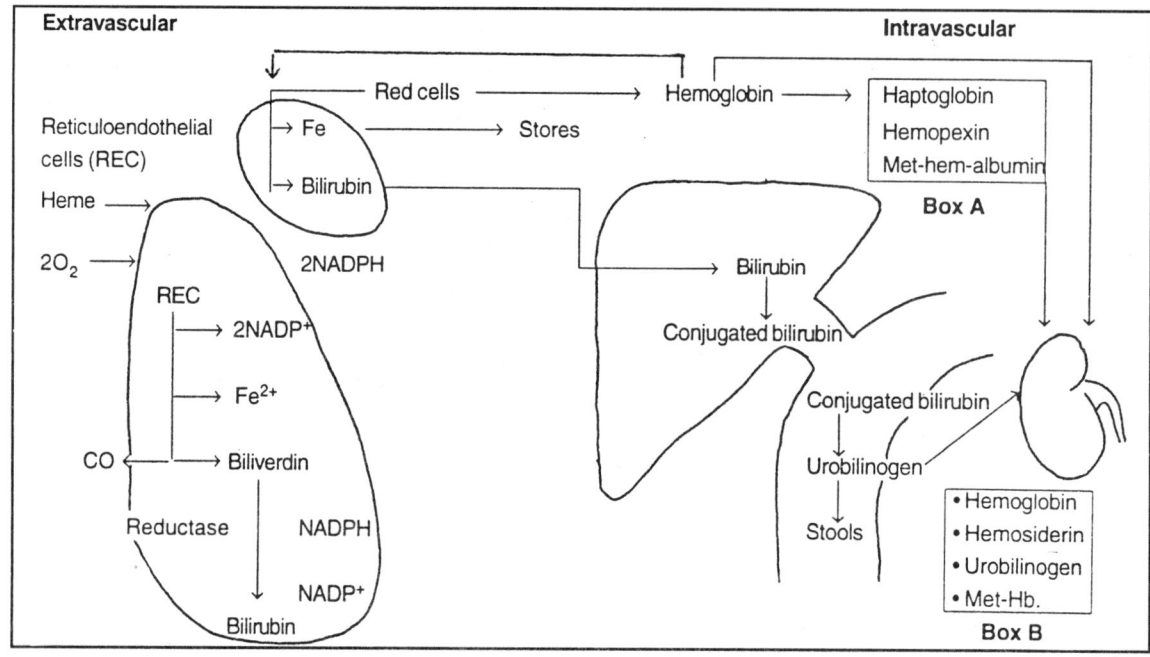

Fig.6.3. Diagnosis of intravascular/extravascular hemolysis.

- In intravascular hemolysis, plasma levels of compounds in box A and urinary excretions of compounds in box B are increased. Hemoglobinuria can lead to oliguria (acute renal failure). In severe cases DIC may occur.
- Common to both types of hemolysis: Increased unconjugated bilirubin in serum and increased urinary excretion of urobilinogen.
- In left part of the figure is shown formation of biliverdin (which changes into bilirubin by a soluble enzyme, biliverdin reductase) by hemeoxygenase system of reticuloendothelial cells.
- Estimations of exhaled CO, blood carboxyhemoglobin level and fecal urobilinogen excretion can be used as measures of hemoglobin breakdown in both forms of hemolysis.

red cell system. These reactions are less severe than those of ABO system (there is no DIC and no complement activation). IgG coated cells are mainly destroyed through phagocytosis by reticuloendothelial (RE) cells of spleen. Complement coated red cells are mainly destroyed in liver in a similar fashion. Some IgG antibodies may activate complement in vivo and cause direct hemolysis. IgG coated red cells can also be destroyed by lymphocytes with FC-receptors. Extravascular hemolysis, commonly, occurs as a chronic process and presents with evidence of stimulated erythropoiesis and increased reticulocyte count (Figs. 6.3, 11.3).

In both intravascular and extravascular hemolysis, bilirubin is the end product. If bilirubin production exceeds capacity of liver to remove it, there occurs accumulation of unconjugated bilirubin in serum and the condition is called hemolytic jaundice. In most

cases (except Rh-immunized new borns), bilirubin levels remain in the range of 3-4 mg/dL as liver is quite efficient in clearing bilirubin from serum. Fever, sepsis and hypoxemia can impair this process in liver. Chronic excessive hemolysis, (hereditary spherocytosis) may result in formation of gall stones.

In Rh-immunized new borns, bilirubin levels can be quite high, especially in premature ones (there is immaturity of bilirubin conjugating system), and can produce kernicterus by entering brain tissue (poor blood brain barrier) and getting deposited in lenticular nucleus of basal ganglia. It produces motor disability and mental retardation. This complication can also occur in severe form of Crigler Najjar syndrome (Fig. 6.2).

Except in early infancy unconjugated bilirubin does not pass into the brain tissue due to blood brain barrier. In new borns, the additional factors which may promote entry of bilirubin into the brain tissue are, prematurity, reduced albumin level, acidosis and increased levels of FFA (increased in fasting state). Anionic drugs like salicylates, sulfonamides also promote the process (Fig. 18.3). Unconjugated bilirubin circulates in blood bound to albumin. The organic anions displace bilirubin from albumin.

Kernicterus is produced in a new born when level of unconjugated bilirubin rises above 20 mg% (at a lower level in premature infants). Severe cases are treated by exchange transfusion (infant should be monitored for hyperkalemia, hypocalcemia, metabolic acidosis and hypoglycemia, during transfusion).

Physiological jaundice (Fig. 18.3)

Jaundice is not present at the time of delivery. Transient rise of unconjugated bilirubin between second and fifth days of life is commonly due to immaturity of hepatic glucuronyl transferase since, after birth, the infant liver is required to eliminate bilirubin (in the absence of placenta). Bilirubin level generally rises to less than 5.0 mg/dL. At times rise may last for several days (upto 2 weeks). Phototherapy forms more soluble isomers of bilirubin which are more easily excreted.

Liver function tests in hemolytic jaundice

Unconjugated bilirubin being water insoluble (circulates with albumin), does not appear in glomerular filtrate and urine. Further, excessive conjugated bilirubin is passed from liver to intestine and increased amount of urobilinogen is formed leading to increased amounts of this pigment in stools (stools are deep brown in colour) and also in urine. In cases of hemolytic jaundice, important biochemical changes are: i) increased level of unconjugated bilirubin in serum; ii) increased excretion of urobilinogen in stool and urine; iii) other LFTs are normal; iv) reticulocytosis. Also see Fig. 11.3.

HEPATIC DISEASES

Hepatitis or acute liver disease

Most commonly, it occurs as viral hepatitis. It may also be caused by toxins (alcohol, paracetamol, bacterial toxins) or may result from shock/septicemia. In all these cases there is both hepato cellular damage as well as cholestasis. Commonly, features like anorexia, fatigue, nausea and mild fever are followed by jaundice. Liver is enlarged and tender.

Viral hepatitis leads to increase in levels of ALT and AST with rise of ALT more than AST. Cholestasis causes increased levels of bilirubin, ALP, 5'-Nucleotidase and γ-GT. Conjugation of bilirubin is also affected and thus levels of both conjugated and unconjugated bilirubin rise in serum (former increases more than latter). Ordinarily, most of the affected liver cells recover and the tests which depend upon liver cell mass (levels of albumin and coagulation proteins (prothrombin time) are not affected. Formation of urea is also not reduced.

The viral agents causing almost all cases of acute viral hepatitis include HAV (hepatitis A virus), HBV, HCV, HDV, HEV and HGV. HAV and HEV have fecal oral transmission. Both infections occur in acute form and are commonly, mild, except that HEV infection can occur in fulminant form in pregnancy. In both these infections, there are no carriers and prognosis is excellent.

HBV infection is mainly transmitted via blood contamination (contaminated needles) but can also be sexually transmitted. The virus can also pass to fetus via placenta. Some times, with hepatitis B virus (DNA) is associated hepatitis D virus (RNA) and results in a severe disease. Hepatitis D virus cannot replicate without hepatitis B virus. HCV is commonly acquired from blood transfusion or drug abuse. It does not cause acute infection. It may cause chronic hepatitis or the carrier state. In HBV infection, chronic hepatitis occurs in 1 to 10% cases (90% in neonates) and the carrier state also occurs.

In HCV infection chronic hepatitis occurs in 50 to 70% cases and the carrier state in 0.5 to 1.0% cases. In chronic HCV infection there may be no symptoms but cirrhosis develops in about 20% cases. Transmission of HGV appears to be similar to that of HCV. It causes acute hepatitis.

Serological investigations help to answer many questions like: i) likely course of the disease; ii) presence of infectivity; iii) development of chronic hepatitis; iv) presence of carrier state (Table 6.2). Also see Figs. 6.4 and 6.5.

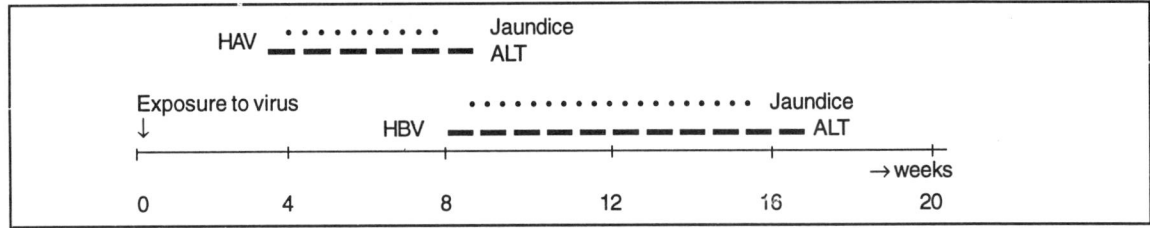

Fig. 6.4. Some features of HAV and HBV infections.

• In viral hepatitis, AST and ALT levels may be >500 units by the time jaundice appears, urine urobilinogen is increased in early icteric period; at peak of the disease it disappears from urine (also from stools); at onset of convalescence urine urobilinogen increases.

- Bilirubinuria occurs before serum bilirubin increases in prodromal period to produce jaundice; during convalescence bilirubinuria disappears while serum bilirubin is still increased. Serum bilirubin is 50-75% direct in early stage; later indirect is proportionately more.

- In acute hepatitis ALT > AST > LD.

• In HAV infection, the period of infectivity (infection by feco-oral route), is roughly related to excretion of HA-Ag in stools. It starts during late incubation period and ends earlier than clearance of jaundice. In fact infectivity diminishes rapidly, once jaundice makes appearance. The disease activity is correlated with presence of anti-HA(IgM). HA-Ag is not measured. Positive anti-HAV-total and negative anti-HAV (IgM) means presence of anti-HAV (IgG) and immunity which is often life long.

- Often runs a milder course, more so in children and there are no chronic carriers.

• In HBV infection (acute) infectivity (blood, saliva, sexual route, placental route) lasts till disappearance of HBs-Ag and appearance of anti-HBs. If HBs-Ag becomes undetectable early, period of activity can be known by the presence of anti-HBc(IgM).

- In 90% of patients (acute hepatitis) HBV resolves within 12 weeks with development of anti-HBs. Relapse usually within one year (↑ ALT) occurs in 20% of such cases.

- <10% of patients have chronic hepatitis (disease for >6 months; ALT and AST >50% above normal):

  -- 70% have benign chronic persistent hepatitis.

  -- 30% have chronic active hepatitis progressing to cirrhosis and liver failure.

  These patients should also be monitored for hepatoma (ultrasound or CT scan and AFT).

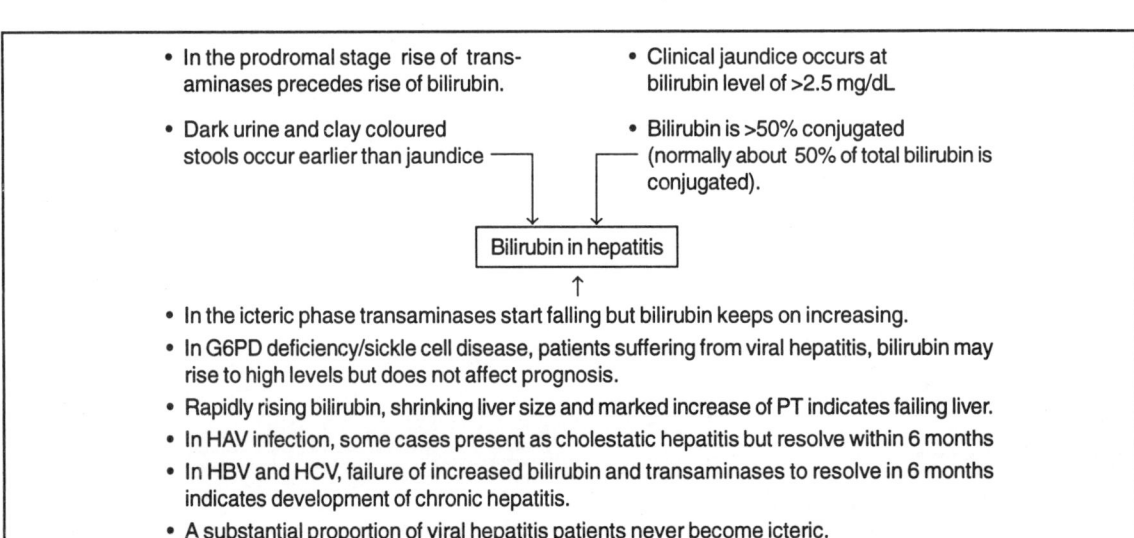

Fig. 6.5. Significance of bilirubin in cases of acute hepatitis.

In some cases of viral hepatitis there is very little hepatic cell dysfunction. Main feature is of cholestasis with increase of bilirubin and alkaline phosphatase. It is a mild hepatic disease but may run a prolonged course. Percutaneous transhepatic cholangiography (PTC) or ultrasound examination may be needed to differentiate the condition from surgical cholestasis (due to stones, neoplasm).

Hepatitis caused by drugs/toxins

Different drugs produce different types of liver disorders. Some result in fatty infiltration/necrosis as a dose related effect (alcohol, acetaminophen, heavy metals), some cause viral hepatitis type disorder (aspirin, halothane, isoniazid) and some cause cholestatic reaction (chlorpromazine, oral contraceptives). *However, a person may have viral hepatitis when he starts taking a drug.* In toxic hepatitis, aminotransferases attain much higher levels than in viral hepatitis.

Alcoholic hepatitis occurs in chronic alcoholics, after a large bout of alcohol. Features resemble those of viral hepatitis but elevations of transaminases and bilirubin are less marked. However, γ-GT is increased out of proportion to ALP, and AST is more than ALT. Alcohol causes damage to mitochondria of hepatocytes and AST is a mitochondrial enzyme. Other alcohol induced changes are also likely to be present.

In a few cases, the attack of hepatitis may be very severe causing rapid liver cell necrosis (fulminating hepatitis) leading to hepatic failure (described later).

Acute liver disease ends up in three ways: Most of the cases resolve, some progress to acute hepatic failure and some lead to development of chronic hepatic failure.

Chronic hepatitis

Chronic hepatitis may or may not follow an attack of acute viral hepatitis. It occurs in 50 to 70% cases of HCV infection and follows only in a small percentage of cases of acute HBV infection. Patients with autoimmune etiology start as chronic

Table 6.2. Serological markers in different forms of viral hepatic disease

Disease from	Infection type				
	HAV	HBV	HCV	HDV	HEV
Acute disease	Anti-HAV-IgM	HBs-Ag/anti HBc-IgM	Anti-HCV	HDV-Ag	Anti-HEV
Infectivity	HAV-RNA[1]	HBs-Ag,HBe-Ag, HBV-DNA[1]	Anti-HCV HCV-RNA[1]	Anti-HDV, HDV-RNA[1]	HEV-RNA[1]
Chronic disease	—	HBs-Ag[2]	Anti-HCV	Anti-HDV	—
Carrier state	—	HBs-Ag[2]	—	Anti-HDV HDV-Ag	—
Recovery	—	Anti-HBs Anti-HBe	—	—	—
Immune state	Anti-HAV-IgG	Anti-HBs Anti-HBc-IgG	—	—	ANTI-HEV[1]

[1] These tests are not available for common laboratory use.

[2] In these patients high infectivity is indicated by presence of HBe-Ag (indicating relative replicative phase); absence of HBe-Ag and presence of anti-HBe means low infectivity.

- Initial testing is done only for HAV and HBV (HBs-Ag, anti-HBc-IgM and anti-HAV-IgM): A patient negative for all the three is tested for HCV. A patient who is anti-HBc-IgM positive but negative for other markers, is followed for appearance of anti-HBs and resolution. If not resolving look for HDV marker. This is generally useful in severe fulminating cases, severe chronic cases, in acute hepatitis like exacerbation in chronic HBV, in areas where HDV is endemic. In following up a patient ALT is used for disease activity.

- Patients HBs-Ag positive or anti-HBc-IgM positive but negative for anti-HBs are vaccinated, or those who are negative for all the three.

- If mother is positive for HBs-Ag the infant must be vaccinated within 12h of birth.

hepatitis. In some cases, starting chronically, neither viral nor autoimmune etiology can be demonstrated. These are called idiopathic or cryptogenic cases.

Chronic hepatitis may be classified according to the etiology, the disease activity or degree of fibrosis. Thus we have chronic hepatitis C, chronic hepatitis B and atutoimmune chronic hepatitis. The terms chronic persistent hepatitis (minimal activity, mild to none fibrosis), chronic lobular hepatitis (mild to moderate activity and mild degree of fibrosis) and chronic active hepatitis (mild, moderate or severe activity, and mild moderate or severe fibrosis) of the previous classification are now reported in terms of activity and degree of fibrosis (as indicated in brackets).

Although, many patients of hepatitis C have no symptoms, a large proportion of these end up in cirrhosis. Most patients of chronic hepatitis (of different etiologies) show fluctuating levels of transaminases, more so those resulting from HCV infection. As in acute hepatitis, there is greater increase of ALT than AST (elevated ALT is often taken as a marker of activity). But once cirrhosis develops, there is greater increase of AST than ALT. ALP may be marginally increased. In more severe cases moderate increase in bilirubin occurs (3 to 10 mg/dL). Hypoalbuminemia and increase of PT occur in severe or end stage cases. In cases of autoimmune etiology, hypergammaglobulinemia is a common finding. Rheumatoid factor may also be commonly demonstrated. In the autoimmune cases, there is often involvement of more than one organ. There may be associated urticaria, migrating polyarthritis, lymphadenopathy, some thyroid disorder, hemolytic anemia and involvement of kidney/lung. These patients are also characterized by relapses and remissions. Chronic hepatitis C cases have been associated with conditions like Sjorgen's syndrome, lichen planus and porphyria cutanea tarda. Hepatocellular carcinoma may occur in cases of viral etiology but not in those of autoimmune etiology.

Interferon therapy is useful in chronic hepatitis of viral etiology and corticosteroids in autoimmune cases.

Cirrhosis of liver

In this disease there is parenchymal damage, fibrosis and nodular regeneration of liver cells. Important causes are given in Table 6.3. Because of large liver reserve, metabolic and clinical abnormalities do not manifest until the disease is quite advanced (more than 80% of liver cells have been destroyed). Liver function tests also remain normal in earlier stages of the disease. Some clinical and biochemical changes are correlated with pathophysiological alterations, in Table 6.4. The patient may present with vague symptoms (Case hisotry 6.2), change in the size of liver, jaundice, ascites, gastrointestinal tract bleed, encephalopathy and a number of other complaints. Diagnostic difficulty may arise when a particular feature presents in isolation.

Biochemical investigations

As already pointed out the liver function tests are normal in earlier stages of cirrhosis. Once the disease is well advanced, albumin and total protein are reduced and prothrombin time is prolonged, because of reduced number of functioning cells. There is rise of both direct and indirect bilirubin and also of ALP, γ-GT and 5-nucleotidase due to distorted bile passages in the liver tissue. Levels of transaminases are variable. In the active stage of the disease, the levels are increased but in the absence of disease activity, the levels are normal. In elevated transaminases, AST is higher than ALT. Ineffective immunoglobulins are also increased. (Table 6.4).

Generally, serum albumin level and prothrombin time are helpful in knowing the severity of the disease. Imaging helps, to know the presence of carcinoma, portal hypertension and ascites. Liver biopsy establishes diagnosis and cause of cirrhosis.

Basis of clinical changes/complications

As the disease progresses and the number of functioning hepatocytes is greatly reduced, a number of abnormalities start manifesting. Besides development of edema and ascites, reduced clotting factors, result in hemorrhages and in severe cases there is

Table 6.3. Causes of cirrhosis

Alcohol abuse:
- Excessive intake of alcohol can cause, fatty liver, alcoholic hepatitis, cholestatic liver disease and mild siderosis, besides cirrhosis.
- Special associated findings are high γ-GT, hyperuricemia hypertriglyceridemia and macrocytosis.
- AST/ALT ratio >1 associated with AST often <300 U/L.
- Increased PT, not corrected by administration of 10 mg/d of vitamin K for 3 days indicates, poor prognosis.

Hepatitis (chronic):
- There is likely evidence of previous infection of HBV/HCV, HDV. In case of cirrhosis following chronic active hepatitis (of autoimmune etiology), one should look for anti-nuclear/anti smooth muscle antibodies.

Toxins/Drugs:
- It is important to look for evidence of liver disease prior to drug intake.

Chronic biliary cirrhosis:
- With progress of the disease there is changing profile of LFTs (cholestatic → hepatic → cirrhotic). Evidence of chronic biliary obstruction (stones: mass lesion).
- For primary biliary cirrhosis, antimitochondrial antibodies, patent bile ducts and liver biopsy.
- Rule out primary biliary cirrhosis in an a symptomatic female (without obesity, alcohol abuse, diabetes mellitus), with elevated ALP.

Hemochromatosis:
- An adult patient presenting with cirrhosis, diabetes mellitus, hypogonadism and skin pigmentation.
- Serum iron and ferritin are increased (iron >200-300 µg/dL; ferritin usually >1000 µg/L), iron binding capacity is reduced. However, the best screening method is estimation of transferrin saturation which is increased (>70%). Ferritin levels may not be affected in early cases and also increase in inflammatory disorders. Diagnosis is confirmed by study of iron in liver biopsy (values in µg/g dry wt. normal 300-1400, symptomatic>6000 : hepatic iron index: µg/g/56 x age : normal <1.0, symptomatic >2, heterozygotes <2). Ferritin levels are used to monitor treatment.

Wilson's disease:
- A young patient (<40 years) presenting with: unexplained disorders of CNS; features of ordinary viral hepatitis; features of chronic active hepatitis; unexplained elevation of aminotransferases, hemolytic anemia with hepatitis or features of cirrhosis. There may be history of Wilson's disease in a near blood relative. Also see the text.

Antitrypsin deficiency:
- Produces liver damage in a neonate and over years progresses to cirrhosis.
- In homozygous state (ZZ) serum ATT level is about 10% of normal and about 60% of normal in the heterozygous state (MZ).

A patient of cirrhosis with a single presenting feature will need careful differential diagnosis:
- Hepatomegaly (malignancy, infiltrative lesions like myelo/lympho proliferative disease, sarcoidosis, amyloidosis, hepatic congestion, and chronic parasitic disease like malaria/kalazar)
- Splenomegaly (myelo/lympho proliferative diseases)
- GIT bleed, ascites, encephalopathy (from other causes).

---

tendency to intravascular coagulation. There is hypoglycemia due to reduced glucose formation in liver. Other metabolic features include hyponatremia, lactic acidosis and hypocalcemia. Tissue hypoperfusion and failure of lactate utilization cause lactic acidosis. Superimposed on acidosis is respiratory alkalosis due to stimulation of respiratory centre by toxins (failure of detoxication by liver). Hypovolemia produced by fluid loss as ascites and presence of toxins in blood may produce hepatorenal syndrome. There is systemic vasodilatation and renal vasoconstriction. GFR is reduced (as in prerenal azotemia) and is better judged by rise of serum creatinine than blood urea since urea synthesis is reduced. Condition is resistant to any treatment.

Important complications of cirrhosis include portal hypertension (which produces portal systemic collateral channels like gastroesophageal varices), splenomegaly, ascites and encephalopathy. A number of factors are involved in ascites of cirrhosis. There is increased hydrostatic pressure in splanchnic capillary bed (due to portal hypertension) and reduced plasma oncotic pressure (due to low plasma level of albumin) and both factors promote formation of ascitic fluid. Distortion of hepatic lymphatics produces increased formation of lymph fluid which increases protein concentration of the ascitic fluid. There is increased central sympathetic stimulation which causes renal vasoconstriction and stimulation of renin angiotensin system increasing aldosterone formation. In kidney there is increased sodium reabsorption both in proximal and distal segments due to increased aldosterone and other factors.

Initial treatment includes bed rest and salt restriction (2g sodium chloride/d). Bed rest increases renal circulation and clearance. Fluid intake is restricted to 1 L/d to prevent hyponatremia. Some aldosterone antagonist (or distal tubule acting diuretic) is also useful. Patient should be monitored for azotemia and hyperkalemia. In severe cases the above management may have to be punctuated with large volume paracentesis.

Encephalopathy is considered separately.

Wilson's disease

In this disease there is impaired excretion of copper with toxic accumulation of metal in liver, brain and other tissues. It is an autosomal recessive disorder (frequency 1:20,000 in general population; frequency of heterozygote carriers is 1:90). Clinical manifestations frequently occur at mid adolescence

Table 6.4. Pathogenesis of certain clinical biochemical features of cirrhosis

Low albumin/protein level/increased PT	Reduced number of functioning hepatic cells
Hyperglobulinemia	Synthesis of ineffective antibodies
Portal hypertension	Sclerosis of sinusoids.
Ascites	Portal hypertension, low serum albumin level.
Raised levels of bilirubin/ALP/ γ-GT; 5 -nucleotidase	Fibrosis of intrahepatic bile passages.
Steatorrhea	Reduced availability of bile salts in the gut
Lactic acidosis	Reduced tissue perfusion because of reduced plasma volume because of edema and ascites (third space losses). Because of reduced plasma volume there is secondary aldosteronism.
Hyponatremia	Because of increase secretion of ADH due to reduced plasma volume.
Increased susceptibility to infection	Defective T-cell function. There is also synthesis of ineffective anti-bodies.
Renal failure (hepato renal syndrome) (systemic vasodilatation with renal vasoconstriction)	Reduced GFR and tubular dysfunction (urine/plasma osmolality ratio <1.2).
Bleeding tendencies	Reduced synthesis of clotting proteins especially those requiring vitamin K for activation. Also reduced platelet number due to sequestration by enlarged spleen and liver. Increased formation of clot inhibitory factors, reduced clearance of activated clotting factors.
Changes in serum bilirubin, transaminases and ALP are inconsistent and not very important in diagnosis	These changes also depend upon the disease etiology

- Progress of disease may be judged from PGA index. It is computed from PT, γ-GT, and apo-A-1 levels.
- As drug metabolism is affected, drugs should be used cautiously, especially in the presence of malnutrition, hypoalbuminemia or prolonged PT.
- Serum ammonia level correlates with severity of encephalopathy, in advanced disease.

(rarely before the age of 6). About half the patients present with hepatic disease, which may be: an episode like that of mild acute hepatitis; acute hepatitis continuining into chronic hepatic disease, insidiously developing chronic liver disease with features like active chronic hepatitis or cirrhosis; fulminant hepatitis. The other half of the patients present with neurological manifestations (tremors, spasticity, rigidity, chorea, dysphagia, dysarthria) and/or bizarre psychiatric manifestations along with the Kayser-Fleischer ring in cornea (copper deposited in cornea). A small percentage of female patients present with amenorrhea or repeated abortions.

Diagnosis is made by showing ceruloplasmin level <200 mg/L along with presence of Kayser-Fleischer ring or by showing copper in liver biopsy >250 µg/g dry liver weight along with low ceruloplasmin level as above. Decreased incorporation of ^{64}Cu in ceruloplasmin is a useful test if hepatic copper is not increased. This test is also useful to rule out other disorders with increased hepatic copper. The test may also be helpful to detect heterozygote carriers.

Normal newborns may show low ceruloplasmin with increased hepatic copper which normalizes in about one year.

Hemochromatosis

This disorder is discussed in Chapter 11. Also see Table 6.3.

α₁-Antitrypsin (ATT) deficiency

It is an autosomal recessive disorder with familial pulmonary emphysema (secondary bronchiectasis also occurs) and liver disease. Incidence of heterozygous state (MS and MZ) is 10-15% of general population (normals are MM) and 1 in 2000 of the homozygous state (ZZ). Purified ATT is available for therapy. Also see Chapter 5 and Table 6.3.

Hepatic failure

It may occur in chronic and relapsing form, in advanced cases of cirrhosis or in acute form in severe (fulminating) cases of viral hepatitis (most commonly, by B and D as well as by E type viruses,

although others can also cause). It may also occur in certain cases of toxin caused hepatitis (paracetamol, halothane and even after a heavy dose of alcohol). Also see Fig. 6.6.

In hepatic failure during fulminant hepatitis, initially there is rapid increase in serum levels of ALT and AST (rise of AST is more than that of ALT) This is followed by marked increase of ALP and bilirubin. Following this, ALT and AST levels come down, as number of viable hepatic cells is greatly reduced, and features like hypoalbuminemia, increased prothrombin time and elevated serum ammonia become dominant. Patient may present with clinical/biochemical abnormalities as in advanced cases of cirrhosis (Table 6.4).

Hepatic failure may produce hypoglycemia (reduced hepatic glucose formation), bleeding tendency, even DIC, electrolyte and pH disturbances (poor hepatic metabolism of aldosterone, accumulation of NH_3) and encephalopathy.

Hepatic encephalopathy

Accumulated ammonia may play an important role in encephalopathic changes. It may have a direct toxic effect on membrane transport processes; it may act by depleting cerebral neurons of ATP (converting α-ketoglutarate of citric acid cycle into glutamate and then glutamine) or by producing intracellular alkalosis (intracellular H^+ combining with NH_3). Other toxins like mercaptans from methionine, short chain fatty acids and phenol have also been implicated. Alternatively, false neurotransmitters (eg; octopamine) resulting from accumulated aromatic/branched chain amino acids might play an important role by displacing natural neurotransmitters from their neuronal sites. Neurotransmission could be inhibited by accumulation of GABA like compound or endogenous benzodiazepines.

Diagnosis

Early changes are sleep disturbances, mood and personality changes. Other features are flapping tremors, rigidity and hyperreflexia and ultimately coma. Breath and urine produce a peculiar smell (fetor hepaticus due to accumulated mercaptans).

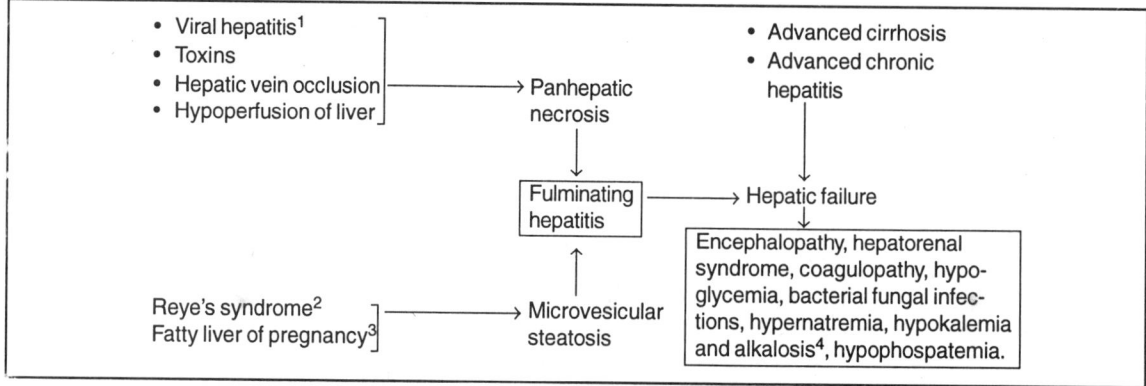

Fig. 6.6. Acute and chronic hepatic failure

---

[1] HBV in presence of HDV or super imposed on chronic hepatitis B; HEV infection in pregnancy; HAV infection occurring in older adults or persons with underlying liver disease.

[2] Reye's syndrome is a rare disorder presenting with acute hepatitis (fulminant) and encephalopathy in children and develops after an infective illness (say chickenpox) and often with additional history of use of aspirin during treatment. There is mitochondrial damage of hepatic cells and presence of acidosis and hypoglycemia along with hepatitis and encephalopathy. Some inherited metabolic disorders may also present with similar features in small children.

[3] Mild intrahepatic cholestasis may occur in third trimester of pregnancy. Rarely, a severe type of fatty liver and failure may develop. Pathological lesion in severe hepatic failure of pregnancy and Reye's syndrome is called microvesicular steatosis with sinusoidal enlargement and cholestasis.

[4] Hypernatremia and hypokalemia are produced because of increased aldosterone levels (poor metabolism in liver). Metabolic alkalosis is produced by hypokalemia and increased NH_3 levels.

The condition may require differentiation from clinical syndromes produced by hypoglycemia, alcoholism, B_1 deficiency and overdose of some sedative. Diagnosis of hepatic encephalopathy is clinical; the laboratory tests have only a supportive role

An important aspect of treatment is to reduce levels of ammonia and other neurotoxins. For this protein intake is reduced (<20 g/d) and adequate intake if calories is ensured (about 300g of glucose/d) to keep endogenous protein breakdown under check. Neomycin is used to keep down the number of intestinal bacteria. Ammonia absorption is reduced by lactulose, a non-absorbable disaccharide which acts as an osmotic laxative. Its metabolism by colonic bacteria results in acidic pH which further reduces NH_3 absorption. The precipitating factors are promptly treated.

Biliary obstruction

Extrahepatic biliary obstruction may be due to gall stones. It may also be caused by carcinoma head of pancreas or lymphoma which block common bile duct at portahepatis. In these conditions of complete

obstruction, both bilirubin and alkaline phosphatase levels increase in serum and urine contains bile salts and pigment but is free from urobilinogen. There is also increase of γ-GT and 5′-nucleotidase. The latter enzyme behaves like biliary tract isoenzyme of ALP. Cholangitis caused by extra hepatic obstruction (Table 6.5) also causes similar changes.

Intrahepatic cholestasis is caused by cirrhosis, cholangitis, gram negative sepsis, hepatitis and drugs. With some of these, liver cell damage is also associated. Also in Dubin-Johnson and Rotor's syndromes, there is cholestasis due to faulty excretion of bilirubin conjugates.

Intrahepatic space occupying lesions are produced by hepatoma or metastases. In these cases often, there is very little biochemical evidence of hepatitis, cellular damage or biliary obstruction. Most commonly there is increase in level of serum alkaline phosphatase. Also, LD (LD5) is generally increased. Increased levels of transaminases, bilirubin and reduced albumin level indicate that tumor is wide spread in liver.

Intrahepatic cholestasis may be restricted or

wide spread. Extrahepatic cholestasis is complete type. The cholestatic liver disease can present with wide variety of features (Tables 6.5 and 6.6).

It is important to differentiate between intrahepatic and extrahepatic cholestasis. The former commonly needs conservative medical treatment while the latter often requires surgical intervention. The liver function test profile is similar in the two cases. History and clinical examination, however, often provide useful information in such cases. Ultrasound, percutaneous or retrograde cholangiographic procedures demonstrate the dilated duct system and the need for surgical intervention.

Retrograde cholangiography may also be used to deliver a stone into the duodenum, in some cases.

For presentations of cases of biliary obstruction, go through case histories 6.3 and 6.5 and see Table 6.6.

Chronic biliary obstruction (primary and secondary biliary cirrhosis)

In primary biliary cirrhosis bile canaliculi and ductules undergo fibrosis in the portal triads. Bile starts entering hepatocytes leading to their necrosis. It is a progressive disorder predominantly affecting women between 40 to 60 years. The disease starts

Table 6.5. Significance of intrahepatic and extrahepatic cholestasis and features of restricted and widespread cholestasis

- It is important to differentiate between intrahepatic cholestasis (viral hepatitis, drug or alcohol induced cholestasis, primary/secondary tumors, primary biliary cirrhosis, intrahepatic cholangitis) and extrahepatic cholestasis (biliary stones, malignancy causing extrahepatic obstruction) by using tests like ultrasound, CT scan or cholangiography, as the management modes are different.
- Important features of restricted intrahepatic cholestasis (cholangitis, primary/secondary malignancy, early primary biliary cirrhosis) are elevated ALP but no increase in serum bilirubin.
- Prolonged widespread cholestasis (extensive cholangitis produced by biliary stones, malignancy causing extrahepatic obstruction, some cases of viral/drug induced liver disease and late primary biliary cirrhosis) produce features as under:
  - Severe jaundice
  - Raised level of ALP
  - Itching due to deposition of bile salts in skin
  - Raised serum cholesterol level
  - Malabsorption of vitamin K and prothrombin deficiency
  - Gradual slow damage of liver cells and increase in level of ALT/AST

- Jaundice caused by malignant obstruction is generally painless and progressive.
- Jaundice associated with biliary stones causes pain and is intermittent.
- In primary biliary cirrhosis early features resemble chronic active hepatitis. Jaundice develops late. Mitochondrial antibodies are seen in majority of patients and serum IgM is usually raised.

Table 6.6. Alternative presentation in post hepatic jaundice

- A patient may present with features (and LFTs) of intrahepatic cholestasis during continuous intake of a drug. History (and dose) of drug intake is very important in such cases.
- A person consults his physician after noting weight loss, consistent pale colour of his stools and deepening yellow colour of his eyes. Liver is enlarged and palpable.
  - Painless deep jaundice with weight loss could be caused by some malignancy (carcinoma head of pancreas or lymph nodes blocking common bile duct at porta hepatis). Jaundice with occult blood in stools may mean carcinoma at some point along bile passage. Radiology and ultrasound could be used to know the cause of obstruction. In case of carcinoma head of pancreas patient may complain of pain radiating to the back. Also liver, gall bladder will be palpable.
- Patient may come with history of non-specific complaint like anorexia, weight loss and anemia. Liver is palpable as firm/hard with irregular mass/masses. LFTs can be variable. The only finding may be increased level of alkaline phosphatase. With extensive multiple secondaries biochemical tests may Indicate both cholestasis and hepatocellular damage. Every effort should be made to look for the primary tumor.

with unexplained pruritis and/or cholestatic pattern of LFTs (marked increase of γ-GT and ALP; bilirubin may also be increased and is useful for knowing prognosis). Circulating IgG (mitochondrial antibody) is detected in more than 90% patients of the disease. Ultrasound will show patency of bile ducts. Liver biopsy is often needed for confirmation of diagnosis.

With progress of the disease the LFT pattern may become as that of hepatitis (as liver cells necrosis occurs due to stagnant bile salts), with increase in levels of transaminases. Finally the chronic cirrhotic pattern develops. The levels of transaminases decrease with decrease of albumin and coagulation factors and increase of ammonia.

Secondary biliary cirrhosis may complicate cases of stones in common bile duct, carcinoma head of pancreas and sometimes hepatitis and sepsis.

One should look for a mass lesion along the course of biliary tree and for stones in common bile duct. Changing profile of LFTs may be as described for primary biliary cirrhosis.

In primary sclerosing cholangitis (more common in men under the age of 45 and often associated with inflammatory bowel disease), there are no antimitochondrial antibodies. The disease, however, shows a characteristic cholangiogram.

To improve fat absorption in all these cases urodeoxy cholic acid is used and dietary fat consists of medium chain triglycerides. Supplements of vitamins A and K, some hydroxylated metabolite of D_3 and Zn are required.

Chronic passive congestion of liver

In congestive heart failure back pressure from right side of heart dilates hepatic sinusoids causing some damage to liver cells. There will be mild rise in aminotransferases and simultaneous increase in serum bilirubin and ALP, in more severe cases. Similar pattern is also seen in infectious mononucleosis in which increase of bilirubin is more marked.

THE GASTROINTESTINAL TRACT

This system is concerned with functions of digestion and absorption of food. Stomach produces gastric juice in which pepsin causes digestion of proteins in acidic medium due to presence of HCl. There is also secretion of intrinsic factor (a glycoprotein) which helps absorption of B_{12} in ileum. Presence of HCl is also important for availability of food iron. Secretion of gastric juice is under nervous (via vagus) and hormonal (gastrin) controls. In gastric disorders, gastric juice analysis has a limited role since procedures like gastroscopy, radiological examination and gastric cytology are more commonly used for diagnosis.

Pancreas has digestive functions as it produces alkaline pancreatic juice containing HCO_3^-, and enzymes for digestion of carbohydrate (amylase), fat (lipase), protein (chymotrypsin, trypsin, elastase, carboxypeptidase) and other nutrients. Bile salts are required for both digestion and absorption of fat. Alkaline reaction of duodenal contents (site of activity of pancreatic juice) is important for pancreatic digestion. In Zollinger Ellison syndrome entry of excessive gastric acid from stomach interferes with pancreatic digestion to produce malabsorption. Pancreas also contains endocrine cells, as large number of microscopic islets, lying between the acinar tissue. Cells secreting insulin, glucagon, somatostatin and gastrin are present in this tissue. Tumors of these cells can produce clinical syndromes. Zollinger Ellison syndrome is produced by a tumor (gastrinoma) of G-cells of endocrine pancreas, duodenum or gastric mucosa (Chapter 16).

Most of nutrient absorption takes place in duodenum and jejunum except that bile salts and B_{12} are absorbed in terminal Ileum. Intestinal malabsorption is discussed in chapter 11. Effects of excessive loss of intestinal fluid (vomiting, diarrhea, loss from fistulae) can also cause water and electrolyte disorders. These are considered in chapter 3. Gut resections produce short gut syndromes. Dysfunction depends upon the segment of the gut and the length resected. Dysfunction is less when resection is done in the region of midgut than in the proximal part or in ileum. The proximal part has an important role in both digestive and absorptive functions. Rapid entry of food into small gut from stomach in gastrojejunostomies produces alimentary hypoglycemia (Chapter 7). In ileal resection problems result from malabsorption of B_{12} and bile salts (Chapter 11).

In gut resections, immediate post operative

problems are loss of fluid and minerals. Their accurate replacement is important. Parenteral nutrition is also needed. As the patient improves enteral nutrition is gradually introduced. Presence of nutrients in the gut promotes adaptive changes, whereby, the handicap of reduced length of gut may be overcome. These changes result from pancreatic and biliary secretions as well as the gut hormones. If resection has been very extensive, permanent parenteral nutrition may be required (Chapter 11).

Diagnosis of gastric pathologies

In establishing diagnosis of gastric disorders, investigative procedure like gastroscopy, radiological examination and gastric cytology are commonly used. Gastric juice analysis, for the same purpose, is done much less frequently. In gastric analysis, there are no well defined normal ranges and only extreme changes could be helpful in diagnosis of disease. Some indications of gastric analysis are: i) to know if patient can secrete gastric juice, in suspected cases of pernicious anemia or ulcerative lesions of stomach; ii) if there are symptoms of duodenal ulcer/marginal ulcer but the ulcer does not show up on x-ray examination; iii) in diagnosis of Zollinger Ellison syndrome; iv) to determine completeness of vagotomy; v) in differential diagnosis of duodenal ulcer.

Gastric function assessment

Assessment of H^+ secretion has a role in diagnosis of gastric disorders. For this purpose a Levine tube (or some other similar tube) is passed through the nose for aspiration of gastric contents over a period of time. Continuous gastric aspiration is preferred, as intermittent suction leads to collection of reduced volume of gastric juice. To a measured portion of total volume, N/10 sodium hydroxide is added to titrate to a pH of 7.0 to 7.4. The end point may be determined with the help of a pH meter or phenol red (colour change from yellow to red). Volume of sodium hydroxide used per litre of gastric juice, gives titratable acidity (mEq/L). Hydrogen ion secretion is expressed as acid output/h. From titratable acidity and the total volume collected

over 1h, hydrogen ion secretion/h, is calculated as follows:

Acid output/h (mEq) = volume of sample × titratable acidity/1000.

Acid output/h is studied first under basal conditions (intubation is done after 12h overnight fast and 8h water deprivation and gastric juice collected by continuous aspiration to collect four 15 min samples for titration). All this is done after aspiration of residual gastric juice in the beginning.

Next, an injection of synthetic pentagastrin (peptavalon) is followed by continuous aspiration of stimulated gastric juice, collected in four 15 min samples, over 1h. In this way maximum acid output is obtained. Anacidity is defined as failure of pH to fall below 6.0 or 7.0 following the stimulation test.

Table 6.7 shows gastric acid secretion in some diseases.

The insulin hypoglycemia test

This test is done to judge completeness of vagotomy in a patient of duodenal ulcer. In the test, after the basal samples have been collected (for 2h), intravenous insulin is given to lower blood glucose to about 50 mg/dL within 30 minutes after the injection. This is followed by collection of samples for next 2h. Vagotomy is said to be complete if the larger/h acid output in the basal 2h samples is more than the larger/h acid output in the post-insulin samples. Alternatively, sham feeding has been used

Table 6.7. Gastric acid secretion in certain conditions

	Acid output (mEq/h)	
	Basal	Stimulated
Normals	0-5	5-20
Achlorhydria	0	0
Gastric cancer	0-5	0-10
Gastric Ulcer	0-5	0.2-15
Duodenal ulcer	0-5	5-30
Zollinger Ellison syndrome	5-70	10-100

- There is no pathognomic range for any disorder except that secretion is very high in Zollinger Ellison syndrome.
- A maximal acid secretion of >40 mEq/h is found in 40% of males with duodenal ulcer but rarely in normals.
- In addition to marked hypersecretion in ZE syndrome, high ratio of maximal to basal acid out put. See Appexdix B.

for stimulation of gastric acid secretion. This is a safer procedure than insulin administration. For sham feeding, the patient chews a sandwitch and then spits out.

Recently, a non-invasive test has been used to assess completeness of vagotomy. The test depends upon production of alkaline tide after food intake, leading to decrease in the urine acid output (increase in pH of urine in 2h or 3h post prandial samples). In post vagotomy cases no increase occurs, in cases of successful complete vagotomy.

Zollinger Ellison syndrome

In this disorder of G-cell adenoma, there is excessive secretion of gastric acid. The disorder may present as peptic ulcer disease resistant to histamine H_2 receptor antagonist therapy or as a case of recurrent ulcer formation. In some cases there is steatorrhea, caused by excessive acid entering duodenum and interfering with the activity of pancreatic lipase.

In this disease serum gastrin levels are increased alongwith hypersecretion of gastric acid. Gastrin levels are increased as HCl is not able to inhibit gastrin secretion. Gastrin secretion is also increased in certain other conditions (Table 6.8). Increased gastrin level and increased secretion of gastric acid

Table 6.8. Disorders with increased gastrin secretion

- G-Cell hypersecretion unresponsive or hyporesponsive to negative feed back.
  - Zollinger Ellison syndrome
  - Duodenal ulcer
- Parietal cells not responsive to gastrin stimulation.
  - Pernicious anemia
  - Atrophic gastritis
  - Gastric carcinoma
  - Gastric ulcer disease
  - Following gastrectomy
  - Omeprazole therapy
- Compensatory gastrin hypersecretion due to loss of some other gastric acid stimulant.
  - Vagotomy
  - H_2 - blocker therapy (long term)

- In Zollinger Ellison syndrome gastrin secretion is not reduced by I/V secretin injection (secretion is reduced in other conditions), or following intragastric acid instillation.

is also found in duodenal ulcer. In this condition, however, gastrin levels are higher than normals in the postprandial state and not in the fasting state.

In duodenal ulcer (male preponderance, acid secretion high, pain relieved by food, vomiting uncommon) as well and in gastric ulcer (acid secretion low or normal, pain after meals, vomiting common), infection with Helicobacter pylori plays an important role in ulcer formation. This infection reduces mucosal resistance, to damage by HCl and also gastric acid secretion is increased via gastrin secretion stimulation. While doing biopsy, for histological demonstration of H. pylori, the biopsy is also subjected to demonstrate ability of the organism to produce ammonia from urea. Biopsy is placed in urea solution and release of ammonia assessed. Radioactive urea breath test may also be done.

In case of Zollinger Ellison syndrome the adenoma is localized by CT, angiography or by estimation of gastrin levels in samples of blood collected from different tributaries of portal vein (during operation).

Zollinger- Ellison syndrome is best treated by resecting the tumor, if it can be localized, otherwise it needs continuous therapy with omeprazole (inhibitor of proton pump).

Treatment of gastric/duodenal ulcers consists of stopping smoking, treatment of Helicobacter pylori infection, and reducing acid secretion by histamine H_2- receptor antagonists (famotidine) or omeprazole. The latter drug promotes more rapid healing than the former.

PANCREATIC DISORDERS

Important disorders of pancreatic exocrine functions are, acute pancreatitis, chronic pancreatitis, pancreatic carcinoma and cystic fibrosis. About 20% of patients of chronic pancreatitis and about 10% of patients of cystic fibrosis may develop diabetes mellitus due to damage to the endocrine portion of pancreas. Cystic fibrosis is discussed in Chapter 11.

Acute pancreatitis

There is acute pancreatic inflammation and escape of pancreatic enzymes from acinar cells into the surrounding tissue. A contact between lysosomal and digestive enzymes in acinar cells might trigger the whole process. Two important predisposing conditions are biliary disease and alcoholism. Other risk factors are mumps, hyperlipidemia, hypercalcemia, drugs (thiazides, corticosteroids, azathioprine and others) and abdominal trauma. Recognition of presence of these factors, through history or laboratory help is often helpful in diagnosis of acute pancreatitis.

There is sudden onset of abdominal pain with some radiation), restlessness, shock, ileus and minimal abdominal findings (unimpressive guarding and tenderness). Serum amylase and lipase levels, studied together, have a high sensitivity and specificity for diagnosis of acute pancreatitis. Study of immunoreactive trypsin is useful to rule out the disorder (see under diagnosis of acute pancreatitis). CT-scan is also useful to visualize inflammed pancreas and also cystic fluid collections.

Diagnosis of acute pancreatitis

The level of serum amylase rises rapidly in an acute attack on first day and then comes down rapidly due to renal excretion of the enzyme. The peak level may be more than 4 times the upper reference limit and the level is normalized in 2 to 4 days, in mild edematous form of the disease. In cases of continued necrosis and in pseudocyst formation, the high levels continue beyond 2 to 4 days. In about 20 % of the cases serum amylase levels may remain in the normal range or remain near normal, especially in lipemic patients due to raised TAG and presence of an inhibitor in serum.

Urinary clearance of amylase is also studied for diagnosis. Normal C_{am}/C_{cr} ratio varies between 1% to 4%. In acute pancreatitis this ratio rises between 7% to 15% (Appendix B). However, in about one third of patients the ratio remains normal and the elevated ratio may also be found in patients of burns, ketoacidosis, renal insufficiency, heart disease and duodenal perforation.

Lipase is considered superior to amylase in diagnosis of acute pancreatitis as it shows greater increase and may remain elevated for upto 14 days after amylase returns to normal. According to one scheme about interpretation of serum amylase and lipase levels: Amylase >2 times the upper normal limit (UNL) and lipase >5 times UNL, means acute pancreatitis: Amylase >2 times UNL but lipase <5 times UNL may be because of renal insufficiency (creatinine >2 times UNL) or late acute pancreatitis/some other abdominal disorder (creatinine <2 times UNL).

Normal level of immunoreactive trypsin (high sensitivity, low specificity for acute pancreatitis) rules out acute pancreatitis but high levels do not confirm the disorder. Elastase-1 has also been found to have high sensitivity and specificity for acute pancreatitis. Increase of the enzyme was also found to be the most useful marker for chronic pancreatitis during painful relapse and cyst formation. Once a good method of estimation is available for this enzyme, it may become an important marker for pancreatic disorders.

Serum amylase levels, also increase (although increase is much less than in acute pancreatitis) in a number of other abdominal emergencies like perforated peptic ulcer (history of ulcer, sudden onset of pain, epigastric tenderness and rigidity, X-ray in erect posture shows gas under diaphragm), biliary colic (right sided upper abdominal pain, gradual in onset with less prostration than acute pancreatitis, tenderness of right upper abdomen, X-ray may show gall stones), acute intestinal obstruction (intermittent intestinal colic, abdominal distension with loud peristalsis followed by ileus and no shock. X-ray examination shows multiple fluid levels) and acute mesenteric thrombosis (pain of gradual onset, elderly person, ileus, bleeding per rectum). Narcotic administration also increases serum amylase level.

Because of upper abdominal pain acute pancreatitis may sometimes require differentiation from myocardial infarction and rarely from dissecting aneurysm of aorta (pain in back and midline, impaired femoral pulsation, shock, restlessness and hematuria).

Management of acute panacreatitis is basically conservative. It consists of relief of pain (not with morphine since it produces spasm of sphincter of oddi), nasogastric aspiration (because of ileus), control of shock, antibiotics (to avoid pancreatic infection), and intravenous calcium gluconate (in case of hypocalcemia). Also read Case history 6.6 and objective type questions.

Chronic pancreatitis

It is a different disease than acute pancreatitis as acute pancreatitis rarely leads to chronic pancreatitis. There is gradual blockade of pancreatic ductal tissue leading to loss of pancreatic tissue (replaced by fibrosis). Etiological factors are alcohol, cholelithiasis (less common), malnutrition and genetic. It is common in middle aged men. There are recurrent attacks of pain (which begins gradually and persists for days) at intervals of weeks or months. There is also steatorrhea, and weight loss. In about 20% patients, diabetes develops. Diagnosis is discussed in Chapter 11.

Amylase isoenzymes

P-type (pancreatic) and S-type (salivary) amylase levels and levels of different isoenzymes of P-type have been used in differentiation of acute pancreatitis from other intrabdominal conditions causing hyperamylasemia, in diagnosis of pancreatic pseudocyst and in other diagnostic problems related to pancreatic diseases. Clinical utility of these studies, however, is limited at present.

Macroamylasemia

It is a benign, acquired state, more common in males above 50 years. Cause is not known. Some paraproteins bind amylase and when present in increased concentration, may cause macroamylasemia. Diagnosis is suspected, in a person, showing high serum amylase levels and C_{am}/C_{cr} ratio less than 1.0%. Serum lipase remains normal. Recognition of this condition is important since it may cause confusion in diagnosis of acute pancreatitis.

About estimations of lipase and amylase

Amylase is one of the most stable enzymes. It is stable for one week at room temperature and for about 6 months when refrigerated. Amylase is a calcium containing enzyme and use of oxalate or citrate can interfere in the estimation. Heparin does not interfere. Hemolysis does not interfere in amylase estimation. One important problem in amylase estimation is that a very large number of methods, not yielding very similar results, are available and different laboratories use different methods. Thus correlation of results from different laboratories becomes difficult.

In acute pancreatitis, lipase rises with amylase but raised lipase levels last longer (for 7 to 10 days). Presence of increased levels for more than 15 days means poor prognosis or development of pancreatic cyst. Lipase is also quite stable like amylase. There is no interference from bilirubin, lipemia or hemolysis, in turbidometric methods. Serum lipase is inhibited by proteins, bile acids and phospholipids but inhibition is reversed by co-lipase. As serum of patient (acute pancreatitis) is deficient in co-lipase, the same must be added to the reagent pack. Calcium is needed for lipase activity but high serum calcium interferes.

PANCREATIC CARCINOMA

A number of tests have been used for diagnosis of pancreatic carcinoma. These include, abdominal ultrasound, CT, ERCP (endoscopic retrograde cholangiopancreatography), tumor markers galactosyltransferase isoenzyme II, CEA, α-fetoprotein, CA 19-9 and pancreatic oncofetal antigen and even the pancreatic function tests. However, no single test has both adequate sensitivity and specificity. Pancreatic carcinoma is usually diagnosed late when metastases have occurred. LFTs may be abnormal in cancer head of pancreas but remain normal in cancers of body or tail.

CASE HISTORY: 6.1

A 30 year old male patient presented with history of anorexia and nausea (for last 5 days). He also noted darkening of the colour of his urine. There was slight tenderness in upper right quadrant, on examination. Bilirubin level was 2.5 mg%. There was no history of alcohol or drug intake. There was no jaundice.

➤ Which liver function tests will have good sensitivity at this stage?

➤ Name the LFTs which reveal extent of hepatocytes involved, the extent of liver cell necrosis and the cholestatic component.

➤ What is importance of serological tests in this case?

➤ What is difference in investigations required in follow up of HAV and HBV cases?

➤ Mention some other presentations of viral hepatitis.

• Before clinical jaundice appears bilirubin starts

appearing in urine and urine should be tested for bilirubin. At early stage, extensive cholestasis has not occurred. Thus sufficient bilirubin is passing into intestine to change into urobilinogen. From this, the fraction absorbed into circulation is mostly excreted in urine as liver fails to resecrete it into bile. Increased excretion of urobilinogen in urine is also a useful test at this stage. Peak levels of ALT/AST also occur early in acute phase. Thus study of these enzymes will be the most sensitive indicator of involvement of hepatocytes in this patient.

- The extent of involvement of liver cells is indicated by ALT/AST levels. A high AST/ALT ratio means that greater number of liver cells will undergo necrosis. Levels of ALP and conjugated bilirubin in serum relate to cholestasis.
- These tests differentiate toxic hepatitis from viral hepatitis and also the nature of virus in case of the latter etiology.
- In HAV and HAE cases, chronic liver disease does not follow acute viral hepatitis. Follow up should be done by urine examination for bilirubin and by studying ALT/AST in serum or only AST. In HBV cases AST/ALT levels should be studied along with serology to follow the case for development of chronic hepatitis. In these cases very long follow up may be required.
- A patient of viral hepatitis commonly presents with jaundice, and features like fatigue and anorexia. A substantial increase in levels of transaminases helps to establish the diagnosis.

5 to 10% cases of HBV infection present with prodromal features like arthralgia, rash and less commonly, proteinuria or hematuria (D/D from SLE, rheumatoid arthritis). Increase of aminotransferases and serological findings help diagnosis.

The patients who remain non-icteric (a substantial number) are diagnosed because of high level of clinical suspicion, increase of aminotransferases and increase of conjugated bilirubin.

A combination of features like shrinking liver size, rapidly rising bilirubin, and marked increase in PT along with signs of confusion, and disorientation indicates fulminant hepatitis. This condition is rare and occurs in hepatitis-B (especially if complicated by presence of hepatitis D) and hepatitis E. In rare cases it may occur in hepatitis A in old individuals.

Also see Case history 6.4.

CASE HISTORY: 6.2

A 44 year old malnourished male presented with history of dull central abdominal pain, weakness and weight loss. Lately, there was anorexia, gradual swelling of abdomen. On examination liver was palpable and firm. Fluid in the peritoneal cavity was demonstrated by shifting dullness. Results of some investigations were as under:

AST 280 U/L, ALT 122 U/L, ALP 320 U/L, bilirubin 10 mg/dL and albumin 2.2 g/dL.

From history, clinical examination and results of biochemical tests, the likely diagnosis is chronic liver disease with cirrhosis (indicated by ascites). Increase of ALT and AST indicates that the disease is active. Raised levels of bilirubin and ALP are due to cholestasis. Reduced liver cell reserve is indicated by reduced level of serum albumin. In such cases a likely intestinal hemorrhage (due to varices) is partly responsible for high bilirubin levels. Hepatic decompensation is further promoted by drugs, hypotension and sepsis. These factors can cause both hepatocyte damage as well as cholestasis.

Alcoholism is a common cause of cirrhosis, and in these cases increase of γ-GT is out of proportion to that of ALP. Chronic alcohol abuse may cause fatty liver (enlarged liver, some increase in levels of ALT/AST but marked increase in γ- GT, while bilirubin level may be in the normal reference range) or cirrhosis. Heavy drinking may cause alcoholic hepatitis. Also see Tables 6.3, 6.4.

Serum albumin level and prothrombin time are useful in following a case of cirrhosis and if encephalopathy develops, serum ammonia levels correlate with progress of the condition. Serum glutamine levels have also been used for this purpose.

Cirrhosis is treated with diuretics and low dietary sodium and infusion of sodium free albumin. Too rapid diuresis may cause encephalopathy and electrolyte disturbances. In patients with alcoholic etiology, abstaining from alcohol is very essential. In case of encephalopathy, protein restriction, and avoiding toxins from gut (gut sterilization, use of laxatives and lactulose) help. Factors which further produce hepatic damage (infection, bleeding from varices and hepatotoxic drugs) should be avoided/managed effectively.

CASE HISTORY: 6.3

A 45 year old obese female presented with colicky pain in upper quadrant of abdomen and jaundice of 2 days duration. There was history of previous several attacks of upper quadrant pain with fever and shivering. She had also noted yellowish colour of her stools and her urine turning dark in colour. Examination revealed that liver was enlarged and tender. Gall bladder was also palpable.

Investigations revealed : ALT 70 U/L, AST 60 U/L, ALP 900 U/L, bilirubin 4.2 mg/dL, and albumin 4.2 g/dL.

Urine was negative for urobilinogen and strongly positive for bile pigment. X-ray showed multiple stones in gall bladder and a stone in the common bile duct area.

Attacks of pain in the upper quadrant with fever and shivering (in the previous history) indicate cholecystitis due to stones in the gall bladder. As one of the stone got impacted in common bile duct, she got the attack of colicky pain of her present illness. Her LFTs are explained by obstruction in common bile duct and also by likely ascending cholangitis.

In the present case there is no difficulty in diagnosis of cause of cholestasis. Cases of secondaries in liver, carcinoma head of pancreas and enlarged glands in the region of porta hepatis can also present with cholestatic jaundice. Excessive intake of some drugs can also cause intrahepatic cholestasis. Brief common presentations in some such cases are given in Table 6.6.

In post hepatic jaundice the important changes are in bilirubin and alkaline phosphatase levels (cholestasis leading to enzyme induction). Alkaline phosphatase level generally rises higher than twice the upper limit of the normal range. If obstruction is complete bilirubin and alkaline phosphatase rise in a parallel manner. In incomplete obstruction rise of alkaline phosphatase is more than that of serum bilirubin. In post hepatic jaundice secondary hepatic cell damage occurs and causes modest increase in level of the transaminases.

In the present case, cholestasis has not yet been able to bring much liver cell dysfunction as is evident from the levels of transaminases and serum albumin.

Gall bladder stones are composed of calcium bilirubinate or cholesterol. Chronic hemolytic disorders (sickle cell anemia) increase incidence of calcium bilirubinate stones. Conjugated bile salts, lecithin and cholesterol are required in balancéd amounts in bile to keep cholesterol in soluble form in bile. Any imbalance can cause formation of cholesterol stones. Incidence is increased in diabetes mellitus and diseases of terminal ileum (impaired bile salt absorption). Cholelithiasis is frequently an asymptomatic discovery during investigations of an unrelated disease. Such stones need not be removed unless person is diabetic. Symptomatic stones should be removed alongwith infected gallbladder. A small stone in common bile duct may pass into duodenum during retrograde cholangiography. Chenodeoxycholic acid is also used orally for dissolution of cholesterol stones.

CASE HISTORY: 6.4

A 30 year old male presented with a mild attack of hepatitis with mild hepatomegaly. There was moderate increase in bilirubin and aminotransferases. A year earlier, he had a similar but more severe attack and moderate increase of AST was seen for more than 4 months after which the patient did not report for follow up.

After an acute attack of viral hepatitis the disease may follow one of the three courses. In majority of cases the hepatic damage resolves. In a few cases it may progress to acute hepatic failure. In certain cases (cases of HBV and HCV infections) chronic hepatitis may result.

In most of the cases that resolve, the process occurs quite smoothly. In some cases mild clinical features (without biochemical evidence) continue for 2 to 3 months, in the form of post hepatic syndrome. In some other cases the cholestatic profile of LFTs, with or without pruritis, continues for a long time (as cholestatic viral hepatitis) after the acute disease is over. In a few case the acute attack of viral hepatitis is followed by attacks of relapsing hepatitis. More commonly, only, there are biochemical relaspses (increase in ALT/AST activity). In all these cases prognosis after an acute viral hepatitis is not altered.

All the above referred problems during resolving stage of viral hepatitis are over by about 6 months. Patient is said to have passed into chronic hepatitis if clinical or biochemical or both types of features continue even after a period of 6 months. Accordingly, the present patient is suffering from chronic hepatitis. It could be case of chronic persistent hepatitis or chronic active hepatitis. In the former, there are no clinical features except slight hepatomegaly in some cases. Bilirubin is normal or slightly raised but there is slight but persistent increase in the levels of transaminases. Prognosis in this case is generally, good. Chronic active hepatitis, on the other hand, generally, leads to cirrhosis. Diagnosis generally needs biopsy study. In active chronic hepatitis cases, it is important to define etiology of the disease, viral or autoimmune. The autoimmune type disorder occurs in remissions and relapses and in each relapse LFT profile is just as in an attack of viral hepatitis. Special features are increase of γ-globulin and presence of smooth muscle and anti-nuclear antibodies. In post viral type there may be very few clinical features. Hepatomegaly is most common. The LFT profile is as in a mild attack of viral hepatitis with moderate increase in bilirubin and AST and minor increase in ALP. Hyperglobulinemia is not seen. Serology may help diagnosis (Table 6.2). In both types hypoalbuminemia and decrease of coagulation proteins occurs when disease is in an advanced stage.

CASE HISTORY: 6.5

A 45 year old woman presented with jaundice. She had history of severe pruritis and fatigue for the previous about one year. Levels of γ-GT and ALP were more than four times the upper limits of the reference ranges while ALT level was only moderately increased. Serum total protein concentration was 8.6 g/dL with albumin concentration of 2.4 g/dL.

In view of high levels of ALP with jaundice the patient appears to have cholestatic jaundice. γ-GT is a marker anzyme for liver disease but increased levels can be caused by some drugs metabolized in liver. History of severe pruritis and high levels of serum globulin (also age and sex of the patient) make primary biliary cirrhosis, a likely diagnosis. Confirmation of diagnosis can come from demonstration of anti-mitochondrial antibodies (present in 95% of cases) or the liver biopsy study. Ultrasound and ERCP will fail to demonstrate dilatation of biliary ducts.

Primary biliary cirrhosis is an autoimmune disease which involves interlobular bile ducts and the granulomatous inflammation spreads from portal tracts to involve liver parenchyma, ultimately leading to cirrhosis and hepatic failure. It is a progressive disease starting with pruritis, (produced by retained bile salts) and jaundice and causing steatorrhea, xanthomatous neuropathy, osteomalacia and portal hypertension, as it progresses. Deficiencies of vitamins A, K and D are produced along with deficiency of calcium. Treatment is unsatisfactory as the disease does not respond to corticosteroids and only symptomatic treatment is possible.

CASE HISTORY: 6.6

A 45 year old man was admitted with severe pain in upper part of abdomen, radiating through back to right iliac fossa. It started following a heavy meal, about 16h before admission. Patient also had repeated vomiting and was not retaining any thing. Except slight tenderness there was no other helpful finding on abdominal examination. Patient was in a state of moderate shock. Serum amylase level was more than 4000 U/L.

Patient was diagnosed to be suffering from acute pancreatitis because of very high level of serum amylase and his clinical picture. On investigation, patient was also found to have mild increase of serum creatinine and reduced levels of calcium and albumin. Blood glucose level was moderately raised.

➤ How to explain the above mentioned biochemical findings of the patient?

• Hypoalbuminemia is explained due to loss of protein rich exudate into peritoneal cavity. Hypocalcemia is explained because of formation of calcium soaps of fatty acids released from fat around inflammed pancreas (by the action of activated lipase), and because of reduced level of serum albumin. Hyperglycemia may be due to the action of glucagon released from inflamed pancreas. Slight increase of serum creatinine is due to renal hypoperfusion because of shock.

An attack of acute pancretitis is considered serious if serum calcium falls below 8.0 mg/dL, serum albumin below 3.0 g/dL and serum creatinine rises above 2 mg/dL.

OBJECTIVE TYPE QUESTIONS

Pick out the wrong statement.

1. Hepatic drug toxicity

i) Acetaminophen produces dose related hepatic toxicity.

ii) Blood level of 300 mg/dL, 4h after acetaminophen ingestion may indicate severe liver damage.

iii) Acetaminophen produces liver cell necrosis.

iv) Halothane produces idiosyncratic hepatic injury, producing specific clinical picture like that of infective hepatitis.

v) Chlorpromazine produces cholestasis with minimal hepatocellular damage.

vi) In idiosyncratic hepatic damage the latent period after drug administration is short.

2. In viral hepatitis

i) A low grade fever is more common in acute hepatitis A and E than hepatitis B and C.

ii) Hepatitis B may start with serum sickness like syndrome.

iii) Very few cases remain unicteric in viral hepatitis.

iv) ALP is normal or there is mild increase.

v) Decrease of albumin is uncommon.

vi) Prolonged PT indicates poor prognosis.

vii) Dark urine and clay colored stools may be noted 1 to 5 days before onset of jaundice.

3. Viral hepatitis (differential diagnosis)

i) History of previous episodes may indicate that the patient has chronic hepatitis.

ii) It may resemble alcoholic hepatitis.

iii) It may resemble toxic hepatitis, following a drug intake.

iv) Viral hepatitis may require differential diagnosis from acute cholecystitis/common bile duct stone.

v) Because of rise of aminotransferases, diagnosis of viral hepatitis in preicteric stage is quite easy.

vi) Passive hepatic congestion due to right ventricular failure may also give rise to clinical picture like that of viral hepatitis.

4. Fulminant hepatic failure

i) There may be severe hyponatremia, hypoglycemia and hypocalcemia.

ii) Failure of formation of glucose from lactate (gluconeogenesis) may produce metabolic acidosis.

iii) Because of ensuing renal failure, blood urea level is increased.

iv) PT is commonly prolonged.
v) Secondary aldosteronism (failure of aldosterone metabolism in liver) may produce hypokalemia and alkalosis.
vi) Certain accumulating toxins may stimulate respiration to produce respiratory alkalosis.

5. Macrovesicular hepatic steatosis (fatty liver)

i) It occurs in alcoholism, diabetes mellitus, protein energy malnutrition and obesity.
ii) Liver may be firm, non-tender and enlarged.
iii) There is minimal hepatic dysfunction.
iv) AST/ALT ratio is greater than 2.
v) Commonly diagnosed by ultrasound, CT or MRI.
vi) In case of uncertainity needle biopsy may help.

6. Reye's syndrome

i) It occurs in children and is associated with hepatic microvesicular steatosis with encephalopathy.
ii) Onset usually follows upper respiratory tract infection.
iii) Cause may be a viral infection.
iv) Exposure to certain drugs especially salicylates may also produce a similar condition.
v) There is severe jaundice.

7. Hepatorenal syndrome

i) It is a serious complication in a patient of cirrhosis or ascites.
ii) There is systemic hypotension, oliguria and worsening azotemia.
iii) It may be precipitated by severe gastrointestinal bleeding, sepsis, paracentesis or vigorous diuresis.
iv) There is greater Na^+ conservation than prerenal azotemia (urine Na^+ less than 5 mmol/L).
v) Vasodilator therapy is quite effective.

8. Chronic hepatitis

i) Does not occur in HAV or HEV infections.
ii) Occurs in HBV, HDV superimposed on HBV and HCV infections.
iii) Chances of chronic hepatitis B following an acute hepatitis B episode greatly decrease with age.
iv) Severity depends upon the type of virus.
v) In contrast to autoimmune hepatitis, in chronic viral hepatitis, hyperglobulinemia and detectable circulating autoantibodies are not seen.

9. Chronic hepatitis

i) The disease may resemble an attack of acute viral hepatitis.
ii) In most cases chronic HBV infection is mild and preceded by a severe acute infection.
iii) Wilson's disease may present as chronic hepatitis, in young adults to be followed by neurological manifestation.
iv) Postnecrotic or cryptogenic cirrhosis and primary biliary cirrhosis may present like chronic hepatitis.
v) It may not be a easy to distinguish between autoimmune and viral cases of chronic hepatitis.
vi) Autoimmune chronic hepatitis may present with many extrahepatic features and circulating autoantibodies as in SLE and rheumatoid arthritis.

10. Hepatic encephalopathy (triggers)

i) Increased dietary protein.
ii) Gastrointestinal bleeding.
iii) Electrolyte disturbances especially metabolic acidosis.
iv) Hypoxia.
v) Use of central nervous system depressants.

11. Hepatic encephalopathy (management, monitoring)

i) Look for any other factor which could impair central nervous system functioning and treat.
ii) Look for any trigger and treat.
iii) Give protein in restricted amount.
iv) Animal protein is better than vegetable protein.
v) Use of lactulose and some broad spectrum antibiotic to reduce formation and entry of ammonia from intestine.
vi) Monitor serum electrolytes and renal function.
vii) Monitor blood glucose and ammonia.

12. Wilson's disease

i) Disease may present in teenage with hepatitis, and in many cases with a renal tubular defect and hemolysis.
ii) Disease may present in an adult with cirrhosis and basal ganglia disturbances.
iii) Some patients of this rare disease may present with fulminant hepatitis.
iv) In this disease there is impaired excretion of copper.
v) Reduced plasma ceruloplasmin level is diagnostic of the condition.

13. α_1-Antitrypsin deficiency

i) In adults, most commonly the disorder results in asymptomatic cirrhosis which may lead to development of hepato-cellular carcinoma.

ii) 15 to 20% of chronic liver disorders (neonatal hepatitis, progressive cirrhosis) in infancy may be caused by α_1-antitrypsin deficiency.

iii) Patients are also prone to develop emphysema in adult life.

iv) Ordinary serum electrophoresis is of no use in diagnosis of the disease.

v) The disease is diagnosed by measurement of α_1-antitrypsin level in serum.

14. Gall stones

i) Commonly composed of cholesterol or bilirubin and calcium salts.

ii) In bile, lecithin and bile salts keep cholesterol in solution.

iii) These can cause biliary colic and predispose to cholecystitis and acute pancreatitis.

iv) It is best to perform prophylactic cholecystectomy for silent gall stones.

v) Ultrasound is better than oral cholecystography in diagnosis of gall stones.

vi) Radiolabeled N-substituted imino-diacetic acid scans are used in diagnosis of acute and chronic cholecystitis.

vii) Analysis of biliary stones is unimportant in diagnosis or surgical management of gall stones.

15. Acute pancreatitis

i) There is acute pain in the abdomen or back, with nausea, emesis, fever, severe prostration in a predisposed individual.

ii) Abdominal tenderness and guarding is unimpressive and there is paralytic ileus.

iii) Serum amylase and lipase are elevated within 24h in most of the cases and remain elevated for more than a week.

iv) If hypertriglyceridemia is there, amylase may appear spuriously, normal.

16. Acute pancreatitis

i) Prior presence of hypertriglyceridemia in a patient of acute pancreatitis is related to hypocalcemia occuring during the disorder.

ii) Blood pressure <90 mmHg signifies poor prognosis.

iii) Oliguria and increasing BUN and serum creatinine, indicate poor prognosis.

iv) Serum calcium <8.0 mg/dL, and serum albumin <3.2 mg/dL also carry poor prognosis.

v) pO_2 <60 mmHg may promote adult type RDS.

vi) Hemorrhagic peritoneal fluid, if found, means bad prognosis.

17. Pancreatic disorders

i) Serum amylase levels are reliable for diagnosis of acute pancreatitis, if levels are three (or more) times the upper normal limit.

ii) Amylase/creatinine clearance ratio is more reliable than serum amylase level in diagnosis of acute pancreatitis.

iii) Level of P isoenzyme is more useful than total amylase activity in diagnosis of acute pancreatitis.

iv) Normal level of immunoreactive trypsin rules out diagnosis of acute pancreatitis.

v) The triad of pancreatic calcification, steatorrhea and diabetes mellitus establishes diagnosis of chronic pancreatitis.

ANSWERS

1. No.(iv). Variable clinical presentations can be produced.

2. No.(iii). A good number of cases remain unicteric.

3. No.(v). Rise of aminotransferases occurs in most systemic viral infections, it is not specific for viral hepatitis.

4. No.(iii). Serum creatinine is increased. Blood urea level may be low due to impaired synthesis in liver.

5. No.(iv). Ratio is >2 in alcoholic cases and <1 in non-alcoholic cases.

6. No.(v). Jaundice is minimal or absent. The major laboratory features are increased PT, transaminases and ammonia along with hypoglycemia, and metabolic acidosis.

7. No.(v). There is poor response to vasodilatory therapy. In general, there is poor response to any therapy. Some patients respond to infusion of salt free albumin. In hepatorenal syndrome, there is renal vasoconstriction along with systemic vasodilatation. There is no pathological renal damage.

8. No.(iv). Severity of disease is judged from histological features as well as from degree of viral replication.

9. No.(ii). In fact majority cases (especially in adults) of HBV infection are not preceded by an episode of an acute infection.

10. No.(iii). Metabolic alkalosis leads to formation of NH_3 from NH_4^+. The former, more readily, enters central nervous system. Hypokalemia produced by alkalosis further stimulates renal NH_3 production.

11. No.(iv). Vegetable protein is preferred over animal protein.
12. No.(v). Low ceruloplasmin levels are also seen in chronic hepatitis and malnutrition. For diagnosis, presence of low plasma ceruloplasmin along with Kayser-Fleischer ring or low plasma ceruloplasmin along with demonstration of increased copper in liver biopsy sample, should be present.
13. No.(iv). The disease is suggested by absence of α_1 globulin in serum electrophoresis (α_1-antitrypsin forms about 90% of this fraction).
14. No.(iv). Only symptomatic ones should be removed.
15. No.(iii). Serum amylase level returns to normal in 3 to 4 days. Pancreatic lipase and pancreatic iso-amylase remain elevated for 7 to 14 days.
16. No.(i). It has a role in triggering the disease. In pancreatitis, formation of calcium soaps in areas of fat necrosis may produce hypocalcemia.
17. No.(ii). This test has many false positives and false negatives and is no better than serum amylase level for diagnosis of acute pancreatitis.

CHAPTER 7

Diabetes Mellitus and Hypoglycemia

Diabetes mellitus may be primary (occuring denovo) or secondary. Secondary diabetes mellitus or impaired glucose tolerance may occur in pancreatic disease (chronic pancreatitis especially in alcoholics, hemochromatosis, cystic fibrosis), hormonal disorders (acromegaly, Cushing's syndrome, pheochromocytoma), with use of drugs (glucocorticoids, phenytoin, thiazide diuretics), in association with certain genetic syndromes (muscular dystrophies, ataxia telangiectasia, Down's syndrome and others), in stressful conditions (severe burns, myocardial infarction and others) and as less well defined cases (impaired fasting glucose, impaired glucose tolerance).

PRIMARY DIABETES MELLITUS

Diabetes mellitus occurs in two major forms; diabetes mellitus type 1, an autoimmune disorder and type 2, a non-autoimmune disorder (Table 7.1). In both disorders, both genetic as well as environmental factors play their roles. In type 2 diabetes mellitus, family history is commonly noted. If a parent of an individual has the disease, his average life time risk of suffering from the disorder is about 38%. Earlier the onset of the disease in the parent, greater the risk to the children. It has an insidious onset and gradually develops over years (Table 7.2). For development of overt disease both reduced tissue sensitivity to insulin and a B-cell defect in secretion

of insulin are required (Table 7.3). Obesity is the major environmental factor required in development of this disorder.

Table 7.1. Classification of primary diabetes mellitus

DIABETES MELLITUS TYPE 1 (autoimmune disorder)

Propensity to DKA (IDDM):

- Common type 1 disorder, patient non-obese with age less than 40 years.

Resistant to DKA (NIDDM):

- Type 1 disorder in non-obese but at an older age, with slow autoimmune damage.

DIABETES MELLITUS TYPE 2 (non-autoimmune disorder)

Resistant to DKA (NIDDM):

- Common type 2 disorder, in obese with age more than 50 years

Propensity to DKA (IDDM):

- A conventional type 2 case becomes vulnerable to stress (to produce DKA) due to decrease of insulin reserve.

MODY (maturity onset diabetes of the young):

- Mild hyperglycemia without ketosis
- Transmitted as autosomal dominant trait.

- Genetic factors are more important in development of diabetes type 2 than diabetes type 1. However, the genes involved (may be a large number) are not known. Genetic factors are better characterized in diabetes type 1 and relate to the genes that control the immune response. And there is enough evidence that diabetes type 1 is an autoimmune disease of B-cells. However, the environmental factors play a more dominant role and thus there is no family history.

Table 7.2. Some important differences between diabetes mellitus type 1 and 2

Type 1	Type 2
There is autommune destruction of B-cells and very little insulin is produced.	Pathogenesis is less well understood. Insulin levels are generally not reduced (see Table 7.3)
Family history not always available.	Family history commonly available.
There is often rapid onset and age of onset is less than 40 years.	Onset is insidious and age of onset is often more than 50 years.
Patient is normal weight or wasted.	Patient is often obese.
Episodes of acute decompensation in the form of diabetic ketoacidosis occur.	Acute decompensation occurs In the form of hyperosmolar coma.
Presence of certain autoantibodies and possiblity of other autoimmune diseases.	No autoantibodies and also relation to no other autoimmune disease.
Insulin levels low to absent and glucagon levels high but suppressible by insulin.	Insulin levels normal to high and glucagon levels high but not easily suppressed.
Complications like diabetic retinopathy, nephropathy and neuropathy in long standing disease.	The same chronic complications also occur in this disorder
	Macrovascular disease is more common in older patients of type 2 than in type 1.

Table 7.3. Pathophysiology and progression of diabetes mellitus type 2

Stage of the disease	Pathophysiological factors		Blood glucose
	Insulin resistance	Insulin secretion	
Potential	Increased	Raised	Normal
Latent	Further increased	Raised	Postprandial increased
Overt	As previous	Reduced from previous level	Overt disease

- In the scheme presented the primary defect in the disease lies in insulin resistance. Insulin resistance produces certain metabolic changes which reduce insulin secretion. These changes include high glucose levels (which may down regulate glucose receptors on B-cells) and increased levels of long chain fatty acids (may interefere with secretion of insulin). Some genetic defect responding to metabolic changes may also be involved.
- Both insulin resistance and reduced secretion of insulin are required for overt disease.
- In an alternative view the primary defect lies in over secretion of insulin (with co-secreted amylin). High insulin levels bring about certain changes which lead to insulin resistance. These changes include: i) increased endogenous fat synthesis (from glucose); ii) increased endogenous fat produces obesity and because of stimulated anabolic reactions there are overnourished liver, adipose tissue and muscle cells which suffer from post receptor defective glucose utilization; iii) increased insulin levels lead to down regulation of insulin receptors. Amylin co-secreted with insulin may produce insulin resistance.
- Glucose resistance is a self perpetuating process as increased glucose levels down regulate glucose transporters.

As already mentioned type 2 disease runs in families but its mode of inheritance is not clear, except in a small subset called maturity onset diabetes of the young (MODY) (Table 7.1). Some genes which have been associated with diabetes mellitus type 2 include those coding for insulin, some mitochondrial components, insulin receptor, glucokinase and glycogen synthase. However, all these genes taken together account for only a small fraction of total patients of the disease. Some patients of the subset called MODY are due to mutation in the glucokinase gene (MODY 2). MODY 1 and MODY 3 are associated with some other mutations. MODY has autosomal dominant inheritance.

In case of diabetes mellitus type 1 (an autoimmune disorder) the genetic factors relate to genes that control the immune response (the HLA-genes). There is increased incidence of HLA-DR3, DR4 and DQ antigens (HLA-antigens DR2 and B7, if present resist the disease). The disease carries genetic susceptibility but the actual autoimmune damage is triggered by viral infection or some non-infectious agent. In the immune directed damage to B-cells, both humoral and cell mediated mechanisms are involved. Most of these patients carry autoantibodies against components of islet cells. Important autoantibodies are islet-cell autoantibodies (ICA), insulin associated autoantibodies (IAAs) and anti-glutamic acid decarboxylase autoantibodies (anti-GADs). Close relatives of patients can be screened for these antibodies to predict their risk for developing the disease. The patients are also likely to have autoantibodies against other endocrine glands (adrenal, parathyroid, thyroid) as well as predilection for certain other autoimmune disorders (as part of PGA syndromes).

In type 1 disorder there is low level of vertical transmission. The genetic predisposition is only permissive. The risk of an individual to develop the disease with first degree relatives having the disorder is as under: If father, the risk is 6%, if mother, it is 2%, if HLA-identical sib, it is 12% and if non-identical sib, the risk is 6%.

Table 7.4. Biochemical basis of certain clinical features of diabetes mellitus

Classical polyuria, polydipsia	Osmotic diuresis
Balanitis/vaginal candidiasis	Glycosuria
Loss of weight	Lipolysis, protein break down
Refractive errors	Osmotic effect of increased glucose concentration in lens.
Hypotension	Loss of Na^+ and water: Acidosis
Orthostatic hypotension/ bladder dysfunction/impotence	Autonomic neuropathy(late complication)
Signs of ischemia in peripheral parts of the body Cardiac arrhythmias/arrest	Vascular thrombosis (late complication) Hypokalemia/hyperkalemia (in DKA)
Hypoxemia in the absence of heart failure/known pulmonary disease	Respiratory distress syndrome (in DKA)
Paresthesia of hand/feet and poor co-ordination	Peripheral neuritis (late complication)

- The catabolic state of muscle and other cells causes leakage of K^+ and phosphate from cells which may be lost in urine producing K^+ and phosphate depletions, which may also contribute to the clinical picture of the patient.

Biochemical basis of clinical features

Hyperglycemia of diabetes mellitus is due to reduced utilization and increased formation of glucose. There is increased glycogenolysis and gluconeogenesis. As renal threshold is exceeded, glycosuria occurs. Osmotic diuresis results in excessive loss of water and electrolytes. Hyperosmolar state causes thirst. Reduced plasma volume may affect circulation.

As glucose is not available for energy, alternative fuel molecules are used. There is increased lipolysis, increased fatty acid oxidation and increased formation of ketones. Increased protein breakdown (muscle and other tissues) diverts aminoacids for formation of glucose and ketones. There is weight loss due to loss of water, glycogen, fat and protein. Muscle protein breakdown leads to loss of body potassium and muscle weakness. Diabetics are also phosphate depleted. Also see Table 7.4.

Insulin resistance is a characteristic of type 2 diabetes and may be associated with other features (Fig. 7.1).

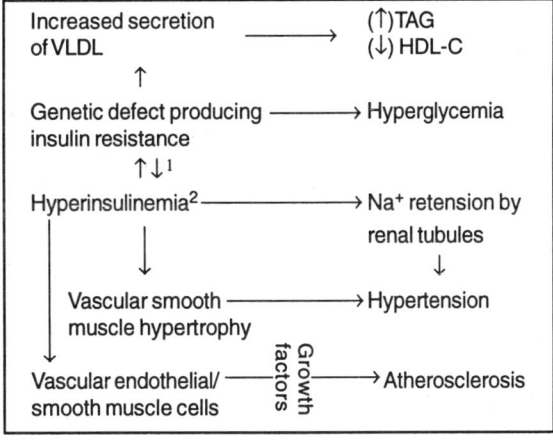

Fig. 7.1. Syndrome of NIDDM and certain associated disorders.

---

[1]Insulin resistance causing hyperinsulinemia or hyperinsulinemia producing insulin resistance in diabetes type 2; see the Text.

[2]Central obesity could be explained by hyperinsulinemia or some other genetic defect.

- Syndrome X includes clinical features of NIDDM, hypertension, central obesity and accelerated atherogenesis.

- Figure shows hyperinsulinemia being responsible for all the features of syndrome X. However, other genetic defects in a closely allied group of genes, are likely to be involved.

Development of ketoacidosis

It is a serious complication, more commonly, encountered in diabetes type 1 and may be precipitated by infection, trauma or some other type of stress. Pathophysiology and clinical features are presented in Fig. 7.2. In stress, insulin secretion is reduced while secretions of hormones which antagonize actions of insulin are increased. There is worsening of hyperglycemia. Low insulin/glucagon ratio promotes ketogenesis. With rise of blood glucose level, there is more severe diuresis. More water than sodium is lost. Thus there is hypovolemia and increase of plasma osmolality. Ketonemia may induce vomiting which further worsens water and electrolyte problems. Hypovolemia impairs renal circulation and may affect tissue perfusion. These changes may add to acidosis produced by ketones. K^+ is released from cells because of acidosis and protein breakdown in muscle.

When GFR is normal this extra K^+ is lost in urine leading to its deficiency but when azotemia occurs reduced GFR leads to hyperkalemia (in presence of K^+ depletion in the body).

Severe diuresis causes depletion of water and sodium but there is more loss of water than sodium. Thus hypernatremia may develop. Increased plasma osmolality, causes movement of water from ICF to ECF, which tends to restore ECF and may produce hyponatremia. Above referred water movement may produce cerebral dehydration and depressed consciousness (Fig. 7.3).

Development of non-ketotic hyperosmolar state

This is more likely to occur in older patients with diabetes type 2. There is no ketosis but plasma glucose level is very high (say 600 mg/dL or more). Insulin level and effectivity are such that excessive

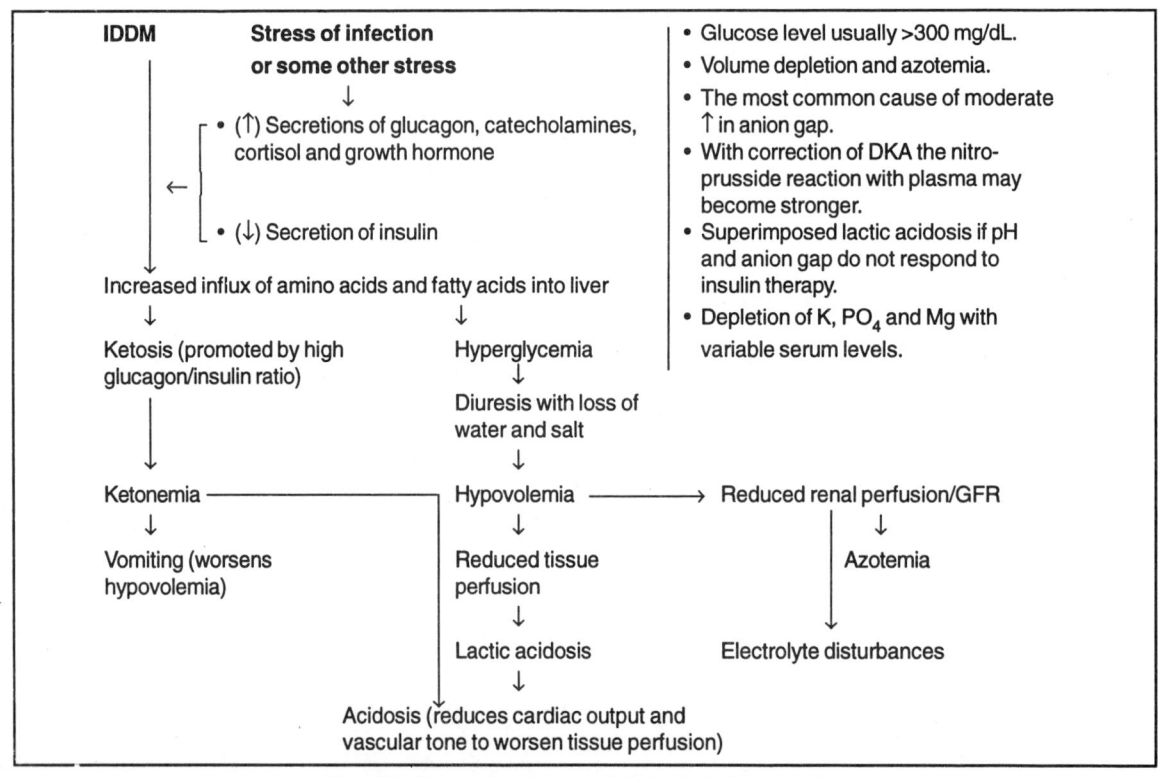

Fig. 7.2. Pathophysiology of diabetic ketoacidosis.

Important features of diabetic ketoacidosis (DKA) are:

- A dehydrated diabetic (tachycardia, postural hypotension) with deep rapid respiration (with fruity odour) and passing into stupor, with history of marked polyuria and polydipsia associated with marked fatigue, nausea and vomiting.

lipolysis and ketogenesis do not occur but glucose formation is greatly increased with impaired glucose utilization. It may be noted that in tissues, different insulin effectivity is required for shifting K^+ into cells, for inhibiting lipolysis (and thus inhibiting ketogenesis) and for glucose transport into cells (for glucose utilization) (Table 7.5).

Non ketotic hyperglycemic coma is precipitated by infections and other conditions which increase secretion of insulin antagonist hormones (glucagon, catecholamines, glucocorticoids and growth hor-

mone) as in case of diabetic ketoacidosis. In addition, conditions causing impairment of renal functions or disturbing water or electrolyte balance, also are likely to precipitate non-ketotic hyperglycemic coma. Thus it may follow use of diuretics or an illness in which water intake of the patient is reduced.

Because of very high blood glucose level, there is marked osmotic diuresis leading to very high serum osmolality and hypernatremia. Because of high serum osmolality, water moves from ICF to ECF, but hypernatremia may persist (Fig. 7.3).

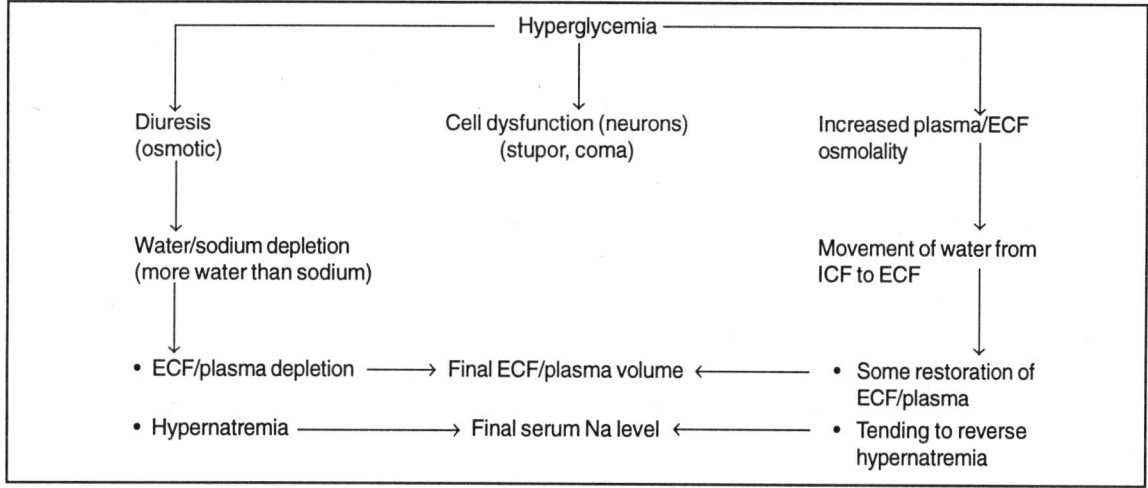

Fig. 7.3. ECF (and plasma) sodium and volume changes in diabetes mellitus.

- In diabetic ketoacidosis there is volume depletion and hyponatremia (commonly). These cases need intravenous normal saline. If a dilute solution is given there is danger of excessive brain cell hydration.
- In cases of non-ketotic hyperglycemia (commonly seen in NIDDM), there is severe hyperglycemia and severe diuresis. These patients often suffer from severe volume depletion and may also have hypernatremia. These patients have less requirement for insulin and are less potassium depleted, compared to cases of diabetic ketoacidosis. Restoration of body water and sodium is the main requirement in these areas.

Table 7.5. Metabolic effects of complete (type 1) and partial (type 2) loss of insulin activity

Path way	Loss of insulin activity	
	Complete loss	Partial loss
Anabolic pathways (glycogenesis, lipogenesis)	Inhibited	Glycogenesis inhibited; Lipogenesis not inhibited
Catabolic pathways (lipolysis, ketogenesis, glycolysis)	Loss of inhibition	No loss of inhibition
Glucose entry into cells	Reduced	Reduced
K^+ entry into cells	Blocked	Reduced

- In partial loss of insulin activity (type 2) as there is no loss of inhibition of lipolysis and ketogenesis, ketoacidosis does not occur, K^+ depletion is less as some K^+ entry into cells is still occuring. Hyperglycemic state occurs as glucose entry into cells is reduced.
- The most characteristic defect of insulin resistance is poor glycogenesis. Uptake of glucose and oxidation to lactate, CO_2 and H_2O are less affected.

Table 7.6. Three serious acute metabolic complications in diabetes mellitus

	Ketoacidosis	Non-ketotic hyperosmolality	Lactic acidosis
Glucose (mg/dL)	High (say 400)	Very high (say 900)	Variable
Sodium (mmol/L)	Hyponatremia	Hypernatremia	Variable (may not be abnormal)
Bicarbonate (mmol/L)	Moderate/severe (say<12.0)	Normal/slightly reduced	Severe (say <10)
Breathing	Hyperventilation	Normal	Hyperventilation
Dehydration	Prominent	Prominent	Not prominent
Smell of ketones	Present	Nil	Nil (only mild ketosis may be there)
Management	Large amounts of soluble insulin: I/V fluids and K$^+$	Large amounts of I/V fluids: insulin in much smaller amounts	Large dose of bicarbonate

- Lactic acidosis occur in a diabetic patient who is seriously ill or has been taking a biguanide. The condition is confirmed by estimation of lactate in plasma.

Table 7.6 compares important features of diabetic ketoacidosis, non-ketotic hyperosmolar state and lactic acidosis.

Lactic acidosis

This complication caused by tissue hypoxia may be associated with diabetes mellitus if the patient is being treated with phenformin (increases anaerobic metabolism) and the patient has renal insufficiency, or when a diabetic patient suffers from a severe infection or cardiovascular collapse. There is no ketoacidosis (unlike diabetic ketoacidosis) and blood glucose level may not be very high (unlike non-ketotic hyperosmolar state). However patient suffers from severe acidosis (Table 7.6).

Late Complications

In uncontrolled diabetes mellitus there is increased glucose utilization in insulin independent pathways, producing pathological changes in tissues, when the condition continues over years. For these changes and the changes causing accelerated atherosclerosis, read under "Following a diabetic for late complications", p.142. Meticulous diabetic control is important to delay these chronic complications of the disease.

SCREENING FOR DIABETES MELLITUS

For the purpose of screening, commonly urine is tested for glucose at random or after a meal. However, glucose may be present in urine, without diabetes mellitus and hyperglycemia, as in renal glycosuria. On the other hand, in old people, renal threshold for glucose may increase and even in the presence of hyperglycemia (and diabetes mellitus), urine may be free from glucose. Thus, presence of glycosuria only suggests that the patient should be tested to confirm diabetes mellitus. Further, absence of glycosuria (especially in old individuals) does not exclude diagnosis of diabetes mellitus. Its confirmation requires estimation of plasma glucose (see below). Indications of estimation of plasma glucose include, presence of glycosuria, strong family history of diabetes mellitus (first degree relations), obesity and pregnancy.

Diagnosis of diabetes mellitus

Presence of glucose and ketones in urine is fairly confirmatory of diabetes mellitus (type 1), in the presence of suggestive features of the disease. However, because of individual variations in renal threshold for glucose and also because ketones alone in urine do not indicate diabetes mellitus, the disease is confirmed by studying plasma glucose levels (Table 7.7). If result of a random or fasting glucose level is equivocal, an oral glucose tolerance test may be helpful (see below). Once diabetes mellitus is confirmed

Table 7.7. Diagnosis of diabetes mellitus

In presence of features suggestive of the disorder:
- Random plasma glucose level >250 mg%
- Fasting plasma glucose level >140 mg%
- Presence of glucose and ketones in urine
- HbA$_1$ level >9%

Even in absence of the suggestive features[1]:
- With the help of oral glucose tolerance test (see the text). In a normal person the fasting level is <115 mg%, 2h value <140 mg% and none of the values >200 mg%. In diabetes 2h value and one more value are more than 200 mg%. Values inbetween those of diabetics and normals indicate impaired glucose tolerance.

---

[1] In the absence of suggestive features of diabetes mellitus random glucose level >250 mg% or the fasting level of >140 mg% must be found at more than one occasions to confirm the disease.

- Even when diabetes mellitus is indicated by presence of glucose and ketones in urine or HbA$_1$ >9%, confirmation needs blood glucose estimation.

---

efforts should be made to characterize the case as one of the specific types (based on clinical features and other aspects: see Table 7.2).

Oral glucose tolerance tests

Before this test, patient should have been on normal intake of carbohydrate for 3 or more days. After taking the fasting blood sample, he is given 75g of glucose in 300 mL of water. He rests and does not smoke during the test. Blood samples are collected half hourly for 2 hours. The patient has diabetes, if 2h and one more value is more than 200 mg% (Table 7.7). Stress of any type (physical, emotional, malnutrition, infection) affects glucose tolerance and makes the results unreliable. Similarly, a large number of drugs (Appendix A) also interfere and need to be discontinued for a few days before the test.

Monitoring a patient during treatment

A good control of blood glucose, during treatment is essential to delay the long term complications of the disease. Patients can do self monitoring at home using test strips. In the initial period, glucose level should be checked, quite frequently (say before each meal and at bed time). Once acceptable control has been achieved, the check has to be less frequent. It may include daily estimation of fasting

plasma glucose level; estimation of plasma glucose level before and after each meal twice a week and a glucose tolerance test done occasionally. The patient should also be educated about warning symptoms of hypoglycemia and such occasions call for checking of glucose level. The overall control, over a period of time, can be monitored by studying level of HbA$_1$ from time to time.

Goals, in terms of blood glucose levels, for a strict diabetic control (which may delay development of late diabetic complications) and for a less strict, but still desirable control, are presented in Table 7.8. The target HbA$_1$ level is about 7% (about 9% in less tight control), or upto 1.5% above the upper normal limit of the laboratory. In cases with tight control, however, risk of episodes of hypoglycemia increases. This tight control is contraindicated in small children (as brain development is affected by hypoglycemia), very old people with significant arteriosclerosis (may also suffer permanent brain injury from hypoglycemia) and in those who are not able to quickly recognize features of hypoglycemia, when these appear.

Table 7.8. Goals in terms of blood glucose levels in diabetes mellitus type 1

Type of control	Blood glucose levels(mg/dL)	
	Preprandial	1h postprandial
Desirable	70 to 100	160
Acceptable	Upto 130	200

- More stringent control (desirable values in the Table) may also be applied to type 2 with the caution that high insulin levels (because of insulin resistance) may aggravate hypertension and atherosclerosis.
- During stringent control in type 1 diabetes chances of hypoglycemia increase, more so if counterregulatory responses are defective.

Other investigations

A known diabetic with severe or long standing disease may present in a semicomatose condition. His clinical state might be because of diabetic ketoacidosis, non-ketotic hyperosmolality, lactic acidosis or even hypoglycemia. The individual complications (the first three) with their diagnosis and principles of management are discussed below. Also see Tables 7.6 and 12.5.

Diabetic ketoacidosis

It is a serious complication, more commonly, encountered in type 1 disease and may be precipitated by trauma or some other type of stress. Pathophysiology and clinical features are presented in Fig. 7.2. Diagnosis is based on history and clinical examination. Urine is examined for glucose and ketones and blood for glucose by a bed side rapid method. For detailed investigations (see below) samples are taken but treatment is started before waiting for the results. The detailed investigations include: plasma glucose, urea, creatinine, ketones, Na^+, K^+ and total CO_2. If total CO_2 is quite low, detailed analysis of acid base status will be needed. Some of these investigations will be needed, repeatedly, during treatment (Table 7.9).

Principles of management include rapid infusion of normal or half normal saline, 8 to 10 U/h of soluble insulin and K^+ supplementation to check excessive gluconeogenesis and to promote glucose utilization in insulin sensitive tissues and thereby to check excessive ketone formation. 5% glucose is added to the regimen when blood glucose falls to about 200 mg/dL. Insulin dosage is scaled down to keep blood glucose between 150-200 mg/dL.

With insulin administration, glucose will start entering the cells which will also facilitate entry of potassium into cells which may produce hypokalemia needing treatment with intravenous potassium. Some potassium may be given as its phosphate salt to restore body phosphate level. This will improve the buffer capacity of plasma. Oxygen delivery to tissues will also improve with increased 2,3 BPG level of red cells. Once GFR and kidney functions improve, acidosis will be taken care of, without any administration of bicarbonate. If however, acidosis is severe (pH <7.1), bicarbonate administration may also be required. Only limited amounts should be used as excessive amounts may produce fluid overload, hypertension and metabolic alkalosis.

Non-ketotic hyperglycemic coma (Table 7.6)

This is more likely to occur in older patients with diabetes mellitus type 2. There is no ketosis and only mild acidosis but plasma glucose is very high (Table 7.6). Severe diuresis leads to extensive water loss and high serum osmolality, causing water to move from ICF to ECF. Treatment is started with normal saline but subsequently more of half normal saline is required in these cases because of excessive loss of water. The precipitating factor should be attended urgently. The urgent need in these cases is normalization of serum osmolality. Insulin requirement is much less than in diabetic ketoacidosis. Requirement for K^+ is also lesser than in diabetic ketoacidosis.

Following a diabetic for late complications

Late complications include diabetic nephropathy, neuropathy and retinopathy. Diabetes mellitus also

Table 7.9. Use of some biochemical parameters during management of a case of diabetic ketoacidosis

Plasma glucose level	Determines the initial dose of insulin
Serum osmolality	Helps to decide whether to start infusion of 0.9% or 0.45% saline
Serum sodium, urea, protein	Are used to assess severity of dehydration
Serum potassium	Helps to decide about potassium administration
Acid base status	Helps to decide about bicarbonate administration (if pH is less than 7.1 bicarbonate should be used).

- Fluid replacement should be gradual to avoid development of cerebral edema. The water deficit is equally borne by ECF and ICF. The latter deficit is corrected by infusing 5% dextrose solution when plasma glucose level falls to about 200 mg/dL.

- A particular level of high plasma glucose requires more insulin administration in the presence of ketoacidosis than in its absence.

- I/V insulin is given in the begnining and once blood glucose level comes down to 250 mg%, S/C insulin (10 units every 6-8h) may be started.

accelerates the process of atherosclerosis and there is special predilection for development of peripheral vascular disease. The biochemical changes that lead to these complications, depend upon increased glucose utilization in insulin independent pathways because of high levels of blood glucose (Figs. 7.4, 7.5). Thus strict control of blood glucose in the disease is very important (Table 7.8) to delay the development of these complications, although, the excellent regulation operative in normal individuals (glucose entering the system via portal circulation, simultaneously, increases appropriate secretion of insulin from the islet tissue) is difficult to achieve.

Diagnosis of above referred complications is mostly, clinical. However, microalbuminuria is considered not only an early predictor of development of nephropathy and hypertension but also a marker of increased mortality from macrovascular disease in diabetes mellitus type 2 (Table 7.10).

Other investigations needed to keep a check for development of chronic complications are total and HDL-cholesterol, TAG, and ECG. The patient should also be watched for peripheral vascular disease. Also read in Chapter 9.

Table 7.10. Urinary excretion of albumin in diabetes mellitus

Type of urine	mg/24h	µg/min	µg/mg creatinine
Normal	<30	<20	<30
Microalbuminuria	30-300	20-200	30-300
Proteinuria (overt)	>300	>200	>300

- First spot urinalysis is performed using a special dipstick (for microalbuminuria). In positive cases detailed analysis is undertaken (in 24h, overnight or 4h urine sample).
- Three samples collected 3 months apart should be tested to know average albumin excretion.
- Fever, congestive heart failure, marked hyperglycemia, marked hypertension and exercise (within 24h) increase the excretion.
- Progression of diabetic nephropathy may be delayed by use of an ACE-inhibitor (to correct renal hemodynamics), protein restriction (about 0.8 g/kg/d) and control of hypertension.

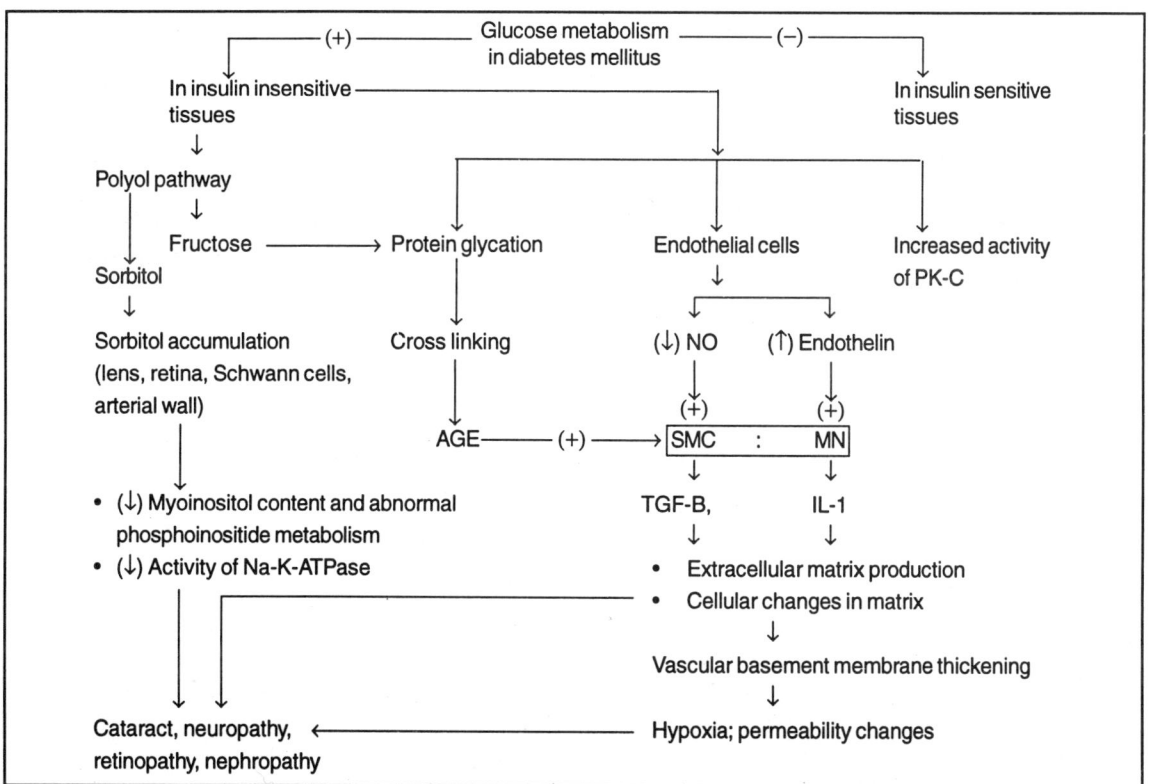

Fig. 7.4. Biochemical basis of late complications of diabetes mellitus.

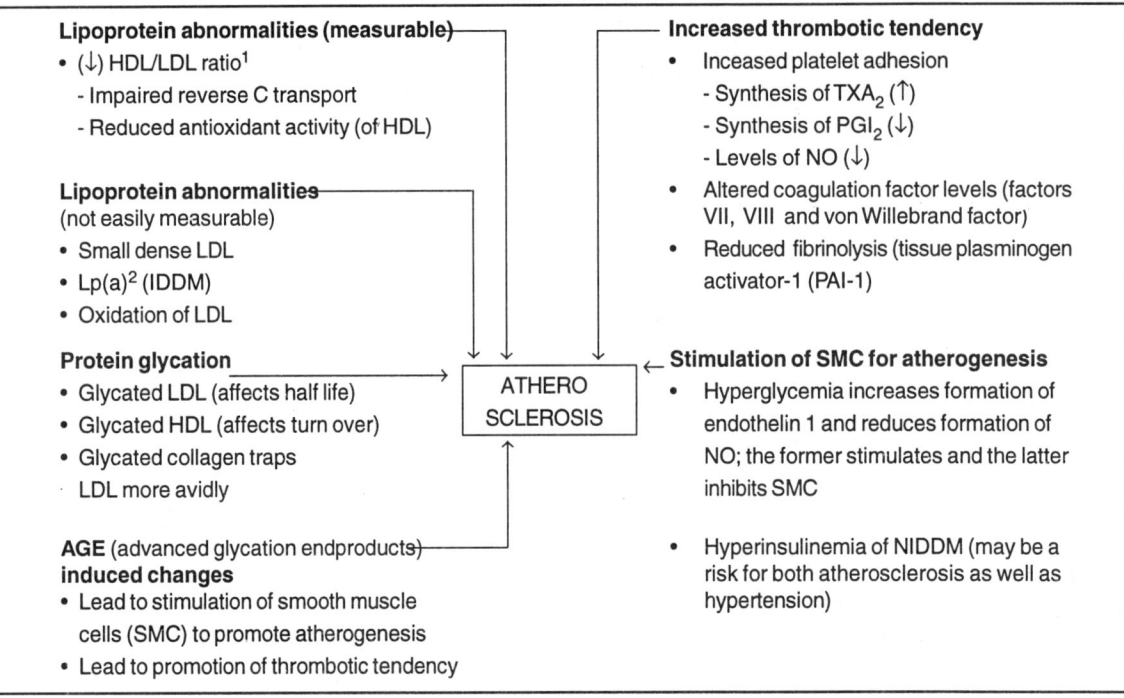

Fig. 7.5. Factors promoting atherogenesis in diabetes mellitus.

[1] In diabetes mellitus, generally, LDL is higher normal and HDL, lower normal. LDL may be increased in IDDM.

[2] Lp (a) is more easily deposited in atherosclerotic lesions compared to LDL. Apo (a) because of extensive homology with plasminogen, acts as its competitive inhibitor to promote thrombosis. It also stimulated SMC in atheroma formation by inhibiting TGF (which inhibits mitogenesis)

HYPOGLYCEMIA

Pathophysiology of hypoglycemia

There are number of counterregulatory responses to hypoglycemia. As insulin secretion ceases in hypoglycemia, secretions of glucagon and epinephrine, followed by those of growth hormone and cortisol increase. Clinical features of hypoglycemia develop only, if inspite of the above regulatory responses, blood glucose level remains low. As blood glucose reaches a low level, increase in cerebral circulation tends to keep up adequate supply of glucose to the brain. The latter response, however, is limited in old age due to atherosclerotic arterial vessels.

The actual blood glucose level at which the symptoms develop is not fixed and depends upon many factors. One such factor is the rate at which blood glucose level falls. In a normal person, if the level comes down rapidly, the catecholamine induced

clinical features (palpitation, tachycardia, anxiety, sweating) start appearing, first, at a level of about 40 mg/dL, to be followed by symptoms related to brain dysfunction (dizziness, convulsions, stupor, coma), at still lower levels of blood glucose. The former set of clinical features constitute the symptoms of hypoglycemia awareness and urgent treatment is required before the second set of symptoms start appearing.

There are three criteria (Whipple's triad) used for diagnosis of hypoglycemia: i) clinical features of hypoglycemia precipitated by fasting; ii) plasma glucose level <45 mg/dL during the attack; iii) prompt relief from symptoms by glucose administration. Repeated episodes of hypoglycemia may lead to behavioural changes and effective disorders.

Hypoglycemia in diabetes

The problem of hypoglycemia, most commonly, arises in a known diabetic (Table 7.11). Quite early

Table 7.11. Some causes of hypoglycemia in a diabetic.

- Inappropriate dose of the drug; inadequate food intake in relation to drug intake; inappropriate level of exercise. Exercise may also increase insulin absorption from the injection site while adequate glucose production in liver may not occur.
- Failure to reduce drug intake after stress is over.
- Diabetic renal disease reduces insulin requirement by increased half life of insulin.
- Delayed emptying of stomach by diabetic autonomic neuropathy, may result in post prandial hypoglycemia.
- It may be drug induced (alcohol, salicylates, β-blockers).
- Lack of predictable uniform response to an antihyperglycemic agent and of counterregulatory process. In patients of type 1 diabetes, natural response to hypoglycemia becomes poor if there is glucagon deficiency. The response is still worse if there is autonomic neuropathy (resulting in poor release of epinephrine). In the latter case the warning symptoms of hypoglycemia will also be missing.
- In patients with tight control of diabetes, one episode of hypoglycemia predisposes to the next by lowering the glucose level required to trigger the epinephrine release (and the warning symptoms).
- It may develop due to adrenal insufficiency as part of polyglandular autoimmune deficiency.
- It may develop in the presence of insulin antibodies from which insulin may dissociate in the fasting state.
- Rarely it may be due to remission in type 1 diabetes.

Table 7.12. Important causes of fasting hypoglycemia.

Due to overutilization of glucose:
- B-cell adenoma/MEN 1
- Islet cell hyperplasia (nesidioblastosis), causes hypoglycemia in late postnatal period.
- Non-pancreatic tumors (fibromas and sarcomas of large size, Wilms tumor of kidney), act by releasing growth factors like IGF-2, IGF-1, TNF-α.
- Drugs like insulin, sulfonylureas.
- Sepsis (there is increased insulin release through sepsis associated cytokines).
- Reduced fat oxidation (if fatty acids or ketones are not available for energy purposes, more of glucose is used)
  - Deficiency of enzymes of fat oxidation (systemic carnitine deficiency).[1]
  - Cachexia with fat depletion.
- Antibodies to endogenous insulin (insulin dissociates from antibodies in fasting state).

Due to reduced glucose production:
- Hormone deficiencies (hypopituitarism, adrenal insufficiency).
- Enzymatic defects in pathways leading to glucose production.
- Substrate deficiency (malnutrition, severe muscle wasting, late pregnancy and also ketotic hypoglycemia of infancy).
- Certain systemic disorders
  - Hepatic congestion
  - Cirrhosis, severe hepatitis
  - Uremia
  - Hypothermia
- Drugs (alcohol, propranol, salicylates)

[1] Reduced oxidation of fatty acids and ketone formation increase glucose oxidation in tissues in systemic carnitine deficiency (hypoketotic hypoglycemia).

in type 1 patients, glucagon response to hypoglycemia is lost. This lowers defense against hypoglycemia. Some patients, subsequently, also lose the catecholamine response. This produces hypoglycemia unawareness, besides, further lowering defense against hypoglycemia. This condition is different from hypoglycemia unawareness produced by autonomic neuropathy in patients with long standing disease. Stringent control of diabetes mellitus with insulin also impairs epinephrine release and may produce hypoglycemia unawareness. If diabetic control is poor, the counterregulatory glucose threshold moves upwards and symptomatic hypoglycemia may occur when blood glucose level is still in the normal range.

Hypoglycemia without diabetes

In non-diabetics, hypoglycemia may be postprandial (reactive) or fasting. In fasting hypoglycemia symptoms appear in the night or early morning or these may be induced by exercise. In the postprandial form, clinical features appear some hours after food intake or ingestion of some drug. Patients with fasting hypoglycemia, especially those with insulinoma (see below), may also exhibit postprandial features but the reactive patients do not present with symptoms in advanced fasting state. Further postprandial or reactive hypoglycemia may occur without any known disease while fasting hypoglycemia always occurs in presence of a disease.

Fasting hypoglycemia

Causes of fasting hypoglycemia are listed in Table 7.12. If only a small amount of glucose (say about 10 g/h) is required for management of a case of recurrent hypoglycemia, reduced glucose production is likely to be the reason, as hypoglycemic

disorders resulting from increased glucose utilization require larger amounts of glucose for management. In general, finding of hypoglycemia, in a person (non-diabetics) without uremia, liver disease, severe malnutrition, malabsorption, or history of alcohol intake, should raise possibilities of insulinoma (single benign adenoma, or multiple tumors as part of MEN-syndrome), non-pancreatic (mesenchymal) tumors, and less commonly enzymatic defects or hormonal deficiencies. Also one should remember, that symptomatic hypoglycemia generally occurs in diabetes mellitus or due to insulinoma or in neonates (described later). In most other cases it is only biochemical hypoglycemia. However, even this type of hypoglycemia can produce brain changes if it occurs repeatedly. This is particularly true in neonates.

The first aim of investigations in a patient with clinical features of fasting hypoglycemia is to rule out insulinoma or some extra pancreatic neoplasm producing the clinical state. If a patient is seen with clinical features of hypoglycemia, his blood sample is collected for estimation of glucose, insulin and/or C-peptide, before giving him glucose (to relieve him of clinical features). If the patient does not present with symptoms the same have to be produced by fasting (Table 7.13). Insulinoma as cause of hypo-

---

Table 7.13. Important tests used in diagnosis of hypoglycemias.

72h fast under supervision:
(patient is fasted for atleast 72h unless symptoms develop and plasma glucose, insulin, C-peptide, and cortisol estimated every 6h)

- For diagnosis of insulinoma one should show inappropriately high insulin (or C-peptide) level for low plasma glucose during an episode of hypoglycemia.
- At plasma glucose level <45 mg/dL, any measurable insulin makes diagnosis of insulinoma, likely (more correctly any level >10 μU/mL)

Extended glucose tolerance test:
(in a 5h glucose tolerance test patient is monitored for hypoglycemic symptoms and blood glucose levels are studied between 2 to 5h)

- In cases of true idiopathic alimentary hypoglycemia biochemical hypoglycemia is demonstrated in the presence of hypoglycemic clinical features. Such cases are rare. Some unknown defect in the absorptive process may be there.
- In functional hypoglycemia clinical features occur when blood glucose level are in the normal range. This condition is also called pseudohypoglycemia or idiopathic post prandial syndrome.
- Prediabetics may also show a late fall in plasma glucose after oral glucose tolerance test without hypoglycemic symptoms.

glycemia can be demonstrated by showing inappropriately high insulin (or C-peptide) level for low plasma glucose level during fasting or an episode of hypoglycemia. Use of C-peptide is better since it is cleared from circulation more slowly than insulin. Moreover, C-peptide only arises from endogenous insulin and not from the exogenous (therapeutic) one. Further, in insulinoma, increased proinsulin (co-secreted with insulin) and its split products produce false, many fold, increase in insulin level (immunoassay of insulin includes these molecules).

The only other disorder which may show inappropriately high insulin (or C-peptide) level for low plasma glucose level in an episode of hypoglycemia is idiopathic hypoglycemia of childhood (see later). Suppressibility of B-cell secretion (demonstrated by C-peptide assay) after insulin induced hypoglycemia may also be used to screen patients of insulinoma (less suppression than in normals). Stimulation tests (more insulin release in insulinoma) using tolbutamide or with glucose are rarely used.

Tumor localization may need imaging studies or transportal vein sampling. 80% of insulinomas are benign, 10% multiple and 10% are malignant. Malignant tumors may also produce other hormones like hCG-β, ACTH, gastrin and glucagon. Treatment is surgical if adenoma can be located, otherwise, long term therapy with diazoxide (inhibitor of insulin secretion) is used. Thiazide is given along with diazoxide because of salt retaining action of the latter drug. Frequent feeding is also used to avoid fasting hypoglycemia.

Non-fasting hypoglycemia (reactive hypoglycemia or post prandial hypoglycemia) (Table 7.14)

Cause is, generally, apparent after history. Important features of different causes are mentioned in Table 7.14. For diagnosis of late hypoglycemia and functional reactive hypoglycemia, a 5h oral glucose tolerance test is used. Use of this test for the former condition has been questioned since many normal asymptomatic persons also show evidence of biochemical hypoglycemia in this test.

Table 7.14. Some important causes of post prandial (reactive) hypoglycemia.

Alimentary hypoglycemia:

Biochemical and clinical hypoglycemia occuring 1.5 to 3h after eating	Rapid absorption of glucose load causes increased insulin release
History of gastrointestinal surgery. Rarely no such history is available (Idiopathic alimentary hypoglycemia).	Give small meals (more frequent) with less carbohydrate and with fiber.

Functional hypoglycemia:

Features resembling those of hypoglycemia 2 to 5h after a meal without appropriately low blood glucose level.	Exaggerated release of catecholamines after a meal
Persons often lean with hyperkinetic personality.	Treatment like that of alimentary hypoglycemia.
Also called pseudohypoglycemia.	

Late hypoglycemia (in prediabetics):

Hypoglycemia ((symptomatic) occuring 4 to 5h after a glucose load).	Defective early release of insulin resulting in exaggerated delayed release of insulin.
As this finding is common (see above) carries no significance in diagnosis.	

Post prandial hypoglycemia seen in infancy:

Galactosemia, fructose intolerance and leucine sensitive hypoglycemia.	In leucine sensitivity cases hypoglycemia occurs in sensitive infants after milk intake.

Neonatal hypoglycemia (transient)

As maternal supply of glucose is stopped at birth, glycogenolysis and gluconeogenesis become important in maintaining blood glucose level, in a neonate. Neonatal hypoglycemia is due to poor glycogen stores and immature enzymes of gluconeogenesis in the newborn. Because of islet cell hyperplasia, newborns of diabetic mothers are more prone to neonatal hypoglycemia. Premature and small for date newborns and newborns with hypoxia also run a greater risk of neonatal hypoglycemia. Neonatal hypoglycemia occurs only in the immediate neonatal period (12 to 18h after birth) and is a short lived abnormality since the relevant enzymes mature in 1 to 2 weeks after birth. Secondary (Fig. 7.6) or idiopathic ketotic hypoglycemia of infancy may also occur quite commonly. Neonatal brain is quite sensitive to hypoglycemic damage and for this reason blood glucose level should not be allowed to fall below 46 mg/dL in neonates.

Hypoglycemia in post neonatal period (persistent) (Table 7.15)

In glycogen storage disease type 1 (von Gierkes disease), there is deficiency of glucose-6-phosphatase and there is fasting hypoglycemia. In hereditary fructose intolerance (deficiency of enzyme fructose-1-aldolase), fructose (or sucrose) admini-

Table 7.15. Important causes of hypoglycemia in infants and children

Transient neonatal hypoglycemia (<2 weeks):
- Maternal reasons (diabetes, toxemia)
- Premature: SGA
- Rhesus immunization
- Asphyxia, hypoxia, sepsis

Persistent neonatal hypoglycemia:
- Endocrine disorders
    - Hypothyroidism
    - Congenital adrenal hyperplasia
    - Anterior pituitary insufficiency
- Inborn errors
    - Glycogen storage disease type I, III, VI
    - Fructose intolerance
    - Galactosemia
    - Organic acid disorders, some amino acid disorders
    - Disorders of fat oxidation including carnitine deficiency disorder
- Increased insulin - glucose ratio
    - B-cell hyperplasia, nesidioblastoma, B-cell adenoma, teratoma

stration causes hypoglycemia (post prandial) along with nausea, vomiting and abdominal pain. Milk ingestion may cause postprandial hypoglycemia in galactosemia. In hypoglycemia of inborn errors, clinical features of hypoglycemia are not common. Inborn errors concerning metabolism of some amino acids and fatty acid oxidation may also be associated with hypoglycemia. In some infants, casein of milk (rich in leucine) can cause hypoglycemia by increasing insulin secretion. This condition, however, is self-limiting and runs in families.

Fig. 7.7 gives a scheme for finding cause of neonatal hypoglycemia.

Use of strips for testing of glucose/ketones

For glucose and ketones both test tablets and test strips are available. Test strips are generally preferred. Test strips for glucose, incorporate glucose oxidase, a peroxidase and a chromogen. If glucose is present, glucose oxidase releases hydrogen peroxide which oxidizes the chromogen. In clinistix strips, O-toluidine is used as the chromogen, and colour change is from pink to purple. Ascorbic acid interferes in the reaction. For ketones (only

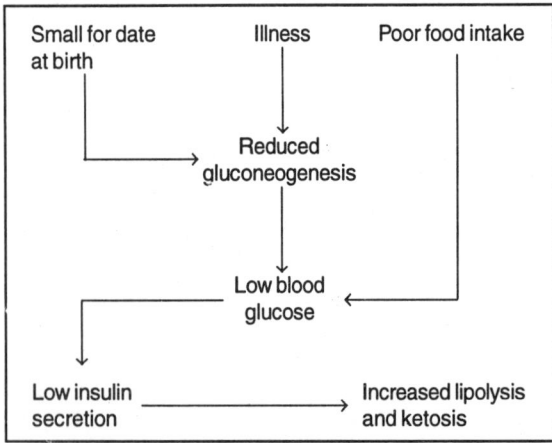

Fig. 7.6. Ketotic hypoglycemia of infancy.

- Treatment of ketotic hypoglycemia requires feeding the infant more frequently.

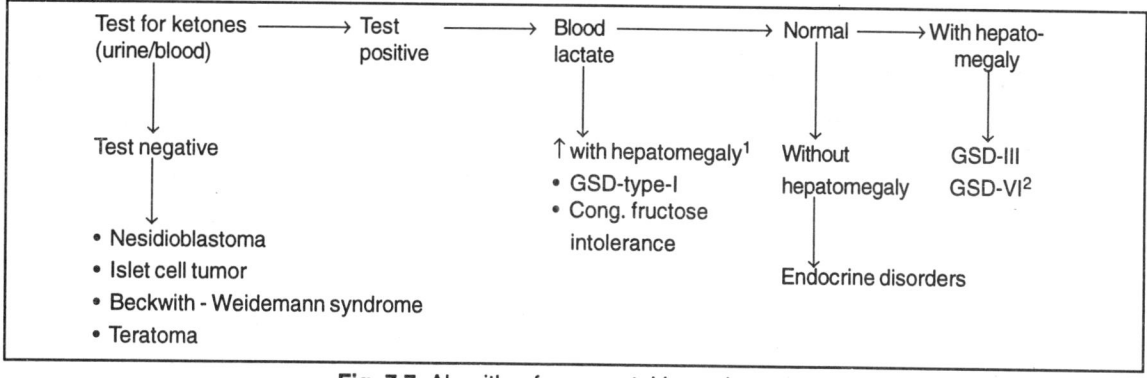

Fig. 7.7. Algorithm for neonatal hypoglycemia.

---

[1] Increase lactate without hepatomegaly means GSD absent.

[2] It is a benign and rare disorder. Another similarly benign but common disorder is hepatic phosphorylase kinase deficiency (formerly VIa or IX). This disorder is X-linked.

- GSD = glycogen storage disease

acetoacetate and acetone react), test is based on the reaction between nitroprusside and acetoacetate/acetone in the presence of alkali. In the presence of severe acidosis (hypoxemia, lactic acidosis) concentration of β-hydroxy butyrate (compared to other ketones) is very high and the test will fail to give correct assessment of level of ketones. The strip tests can be used for urine, blood and plasma, to evaluate glucose and ketones, semiquantitatively. The colour obtained can be interpreted, visually (by comparing with a colour chart) or using a reflectancemeter or a colorimeter. Both venous and capillary samples can be used in these tests.

While using these strips, the instructions of manufacturers should be followed, strictly. Strips should not be out-dated and should be properly stored (protected from humidity, air and excessive heat). If the strip method shows blood glucose level of 300 mg% or more, the correct level needs to be confirmed by the use of a more accurate method. Strips measure the metabolite content of fluid absorbed into the strip from the blood sample; less fluid enters if hematocrit is high and more if it is low.

More accurate enzymatic laboratory methods are used both for glucose and ketones. For ketones, these methods are cumbersome and not much used for patients.

Microalbuminuria (Table 7.10)

It is tested in an overnight, timed, urine sample. Immunological methods are used for protein assay in urine. Alternatively, TCA (trichloracetic acid) precipitate is dissolved in sodium hydroxide and albumin level estimated by the biuret method. In microalbuminuria the patient excretes 20 to 200 μg of protein per minute. As the condition progresses microalbuminuria changes into albuminuria (the heat coagulation test becomes positive) and features of nephrotic syndrome and azotemia start developing.

Glycosylated hemoglobin (HbA$_1$)

Glycosyated hemoglobin is formed by reaction of hemoglobin with glucose (HbA$_{1c}$), glucose 6-PO$_4$ (HbA$_{1a}$), and fructose 6-PO$_4$ (HbA$_{1b}$). Control of glycemia in diabetes mellitus is best correlated with levels of HbA$_{1c}$ but commonly used methods estimate total glycosylated Hb called HbA$_1$ (HbA$_{1c}$ + HbA$_{1a}$ + HbA$_{1b}$). Level of HbA$_1$ hemoglobin indicates average blood glucose level over the previous 8 to 12 weeks, the period related to average life span of different populations of red cells, at any one time. Normally this level is less than 7% and rises to 12 to 25% if the control of glycemia (in diabetes mellitus) is poor. Serum fructosamine is formed by non-enzymatic glycosylation of serum proteins (mostly albumin). Its serum level indicates average glucose level over previous 2 weeks, because of shorter half life of serum albumin. Reference range is 2.4-3.4 mmol/L (fructosamine - albumin ratio 54-86 μmol/g). It is not a popular parameter. Fructosamine and HbA_1 are not useful in gestational diabetes.

In the above account term glycosylated Hb has been used for non-enzymatic addition of hexoses. More strictly glycosylation means enzymatic addition of hexose and glycation means non-enzymatic addition.

CASE HISTORY: 7.1

A 25 year old female was brought to hospital in a drowsy state and with deep rapid breathing. She had 48h history of abdominal pain and vomiting. She was a known diabetic and had recently suffered from an attack of malaria. Urine was strongly positive for glucose and ketones.

➤ What is cause and implications of vomiting?
➤ What are important investigations required in the case and how will these guide management of the case?
➤ Name two other serious acute biochemical complications encountered in patients of diabetes mellitus.
➤ What is significance of raised amylase level in such cases?
➤ After this patient comes out of her acute metabolic decompensation, which biochemical test can be done to screen her for chronic complications?

• Vomiting is produced by stimulation of chemoreceptor trigger zone (which in turn stimulates the vomiting centre in medulla) by ketones and it further worsens water and electrolyte disturbances.
• Table 7.9 indicates the important investigations and their implication in management. It may, however, be mentioned that treatment is started without waiting for the results of the detailed investigations, once approximate, level of blood glucose is known (using a bed side method).
• The two other acute biochemical complications are, diabetic non-ketotic hyperosmolar state and lactic acidosis. In the former condition, plasma glucose level may be two times or even higher than that in diabetic ketoacidosis. This leads to much larger free water loss due to more severe diuresis, leading to higher serum osmolality, serum sodium and serum creatinine, than in

diabetic ketoacidosis. Table 7.6 compares biochemical changes in the three conditions.
• Serum amylase is often raised in patients of diabetic ketoacidosis and can be cause of misdiagnosis. However, levels are not that high as in acute pancreatitis (similar increase of amylase can also occur in intestinal obstruction, cholecystitis and perforated duodenal ulcer). In all these conditions, levels rarely rise above 3 times the upper reference limit. Abdominal pain of diabetic ketoacidosis may be due to gastric distension or stretching of hepatic capsule.
• Diagnosis of late diabetic complications is, mostly, clinical except for diabetic nephropathy. Microalbuminuria gives an early indication of diabetic nephropathy.

CASE HISTORY: 7.2

The patient of case history 7.1, after successful management of her acute episode, again reported to hospital (after a period of 6 months) with complaints of amenorrhea and repeated hypoglycemic episodes. Comment on her clinical features.

The patient has diabetes mellitus type 1 which is an autoimmune disorder. Such patients may also suffer from autoimmune damage of other endocrine glands (PGA syndromes; Chapter 16). Thus she might have developed pituitary and/or adrenal failure which would explain her amenorrhea as well as her increased sensitivity to insulin. Alternatively, it can happen in early pregnancy when lot of glucose is diverted for fetal utilization. However, as pregnancy progresses, some placental hormones reduce insulin sensitivity.

CASE HISTORY: 7.3

A lady reports to her doctor that her husband is often quiet, uncommunicative and feels unconcerned about rest of the family, when he comes from the office or when he gets up in the morning. He, however, immediately cheers up after a cup of tea, and starts behaving normally. This has been noticed about him over the past few months and condition has been gradually deteriorating.

With this type of history, the patient needs to be investigated for hypoglycemia of insulinoma. Diagnosis is made by demonstrating hypoglycemia and high insulin level when symptoms are present (insulin level is not appropriately low to the low level of plasma glucose). Fasting clinical hypoglycemia can occur in certain other conditions (Table 7.12) but in these disorders insulin levels are appropriately reduced to the low glucose levels. In a few cases of insulinoma, confirmation of diagnosis may require demonstration of inappropriate C-peptide level during induced hypoglycemia (see

Table 7.13). Most of the times, the tumor is benign and about 10% of benign tumors are associated with adenomas of other endocrine glands. A benign tumor needs resection. For malignant tumors when resection is not possible, streptozotocin (along with doxorubicin) is used which specifically, destroys the B-cells.

CASE HISTORY: 7.4

A known diabetic developed a serious pyogenic infection. His family doctor, while treating him for the infection, increased his daily dose of insulin. The infection healed over a period of about 2 weeks. But now the patient reported with frequent episodes of clinical hypoglycemia.

Infection, trauma and many other stresses increase insulin requirement of a diabetic patient. It is for this reason that dose of insulin had to be increased in this patient during his pyogenic infection. But the dose should have been reduced with clearing of the infection. This was however, not done and explains the new complaints of the patient. Insulin requirements of a diabetic change under different physiological and pathological conditions. A diabetic person should be informed about these facts. An identification card carried by a diabetic about his disease can also be helpful in emergency situations.

OBJECTIVE TYPE QUESTIONS

Pick out the wrong statement

1. Diabetes mellitus

i) Type 2 diabetes mellitus is more common than type 1.
ii) Type 2 disease shows familial aggregation.
iii) Pathogenesis of type 2 disease is less well understood.
iv) The major environmental factor in type 2 disease is obesity.
v) Close relatives of a patient of type 2 disease can be screened for anti-GADs to know their risk for developing the disease.

2. Glycosylated hemoglobins

i) Glycosylated hemoglobins are called fast hemoglobins due to their faster migration (than hemoglobin) in column methods.
ii) In the column methods the different glycosylated hemoglobin fractions obtained are called hemoglobins, A_{1a}, A_{1b}, A_{1c} and Pre-A_{1c}
iii) HbA_1 (HbA_{1a}+HbA_{1b}+HbA_{1c}) means total of fast hemoglobins.
iv) Hemoglobin A_{1c} is the most abundant of the fast

hemoglobins and is used to monitor long term diabetic control.
v) Levels of pre-A_{1c} change quite rapidly and if included with A_{1c}, will interfere in proper interpretation.
vi) In the column methods, there is no interference from abnormal hemoglobins.

3. Monitoring of diabetic control

i) In olden times frequency of nocturia was used to monitor diabetic severity.
ii) It may be done by preprandial study of urine for glucose.
iii) Self monitoring may be done by studying capillary blood glucose.
iv) Level of glycosylated hemoglobin indicates glycemic control over about past 2 months
v) Serum fructosamine measures nonlabile glycated serum proteins and indicates glycemic control over about previous 2 weeks.
vi) There is no biochemical parameter to predict onset of late complications.

4. Glucose tolerance test

i) It is indicated in borderline fasting or postprandial blood glucose level.
ii) It is indicated if the patient shows persistent glycosuria.
iii) It is needed during pregnancy if there is glycosuria or if there is family history of diabetes mellitus or if the woman had unexplained fetal loss.
iv) Test is equally sensitive whether glucose load is 50g or 100g.
v) It should not he done immediately after a severe illness.

5. Diabetic ketoacidosis

i) 2,3 BPG deficiency shifts the O_2 dissociation curve to the left.
ii) Acidosis in the presence of 2,3 BPG deficiency maintains the normal shape of the O_2 dissociation curve.
iii) If acidosis is treated rapidly, 2,3 BPG deficiency would shift the O_2 dissociation curve to left.
iv) Poor release of O_2 would promote anaerobic glucose metabolism, increasing formation of lactic acid.
v) In treatment of acidosis, if HCO_3^- is raised to normal level, alkalosis may occur with metabolism of ketones to HCO_3^-.
vi) The best way to follow the treatment is to repeatedly study ketone level in plasma.

6. Diabetic ketoacidosis

i) Normal ratio of β-hydroxy butyrate to acetoacetate in plasma is 3:1.

ii) Ratio of β-hydroxy butyrate to acetoacetate may rise in diabetic ketoacidosis to 8:1 in the presence of severe hypoxia or circulatory collapse.

iii) In such cases of circulatory collapse, ketoacidosis may be masked.

iv) Ketone reagent strips are commonly used for semiquantitative analysis of plasma for ketones.

v) In most cases of diabetic ketoacidosis a 1:10 dilution of plasma gives a strong positive reaction on ketone strips.

7. Ketoacidotic/hyperosmolar coma

i) Hyperosmolar coma is more common in elderly patients of NIDDM

ii) There is more severe volume depletion in hyperosmolar coma than in coma due to diabetic ketoacidosis.

iii) Patients of hyperosmolar coma require large amounts of I/V fluids to establish circulation and urine flow.

iv) K^+ may be needed early in diabetic ketoacidosis than hyperosmolar diabetic patients.

v) In a diabetic patient if plasma HCO_3^- is 10 mmol/L and plasma ketones are not elevated, lactic acidosis will be the likely diagnosis.

8. Hypoglycemia in diabetes mellitus

i) The most important counterregulatory hormone to insulin is glucagon.

ii) GH and cortisol are involved only if hypoglycemia is prolonged (prolonged fasting).

iii) Release of epinephrine in hypoglycemia is important since it produces the warning symptoms during hypoglycemia.

iv) One episode of hypoglycemia in a diabetic patient lowers threshold for epinephrine response during the next episode of hypoglycemia.

v) Hypoglycemia unawareness is a feature of diabetic patients with autonomic neuropathy not seen in other cases.

9. Somogyi phenomenon

i) It is rebound hyperglycemia following an episode of hypoglycemia (wide fluctuations in blood glucose level in a diabetic on insulin).

ii) It may occur if patient is getting more than required amount of insulin.

iii) Patient may have excessive hunger and gain in weight.

iv) In a controlled diabetic if there is regular early morning rise in blood glucose, somogyi phenomenon can be the only cause.

v) Somogyi phenomenon, generally, occurs in children and not in adults.

10. Late complications of diabetes mellitus

i) In insulin insensitive tissues, glucose changes into sorbitol and accumulates as a tissue toxin.

ii) High level of glucose in blood and tissues causes protein glycation.

iii) Glycosylated proteins form cross linked proteins called advanced glycation end products (AGE).

iv) Both the above processes are involved in micro and macro vascular complications of diabetes mellitus.

v) Microvascular and macrovascular changes are equally common in NIDDM and IDDM.

ANSWERS

1. No.(v). Close relatives of a patient of type 1 disease are screened for GAD antibodies to know their risk for developing the disease.

2. No.(vi). With most column methods methemoglobin, hemoglobin F, and hemoglobin Wayne co-elute with glycosylated hemoglobins. Hemoglobin F or methemoglobin can interfere in electrophoretic measurement of glycosylated hemoglobins.

   To avoid interference from hemoglobin pre-A_{1c} red cells should be washed with saline prior to estimation. Reliability of glycosylated hemoglobin is also reduced in uremia.

   Levels of hemoglobin A_{1c} correlate best with the diabetic control, although most of the methods estimate hemoglobin A_1.

3. No.(vi). Microalbuminuria is used as an early indicator of diabetic nephropathy and other late complications.

4. No.(iv). Higher loads increase sensitivity and reproducibility but often lead to nausea and vomiting which invalidates the results.

5. No.(vi). The best way to follow the treatment is to monitor pH (it should rise) and anion gap (it should reduce). HCO_3^- may be low because of Cl^- (NaCl) used in treatment. If pH and anion gap do not change, it may indicate insulin resistance. In the test for ketones, colour is produced by acetoacetic (and acetone) and not β-hydroxy butyrate. As acidosis is treated more acetoacetate will form from β-hydroxy butyrate and the intensity of colour in the test for ketones may not decrease.

6. No.(v). Undiluted plasma gives strongly positive result in starvation ketosis. A strong reaction at a dilution higher than 1:1 is considered as an evidence of diabetic ketoacidosis.

7. No.(iv). K^+ enters cells readily in the absence of acidosis.

8. No.(v). Besides autonomic neuropathy, it also occurs if catecholamine response to hypoglycemia is lost and it may occur quite early in course of IDDM.

9. No.(iv). It occurs more commonly because of dawn phenomenon (resulting from nocturnal surge of growth hormone). To differentiate between the two, blood glucose is measured at 3 AM (high level would indicate dawn phenomenon). A patient showing dawn phenomenon needs more insulin and patient showing Somogyi phenomenon needs reduction in insulin dose.

10. No.(v). Macrovascular complications are more common in old patients of NIDDM.

CHAPTER 8

Porphyrias, Hyperuricemia and Gout

PORPHYRINS

The porphyrins are intermediate products in heme biosynthesis (Fig. 8.1). ALA-synthase is the rate-limiting step and needs pyridoxal phosphate as a coenzyme. ALA, next, undergoes a condensation reaction to form porphobilinogen (PBG) by the enzyme ALA-dehydratase. This enzyme is present in high concentrations, both in hepatic and bone marrow cells. Next, PBG deaminase (also called hydroxy methyl bilane (HMB) synthase or uroporphyrinogen I synthase) forms a linear structure called polypyrrole (or hydroxymethylbilane) by condensing four PBG molecules. This is followed by formation of uroporphyrinogen III by cyclization of the linear structure by the action of uroporphyrinogen III synthase (commonly called co-synthase) and abbreviated as URO-synthase in Fig. 8.1. Further reactions are shown in Fig. 8.1. In the absence of uroporphyrinogen III synthase, type I compounds (uroporphyrinogen I and coproporphyrinogen I) are synthesized (non-enzymatic formation of uroporphyrinogen I from polypyrrole) and corresponding oxidation products (uroporphyrin I and coproporphyrin I) are detectable in urine/feces. Finally, in the normal pathway (Fig. 8.1) protoporphyrin IX incorporates ferrous iron to form heme.

The pathway is regulated differently in liver and bone marrow. In liver there are two forms of the regulatory enzyme. ALA synthase, inducible and non-inducible. Free heme regulates (negative feedback effect) synthesis and mitochondrial trans-location of non-inducible ALA synthase. The inducible enzyme is induced by many of the drugs which are known to induce cytochrome-P450 in endoplasmic reticulum of the liver cells.

Entry of iron into the erythroid cells and heme synthesis are coordinated processes. Hypoxia and certain growth factors (IL-3, erythropoietin) stimulate the process in bone marrow.

PORPHYRIAS

This is a group of inherited and acquired disorders characterized by abnormalities of activities of specific enzymes of the pathway of heme biosynthesis. There is excessive formation of porphyrins and/or porphyrin precursors. The specific enzymatic blocks (Fig. 8.1) cause decrease in synthesis of specific porphyrins and heme, resulting in stimulation (in liver) of the regulatory enzyme ALA-synthase (and of the pathway) due to loss of the feed back inhibitory effect. Some metabolites accumulate.

Porphyrias are hepatic or erythropoietic. In hepatic porphyrias the major site of excessive porphyrin production is liver and in erythropoietic, the erythroid tissue (Fig. 8.1). Porphyrias are also classified as acute and chronic. In acute porphyrias the stimulated pathway leads to excessive formation of ALA and porphobilinogen (PBG) with or without other porphyrins. In chronic porphyrias increased formation of porphyrins occurs but not of ALA and PBG. Accumulation of ALA and PBG results in neuro-visceral presentation while accumulation of

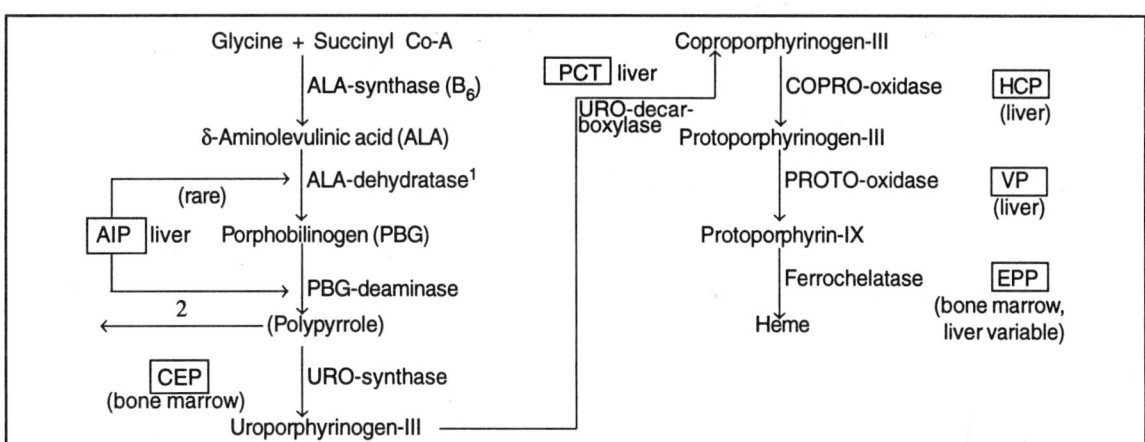

Fig. 8.1. Outline of the pathway of heme synthesis also indicating thedefective enzymes in different porphyrias.

---

[1] In rare cases AIP type presentation may occur with defective ALA-dehydratase.

[2] If URO-synthase activity is reduced, polypyrrole changes into type 1 porphyrinogens.

- **AIP (Acute intermittent porphyria):** For diagnosis, urinary ALA and PBG (increased during the attack) and erythrocyte PBG-deaminase (inbetween the attacks and in asymptomatic heterozygotes) are evaluated. Heterozygotes can also be identified by RFLP studies in families in which preliminary data on their disorder exists.
- **HCP (Hereditary coproporphyria):** Coproporphyrin increased markedly in urine and feces, more so if case is symptomatic. Increased ALA and PBG during an acute attack. Enzyme study is not widely available.
- **VP (Variegate porphyria):** Increased copro and proto porphyrins in feces and coproporphyrin in urine in the symptomatic and urinary ALA and PBG in acute attacks.
- **PCT (Porphyria cutanea tarda):** Increased uroporphyrin and 7-carboxylate porphyrin in urine and isocoproporphyrin in feces. Urodecarboxylase activity reduced in red cells and cultured fibroblasts.
- **CEP (Congenital erythropoietic porphyria):** Decreased activity of URO-synthase increases synthesis and excretion of type 1 porphyrins. Confirmation by demonstrating low enzyme level in red cells. For prenatal diagnosis enzyme activity is studied in cultured amniotic fluid cells or porphyrin levels in amniotic fluid.
- **EPP (Erythropoietic protoporphyria):** Increased protoporphyrin levels in feces and red cells. Ferrochelatase activity in cultured lymphocytes and fibroblasts is reduced. In lead poisoning, too, there is inhibition of red cell ferrochelatase activity. This results in marked elevation of erythrocyte Zn protoporphyrin (ZPP). Only metal free protoporphyrin accumulates in EPP.

porphyrins (in cutaneous tissue) results in cutaneous photosensitivity. If excessive accumulation of both types of compounds occurs, it causes both cutaneous and neurovisceral manifestations.

Acute intermittent porphyria (AIP)

It is the most common of the inherited porphyrias. The defective enzymes are shown in Fig. 8.1. It is transmitted as an autosomal dominant trait but affects three females to every two males, meaning, thereby, that the disease has some relation to female sex hormones. Further condition seldom manifests before puberty. Acute intermittent porphyria occurs in the form of acute attacks with long periods of remission in between.

Typical attack presents with abdominal colic,

ileus and reduced bowel sounds, behaviour changes and less commonly with peripheral neuropathy. Abdominal symptoms are neurologic and not inflammatory since there is no abdominal tenderness, no fever or leukocytosis. Neuropathy is mostly motor and sensory changes are much less prominent. An attack may be precipitated by infection, fasting or some drug (alcohol, barbiturates, sulfonamides). For diagnosis see below and also see Fig. 8.1.

Symptomatic treatment may need some narcotic analgesic and phenothiazine (for nausea, anxiety). Intravenous hematin or heme-albumin produces recovery from the attack.

Diagnosis

In AIP and other acute porphyrias (which also

present as acute attacks), diagnosis requires demonstration of increased excretions of ALA and PBG in urine during an attack. Urine should be screened for PBG in any patient suffering from unexplained abdominal pain (especially in the presence of behaviour changes or psychosis or peripheral neuritis). Relation of an acute attack to certain drugs should be borne in mind. For screening of persons at increased risk (family members), it is best to look for PBG in urine in AIP, fecal porphyrins in VP and HCP. Alternatively defective enzyme can be measured (Fig. 8.1). In all the three acute disorders some commonly used drug may produce a serious illness.

Lead intoxication

Many manifestations of lead intoxication (abdominal pain, constipation and features of neuropathy) are similar to those of acute porphyrias and erythropoietic protoporphyria (EPP, Appendix 8.1). Lead inhibits ALA dehydratase, ferrochelatase and coproporphyrinogen oxidase (Fig. 12.1).

In lead intoxication, there is marked increase of erythrocyte Zn protoporphyrin (ZPP). In erythropoietic porphyria metal free protoporphyrin accumulates in erythrocytes. Screening for lead intoxication can be done by determination of ZPP in circulating red cells. ZPP is extracted in acetone followed by quantitation with a hematofluorometer. In the extraction procedure Zn remains attached to porphyrin and thus it is possible to differentiate lead poisoning from EPP. ZPP level should be expressed in terms of hemoglobin level of the sample. This avoids interference of anemia. If the test indicates presence of lead toxicity, confirmation, by estimation of lead in blood, is recommended.

ANALYTICAL NOTE

In an acute attack of porphyria (abdominal pain) the Waston-Schwartz test is used to screen urine for PBG. This compound (PBG) condenses with p-dimethylaminobenzaldehyde in HCl (Ehrlich's reagent) to form a magenta coloured complex. Fresh sample of urine protected from light, should be used for this test. The test is positive only when PBG level in urine is 3 to 5 times higher than the normal. Besides PBG, the test also gives a semiquantitative

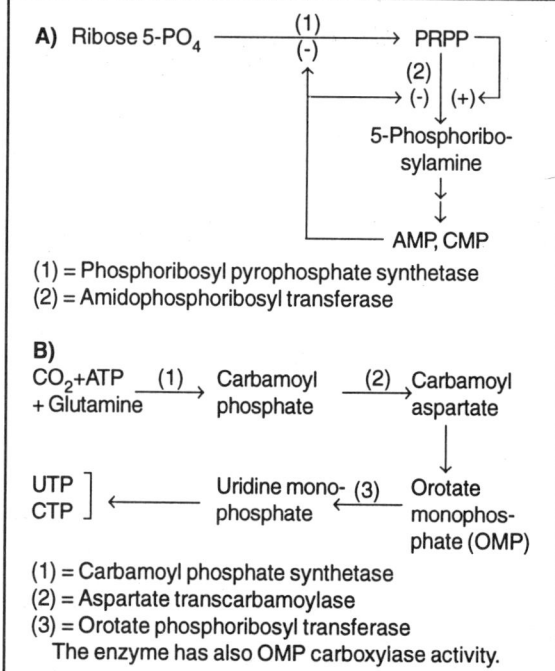

(1) = Phosphoribosyl pyrophosphate synthetase
(2) = Amidophosphoribosyl transferase

B)
(1) = Carbamoyl phosphate synthetase
(2) = Aspartate transcarbamoylase
(3) = Orotate phosphoribosyl transferase
  The enzyme has also OMP carboxylase activity.

Fig. 8.2. Feedback regulation of purine and pyrimidine biosynthetic pathways.

- Overactivity of PRPP synthetase causes hyperuricemia.
- Defect in orotate phosphoribosyl transferase causes orotic aciduria in which an infant suffers from megaloblastic anemia, orange coloured urine and orotic acid stones.

estimate of urobilinogen in urine. Normal urine contains only a small amount of the urobilinogen.

Porphyrins are coloured (because of presence of methenyl bridges) while porphyrinogens are colourless as they lack these linkages. All porphyrins have an intense absorption band near 400 nm (Soret band). When solutions of porphyrins are irradiated with light of this wave length, all free porphyrins exhibit an intense red fluorescence. This is used for screening urine, blood or feces for porphyrins. PBG and uroporphyrin are excreted only in urine (because of water solubility). Protoporphyrin is only excreted in bile (and feces) while coproporphyrin although mainly excreted in bile also appears in urine. For screening purpose, porphyrins are first extracted into an organic solvent (say acetic acid-ethyl acetate) and then reextracted into HCl. For irradiation, an ultraviolet source is used.

Examination of fluorescence spectrum of

porphyrins in plasma at neutral pH (saline diluted plasma) is used to differentiate VP from other porphyrias especially PCT (Appendix 8.1).

After prior purification, fluorometric methods can be used for quantitative analysis.

HPLC is commonly used for rapid identification and quantitative estimation of porphyrins in urine, blood and feces.

BIOSYNTHESIS AND DEGRADATION OF PURINE AND PRYIDINE NUCLEOTIDES

For endogenous synthesis of nucleic acids, the required purine and pyrimidine nucleotides are provided by de-novo synthesis (Fig. 8.2). During normal cell turnover, cell lysis results in breakdown of nucleic acids to nucleotides. The purine nucleotides are catabolized to uric acid (Fig. 8.3) and pyrimidine nucleotides to β-alanine, β-amino isobutyric acid, ammonia and CO_2. Some of the breakdown products may also be reused in formation of nucleotides (Fig. 8.3).

In the de-novo pathway for purines, purine nucleotides and not free purines are synthesized and the main pathway ends with formation of inosine monophosphate (IMP), which is next converted into other purine nucleotides. On the other hand the de-

novo pathway for pyrimidines, first gives rise to orotic acid which undergoes phosphoribosylation to orotidine monophosphate (OMP) which is decarboxylated to UMP by the same enzyme (Fig. 8.2). UMP can be converted into other pyrimidine nucleotides. Hereditary defect in orotic acid phosphoribosylation gives rise to the disorder of orotic aciduria. In the two pathways the nucleotide end products produce feedback inhibition of the first two enzymes of the respective pathway (Fig. 8.2).

Hyperuricemia and gout are discussed below while important features of other disorders related to the pathways are summarized in Appendix 8.3.

URIC ACID AND HYPERURICEMIA

In human body catabolism of purines produces uric acid. Body uric acid pool is about 1200 mg. It derives uric acid from catabolism of dietary and endogenous nucleoproteins and direct transformation of synthesized purine nucleotides (Figs. 8.2 and 8.3). Most of uric acid is lost from the body by excretion in urine and a small amount is excreted into gut where it is degraded by intestinal bacteria. 98% or more of uric acid present in glomerular filtrate is reabsorbed in proximal tubules. This is followed by tubular secretion of uric acid. In the second phase of tubular

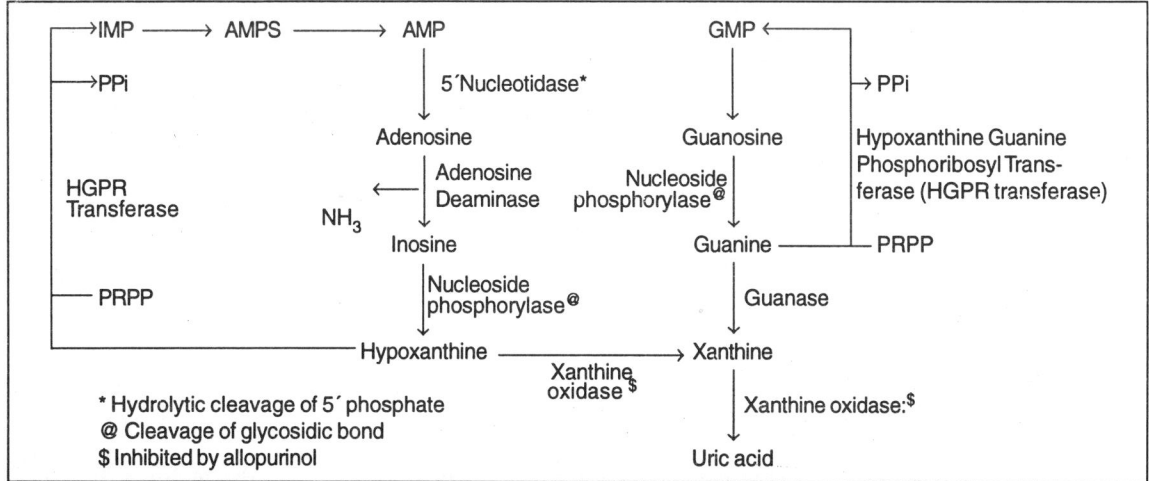

Fig. 8.3. Catabolism of purine nucleotides. Note that due to absence of enzyme adenase from animal tissues deamination takes place at the level of corresponding nucleoside or nucleotide. Note three inborn errors related to this pathway: adenosine deaminase deficiency, purine nucleoside phosphorylase deficiency and HGPRT deficiency.

reabsorption, about 40% of the secreted uric acid is reabsorbed. Uric acid that appears in urine, is only a little more than 60% of the secreted component.

The normal reference interval for uric acid is likely to vary depending upon the analytical method, the race, sex, age and also on social and geographical factors. The level in children is about 1 mg/dL less than adults. Urinary excretion of uric acid, in patients of hyperuricemia may help finding the cause (see below). Also see Fig. 8.4 & Appendix B.

Hyperuricemia and gout

Hyperuricemia is defined as blood uric acid level of >7.0 mg/dL. Above this level, risk of developing gout or urolithiasis is increased. Gout is hyperuricemia associated with acute arthritis (generally monoarthritis) and there is rapid response to the drug colchicine. The first metatarsophalangeal joint is most commonly involved (other joints at risk are of hand and feet and the ankle joint). Joint is tender and severly painful and there are associated fever, leukocytosis and raised ESR. The attack is self limited and may clear in about 10 days. Table 8.1 shows certain features and investigations which may help diagnosis.

Most patients of gout have hyperuricemia but most patients of hyperuricemia do not have gout. The two terms are not synonymous, although hyperuricemia is one important factor in development of gout/gouty nephrolithiasis. Gout is more common in patients of primary hyperuricemia. Hyperuricemia is called primary when its cause is not known (primary hyperuricemia: Appendix 8.2). In 75 to 90% of such patients there is reduced fractional excretion of uric acid and in 10 to 15%, hyperuricemia is caused by overproduction. Gout is uncommon if a known kidney disease is responsible for hyperuricemia, except in polycystic kidney disease.

Patients of gout should be investigated for hyperlipidemia and myeloproliferative disorders. If gout and severe hyperuricemia is encountered in a young patient, the enzymatic defects should be looked for (Appendices 8.2 and 8.3).

Acute gouty arthritis is produced by interaction between sodium urate crystals and different cells like polymorphnuclears, mononuclears and synovial lining cells. The activated cells release a host of mediators which produce local inflammation and tissue destruction and general reactions. The precise mechanism that initiates and attack of acute

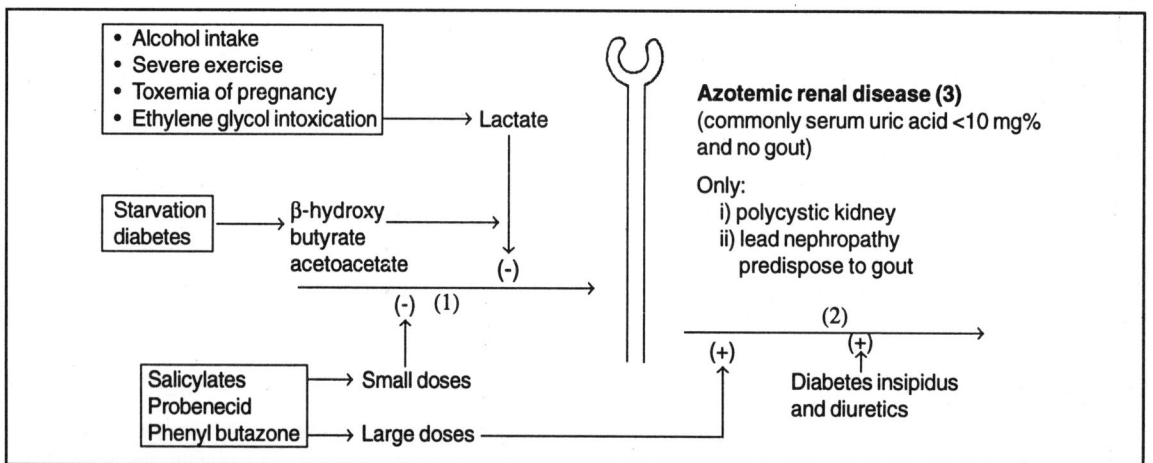

Fig.8.4. Some secondary causes of hyperuricemia in which urinary excretion of urate is modified.

(1) Secretion of urate. Note that a number of drugs in small doses, lactate, acetoacetate and hydroxybutyrate inhibit urate secretion to produce hyperuricemia.

(2) Reabsorption of urate. Diuretics and diabetes insipidus act by producing hypovolemia.

(3) In azotemic renal disease hyperuricemia is caused by reduced GFR and by increasing its reabsorption (not shown). Gout is not common in these disorders except in lead encephalopathy and polycystic kidney.

Table 8.1. Diagnosis of gouty arthritis

- Most patients of hyperuricemia, particularly those with secondary hyperuricemia do not develop gouty arthritis.
- Gouty arthritis is usually associated with primary hyperuricemia (runs in families, but mode of inheritance is not certain).
- Commonly occurs in men over 40. In females it may occur, only after menopause.
- Gout is commonly associated with a particular personality (high IQ, obesity, hypertension, increased alcohol intake and hyperlipidemia).
- It is generally monoarthritis which rapidly responds to colchicine or NSAIDs.
- X-ray examination is not helpful in early cases but shows punched out erosions later.
- Diagnosis is confirmed by demonstrating crystals of monosodium urate inside cells or free in synovial fluid. For this a wet smear of synovial fluid is examined . The compensated polaroscopic examination of a wet smear of joint aspirate is done. Crystals are negatively bifringent and needle like.

arthritis is not understood. An attack may be precipitated by trauma, sudden change in plasma uric acid level, infection, severe exercise, surgery or some other stress. Entry of certain proteins into the synovial fluid may have roles in initiating (IgG) and terminating (apo-B from lipoproteins) the attack. Acute attack is treated with use of anti-inflammatory drugs like NSAIDs and colchicine. Once the acute phase is over, some drug should be used to reduce serum uric acid level. Two types of drugs are used: i) which inhibit xanthine oxidase to reduce uric acid formation (allopurinol); ii) the uricosuric drugs (salicylate, probenecid). Their indications are presented in objective type questions.

Hyperuricosuria from dietary purine excess or from endogenous overproduction and low urine pH promote formation of stones (also see below) that are pure uric acid or mixed calcium oxalate and uric acid stones. To prevent nephrolithiasis, urine volume should not be allowed to fall below 2 L/d and it should be kept alkaline with the use of sodium bicarbonate or acetazolamide.

Gout and renal disease

Uric acid renal stones occur in 10 to 20% cases of gouty arthritis. These stones may, however, form even before arthritis. *Uric acid nephropathy* (uric acid precipitates to block collecting ducts), which

produces acute renal failure and *urate nephropathy* (deposits of sodium monourate in renal interstitial tissue, producing renal insufficiency) are less common. The latter condition is often associated with pyelonephritis. Urinary uric acid/creatinine ratio can be used to distinguish between acute renal failure with reduced urine output; produce by uric acid nephropathy (ratio >1.0) and that due to other causes (ratio <1.0). Uric acid nephropathy mostly depends upon serum/urine uric acid levels (and pH of urine), without susceptibility to gout.

Asymptomatic hyperuricemia

Important causes are given in Appendix 8.2. As already pointed out, hyperuricemia may be associated with gouty arthritis or renal disease but asymptomatic hyperuricemia as such, neither reduces renal function nor does it influence progression of an existing renal disease. Hyperuricemia is commonly associated with obesity, hypertension, diabetes and hypercholesterolemia and control of these associated disorders leads to decrease in plasma level of uric acid. However, hyperuricemia is not a risk factor for atherosclerosis. Asymptomatic hyperuricemia does not require treatment but its cause should be found out, which may need treatment.

HYPOURICEMIA

This condition is less common and generally, harmless. It is produced by congenital or acquired renal tubular transport defects. Important conditions are Fanconi syndrome, Wilson's disease, multiple myeloma and heavy metal toxicity. It may be produced by uricosuric drugs and total parenteral hyperalimentation. It may also be associated with certain malignancies, cirrhosis and diabetes mellitus. It is also a feature of a rare congenital condition of xanthine oxidase deficiency (or combined deficiencies of xanthine oxidase and sulfite oxidase) which may lead to formation of xanthine stones. Hypouricemia also results from purine nucleoside phosphorylase deficiency (Appendix 8.3). In a severe liver disease there is inhibition of conversion of xanthine to uric acid and hypouricemia may result. Hypouricemia may need no treatment but calls for finding the cause of the condition.

Appendix 8.1. Features of some porphyrias

ACUTE PORPHYRIAS
(accumulation and increased urinary excretions of PBG and ALA; leading to neurovisceral presentation):

Acute intermittent porphyria (AIP) (autosomal dominant occurs at adolescence):
* See the text.

Hereditary coproporphyria (HCP) (autosomal dominant, very rare, occurs in young adults):
* The affected patients may be asymptomatic or may present (after puberty) with neurovisceral symptoms, milder than as seen in AIP.
* Photosensitivity features (may also occur as in PCT and VP).
* Corproporphyrin III is almost always present in feces. Coproporphyrin, ALA and PBG appear in urine during an attack.
* Enzyme studies in red cells, liver tissue.

Variegate porphyria (VP) (autosomal dominant, occurs in young adults):
* Important disease in Whites in South Africa (high incidence).
* Presentation is variable. There may be cutaneous lesions and patient may also suffer from acute attacks.
* Skin lesions of VP, HCP and PCT can not be differentiated by clinical examination or skin biopsy study.
* Enzyme level in cultured fibroblasts, liver tissue, lymphocytes.
* VP can be easily differentiated from other porphyrias by examination of fluorescence emission spectrum of porphyrins in plasma at neutral pH. This is especially true for differentiating VP from PCT.

CHRONIC PORPHYRIAS
(no increased urinary excretions of PBG and ALA and no acute attacks; main feature is photosensitivity.)

Porphyria cutanea tarda (PCT) (autosomal dominant, starts in middle age):
* The most common porphyria in Europe and U.S.; may occur in sporadic/toxic forms (URO-decarboxylase activity reduced in liver but not in red cells and other tissues) and familial form (URO-decarboxylase activity reduced in all tissues).
* Hepatic URO-decarboxylase activity is reduced by alcohol, iron, estrogens and various chemicals (hepatotoxic).
* There is skin photosensitivity(see under VP)
* All patients have liver disease which can be cause or effect (or both) of the disorder.
* Treatment includes avoiding sensitizers and repeated phlebotomy to reduce liver iron load which inhibits the enzyme.

Erythropoietic protoporphyria[1] (EPP) (autosomal dominant):
* The second most common of the porphyrias.
* It may occur in early life or in adulthood and presents with skin photosensitivity. It may also produce chronic liver disease by accumulation of protoporphyrin in liver. Gall stones may also form.
* Feces are fluorescent because of elevated levels of protoporphyrin and coproporphyrin.
* Oral administration of β-carotene improves tolerance to light. Blood transfusion or intravenous heme therapy also helps (to suppress erythropoiesis; to inhibit hepatic synthesis).

Congenital erythropoietic porphyria (CEP) (autosomal recessive):
* Very rare disorder, in which a neonate shortly after birth presents with red coloured urine, hemolytic anemia and severe cutaneous photosensitivity. Teeth have reddish brown color and show fluorescence.
* Red coloured urine is due to excessive excretion of coproporphyrin and uroporphyrin (mainly type 1) in urine.

[1] Fluorescence microscopy or viewing protoporphyrins extracted into HCl (first extracted from blood into ether, acetic acid and next reextracted into HCl) in UV light, are used as screening tests to differentiate between EPP, lead toxicity and CEP.

- AIP, HCP, VP and PCT are hepatic porphyrias; EPP and CEP are erythropoietic.

Appendix 8.2. Important causes of hyperuricemia

Primary idiopathic hyperuricemia:

• Great majority of these patients are males (above 40 years) and suffer from reduced uric acid clearance. Runs in families. Inheritance may be autosomal dominant with incomplete penetrance or it may be a polygenic disorder.

Inborn errors causing hyperuricemia:

• HGPRT deficiency.
• PRPP synthetase overactivity due to mutant enzyme.
• Glycogen storage diseases types I*, III, V, VII.
• Fructose 1-PO$_4$ aldolase deficiency*.

Increased nucleic acid turnover:

• Lymphoproliferative, myeloproliferative disorders and other widely disseminated malignant neoplasms.
• Psoriasis, hemolysis, rhabdomyolysis.
• Use of chemotherapy and ionizing radiations for tumors.

Reduced uric acid excretion by increased organic acid excretion in urine or some ofther mechanism

• Diabetic ketoacidosis, lactic acidosis (alcohol*, severe exercise, toxemia of pregnancy, ethylene glycol intoxication).
• Sarcoidosis, hypothyroidism, down's syndrome, hypertension, hyperparathyroidism, lead intoxication.

Increased ATP expenditure causing increased nucleotide degradation:

• This mechanism operates in * marked causes.
• In alcoholics, lactic acidosis also promotes hyperuricemic.

Hypovolemia increasing tubular reabsorption of urate:

• Diuretics and diabetes insipidus.

Renal diseases:

• See objective type questions.

Drugs:

• See Appendix A.

- The most common causes of secondary hyperuricemia include, renal failure, ketoacidosis, lactic acidosis, toxemia of pregnancy and use of diuretics.
- Hyperuricemia also has a positive relationship with hyperlipidemia, obesity, atherosclerosis, hypertension (in hypertension cause may be reduced renal blood flow and increased vascular resistance), social class, exercise and achievement oriented behaviour.
- Increased ATP degradation also increases uric acid production by reducing feed back inhibition of the de-novo pathway because of lower levels of nucleoside mono-phosphates.

Appendix 8.3. Important features of certain genetic disorders related to metabolism of purine/pyrimidine nucleotides

Lesch Nyhan syndrome

• X-linked recessive disorder. As hypoxanthine and guanine are not utilized for nucleotide synthesis more of these change into uric acid.
  - Patient presents with neurological abnormalities (unrelated to high uric acid level in body fluids (spasticity, choreoathetosis, mental retardation).
  - Gouty arthritis and nephrolithiasis.
• Increased phosphoribosyl pyrophosphate synthetase activity (X-linked)
  - Gouty arthritis and nephrolithiasis.
• Adenine phosphoribosyl transferase deficiency
  - As adenine is not utilized for synthesis of nucleotides. It is converted into xanthine and 2,8 dihydroxy adenine.
  - Frequency of heterozygous state is 0.4 to 1.1 per 100.
  - Nephrolithiasis (2,8 dihydroxy adenine stones).

Orotic aciduria
(Orotic acid phosphoribosyl transferase deficiency; the enzyme includes activity of OMP-decarboxylase)
  - Infant suffers from megaloblastic anemia, orange coloured urine and orotic acid stones.

Adenosine deaminase deficiency
(Toxic metabolites accumulation causes inhibition of cell replication)
  - There are associated abnormalities in ribs, pelvis and scapula.
  - First there is deficiency of T-cells followed by that of B-cells as well.
  - The condition is responsible for 25% of all cases of combined T and B cell deficiency.

Purine nucleoside phosphorylase deficiency(PNP deficiency)
(Immune disorder with deficiency of only B-cells)
  - There is associated red cell aplasia.
  - In ADA deficiency and PNP deficiency the enzyme activities are studied in red cell lysate. Screening test is also available requiring dried sample of blood on filter paper.

Hereditary xanthinuria
(There is deficiency of xanthine oxidase)
  - Many patients are asymptomatic
  - Xanthine stones (in kidney) may form

Myoadenylate deaminase deficiency
(Formation of IMP from AMP is affected)
  - Patient may present with myopathy.

Adenylosuccinate lyase deficiency
(This enzyme is involved in bio-synthesis of purines)
  - Patient presents with psychomotor deficiency.

OBJECTIVE TYPE QUESTIONS

Pick out the wrong statement

1. Porphyrias

i) Liver and erythropoietic tissue are two major sites for porphyrin synthesis.

ii) Same regulatory mechanisms operate in liver and erythropoietic tissue to regulate the process.

iii) In acute porphyrias defect lies in hepatic synthesis.

iv) In acute porphyrias ALA or ALA and PBG excretions increase in urine.

v) Excretion of type 1 porphyrins occurs in porphyria with block in URO-synthase (in CEP).

2. Acute intermittent porphyria (AIP)

i) AIP behaves like an autosomal dominant disorder.

ii) Patients become symptomatic when exposed to factors which increase production of porphyrin precursors.

iii) Urinary excretions of PBG and ALA increase during an attack and become normal subsequently.

iv) It is not possible to identify the patient unless he is in an attack.

v) For management it is important to identify the precipitating factor/factors.

3. Acute intermittent porphyria

i) An acute attack of AIP may be provoked by alcohol and certain drugs including steroids.

ii) An acute attack may be provoked by infection or surgery.

iii) An acute attack may be provoked by a weight reducing diet.

iv) Seizures in acute attacks of AIP can be easily controlled with phenytoin.

v) Infusion of heme (as heme albumin or heme arginate) may be used to control an attack.

4. Porphyria cutanea tarda (PCT)

i) The defective enzyme is hepatic uroporphyrinogen decarboxylase (URO-decarboxylase).

ii) It is the most common porphyria.

iii) Like other hepatic porphyrias urinary excretions of ALA and PBG are increased.

iv) Finding of increased excretion of isocoproporphyrin in feces is diagnostic of PTC.

v) There is increased risk for hepatocellular carcinoma.

5. Erythropoietic protoporhyria

i) It is caused by partial deficiency of ferrochelatase.

ii) Exposure to sun causes more severe symptoms (redness, swelling, itching, burning sensations) than actual skin lesions.

iii) Urinary level of protoporphyrin is increased.

iv) Ferrochelatase activity is reduced in cultured fibroblasts and lymphocytes.

v) Lead intoxication can also inhibit ferrochelatase.

6. Variegate porphyria

i) It resutls from deficiency of protoporphyrinogen oxidase (PROTO-oxidase).

ii) it is quite common in Whites of South Africa.

iii) Plasma porphyrins are increased especially, when there are skin lesions.

iv) The skin lesions of VP, PCT and HCP are of different nature and can differentiate the three conditions.

v) The drugs which provoke AIP may also provoke VP.

7. PCT AND CEP

i) Three important features of CEP are hemolytic anemia, skin lesions and red coloured urine.

ii) In PCT, skin sensitivity is the major feature.

iii) Both PCT and CEP are equally common.

iv) PCT may require phlebotomy as iron induces hepatic URO-decaboxylase deficiency.

v) CEP may require blood transfusion because of hemolytic anemia.

vi) In PCT isocoprophyrins increase in feces.

vii) Red coloured urine in CEP is due to excretion of uro and coproporphyrins, mainly type 1.

8. Renal involvement in hyperuricemia/gout

i) In uric acid nephropathy, uric acid is deposited in renal interstitial tissue.

ii) Uric acid nephropathy can cause reversible acute renal failure.

iii) Urinary stones, in patients of gout, are not always composed of uric acid.

iv) In gout, kidney stones may be composed of calcium phosphate, calcium oxalate or of these salts mixed with uric acid.

v) Uric acid stones can develop in gout, before arthritis.

9. Asymptomatic hyperuricemia

i) Ordinarily, it is not treated, simply, for fear of developing renal damage or uric acid stones.

ii) It does not alter progression of existing renal disease.

iii) It is not an independent risk factor for athero-sclerotic disease.

iv) If associated with problems like hypertension, obesity, diabetes and hypercholesterolemia, there is need of treating these and not hyperuricemia.

v) Gouty arthritis is as common in hyperuricemia due to chronic renal failure as in primary hyperuricemia.

10. Diagnosis of acute gouty arthritis

i) The triad of acute monoarticular arthritis, hyperuricemia, and a quick response to colchicine is a good evidence for gouty arthritis.

ii) A definitive diagnosis requires demonstration of intracellular sodium urate crystals in synovial fluid.

iii) While using a hypouricemic drug the goal should be to reduce uric acid level to about 7.0 mg/dL.

iv) Diet should take care of obesity, hyperlipidemia, diabetes mellitus and hypertension.

11. Hyperuricemia/gout

i) Hyperuricemia is serum urate concentration >7.0 mg/dL.

ii) If hyperuricemia is found, its cause should be found out and treated.

iii) Urinary excretion of 800 mg/d is taken as the cut off level (person on regular diet) to decide about overproduction, as cause of hyperuricemia.

iv) In acute uric acid nephropathy the ratio of uric acid to creatinine in any urine sample is <1.0.

v) Acute uric acid nephropathy may require differ-entiation for acute renal failure from other causes.

12. Allopurinal in gout/nephrolithiasis

i) Patients at risk for acute uric acid nephropathy.

ii) When hyperuricemia is due to reduced excretion of uric acid.

iii) In presence of renal insufficiency (creatinine clearance <80 mL/min).

iv) Patients with nephrolithiasis (any type) and uric acid excretion >600 mg/d.

v) In old age or if uricosuric drugs can not be taken.

13. Primary gout

i) Although of genetic origin, fewer than one third of all patients have family history.

ii) It may be an autosomal dominant trait with incomplete penetrance.

iii) Close relatives, if not suffering from gout may show hyperuricemia.

iv) 90% of all patients of gout are males.

v) In >75% of these patients there is evidence of increased production of uric acid but cause is not known while in <15% there is decreased fractional clearance of uric acid when creatinine clearance is not reduced.

14. The alkaline phosphotungstic acid reduction method (urate estimation)

i) In the protein precipitation step, uric acid co-precipitates with uric acid.

ii) Occurence of turbidity during colour formation.

iii) Interference may occur from ascorbate, homogentisic acid, thiols and glucose (at higher plasma levels).

iv) Beer's law is not obeyed over the desired range of concentration of uric acid in plasma.

v) With suitable modifications, however, the above problems have been overcome and the modified method has become the most specific method for uric acid estimation.

vi) Uric acid is stable both in urine and serum, at room temperature, for about three days.

15. Urate retention in renal disease

i) It is caused mainly by reduction of GFR.

ii) Plasma urate level seldom increases above 10 mg/dL, probably because of increased gastrointestinal secretion and uricolysis.

iii) Clinical gout is uncommon in renal disease.

iv) Lead nephropathy is associated with gout in about 50% of cases.

v) In polycystic kidney gout may occur before the deteriorating renal function produces azotemia.

ANSWERS

1. No. (ii). different regulatory mechanisms operate in liver and the erythroid tissues.

2. No. (iv). Latent heterozygotes can be identified by studying level of PBG-deaminase in erythrocytes. This can also be done by RFLP studies in families with preliminary data on their disorder.

3. No. (iv). Almost all antiseizure drugs may worsen AIP; bromide is an exception.

4. No. (iii). PCT does not produce syndrome of acute porphyria and does not produce increased urinary excretions of the ALA and PBG.

5. No. (iii). Protoporphyrin levels are increasd in circulating red cells, plasma and feces but not in urine.

6. No. (iv). Not distinguished by clinical examination or biopsy of skin lesions. The three conditions must be distinguished by assay of

porphyrins and porphyrin precursors in blood urine and feces.

7. No. (iii). PCT is the most common of the porphyrias; EPP is next only to PCT in frequency. CEP is rare.

8. No. (i). Large amounts of uric acid crystals are deposited in renal collecting ducts. On the other hand in urate nephropathy (rare) sodium monourate crystals are deposited in renal interstitium to produce renal insufficiency.

9. No. (v). Gouty arthritis is very uncommon in hyperuricemia of chronic renal failure, except in cases of polycystic disease of kidney, in which its prevalence may be more than 20%.

10. No. (iv). Uric acid level should be reduced to about 5.0 mg/dL (below the saturation point of 6.8 mg/dL) so that the urate crystals start dissolving leading to reduced uric acid pool.

11. No. (iv). In most forms of acute renal failure with reduced urine output, uric acid to creatinine ratio is less than 1.0 as urinary level of uric acid is normal or reduced. This ratio is >1.0 in acute uric acid nephropathy.

12. No. (ii). When hyperuricemia is due to reduced excretion, there is indication of use of some uricosuric drug (other requirements are absence of urolithiasis, absence of renal insufficiency and age of the patient <60 years).

13. No. (v). It is the other way round. Reduced fractional clearance of uric acid is more common a cause than increased production.

14. No. (v). The most specific method is one which is based on oxidation of uric acid to allantoin by the enzyme uricase.

15. No. (i). Greater role is played by reduced secretion of uric acid than reduced GFR.

CHAPTER 9

Lipoproteins and Lipoprotein Disorders

LIPOPROTEIN STRUCTURE AND METABOLISM

Hydrophobic molecules of cholesterol (C) and triglycerides (TAG) are transported in plasma as lipid protein complexes called lipoproteins. In the peripheral part of these macromolecules lie phospholipids (PL) (with their polar heads facing aqueous plasma) and certain special proteins called apolipoproteins. These proteins lie interspersed between the surface PL molecules and perform functions like serving as ligands for receptors, as enzyme activators, as enzyme inhibitors and others.

Lipoproteins are analyzed by ultracentrifugation, in which these separate according to their densities and by electrophoresis in which these separate according to their charge (Table 9.1).

Apolipoproteins and their functions are given in Table 9.2.

Metabolism of lipoproteins

Lipoproteins carry exogenous or dietary lipids from intestine (chylomicrons) and endogenous lipids from liver (VLDL) to different tissues. In this way dietary TAG is distributed to tissues for energy purposes and to adipose tissue for storage. VLDL arising from liver carries TAG synthesized from carbohydrate or from FFA coming from adipose tissue. LDL arises from VLDL and carriers C synthesized in liver for use in other tissues. HDL collects C from tissues and lipoproteins, changes it into CE (cholesterol ester) for disposal in liver. Important reason for interest in metabolism of lipoproteins arises from their relation to atherosclerosis.

Table 9.1. Some properties of human lipoproteins

Lipoprotein (% of protein)	Electrophoretic mobility	Density	Lipid composition (TAG/C/PL) %
Chylomicrons (1-2)	Remain at origin	1.006	(80-95/2-7/3-9)
VLDL (7-10)	Pre-beta	1.006	(55-80/5-15/10-20)
IDL	Beta	1.006-1.019	(20-50/20-40/15-25)
LDL (about 20)	Beta	1.019-1.063	(5-15/40-50/20/25)
HDL (about 33)	Alpha	1.063-1.21	(5-10/15-25/20-30)
Lp* (a)	Pre-beta	1.04-1.08	

* This lipoprotein is formed by linking of apoprotein (a) with apo-B-100 of LDL. Apoprotein (a) has homology with plasminogen and is a glycoprotein different from apo-A proteins.

- A subspecies of LDL called small dense LDL contains more TAG than LDL.

- Both Lp (a) and small dense LDL are more atherogenic than LDL.

Table 9.2. Different apolipoproteins, their features and functions

A-I (29 KD, 243-245 aa) Major component of apoprotein part (75%) of HDL	Synthesized in liver and intestine. Impaired synthesis causes HDL deficiency. Activator of LCAT. Ligand for HDL receptors.
A-II (17.4 KD, 154 aa) 20% of apoprotein part of HDL	May be activator of HTGL
A-IV (44.5 KD) In small amounts present in HDL and chylomicrons.	May be a cofactor for LCAT. May facilitate transfer of apo-CII to chylomicrons/VLDL
B-100 (512.7 KD, 4536 aa) Forms 10% of VLDL and 90% of LDL	Ligand for LDL receptor (apo-B100, apo-E)
B-48 (240.8 KD) Forms almost 100% of apoprotein part of chylomicrons.	Same gene forms apo-B100 and apo-B48. For B48 the m-RNA is prematurely terminated. The part of B100 which acts as ligand for LDL receptor lies in carboxy terminal third of B100 and is missing in B48.
C-I (6.6 KD, 57 aa) Minor constituent of HDL and VLDL.	May activate LCAT.
C-II (8.9 KD, 78 or 79 aa) Forms 5 to 10% of VLDL protein and 2% of HDL protein.	It is a potent activator of LPL. Its absence is responsible for some cases of familial hyperchylomicronemia.
C-III (8.8 KD, 79 aa) It is a major component of VLDL protein (25 to 30%) and main form of apo-C in HDL	It inhibits lipolysis in triglyceride rich lipoproteins and may be involved in delaying clearance of remnant particles.
D(32 KD) It is a minor apo-lipoprotein. It is a minor constituent of HDL protein.	It can activate LCAT by acting as a specific carrier of lysolecithin.
E(34 KD, 299 aa) It is found in different lipoproteins except LDL. Also present in remnants.	Along with apo-B100 it is a ligand for LDL receptor and alone it is ligand for LRP (LDL related receptor protein).

- CETP (cholesterol ester transfer protein) helps transfer of CE from HDL to VLDL and IDL, in exchange for TAG.
- Apo-C-I, C-II and C-III are associated with all lipoproteins except LDL.
- Apo-A-I is the major apo-lipoprotein of HDL.
- Apo-A-I and apo-B as such are becoming important in predicting risk to CAD.

Chylomicrons and VLDL (Fig. 9.1)

Both lipoproteins transport TAG to tissues, chylomicrons from intestine (exogenous TAG) and VLDL from liver (endogenous TAG). Chylomicrons are secreted with apo-B-48, apo-A-I, apo-A-II, apo-A-IV, apo-C-II, apo-C-III and apo-E while VLDL particles are secreted with apo-B-100, apo-C-II, apo-C-III and apo-E. Some part of quota of apo-C-II, apo-C-III and apo-E, of these lipoproteins is acquired in circulation from HDL.

Chylomicrons and VLDL unload their TAG in tissues (muscle, adipose tissue) with the help of LPL (lipoprotein lipase) activated by apo-C-II. After unloading TAG, chylomicrons change into chylomicron remnants and VLDL into IDL. As these smaller particles are being formed, lipid exchanges occur between these particles and HDL. TAG and PL pass to HDL while cholesterol ester passes in the reverse direction (Fig. 9.2). CETP

(cholesterol ester transfer protein) catalyzes this lipid transfer. Fig. 9.2 also shows transfer of certain apoproteins from HDL to chylomicrons and VLDL and then back to HDL.

Chylomicron remnants are finally completely metabolized in liver. IDL is, partly, taken up like chylomicron remnants and completely metabolized. The rest of IDL is changed into LDL by loss of TAG with the help of HTGL (hepatic triglyceride lipase) in hepatic sinusoids (Fig. 9.1).

LDL

LDL arises from VLDL as shown in Fig. 9.1. About two thirds is metabolized in liver and the rest in extra hepatic tissues. It is bound on LDL receptors and internalized and then exposed to lysosomal enzymes. Apo-B-100 is completely degraded, and CE hydrolysed and LDL receptor is recirculated to cell membrane for reuse. Free cholesterol (C)

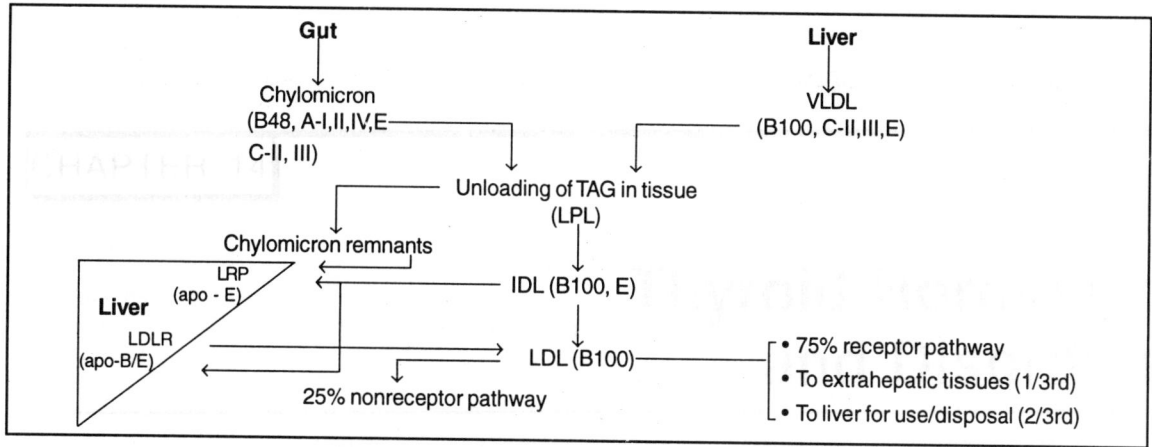

Fig. 9.1. Metabolism of chylomicrons and VLDL.

- Some VLDL may arise in intestine and is metabolized like chylomicrons.
- Apo-E as well as apo-B100 are ligands for LDLR (LDL-receptors). These receptors can bind, IDL and LDL. Only apo-E is the ligand for LRP (LDL-related protein). It can bind IDL and chylomicron remnants.
- About 50% of IDL is completely metabolized in liver and the rest 50% changes into LDL.
- Some workers believe that after unloading of TAG, VLDL changes into VLDL remnants. Some of these remnant particles are completely metabolized in liver, like chylomicron remnants, others change into IDL with the help of HTGL (hepatic triglyceride lipase) in hepatic sinusoids. IDL then changes into LDL explaining intravascular formation of LDL.

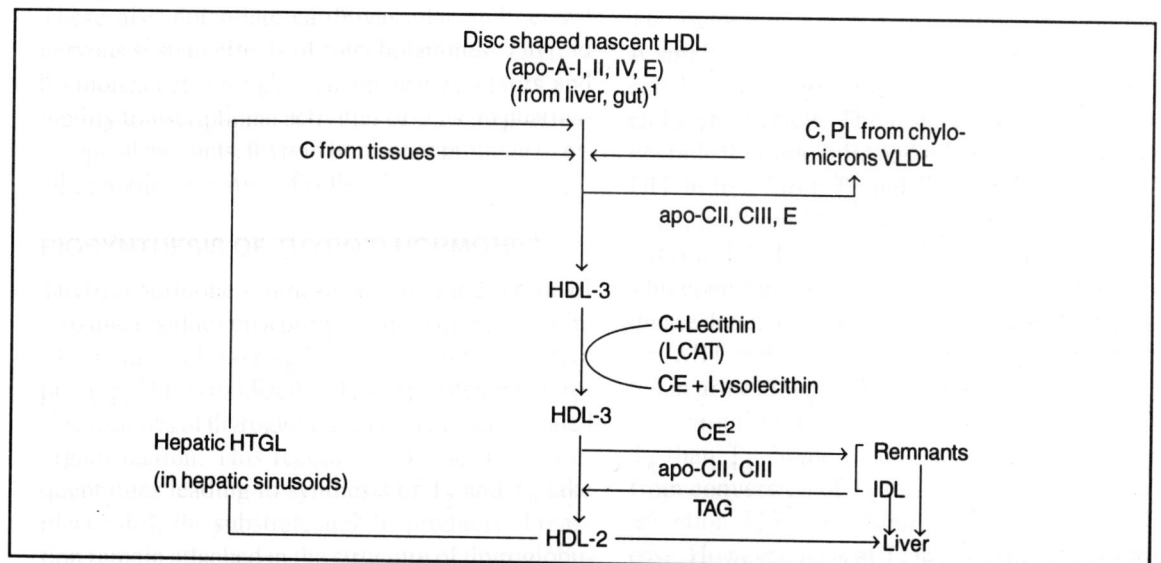

Fig. 9.2. Metabolism of HDL.

---

[1]The C apoproteins can be added to HDL after their secretion as PL - complexes or by transfer from TAG rich lipoproteins. HDL may also arise denovo in circulation from surface components (C, PL, A-I, A-II, C-I, C-II, C-III of TAG rich lipoproteins, as these are catabolized). Efflux of excess C from foam cells (in vessel wall) along with apo-E also results in secretion of HDL.

[2]Transfers of CE and TAG are mediated by CETP.

- Apo A-I is important to maintain integrity of HDL particles and responsible for its anti-atherogenic function.
- Apo A-I and A-II arise both from liver and intestine, A-IV is synthesized in intestine.

produced is used by the cell for membrane synthesis, steroid synthesis (in steroid hormone secreting cells) and other purposes. Some is reesterified by microsomal acyl cholesterol acyl transferase (ACAT) for storage; for use it can be hydrolyzed by a neutral cholesteryl ester hydrolase (CEH). Free C in the cell can reduce its denovo synthesis by inhibiting HMG-CoA reductase (Fig. 9.3). Finally, any surplus C is transferred to the surface of cell membrane to be collected by HDL for final disposal in liver.

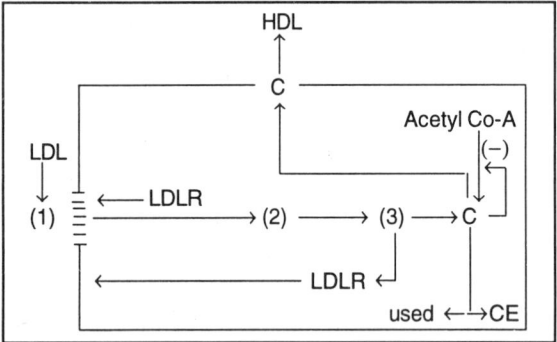

Fig. 9.3. The receptor pathway of LDL in extrahepatic tissues.

---

(1) Uptake of LDL at LDL-receptor (LDLR)
(2) Endocytosis and formation of endosome (it contains LDL + LDLR).
(3) Hydrolysis in endolysosome.
  - Released LDLR is recycled.
  - Released C is used in the cell.
  - Denovo C synthesis is inhibited.
  - Some C is stored as CE with the help of acyl Co-A cholesterol transferase (ACAT)
  - Surplus C is passed on to cell membrane for take up by HDL.

In liver cells, there is excretion of LDL-C as such and after its conversion to bile salts. It is also reused in VLDL biosynthesis. This helps to keep serum C in the normal range. In hypothyroidism there is reduction of LDL receptors on liver cells and it leads to increase in level of serum C. Also many drugs used for lowering serum C level act by inducing LDL receptors, on hepatic cells.

About role of LDL, some modified forms of LDL and other lipoproteins, in atherogenesis, read under "hyperlipidemia and atherogenesis".

HDL

Nascent HDL is synthesized in liver and intestine, composed mostly, of phospholipid and apo-A-I, apo-A-II and apo-A-IV. The apo-C-II and apo-C-III are added subsequently or received from other lipoproteins. It receives C from cells and also from other lipoproteins (Fig. 9.2). The enzyme lecithin-cholesterol-acyl-transferase (LCAT) esterifies C to CE and in this form this lipid is transported back to liver, either directly (by HDL) or by transfer to other lipoproteins (IDL, chylomicron remnants) on their way to liver. This is called reverse cholesterol transport.

During their metabolic cycles, there is exchange of lipids and apoproteins between HDL and TAG rich lipoproteins (Fig. 9.2). HDL is anti-atherogenic because of its role in reverse C transport. Other reason for anti-atherogenic role may be, ability of HDL to remove C directly from foam cells (which secrete apo-E containing lipid particles, which may themselves be HDL particles). HDL also protects LDL from oxidation and also low HDL state is commonly associated with increase of apo-B lipoproteins.

HDL cycle is shown in Fig. 9.2. Increased CETP activity in hyperglyceridemia interferes in this cycle and may promote atherogenesis (Fig. 9.4).

DISORDERS OF LIPOPROTEIN METABOLISM

A large number of clinical disorders are related to abnormalities of metabolism of lipoproteins. The most significant one is atherosclerosis, leading to coronary artery disease (CAD) and other diseases. Other clinical conditions, not related to atherosclerotic process are acute pancreatitis, hepatic steatosis, certain skin lesions (xanthomata, xanthelasmata and others) and certain neurological and ocular disorders. Lipid disorders may be primary or because of presence of certain other diseases (secondary lipoprotein disorders). Many drugs also produce lipid abnormalities. Once a patient is known to have a lipid disorder and for some other disease, needs a prolonged drug therapy, the drug should be chosen carefully, with respect to its effect on plasma lipids.

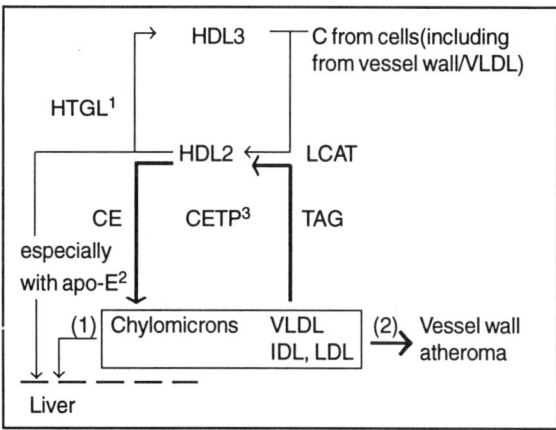

Fig. 9.4. Hypertriglyceridemia interference in reverse cholesterol transport; low HDL-C and atherogenesis.

---

[1] Conversion of HDL2 to HDL3 during circulation through liver. HTGL unloads TAG.

[2] HDL2 may also be completely metabolized in liver.

[3] Hypertriglyceridemia increases CETP activity.

- Hypertriglyceridemia increases exchange of lipids between HDL2 and apo-B lipoproteins. The CE-enriched lipoproteins are then diverted to vessel wall (instead of liver). However, chylomicrons and their remnants may not be able to enter vessel wall (because of large size), thus excluding, atleast, hypertriglyceridemia of familial LPL deficiency as a risk for CAD.

- Factors in relationship between hypertriglyceridemia and low HDL levels include, increase CETP-mediated transfer of CE from HDL to VLDL (and other lipoproteins), shift of phospholipids, C-II and C-III from HDL to VLDL (and other lipoproteins) and increased fractional clearance of CE-poor HDL.

- Reverse C transport means: C from cells → HDL → HDL (CE) → apo-B lipoproteins → liver. Hypertriglyceridemia interference in the process causes shift of CE back into cells (reduced process (1) increased process (2)).

Secondary causes of lipid disorders (Table 9.3)

Diabetes mellitus

In IDDM, if the glycemic control is poor, there is increased production of VLDL (increased FFA influx into liver) and reduced VLDL disposal (LPL inhibition by insulin deficiency: increased apo-C-III content of VLDL). There is increase of both VLDL and LDL-C and HDL-C is reduced. A good glycemic control normalizes VLDL, TAG and LDL-C and also increases HDL-C. In NIDDM with presence of obesity and insulin resistance, there is increase of VLDL and TAG and HDL-C is reduced. In

the presence of an associated familial lipoprotein defect, hypertriglyceridemia becomes marked and even risk to acute pancreatitis may be there. LDL-C may not increase although LDL is of small dense type. In families of patients of NIDDM, some members may show only, hypertriglyceridemia, some only diabetes and some both diabetes and hypertriglyceridemia. In NIDDM glycemic control is less effective in normalization of lipid levels especially HDL-C. Weight control may be more effective.

In most diabetics plasma lipid levels are in the normal range but atherogenesis is increased. This may be because of some subtle lipoprotein abnormalities adding to the atherogenic effect of some other factors present in NIDDM (Fig. 7.5). Thus hypertriglyceridemia of diabetes always needs careful management.

Hypothyroidism

Hypothyroidism causes hypercholesterolemia by reducing LDL metabolism by the receptor pathway. Besides increase of total C, there is increase of LDL-C and apo-B. Total-C/HDL-C and LDL-C/HDL-C ratios also increase. In thyroid hormone deficiency, LPL activity is also reduced leading to hypertriglyceridemia. Hypothyroidism is known to exacerbate lipidemia of dysbetalipoproteinemia. The above referred lipid abnormalities are seen even in subclinical form of hypothyroidism. Thus in any lipid abnormality, it is important to determine T_4 and TSH levels to diagnose subclinical hypothyroidism, which can produce almost any lipid abnormality.

Obesity

Obesity especially central obesity (or abdominal obesity) is related to hypertension, hyperinsulinemia, diabetes type 2 and blood lipid disorders (↑TAG, ↑C). Obese subjects have increased rates of synthesis of bile acids and C. Although there is increase of C, HDL-C is reduced. With loss of weight there is decrease of TAG and C levels and increase of HDL-C. Exercise gives additional benefit over and above that produced by loss of weight.

Pregnancy and lactation

During pregnancy total-C may increase by 50%

Table 9.3. Some important secondary hyperlipidemias

Diabetes mellitus:

↑VLDL ± ↑ Chylomicrons, ↓HDL: ↑TAG. Diabetes treated with insulin will metabolize VLDL to LDL, causing normalization of VLDL but initial increase of LDL (β-shift). Also see the text.

Hypothyroidism:

↑ LDL, ±↑ VLDL: ↑C, ±↑ TAG, even in subclinical hypothyroidism (↑TSH, nT_4). Also see the text.

Nephrotic syndrome:

Increased VLDL synthesis which is coupled to albumin synthesis, LDL formation also increases from VLDL. There is reduced TAG hydrolysis due to low albumin to accept FFA. There is loss of HDL in urine. ↑LDL, ±↑VLDL, ↓HDL: ↑C, ↑±TAG. There is also increase of Lp(a). Associated hypertension and increased clotting tendency further accelerate atherosclerosis.

Uremia:

There is reduced activity of LPL and insulin resistance may increase adipose tissue lipolysis and increased entry of FFA into liver (VLDL synthesis): ↑VLDL, ↑TAG. There is low LDL-C and TAG enrichment of HDL and LDL (reduced activity of HTGL).

Obstructive liver disease:

• Due to obstruction there is entry of biliary lecithin into plasma which reacts with free C, albumin and apo-C to form LpX. This lipoprotein has density in LDL range but LpX does not react with LDL receptors. This condition is thus resistance to drug treatment. Total-C is increased.

Obesity:

There is often increased TAG and reduced HDL-C. Those with elevated waist-hip ratio (abdominal obesity) have increased total-C and increase of small dense LDL, increased TAG and increased apo-B. It may be a part of a syndrome comprising, upper body obesity, glucose intolerance, hypertension and hypertriglyceridemia. There is increased incidence of CAD. Also see the text.

Alcoholism:

Acetate from alcohol spares FFA from oxidation, increased amounts of which are diverted to TAG and VLDL synthesis; increased level of NADH also stimulates FFA synthesis. There is increase in levels of VLDL and TAG. If an alcoholic has genetic hyperlipidemic background there will be increase of chylomicrons also and very high levels of TAG. Even risk to acute pancreatitis may develop. HDL-C level is increased as there is stimulated apo-A-I synthesis and inhibition of CEPT.

- β-Adrenergic blocking agents increase VLDL and TAG and reduce HDL.
- Hypothyroidism is responsible for 2% of all cases of hyperlipidemias and is, second, only to diabetes as a cause of secondary hyperlipidemia.

and TAG by about 100%. Increase is still more in cases of pre-eclampsia. At six weeks postpartum the lipid levels normalize. Increased level of cholesterol, during pregnancy does not increase risk for CAD. If a woman is suffering from mild familial hypertriglyceridemia or some other genetic disorder of TAG removal, quite high levels of TAG may be attained in third trimester of pregnancy. Further her triglyceridemia will go on worsening with repeated pregnancies. At some stage it may become a risk for acute pancreatitis. Some other secondary hyperlipidemias are summarized in Table 9.3.

Primary hyperlipoproteinemias

Most of the primary disorders are polygenic in which the genetic defects are not clearly defined and also the phenotypes result from interaction between the genetic and the environmental factors. The primary disorders may be grouped in different ways. For present discussion, these are being grouped as disorders causing hypercholesterolemia, hypertriglyceridemia and mixed hyperlipidemia. Important features are summarized in Table 9.4.

Disorders causing hypercholesterolemia

Familial hypercholesterolemia

There is selective increase of LDL (and LDL-C) right from birth and levels increase during childhood and adolescence and in heterozygous adults

Table 9.4. Common forms of primary hyperlipoproteinemias

Disorders (modes of inheritance)	Lipoprotein increased (TAG/Total-C mg/dL)	Phenotype[1]	Remarks
Disorders causing hypercholesterolemia:			
Familial hypercholesterolemia (AD)	LDL (Total-C:275-500 in heterozygotes, >500 in homozygotes)	IIa (plasma clear)[2]	*(relatively common)* Early vascular disease Tendon xanthomata
Familial apo-B-100 defect (AD)	LDL (Total-C:275-500 in heterozygotes) (often less than above disorder)	IIa	*(less common than above)* Probably same as above but often less severe
Polygenic hypercholesterolemia	LDL (Total-C:275-350)	IIa	*(more common than first)* Risk to vascular disease No tendon xanthomata
Disorders causing hypertriglyceridemia:			
Familial lipoprotein lipase deficiency (AR)	Chylomicrons (TAG:>750)	I, V (plasma milky)	*(rare)* Risk to pancreatitis, abdominal pain, hepatosplenomegaly.
Familial apo-CII deficiency	As above	As above	*(very rare)*
Familial hypertriglyceridemia (AD)	VLDL (TAG: 250-750) TAG-enriched VLDL	IV (plasma cloudy)	*(most common)* Risk to vascular disease may be there.
Disorders causing mixed hyperlipidemia:			
Familial combined hyperlipidemia (AD)	VLDL and/or LDL (reduced HDL) (TAG:250-750, Total-C: 250-500) Greater no. of VLDL particles	IIb (plasma turbid)	*(quite common)* Risk to vascular disease
Familial dysbeta-lipoproteinemia (AR)[3]	VLDL, IDL (normal LDL, reduced HDL) C-enriched VLDL. (TAG:250-500, Total-C 250-500)	III (plasma turbid)	(relatively common) Risk to vascular disease Palmar, tuboeruptive xanthomata.

[1] Phenotype V (milky plasma; on standing supernatant creamy, infranatant milky; ↑ chylomicrons, ↑ VLDL, total-C 250-500 mg/dL; LDL-C not much ↑; HDL-C ↓, TAG markedly ↑) is rare infamilial form but common in secondary forms (when a secondary cause of hypertriglyceridemia complicates FCH or FHT or when two causes of hypertriglyceridemia exist together).

[2] In the standing plasma test (observing plasma after keeping it at 4°C, overnight), type I (creamy layer at top, clear underneath), type IIa (all clear), type IIb and III (no creamy layer, clear to turbid), type IV (plasma cloudy and unchanged on standing) and type V (see above).

[3] Disease expression requires homozygosity for apo-E_2 and presence of some other factor causing hyperlipidemia.

- FCH may present with only increased TAG level (D/D Familial hypertriglyceridemia) or with only increase of total-C (D/D polygenic hypercholesterolemia). But commonly, both FCH and familial dysbetalipoproteinemia present with increased TAG as well as total-C.

- As VLDL and chylomicrons are competing substrates for LPL, any condition causing high levels of VLDL will increase level of chylomicrons as well (also vice versa).

serum C levels are generally higher than 350 mg/dL. There is early coronary artery disease (CAD). In about 30% cases, CAD occurs before the age of 40 years. A high serum C level in the absence of significant hypertriglyceridemia is highly suggestive of the diagnosis. The family should also be screened for the disorder. Lipid deposits in the form of tendon xanthomata, xanthelasmata, and arcus senilis are also commonly seen. The tendon xanthomata are quite specific.

The disorder is caused by LDL receptor defect. Defect may relate to receptor protein synthesis, its intracellular transport, receptor clustering, its binding to LDL or its recycling. An allied disorder is caused by defective apo-B-100 which does not allow proper binding to its receptor (it produces a relatively milder disorder).

Familial hypercholesterolemia needs drug treatment (Appendix 9.1). Useful drugs are bile salt sequesters, nicotinic acid and HMG-CoA inhibitors. The drugs in the last group have very few side effects. Some patients of FCH (see below) may also present with the same phenotype as in familial hypercholesterolemia.

Polygenic hypercholesterolemia

This condition is much more common than familial hypercholesterolemia. In these patients, multiple genes interact with environmental factors to produce the disorder. Unlike the familial disorder (see above) plasma C levels are not very high (<350 mg%) and patient greatly benefits from dietary management.

In patients of high LDL-C, before diagnosis of familial hypercholesterolemia, polygenic hypercholesterolemia should be ruled out. Also looking for hypothyroidism or nephrotic syndrome (urine examination for protein) may also be rewarding as the two conditions result in increased LDL-C.

Disorders causing hypertriglyceridemia

In one group of patients, hypertriglyceridemia is produced because of poor activity of LPL and failure to metabolize exogenous TAG (familial chylomicronemia), with accumulation of chylomicrons in plasma. In the second group there is increased synthesis of TAG enriched VLDL particles which are not properly metabolized by LPL (familial hypertriglyceridemia), resulting in accumulation of VLDL in plasma. Lipidemia is worsened, in this group of patients, if some additional factor increases FFA influx into liver (obesity, impaired effectiveness of insulin, alcoholism).

Chylomicrons and large VLDL particles fail to enter arterial vessel wall and thus familial chylomicronemia is considered free from risk of atherogenesis while in familial hypertriglyceridemia (FHT) this risk is considered doubtful, although any delay in clearing of VLDL and remnants may generate more atherogenic LDL and remnants and in addition, may lead to decrease in HDL level (Figs. 9.4, 9.5).

Familial chylomicronemia (Familial LPL deficiency)

In this disorder LPL activity is reduced because of enzyme defect or defect in its activator, apo-C-II. As there is poor disposal of chylomicrons, in the standing plasma test (Table 9.4), there is creamy layer with clear plasma underneath. Serum TAG levels are very high (often >1000 mg/dL). VLDL is normal or increased (especially in pregnancy due to high levels of estrogens). Total-C may be increased slightly but not LDL-C; HDL-C may be normal or reduced. Post heparin lipolytic activity of plasma is absent. In cases of coenzyme deficiency (apo-C-II), the same can be demonstrated by isoelectric focussing of proteins of VLDL.

The disorders are present from birth and may be recognized in early infancy or in adulthood with an attack of acute pancreatitis or by the presence of lipemic serum. Other clinical features include, eruptive xanthomas (yellowish papules with erythematous bases) lipemia retinalis and hepatosplenomegaly. Risk of CAD is not increased. Acute pancreatitis is caused by release of FFA and lysolecithin in capillary bed of pancreas (from lipoproteins); FFA lyse parenchymal cell membranes, when binding capacity of albumin is exceeded.

Treatment lies in reducing amount of fat in diet but maintaining required intake of essential fatty acids and fat soluble vitamins.

Familial hypertriglyceridemia (Endogenous)

Hypertriglyceridemia may occur as a familial disorder or more commonly, as secondary lipid disorder in diabetes, obesity, alcoholism, hypothyroidism, uremia and with the use of oral contraceptives. The familial disorder is probably inherited as autosomal dominant trait with reduced penetrance.

Phenotype is that of WHO type IV and there is increase in plasma VLDL and TAG. LDL-C is normal and HDL-C normal or low (Table 9.4). Condition is mild unless complicated by another lipidemia producing condition (see above). In latter cases, WHO phenotype V may be produced. In such cases risk of pancreatitis may develop and patients should be treated with both diet and drugs (like nicotinic acid and fibrate). Ordinarily, only dietary treatment in enough.

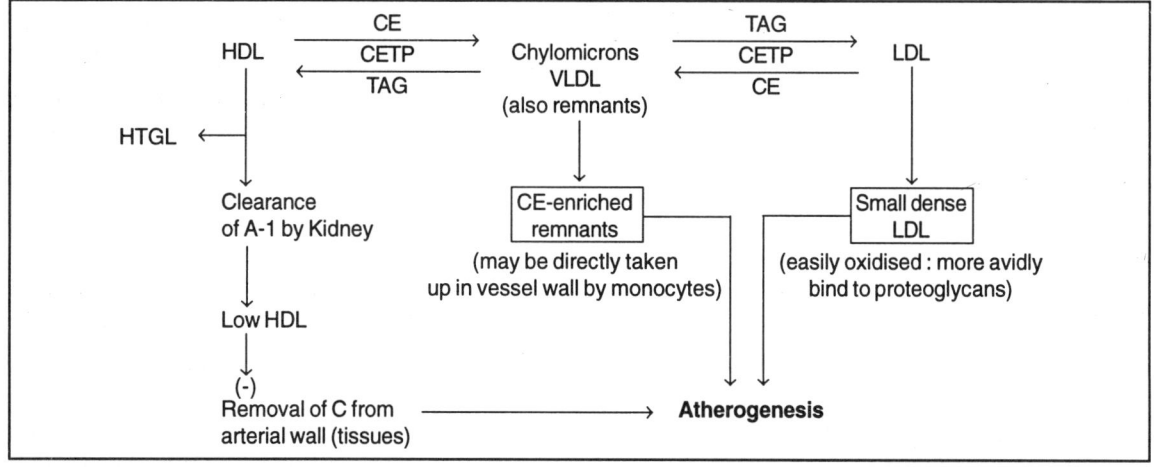

Fig. 9.5. Atherogenesis promoted by delay in clearing of apo-B lipoproteins from circulation.

- Any delay in clearance of TAG rich particles in plasma promotes the above reactions causing atherogenesis (occurs in apo-B, lipoprotein genetic abnormalities).
- Low apo-A (HDL) and the small dense LDL levels may also be determined genetically.
- In familial chylomicronemia the retained particles are too large to enter vessel wall (no risk of premature atherosclerosis). In familial hypertriglyceridemia such a risk is doubtful.

Although, risk of CAD is considered controversial in familial hypertriglyceridemia (FHT), in some studies 5 to 15% of myocardial infarction survivors were found to have this disorder. These patients were frequently overweight, had low HDL-C, and many also had male type obesity, insulin resistance, type 2 diabetes and hypertension. This disorder (may be a subgroup of FHT) was named familial dyslipidemia. In FHT, however, LDL-apo-B is not increased.

Disorders with mixed lipidemia

Familial combined hyperlipidemia and familial dysbetalipoproteinemia are disorders which cause increased levels of total C and TAG in plasma. In the latter disorder, there is accumulation of remnant particles both from exogenous and endogenous pathways, as their disposal is impaired. The former disorder is a heterogeneous group in which there may be increased synthesis of apo-B-100 and/or defective clearance of VLDL. A variable lipoprotein phenotype is produced. HDL levels are reduced in both types of disorders. A delay in clearing of remnants from plasma can promote atherogenesis (Fig. 9.5).

Familial combined hyperlipidemia (FCH)

In this disorder patients may have increased levels of both VLDL and LDL (combined hyperlipidemia) or only one of the two. Further lipoprotein pattern of a given patient is different from that of his family members and also the pattern changes from time to time. The disorder is not fully expressed until adulthood. Tendon and tuberous xanthomas are not part of clinical presentation of this disorder.

A number of variants of this disorder have been reported. These are all characterized by small dense LDL particles (Fig 9.5), and include hyperapo-B (discussed separately), LDL subclass pattern B, familial dyslipidemic hypertension, and syndrome X. Besides small dense LDL these syndromes also share other features like hyperinsulinism, glucose intolerance (or diabetes type 2), hypertension and low levels of HDL (especially when TAG level is high). Some of these features are also present in common patients (besides variants) of FCH. Most patients of FCH have reduced levels of HDL.

The main genetic defect in FCH and its variants is increased production of apo-B-100. Other defects which could contribute towards/produce the phenotype of the disorder are, increased production of apo-C-III (which inhibits LPL activity), defective formation of apo-A-IV (which helps transfer of apo-C-II to chylomicrons. Table 9.5 Compares some features of FHT and mixed lipidemias.

As risk of CAD is significantly increased in these patients, they should be treated vigorously with diet and drugs.

Dysbetalipoproteinemia

In this disorder plasma VLDL (β–VLDL) is unusual and increased; (LDL-C and HDL-C are low or normal). β–VLDL is enriched in C and the ratio of VLDL-C to total TAG is higher than 0.3. Its electrophoretic mobility is that of β-lipoprotein rather than pre-β-lipoprotein. Plasma levels of C and TAG are approximately same when expressed as mg/dL; both lipids being increased. Marked lipidemia and clinical features are delayed until adulthood. Patients have tuberous xanthomas (on extensor sides of elbows and knees) and planar xanthomas (of palmar creases). Patients are often, obese, diabetic, hypertensive and hyperuricemic. Atherosclerotic diseases of coronary artery and peripheral vessels, occur, commonly.

In this disorder, remnant particle metabolism is impaired because of defective iso-form of apo-E (named apo-E2). The disorder is produced by apo-E2/2 phenotype. One percent population has apo-E2/2 phenotype but disease prevalence is only 1:2000. Thus some other lipid defect must be present for disease expression. Often patients have obesity, diabetes, alcoholism or hypothyroidism. For diagnosis see under investigations. Treatment is dietary (low saturated fat, low cholesterol and no alcohol). Drugs may also be needed (Appendix 9.1).

Familial hyperapobetalipoproteinemia (Hyper-apo-B)

In familial combined hyperlipidemia (vide supra)

Table 9.5. Comparing features of FCH, FHT and dysbetalipoproteinemia

Familial combined hyperlipidemia (FCH)	Familial hypertri-glyceridemia (FHT)	Familial dysbeta-lipoproteinemia
↑ apo-B Synthesis (↑no. of VLDL)	TAG rich VLDL (poor disposal by LPL)	┌────── β-VLDL ──────┐ VLDL IDL Remnants ↓(-) ← apo-E$_2$/2 →(-) ↓ Final disposal LDL
Phenotype IV ↔ IIb ↕ ↕ V IIa	Phenotype IV ↔ V	Phenotype III
Phenotype varies in the patient and variable in his family	Phenotype IV may worsen to type V	Phenotype expression needs a complicating hyperlipidemia factor
Total-C, TAG moderately ↑. ↑LDL-C, ↓HDL-C	Total-C (N), TAG (<350 mg%) LDL-C (N), ↓HDL-C	Total-C & TAG moderately ↑ N/↓ LDL-C, ↓HDL-C, ↑IDL-C
Diet control, weight loss may change phenotype IV to IIb or IIa. (Flip-flop pattern)	In type V, eruptive xanthomas (diet control, weight loss converts type V to type IV)	Palmar and tuberous xanthomas (not seen in FCH)
Confirmation may require LDL apo-B study		Confirmation may require electro-phoresis and study of isoforms of apo-E

- Any condition in which disposal of VLDL is delayed there is increased exchange of TAG and CE between VLDL and HDL, increasing CE content of VLDL.
- In FHT risk of CAD is controversial. A subclass called dyslipidemia carries increased risk for CAD (see text).
- FCH and familial dysbetalipoproteinemia are mixed lipidemias. TAG, total-C ratio lies between 1 to 3. In the latter disorder this ratio is commonly 1.

there is increased production of apo-B-100 accompanied with increased secretion of VLDL. In the present disorder plasma levels of apo-B are increased without increased plasma level of VLDL. Risk of CAD is increased.

Familial hyperalphalipoproteinemia

Mutations of CETP gene lead to presence of certain CETP proteins in Japanese and cause hyper-α-lipoproteinemia and longevity. In these patients total-C, apo-A-I and HDL-C are increased, LDL-C is normal and TAG is low or normal. There is decreased risk of CAD.

Familial lipoprotein (a) excess

Lipoprotein (a) particle is LDL with one molecule of apo (a) attached to it. Apo (a) has some structural homology with plasminogen. Increased level of this lipoprotein is a heritable trait, and causes premature coronary artery disease. Measurement of lipoprotein (a) is commercially available.

Familial Hypo-α-lipoproteinemia

Severe deficiency of HDL is rare and is found either due to some abnormality in apo-A-I, A-IV, C-III gene complex or when fractional catabolism of HDL is increased (Tangier disease, LCAT deficiency). In Tangier disease besides low HDL, there are other lipid abnormalities. Total C is reduced and TAG, moderately, raised. There is storage of CE in tissues. There is, thus, enlargement of tonsils, adenoids, and spleen. Risk of CAD is slightly higher but not to the extent, expected from loss of protective effects of deficient HDL.

LCAT deficiency is a rare disorder in which plasma CE level is very low but levels of C and TAG are raised. As LCAT is important in normal metabolism of lipoproteins, plasma contains abnormal lipoproteins in this disorder. There is high concentration of nascent HDL. Plasma contains an abnormal subfraction of LDL called lipoprotein X (Lp-X) which is also found in patients of cholestasis (Table 9.3). VLDL is also abnormal (migrates differently on electrophoresis). The abnormal lipoproteins are deposited in glomeruli (causing renal damage), in RBC membrane (reducing their life

span) and these also produce premature atheromas in large arteries.

Mild deficiency of HDL (due to decrease of apo-A-I production or enhanced fractional catabolism) is common in patient of familial combined hyperlipidemia and other familial hyperlipidemias. It has been postulated that familial combined hyperlipidemia, familial dyslipidemia, familial hyperapobetalipoproteinemia, and familial hypoalphalipoproteinemia may be variants of the same disorder in which there is increased secretion of apo-B containing lipoproteins and increased catabolism of apo-A-I containing lipoproteins. Phenotypic abnormalities are brought out by an atherogenic diet and there is also predisposition to central obesity, and increased risk of CAD.

Abetalipoproteinemia

There is failure to secrete apo-B and therefore chylomicrons, VLDL and LDL are absent from plasma. There is failure of fat absorption. If the child survives, he or she suffers from many neurological defects (attributable to malabsorption of vitamin A and E). Serum lipids are very low and only HDL is present. It is extremely rare autosomal recessive disorder. Patients are treated with fat-soluble vitamins.

Familial hypobetalipoproteinemia

This disorder (autosomal dominant) is because of defects at the apo-B locus, leading to reduced formation of apo-B or formation of truncated gene products. In the homozygous state for null alleles condition appears like abetalipoproteinemia. Compound heterozygous patients present with a milder disease. Patients are treated with vitamin E. There may be decreased risk to CAD.

Hyperlipidemia and atherogenesis

As already mentioned hyperlipidemias are related to a number of human disorders including atherosclerosis. Atherosclerosis is a complex process involving lipid factors, factors related to thrombotic process and other factors. The lipid factors may be measurable and amenable to management, measurable but not amenable to management and neither measurable (at present) nor amenable to treatment (Fig. 7.5).

LDL-C has a direct relation to atherogenesis and CAD. The same cannot be said for total-C since it also includes HDL-C. Thus when total-C levels is modestly high ($\approx$260 mg%) it is advisable to measure HDL-C, (levels of which are inversely related to atherogenesis). However, when total-C levels are higher, these are due to LDL-C since HDL-C can almost never contribute more than 120 mg% to total-C except in obstructive liver disease.

LDL-C is atherogenic since LDL particles can readily penetrate into arterial intima. VLDL (especially large particles) cannot penetrate the vessel intima and may not be atherogenic. In case, however, elevated VLDL leads to increase of IDL (which can penetrate vessel intima), atherosclerosis will be promoted.

Oxidative modification of LDL in the arterial wall promotes the atherogenic process in so many ways (endothelial cells, monocyte-macrophages and smooth muscle cells cause this oxidation). As apoprotein is modified its uptake at LDL-receptor is reduced and uptake by the scavenger pathway is increased, causing formation of foam cells. In addition, the oxidatively modified LDL in the vessel wall stimulates secretion of a number of cytokines and growth factors by endothelial cells, smooth muscle cells and monocyte derived macrophages. This results in recruitment of more monocytes in the lesion area and proliferation of smooth muscle cells. The activated smooth muscle cells synthesize and secrete increased amounts of extracellular matrix which is part of the atherosclerotic lesion. In animal models, treatment with antioxidants has been shown to reduce the extent of atherosclerosis.

Lp (a) found in some cases of hyperlipidemia, is more atherogenic than LDL. Increased atherogenesis may be related to capacity of Lp (a) to inhibit thrombolysis or it may be because it binds more avidly to matrix in vessel wall. Lp (a) levels can be studied electrophoretically.

A subspecies of LDL called small dense LDL is also more atherogenic than LDL. Conditions associated with this lipoprotein have high level of TAG (Fig. 7.5, 9.5). Estimation of this lipoprotein for clinical purposes is not possible as yet.

Very high TAG levels, say >800 mg/dL (due to chylomicrons or TAG enriched VLDL) do not contribute to atherogenesis (as the lipoprotein particles causing hypertriglyceridemia cannot enter vessel wall due to their large size). This is especially true if HDL is not low. On the other hand, even lower TAG levels (250 to 500 mg/dL) in the presence of increased levels of LDL, IDL, C-enriched VLDL (in FCH, dysbetalipoproteinemia) promote atherogenesis.

Besides lipid abnormalities (see above), some other controllable risk factors for atherogenesis are, hypertension, diabetes, smoking, hemostatic factors (hyperfibrinogenemia, hyperhomocysteinemia), sedentary life (moderate exercise increase HDL-C, lowers blood pressure and reduces blood clotting tendency) and obesity. Presence of family history increases likelihood of atherogenesis. Women in the reproductive years of life are protected. Homozygous deletion mutant (DD) of angiotension converting enzyme has also increased risk. Excessive free radical production may also predispose to atherogenesis. In smokers, there is increased fibrinogen level and in animal studies, smoke has been associated with increased endothelial permeability, platelet aggregation, platelet production of TXA_2 and mitogenic activity of smooth muscle cells in culture.

Lipoprotein risk factors in women

Estrogens in women in reproductive period of life are highly protective against the atherosclerotic process. Estrogens lower LDL-C levels and act as an anti-oxidant to reduce LDL uptake by the arterial wall. They may also act by decreasing platelet adhesiveness (in the atheromatous plaque) and by influencing local prostacyclin and thromboxane levels.

LDL-C is an equally potent risk factor in women as in men but low HDL-C is more potent predictor of risk for CAD in women than in men. Same is true about TAG levels which are more strongly indicative of risk for CAD in women. Weight loss in women may not increase HDL-C (in men there is increase of HDL-C) and LDL-C remains, relatively, unaffected. All these different observations in women (compared to men) are possibly due to much higher levels of estrogens. Diabetic women have more favourable lipoprotein pattern than men. Higher waist to hip ratio leads to lower HDL-C and higher LDL-C, and higher risk of CAD. This relationship is stronger in women than men.

Women tolerate oral contraceptives well and these do not increase risk for CAD (except for women who smoke also). Combination of smoking and use of oral contraceptives greatly increases risk for CAD. Premenopausal women tolerate atherogenic lipids better than men.

For the purpose of treatment the lipid lowering drugs are discouraged in premenopausal women and dietary treatment is preferred. In post menopausal women in selected cases estrogen therapy may be tried to lower LDL-C and raise HDL-C before other drugs are used.

INVESTIGATIONS

Incidence of CAD and other atherosclerosis related disorders can be reduced if people, in general, receive timely advice on risk factors for these disorders, including the atherogenic lipids. However, some individuals/patients need to be investigated and treated on priority. These include: i) patients with clinical evidence of CAD or some other atherosclerotic disorders; ii) if there is an accompaniment of a lipid disorder like xanthelasma or tendon xanthomata, lipemic plasma or corneal arcus at an age of less than 40 years; iii) patients having a disease which can cause secondary hyperlipidemia; iv) if more than two risk factors for CAD are present, although there is no CAD; v) those with family history of CAD.

Besides these priority patients, it is advisable that all adults also get themselves screened for lipid disorders. For screening, total-C, TAG and HDL-C levels are estimated (Table 9.6). Next, those with total-C of 200 mg/dL to 239 mg/dL, and with less than two risk factors (HDL-C <35 mg/dL is also taken as a risk factor) are given information on dietary modification, physical activity and risk factor reduction. Those with total-C of 240 mg/dL or more or those with total-C of 200 to 239 mg/dL but with two major risk factors or those with clinical evidence

of CAD (or any other atherosclerotic process) are chosen for estimation of LDL-C and other investigations (to establish any primary lipoprotein abnormality) and treatment, as described below.

If lipid abnormality is found, carefully exclude any secondary cause of hyperlipidemia and if present, treat it. If no secondary cause is found, the individual is put on a hyperlipidemia management diet for a period of 3 months. If hyperlipidemia persists, he is investigated for his primary lipoprotein disorder and treated depending upon the level of his LDL-C.

Investigating for a secondary cause of hyperlipidemia

Important secondary causes are hypothyroidism, diabetes mellitus, excessive alcohol intake, cholestatic liver disease and nephrotic syndrome. Some of these causes can only be discovered after investigations. Every case of hyperlipidemia should be investigated for hypothyroidism by estimating TSH and T_4, since subclinical hypothyroidism can produce lipid abnormalities. Excessive fat intake also can increase plasma lipid levels.

Blood sample

Blood sample should be taken after an overnight fast of 12 to 14h since after a fat containing diet there is increase of TAG and that in turn, causes decrease of both HDL-C and LDL-C (because of CETP activity).

Before investigations, the patient should have been free from all drugs for previous 2 weeks. Stress of any serious illness can also alter plasma lipids. Thus, lipid investigations should be undertaken only 3 months after myocardial infarction, a major surgical operation or any other serious illness. After myocardial infarction, a sample taken within 12h, is unaffected by the event and may be useful to indicate the lipid values prior to the episode. Prolonged application of tourniquet also alters plasma volume and levels of plasma lipids (Chapter 1).

The procedure to arrive at the diagnosis of primary lipoprotein disorder of the patient, primarily depends upon, the clinical presentation of the disorder, the results of the standing plasma test and plasma levels of total-C and TAG. Generally, it is possible to define the primary lipoprotein abnormality by the investigations mentioned above (Tables 9.4, 9.5). At times, a few other investigations may also be needed. Some times diagnosis of familial dysbetalipoproteinemia may require knowledge of VLDL-C/plasma TAG ratio. This ratio lies between 0.1 to 0.25 (mass/mass) in normals while in familial dysbetalipoproteinemia the ratio is more than 0.3. Electrophoretic study of plasma lipoproteins is of limited value in diagnosis and only occasionally used. Ultracentrifugal fractions of d<1.006 kg/L and d>1.006 kg/L are studied electrophoretically (agarose gel electrophoresis is preferred) for diagnosis of β-VLDL and Lp(a), respectively. In ordinary electrophoresis of plasma proteins, Lp(a) would overlap VLDL and β-VLDL would overlap LDL. Increased levels of Lp(a) in white races (but not in American and African Blacks) has been reported as a risk factor for CAD.

Occasionally, studies of apo-A, apo-B or apo-E may be needed. In some studies it has been demonstrated that apo-A-I and apo-B (more so the latter) are better predictors of the atherosclerotic process than HDL-C and LDL-C. These two apoproteins can be studied by immunoassay methods. In practice, however, the apoprotein studies are not required except in some cases to demonstrate absence of E-3 and E-4 isoforms of apo-E, in confirmation of diagnosis of dysbetalipoproteinemia. The study needs electrofocussing of TAG rich fraction of plasma.

Result variations in lipid analysis

A number of factors affect plasma lipid levels. These include, age, sex, season, posture, period of venous occlusion, food intake (effect will also depend upon the caloric content, the amount of fat and cholesterol), drugs, pregnancy and a number of clinical conditions.

A person interpreting results of plasma lipids should be conversant with uncertainties of these measurements. For example a laboratory operating with CV of 3% and bias of 3% will have total error of 8.9% (1.96 (% CV) + % bias). Further, lipoprotein-C results are more variable than results

of total cholesterol (as more number of steps are involved in the former estimation). It should also be understood that a number of factors other than analytical (see above) can effect the results and due attention should have been paid to such factors while sample is collected for analysis. One should also be familiar with large physiological variations of levels of cholesterol, TAG and lipoproteins. CV of physiological variations within an individual averages about 6.5%, but can be higher in certain individuals. Thus, when serial samples from an individual are measured, in 95% of the samples there will be variation of 13% above or below his mean value. As physiological variation is much higher than the analytical variation, measurements must be made in several samples taken at weekly intervals to establish the person's usual lipoprotein concentration. (In practice at least two samples should be analyzed and mean of the two is used to define the patient's lipid status. If the two samples give quite variable results the analysis of third sample may become necessary).

Desk top analysis of lipids

Some of the instruments are based on dry chemistry analysis, and use reagent impregnated strips or slides. The sample (about 20μl) diffuses into reagent containing zone (and dissolves reagents) where the enzymatic reaction occurs. At the end of the incubation period, concentration is worked out from the reflectance measurement. In some instruments total-C, HDL-C and TAG can be measured from a single sample. Some analyzers use reagent solutions and finally absorbance measurements are done.

When these instruments are operated by experienced operators and properly calibrated, the results are reasonably accurate and precise. A dry chemistry test for cholesterol for home use is also available. In measurements, finger prick samples give more variable results than the venous samples.

MANAGEMENT OF HYPERLIPIDEMIA

Treatment of a lipid disorder aims at correcting the abnormal lipid levels, since these predispose to atherosclerosis, pancreatitis and other pathological

Table 9.6. The desirable and high levels of total-C and TAG in plasma in adults without evidence of CAD

	Total-C (mg/dL)	LDL-C (mg/dL)	TAG (mg/dL)	HDL-C (mg/dL)
Desirable	< 200	< 130	< 200	> 60
Border line high	200-239	139-159	200-400	35-60
High	≥ 240	≥ 160	400-1000	<35
Very high			>1000	

- HDL-C of <35 is a risk factor and >60 is a negative risk factor.
- Levels of total-C and HDL-C decide need for further investigations. If total-C is <200 mg especially with HDL-C >35 mg/dL, only awareness on diet and risk factors is required and no further invetigations are undertaken (more details in the text).
- Need for treatment with diet or with diet and drug is decided by the levels of LDL-C. The treatment goals are also decided by the LDL-C levels.
- Although HDL-C level less than 35 mg/dL is considered as an independent risk factor for CAD, no specific treatment is available to increase this level. Many drugs, however, which lower LDL-C also tend to increase HDL-C.
- If only TAG level is increased and LDL-C is not high, TAG level must be brought down to less than 400 mg% to reduce risk for development of acute pancreatitis, hepatomegaly and hepatic steatosis.
- In certain specific cases, ↑ of both LDL-C (or IDL-C) and TAG (as in FCH and dysbetalipoproteinemia), along with treatment of LDL-C, the TAG levels are also brought down to <200 mg/dL to reduce risk for CAD (in these cases high TAG levels become independant risk factor for CAD.

changes in the body. Commonly the abnormal LDL-C and TAG levels are treated without bothering about the actual primary disorder. The lipoprotein disorder, however, may become important, some times. For example reduced intake of calories as fat is useful in disorders of exogenous pathway and reduced caloric intake as carbohydrate is useful in disorders of endogenous lipoprotein pathway. Risk for CAD is also better defined by the precise lipoprotein abnormality than simple LDL-C level.

LDL-C is a better predictor of risk for CAD than total-C. As already mentioned the treatment goals to reduce risk of cholesterol to atherosclerosis are related to LDL-C and not total-C (Table 9.6). At present there are no such goals for lowering plasma TAG levels. Generally, however, when high TAG levels are brought down to less than 400 mg%, risk for acute pancreatitis is greatly reduced. Further, in cases where TAG levels are between 250 to 500 mg%, although there is very little risk for acute pancreatitis, the added risk for CAD may or may not be there. This is decided by the level of LDL-C or presence or absence of increased IDL. TAG levels of 250 to 500 mg/dL, if due to dysbetalipoproteinemia or FCH, become an independent risk factor for CAD. Presence of central obesity, hypertension, insulin resistance and low HDL-C levels (even in the absence of increased LDL-C)

make high TAG level, an independent risk factor for CAD. The same is also true in diabetes mellitus. In all these cases where high TAG levels are an independent risk factor for CAD, if levels are brought down to less than 200 mg%, the risk to CAD is much reduced. In diabetes with atherosclerotic disease the target value during lowering of TAG is 150 mg% or less.

Low HDL-C is considered as an independent risk factor for CAD. However, no specific treatment is prescribed in that connection. Generally, however, dietary changes and many drugs which lower LDL-C (especially gemfibrozel and niacin) also increase HDL-C. Other factors which tend to increase HDL-C are exercise, loss of excessive weight and stopping smoking.

In many subjects with mild to moderate hyperlipidemia, control of diet alone will be sufficient to normalize the lipid abnormalities. If some drug has to be used it should be used on a proper foundation of diet control. In children drugs are not used except in case of familial hypercholesterolemia with presence of other risk factors (cholestyramine is the drug of choice). Drug treatment should be avoided in pregnancy.

Restriction of calories

Calories should be reduced to have weight close to

the average of the desirable body weight for the height (severe weight loss is undesirable as it may increase plasma-C level). Obesity, especially, central obesity (increased waist to hip girth ratio) is an independent risk factor for CAD. Besides, excessive body weight increases LDL-C and TAG and reduces HDL-C. It also leads to increase in both systolic and diastolic blood pressures. Moderate exercise, besides helping to reduce body weight, has other protective effects for CAD, which include: i) ↓ in process of atherosclerosis of CAD; ii) ↓ in risk of thrombosis; iii) ↑ in myocardial metabolic capacity/mechanical performances; iv) ↑ in cardiovascular capacity; v) reduced vulnerability to ventricular fibrillation. Exercise has an additional HDL-C increasing effect besides that realized through weight reduction.

Fat intake

Saturated fatty acids down regulate hepatic LDL - receptors and thus tend to increase plasma C levels. However, stearic acid and medium chain fatty acids are free from this effect (out of common fatty acids of neutral fat). PUFA (polyunsaturated fatty acids) do not increase plasma C levels but may reduce HDL-C slightly when taken in excess (>13% of total calories), more so in men and are potentially carcinogenic as these increase production of oxygen free radicals. Monounsaturated fatty acids or MFA, present in olive oil, high oleic safflower and sunflower oils, peanut and canola oils, do not increase LDL-C and in addition raise HDL-C.

In lowering of TAG levels, reduction of total caloric intake plays a greater role than varying the source of calories. For example for lowering of TAG levels from higher to less than 500 mg%, a marked restriction of fat and calories is required, along with increased exercise (to reduce adipose tissue mass). Alcohol and refined carbohydrates should be restricted. Fat should be in the form of some vegetable oil rich in PUFA and MFA and carbohydrtaes should be used in the form of complex carbohydrates.

Some physicians prefer to obtain more calories from fats in phenotypes IV and V (abnormalities of endogenous lipoprotein pathway) while reducing calories from carbohydrates. In such a situation, long chain fatty acids (saturated, cis-monounsaturated, polyunsaturated) should be used instead of medium chain fatty acids which tend to increase TAG levels like carbohydrates. This regemin is suitable for lean individuals but should not lead to increase in weight. PUFA (n-3) from fish oils are also useful in lowering TAG levels but these may increase LDL-C. These should not be used in diabetes as these may worsen the diabetic control. Fish oils have to be used as a drug (3 to 7 g/d) as small amounts are not effective.

For lowering of LDL-C, NCEP recommendations are given in Table 9.7. From practical stand

Table 9.7. NCEP recommendations for dietary management of high LDL-C levels

Dietary item	Step 1 diet	Step 2 diet
Total-fat	<30% calories	0% calories
Fatty acids		
- Saturated	<10% calories	<7% calories
- Polyunsaturated	<10% caloreis	≤10% calories
- Monounsaturated	10-15% calories	10-15% caloreis
Carbohydrates	50-60% calories	50-60% calories
Protein	10-20% calories	10-20% calories
Cholesterol	<300 mg/dL	<200 mg/dL

- LDL-C levels for starting dietary treatment, drug treatment and as goals of treatment in the three groups (no CAD and <2 risk factors; no CAD and 2 or more risk factors; and with CAD) are, respectively, ≥160, ≥190, <160;   ≥130, ≥160, <130; >100, >130, <100 (mg/dL).

- Step 1 diet may lower LDL-C by 8-10% and step 2 by another 5 to 7% although there are great individual variations. For drugs see Table 9.5.

- NCEP = National Cholesterol Education Program (USA)

point one should reduce intake of whole milk dairy products, egg yolk, red meat, palm oil, coconut oil and in their place increase intake of fresh fruits, vegetables, complex carbohydrates (especially whole grain products) and low fat dairy products. Fat should be obtained from sources of low saturated fat (bran, nuts and olive oil).

Besides diet, lifestyle also influences the athero-sclerotic process. Thus along with a healthy diet (with respect to risk for CAD) a healthy lifestyle (moderate physical activity/exercise, no smoking, periods of relaxation, avoiding social isolation, avoiding work related stress especially high demand low decision attitude) should be adapted as part of enjoyable life. Diet itself has influence on three important risk factors, body weight, lipid profile and hypertension.

Appendix 9.1. Drugs for lowering plasma lipids.

TO LOWER ONLY LDL-C

Bile acid binding resins:

• Cause loss of bile acids in stools.	↓LDL-C	Causes malabsorption.
• ↑Hepatic LDL-receptors	↑HDL-C and TAG	Also use soluble fiber (adds to LDL-C loss).

Probucol:

• Precise mechanism of action remains elusive. May be increasing nonreceptor mediated catabolism of LDL-C.	↓ LDL-C by 10-20% (like fibrates)	
• Has additional antioxidant action.		

TO LOWER LDL-C & TAG AND TO INCREASE HDL-C

Fibrates:

Precise mechanism of action not known. May be

• ↑LPL activity	↓↓↓TAG (VLDL)	Long term risk of cholelithiasis.
• ↓VLDL synthesis	LDL-C (variable)	May cause myositis.
• ↑LDL catabolism	↑↑ HDL-C	Monitor with LFTs.

HMG-CoA reductase inhibitors:

• ↓ cholesterol synthesis	↓↓ TAG (VLDL)	Drugs of choice in dysbeta-
• ↑LDL receptors (hepatic)	↓↓↓LDL-C	lipoproteinemia; preferred over
	↑ HDL-C	resin in cases with very high LDL-C and in high risk ones.

Nicotinic acid:

• Precise mode of action not known.	↓↓↓TAG (VLDL)	Inexpensive drug; not used in
• Probably acts by reducing synthesis of VLDL (by reducing influx of FFA into liver) and LDL	↓↓LDL-C	diabetes (worsens diabetic
	↑↑ HDL-C	control). Also not used in patients of hyperuricemia renal, liver and peptic acid disease

---

- In case of high LDL-C and TAG <200 mg%, use cholestyramine (alongwith soluble fiber). Add lovastatin if necessary.

- In hypertriglyceridemia and FCH (main increase of VLDL and TAG, with or without increase of LDL-C), nicotinic acid is the drug of choice if it can be tolerated, otherewise use fibrate. Any increase in LDL-C as such or if caused by drug may need additional use of small amount of cholestyramine.

- PUFA (n-3) from fish oils are also useful in lowering TAG levels in hyperlipidemic patients except in diabetics since the diabetic control is worsened.

- In dysbetalipoproteinemia, drug of choice is some fibrate although, HMG-CoA inhibitors can also be used.

CASE HISTORY: 9.1

In a 32 year old obese woman, taking oral contraceptives, during routine investigations, plasma appeared turbid (sample was taken after an overnight fast). In the standing plasma test, a thin creamy layer was seen over the turbid plasma. Levels of serum C and TAG were 190 and 700 mg/dL, respectively. She was advised to stop the use of oral contraceptives. After about 3 months, serum TAG was reduced to 350 mg/dL.

The patient is likely to be a mild case of familial hypertriglyceridemia, although, obesity itself could also contribute to the lipid profile of the patient. Incidence of this familial disorder is 1 in 600, in normal population. Generally, TAG level is not very high and lipoprotein phenotype is WHO type IV. However, in the presence of some secondary cause (obesity, use of alcohol, oral contraceptives, therapeutic glucocorticoids, diabetes mellitus), TAG level may become very high and lipoprotein phenotype becoming WHO type V. Eruptive xanthomas may make their appearance and risk of pancreatitis is also increased. Risk of CAD in such cases is controversial and may depend upon the level of HDL-C, presence or absence of small dense LDL, insulin resistance and certain clinical features like hypertension. The patient under reference needs dietary treatment and alternative method of contraception. Oral contraceptives lead to worsening of an already existing lipid disorder, as in the present case. In normal women, however, oral contraceptives are tolerated quite well.

WHO phenotype V can also be produced in a severe case of FCH but in that case LDL-C will be increased. FCH has increased risk for CAD while phenotype V produced in familial hypertriglyceridemia may be free from this risk. This phenotype can also occur in apo-C-II deficiency cases of primary chylomicronemia. Apo-C-II deficiency may also produce phenotype I (produced by familial deficiency of LPL).

Familial LPL deficiency is a rare disorder which presents with features like eruptive xanthomata (crops of itchy yellowish pappules with erythematous bases), hepatomegaly, lipemia retinalis and recurrent abdominal pain. Ultimately acute pancreatitis may occur. In cases of familial LPL deficiency (phenotype I) if fat is restricted to about 10 g/d for 3 to 5 days, TAG level may fall sharply (say from 1000 mg to about 400 mg/dL).

Type V phenotype may also result in an obese person suffering from uncontrolled diabetes (presence of two secondary causes of hypertriglyceridemia). Proper control of diabetes will sharply reduce TAG level but may increase LDL-C.

CASE HISTORY: 9.2

A 42 year old patient consulted his physician because

of his arcus senilis and xanthelasma (small yellowish grey plaques around eyes). His BP was in the normal range and his ECG record was also normal. Serum C level was 310 mg%, and TAG in the normal range.

> ➤ What is the significance of xanthelasma and arcus senilis in the patient?
> ➤ How to investigate this patient?
> • Arcus senilis is quite suggestive of some lipid disorder but it may be present in many individuals without any lipid abnormality. Xanthelasma is suggestive of hypercholesterolemia, especially when present in an individual below the age of 40 years. In older people it may be found without such abnormality. Tendon xanthomata, however, are pathognomic of familial hypercholesterolemia. Eruptive xanthomata indicate hypertriglyceridemia. Xanthomas are deposits of fatty material in the skin, subcutaneous tissue and tendons.
> • With total-C of 310 mg/dL and TAG in the normal range, presence of FCH or dysbetalipoprotinemia is unlikely. Two important conditions that need to be considered are polygenic hypercholesterolemia and familial hypercholesterolemia.

In polygenic hypercholesterolemia (condition is more common than familial hypercholesterolemia) total-C level is commonly <350 mg%. The family study will show continuous distribution of total-C with high mean value. Dietary management greatly benefits the patient.

In cases of familial hypercholesterolemia total-C level is generally >350 mg%. In the family study there will be bimodal distribution of total-C levels (normals and heterozygotes). In this condition there is premature atherogenesis and history of premature CAD in the family. The heterozygous form occurs with a frequency of 1 in 500 in normal population. Homozygous form of the disorder is more severe but rare. Tendon xanthomata are pathognomic of familial hypercholesterolemia. The disorder results from LDL receptor defect. In about 5% of families, however, defect lies in apo-B-100 and not in LDL receptors. In these families tendon xanthomata are often not seen and LDL-C levels only modestly increased.

In the present patient, although, ECG is normal the patient should be kept under observation. He should be put on strict dietary treatment and reinvestigated after one month. If the patient has polygenic disorder his total-C should greatly improve.

CASE HISTORY: 9.3

A 48 year old diabetic presented with complaints of intermittent claudication. He had yellowish papules with erythematous bases (eruptive xanthomas) over buttocks and elbows. Linear fatty structures were also present on creases of his palms. In standing plasma test, turbidity was seen without the creamy layer over the top. Serum C and TAG levels were 310 mg/dL and 270 mg/dL, respectively. None of the children had an abnormal lipid profile.

The lipid profile of the patient could be produced by familial combined hyperlipidemia or familial dysbetali-poproteinemia. Presence of palmer and tuberous xan-thomas suggested the latter condition (which needs homozygosity for apo-E2 and presence of some factor promoting hyperlipidemia for disease expression). Diabetes could have helped the disease expression in this case. Although diabetes itself, can also produce increase of plasma VLDL level and if it is poorly controlled, some rise of LDL but serum C level of 310 mg/dL is generally not expected as a simple secondary lipid abnormality in diabetes mellitus.

In the patient diabetes should be first controlled with insulin and then plasma lipids restudied. Confirmation of dysbetalipoproteinemia requires demonstration of band of β-VLDL by electrophoresis. Treatment will depend upon the serum C and TAG levels found after control of diabetes mellitus. This condition responds to treatment quite well.

Familial dysbetalipoproteinemia is an uncommon condition (occurring in about 1/2000 of the population) compared to FCH. Both the conditions show increased risk for CAD. In both conditions patients are often over-weight/obese, hypertensive and may also have diabetes and gout. As already said, a superimposed primary or secondary lipid disorder is required for lipid abnormality and disease expression of familial dysbetalipo-proteinemia.

In FCH, tendon and tuberous xanthomas do not occur. However, corneal arcus and xanthelasma may be seen. Two important features of FCH are, changing lipid profile of the patient and great variability of lipid profile between the patient and his different family members. Because of changing lipid profile, FCH may present for differential diagnosis from, familial or polygenic hyper-cholesterolemia (↑ total-C/↑ LDL-C, with VLDL and TAG in normal range), from familial hypertriglyceridemia (↑VLDL/↑TAG; and total-C in the normal range) and familial dysbetalipoproteinemia as in the present case.

It may be added that management of primary lipoprotein disorders is mostly guided by total-C, LDL-C and TAG levels. Precise knowledge of the lipoprotein disorder, however, helps to correctly define the risk to CAD.

OBJECTIVE TYPE QUESTIONS

Pick out the wrong statement.

1. LDL

i) It arises from metabolism of VLDL.

ii) It is associated with apo-B-100.

iii) Major fraction of LDL is metabolized in extra-hepatic tissues

iv) Oxidized LDL is more atherogenic than LDL.

v) Small dense LDL is more atherogenic than LDL.

2. Atherosclerosis

i) Increased levels of LDL-C and apo-B are risk factors for atherosclerosis.

ii) The scavenger pathway is responsible for promoting atheroma formation.

iii) Oxidized LDL is a ligand for the scavenger pathway.

iv) VLDL and IDL have the same atherogenic potential.

v) HDL can mediate removal of CE from foam cells in the atheroma.

3. HDL

i) Low HDL-C level is an independent risk factor for atherosclerosis.

ii) Primary HDL deficiency is more common than secondary HDL deficiency.

iii) Increased CETP mediated transfer of CE from HDL to VLDL occurs in hypertriglyceridemia making HDL poor in CE.

iv) There is increased fractional clearance of CE-poor HDL.

v) Increased shift of phospholipid, C-II, C-III from HDL to VLDL also increases HDL clearance.

4. Primary hyperlipoproteinemias

i) A high serum C in the absence of significant hypertriglyceridemia is highly suggestive of diagnosis of F. hypercholesterolemia.

ii) The tendon xanthomas are quite specific for the disorder.

iii) Polygenic hypercholesterolemia is more common than F. hypercholesterolemia.

iv) Both F. hypercholesterolemia and polygenic hyperchoelsterolemia need drug treatment.

v) Familial combined hyperlipidemia is also an important cause of hypercholesterolemia.

5. Diabetes mellitus

i) Hyperglycemic control in IDDM normalizes lipid abnormalities quite effectively.

ii) Weight loss in NIDDM is more effective than glycemic control in normalizing lipid abnormalities.

iii) With slight lipid abnormalities in NIDDM there is no increased risk to atherosclerosis.

iv) LDL-C levels are often in the normal range in NIDDM.

v) Risk for atherosclerosis is more in NIDDM than IDDM.

6. Pregnancy

i) In pregnancy total-C may increase by about 50% and TAG by about 100%.

ii) Increase in levels of TAG and total-C are more in presence of pre-eclampsia.

iii) At about 6 weeks postpartum the lipid levels normalize.

iv) High total-C level in pregnancy is a risk for atherosclerosis.

v) High TAG levels in pregnancy may form risk for acute pancreatitis.

7. Diagnosis

i) Lipid abnormalities may be due to abnormalities in specific lipo-proteins.

ii) Diagnosis of lipid abnormalities depends upon TAG and total-C levels.

iii) HDL-C is measured in supernatant after precipitation of VLDL and LDL.

iv) VLDL-C is calculated as TAG/5 (both values expressed as mg/dL), at all plasma TAG levels.

v) LDL-C is found out by difference.

vi) Ratio of β-VLDL-C to TAG in dysbetalipoproteinemia is >0.3.

8. Investigations

i) A secondary cause of hyperlipidemia should be first excluded.

ii) If no secondary cause is found, patient should be put on hyperlipidemia management diet for about 3 months.

iii) If hyperlipidemia persists after the dietary treatment, the patient should be investigated for diagnosis of specific lipoprotein abnormality.

iv) Lipoprotein electrophoresis will have to be used to find out the specific lipoprotein abnormality.

v) Stress of a serious disease leads to modest changes in plasma lipids.

9. Investigations

i) The history, clinical examination along with plasma TAG and total-C levels are generally enough to arrive at diagnosis of a primary lipoprotein abnormality.

ii) Decision on type of management is based on levels of LDL-C.

iii) Treatment goals are also related to LDL-C levels.

iv) In some individuals a modest increase in total-C may be due to increase of HDL-C.

v) Low HDL-C is an independent risk factor for atherosclerosis.

vi) Patient with low HDL-C should be advised to take some drug which specifically increases HDL-C.

10. The TAG levels

i) Plasma TAG levels above 500 mg/dL form a risk factor for acute pancreatitis.

ii) TAG levels reduced to less than 400 mg/dL reduce the risk for acute pancreatitis.

iii) High plasma TAG levels in familial lipoprotein lipase deficiency do not form a risk for atherosclerosis.

iv) In no primary lipoprotein abnormality, high TAG is an independent risk factor for atherosclerosis.

v) In NECP (National Cholesterol Education Programme) recommendations there are no set goals mentioned for lowering of high plasma TAG levels.

ANSWERS

1. No.(iii). Two thirds of LDL is metabolized in liver and only on third in peripheral tissues.

2. No.(iv). IDL is CE enriched and more atherogenic.

3. No.(ii). Secondary HDL deficiency is more common.

4. No.(iv). Polygenic hypercholesterolemia is more common and generally, managed by dietary treatment.

5. No.(iii). Even with subtle lipid abnormalities risk for atherosclerosis is increased in NIDDM.

6. No. (iv). High total-C level in pregnancy has no risk for atherosclerosis.

7. No.(iv). This calculation is valid only upto TAG level of 400 mg/dL. At higher levels ratio of TAG to VLDL-C is >5.

8. No.(iv). Electrophoresis of plasma lipoproteins has only limited value in diagnosis.

9. No.(vi). At present no drug is available which can specifically increase HDL-C level.

10. No.(iv). TAG levels between 250 to 500 mg/dL if due to dysbetalipoproteinemia or FCH form an independent risk factor for atherosclerosis.

CHAPTER 10

Parathyroid Hormone, Vitamin D and Bone

CALCIUM AND PHOSPHATE HOMEOSTASIS

Major amounts of these ions lie in bones. About 15% of phosphate and about 1% of calcium lie in soft tissues. Balance of these two ions in the body, greatly, depends upon their absorption from intestine and excretion in urine.

Absorption of calcium is reduced by excess of dietary oxalate (forms insoluble calcium oxalate) and steatorrhea (fatty acids form insoluble calcium soaps). Vitamin D status of the body is single most important factor which determines fractional absorption of calcium from the intestine. Normal fractional absorption of dietary calcium is 30 to 50%. It is increased by vitamin D but reduced by increased load of dietary calcium. In cases of idiopathic hypercalciuria the effect of dietary load of calcium on calcium absorption is lost (see later).

Normally, about 98% of filtered calcium is reabsorbed. The reabsorbed fraction depends upon vitamin D, parathyroid hormone (PTH) and presence of nonabsorbable anions in the filtrate. The loop diuretics increase urinary excretion of calcium while thiazides reduce calcium excretion. An efficient endocrine control over absorption and excretion of calcium regulates ECF calcium. Daily turnover of calcium in an adult is shown in Fig. 10.1.

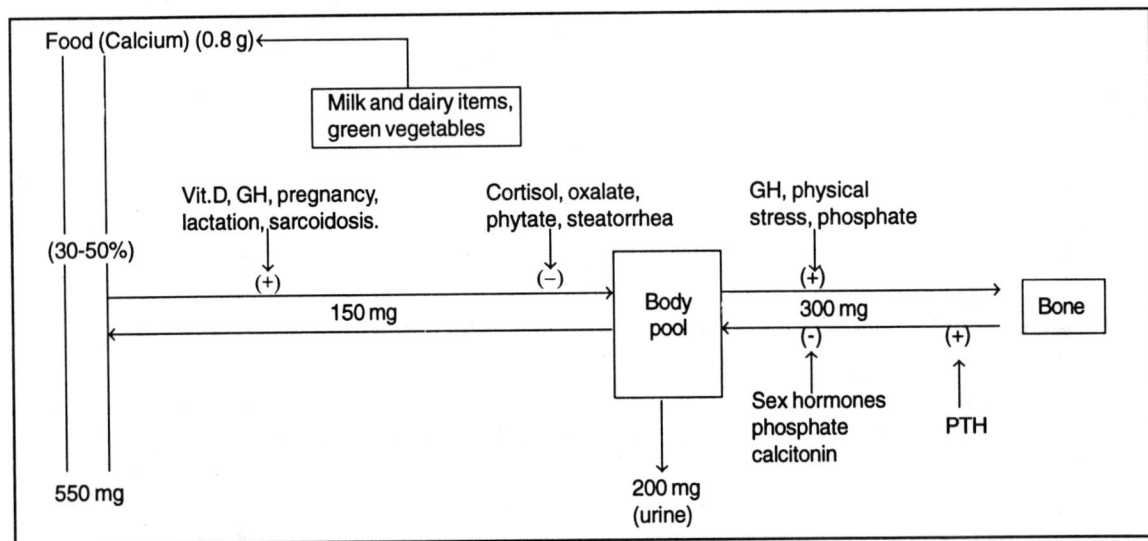

Fig.10.1. Normal daily turn over of calcium.

Vitamin D is also important in absorption of dietary phosphate by a mechanism which is independent of calcium absorption. Phosphate absorption is reduced by heavy metal cations (Al^{+3}, Mg^{+2}, Ca^{+2}) but unlike calcium absorption, it is not reduced by increased dietary load of phosphate. Fractional absorption of phosphate from intestine is greater than that of calcium (70 to 80%).

Kidney reabsorbs a smaller fraction of filtered phosphate than calcium (85 to 95%). Vitamin D promotes renal reabsorption of both calcium and phosphate while PTH increases reabsorption of

calcium but reduces that of phosphate. Daily turnover of phosphate and magnesium in a normal adult is shown in Fig. 10.2. Magnesium is discussed on page 198. Fig.10.3 compares homeostatic mechanisms for serum levels of calcium and phosphate.

Normal reference range for serum calcium is 9.2 to 11 mg%. About half of serum calcium is protein bound (mostly to albumin) and the rest half is unbound or free. What is physiologically significant is the unbound calcium but what is generally measured in the laboratory is the total calcium. Further, it is the unbound calcium which is regulated,

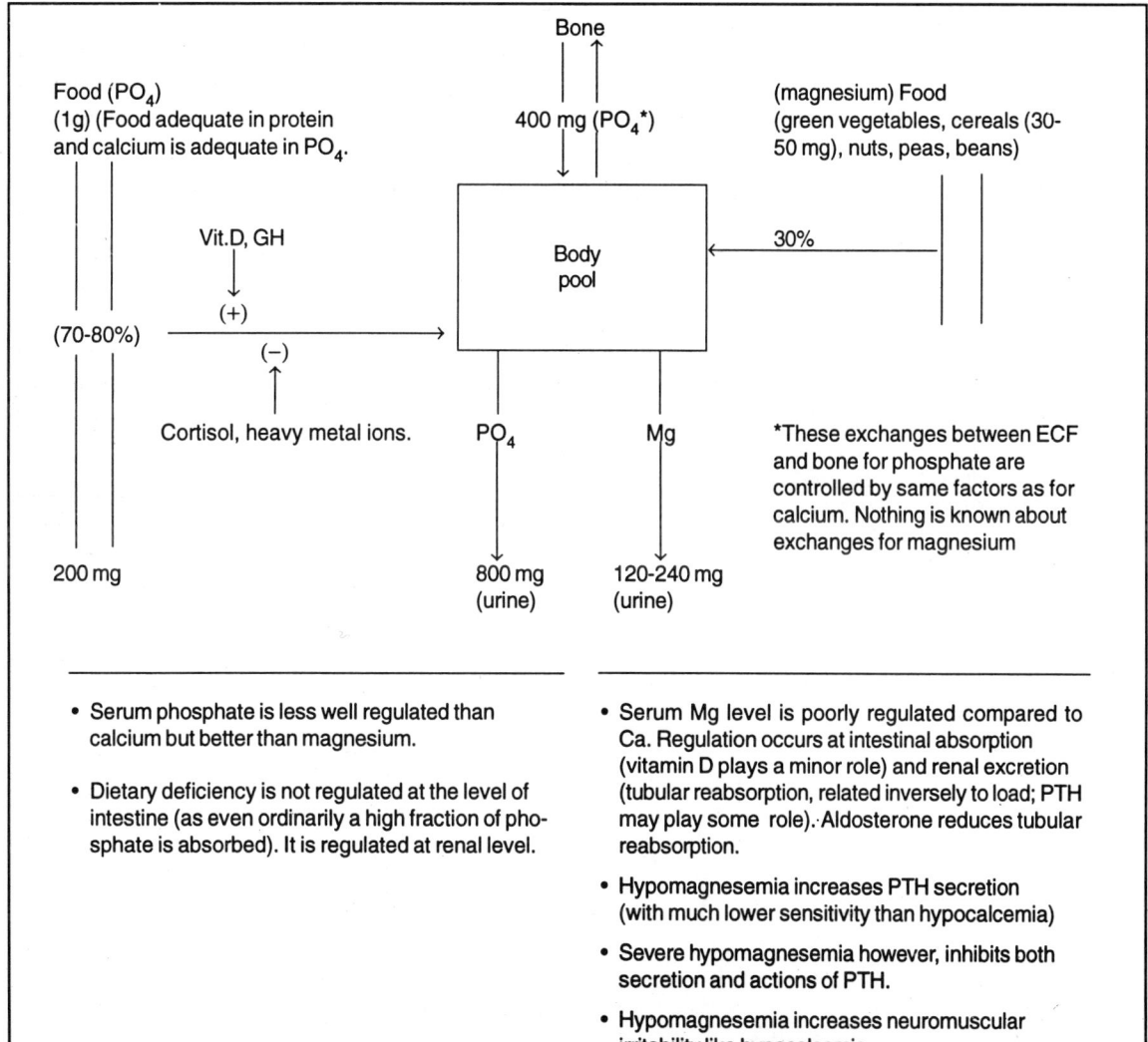

• Serum phosphate is less well regulated than calcium but better than magnesium.

• Dietary deficiency is not regulated at the level of intestine (as even ordinarily a high fraction of phosphate is absorbed). It is regulated at renal level.

• Serum Mg level is poorly regulated compared to Ca. Regulation occurs at intestinal absorption (vitamin D plays a minor role) and renal excretion (tubular reabsorption, related inversely to load; PTH may play some role). Aldosterone reduces tubular reabsorption.

• Hypomagnesemia increases PTH secretion (with much lower sensitivity than hypocalcemia)

• Severe hypomagnesemia however, inhibits both secretion and actions of PTH.

• Hypomagnesemia increases neuromuscular irritability like hypocalcemia.

Fig.10.2. Normal phosphate and magnesium balances.

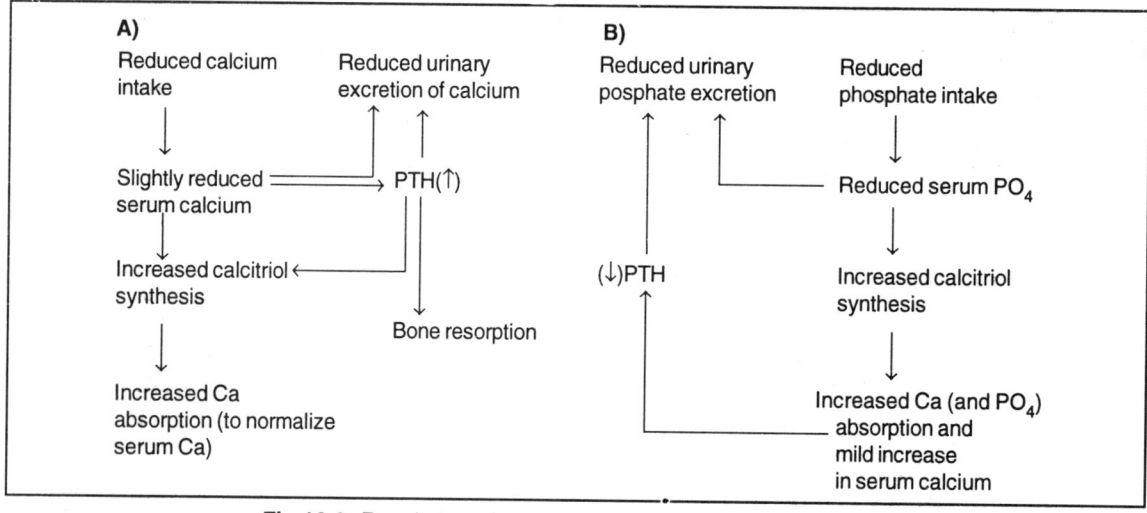

Fig.10.3. Regulation of serum calcium and phosphate levels.

- Variations in dietary intake of calcium are mainly adjusted at the level of intestinal absorption of calcium. These do not much effect the urinary excretion. Both PTH and calcitriol are involved in regulation.
- Variations in dietary intake of phosphate are mainly adjusted by varying urinary loss.
- Bone resorption to normalize serum calcium level in hypocalcemia becomes important if deficiency is prolonged, if calcium requirement is high and in old age (in the last case increased intestinal absorption fails to occur adequately).

mostly, by PTH and calcitriol. It is therefore important that we should be able to interpret the reported total calcium in terms of unbound calcium (see under diagnosis of hypocalcemia).

A decrease in concentration of free calcium increases neuromuscular irritability to cause tetany. As will be described later. Hypomagnesemia and alkalosis decrease threshold for tetany while hypokalemia and acidosis increase the threshold. Increase in concentration of free calcium leads to anorexia, nausea, constipation, hypotonia and depression. Even coma may occur. Persistent hypercalcemia particularly, when associated with increased serum phosphate level may lead to deposition of calcium phosphate in soft tissues (walls of blood vessels, cornea, renal parenchyma and other places).

Normal reference range for serum phosphorous (inorganic) in adults is 2.3 to 4.7 mg% and in children it is higher (4.0 to 7.0 mg%). Higher phosphorous levels in children are related to their higher levels of GH. Children are in positive balance of both calcium and phosphate while adults are in balance of these ions.

Chronic hypophosphatemia may impair growth of children. Oxygen delivery in tissues is affected because of low levels of 2, 3 BPG and ATP in red cells. Hemolytic anemia may result from reduced ability of red cells to deform while passing through capillaries. It may also reduce $Ca^{+2} \times PO_4^{3}$ ion product which is important in process of matrix calcification. Acute and severe hypophosphatemia may produce myopathy which may be associated with increased level of CPK in serum and rhabdomyolysis. Hyperphosphatemia maintained for long periods may result in ectopic calcification (seen in vitamin D intoxication and severe untreated cases of chronic renal failure). Also see Appendix B.

BONE FORMATION AND BONE RESORPTION

Bone contains about 99% of total calcium, 90% of total phosphate and 55% of total magnesium. Bone minerals are present as hydroxyapatite crystals $[Ca_{10} (PO_4)_6 (OH)_2]$. Bone minerals form 70% of bone weight and rest is formed by organic matrix of bone called osteoid. Collagen is the main constituent of collagen fibers of osteoid. During bone resorption collagen is also degraded and certain degradation products are released (hydroxyproline, pyridinoline (Pyr) and deoxypyridinoline (D-Pyr), hydroxylysine and its glycosides) and act as markers of bone resorption. As will be indicated below, osteoblasts play an important role in bone formation. When these cells are active, they release alkaline phosphatase (the precise role of this enzyme in bone formation is not known) and osteocalcin (which is partly incorporated into matrix) into circulation. Plasma levels of alkaline phosphatase, type 1 procollagen carboxy terminal peptides and osteocalcin are used as markers of osteoblastic activity and bone turnover rate.

Both bone formation and bone resorption are processes mediated by certain bone cells. Cells present in bone are osteoblasts, osteocytes and osteoclasts. Osteoblasts arise from osteoproginator cells which, in turn, arise from mesenchymal cells of bone connective tissue and appear on bone surfaces in the area of bone formation. Osteoblasts synthesize the matrix constituents and are then involved in osteoid mineralization. After completing their functions they change into relatively inactive cells called osteocytes. Osteoclasts are multinucleated cells derived, probably, by fusion of circulating monocytes (or from bone marrow monocyte precursor cells) and are involved in bone resorption.

Bone formation consists of two processes, osteoid formation and matrix mineralization. Osteoid is formed by the activity of osteoblasts under the influence of a number of hormones (insulin, GH, sex hormones and thyroid hormones) and growth factors (TGF-β, IGF-I, IGF-II, morphogenic proteins, PDGF, FGF) (Fig. 10.4). Matrix mineralization consists of mineral nucleation and rapid calcification after nucleation. Matrix nucleation is an ill understood process which involves prior hydrolysis of pyrophosphate/degradation of certain glycoproteins at the site of nucleation. Both osteoblasts and calcitriol may also play roles in process of nucleation. Rapid calcification after nucleation depends upon $Ca^{+2} \times PO_4^{-3}$ ion product in ECF

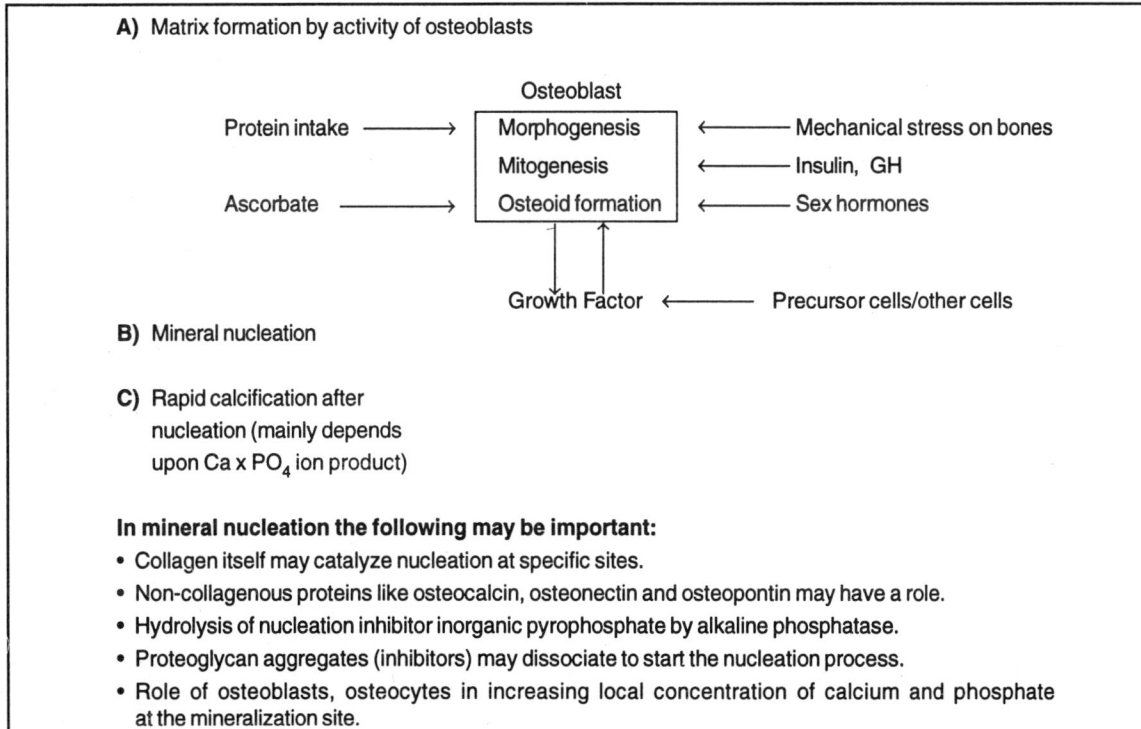

Fig.10.4. Steps in bone formation.

(which determines $Ca^{+2} \times PO_4^{-3}$ ion product in metastatic solution bathing matrix). Calcitriol is responsible for maintaining normal ion product in ECF.

Bone resorption is mediated by osteoclasts. PTH acts on osteoblasts to release certain factors which stimulate osteoclasts for bone resorption (Fig. 10.5). Calcitriol is also required for the bone resorption activity of PTH. In severe deficiency of vitamin D, PTH fails to accomplish bone resorption. Calcitonin blocks the bone resorptive activity of osteoclasts.

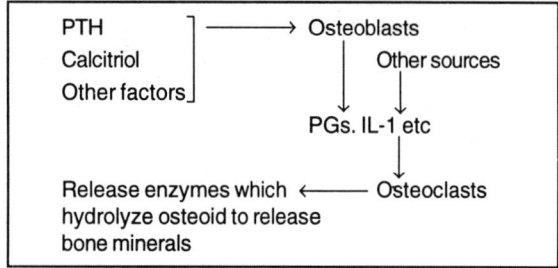

Fig. 10.5. Process of bone resorption.

- Squamous cell and renal tumors produce and secrete parathyroid hormone related peptide (PTHrP) which causes bone resorption by acting like PTH.
- Leukemia, lymphoma, multiple myeloma and carcinoma breast produce bone resorption by local action of released mediators (IL-1, tumor necrosis factor, PGs of E series).

REGULATION OF SERUM CALCIUM LEVEL

It has already been pointed out that level of unbound calcium in serum is efficiently regulated by a fine endocrine control over absorption (from intestine) and excretion (renal) of calcium (Fig. 10.6), by parathyroid hormone (PTH) and calcitriol (activated form of vitamin D).

Hypocalcemia is a stimulus for secretion of PTH from two pairs of parathyroid glands located on posterior surface of thyroid gland. Change in secretion of PTH is brought about not only by changing the rate of hormone synthesis but also by varying the rate of hormone degradation (Fig. 10.7). A reliable immunometric assay for intact hormone molecule is now available. There is linear correlation between plasma PTH levels and calcium levels in the range 4.0 to 10.5 mg/dL. This means that in cases of hypercalcemia (plasma level >10.5 mg/dL) due to causes other than hyperparathyroidism, there will hardly be any PTH in plasma.

Fig. 10.6 shows actions of PTH to increase level of serum calcium. In kidney it increases reabsorption of calcium and reduces reabsorption of phosphate. As the renal action of PTH involves activation of adenylate cyclase, increase in urinary

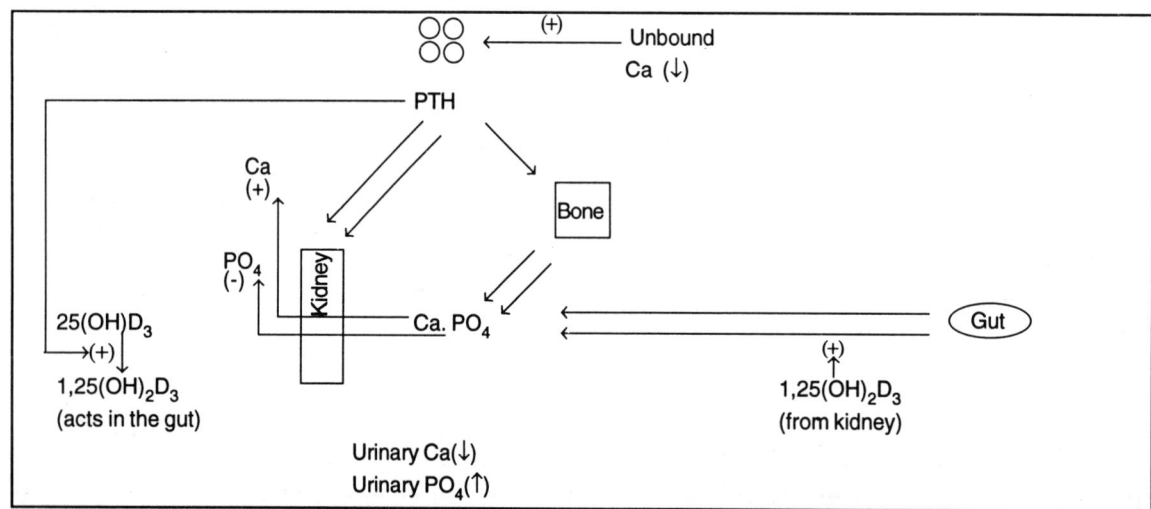

Fig.10.6. The three sites of action of PTH (bone, intestine, kidney).

- Normally low serum calcium is normalized by renal and intestinal actions of PTH. Bone resorption becomes important when hypocalcemia is prolonged or in old age when intestinal absorption falls.
- Both PTH and calcitriol are important in regulation of serum Ca. There is linear correlation between plasma PTH and Ca levels in the range of 4.0 to 10.5 mg%. Thus there will he hardly any active PTH in plasma if Ca level is > 10.5 due to some non-PTH cause.

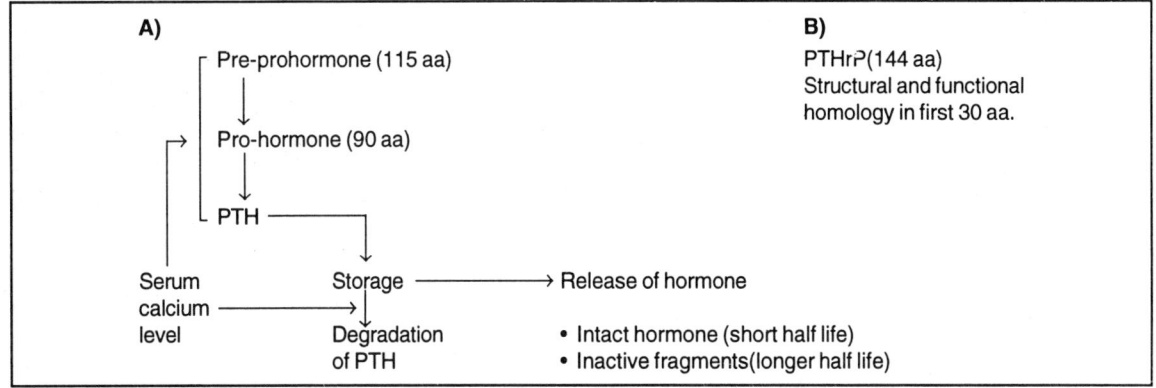

A)

Pre-prohormone (115 aa)

↓

Pro-hormone (90 aa)

↓

PTH

Serum calcium level → Storage → Release of hormone

Storage ↓ Degradation of PTH

B)

PTHrP(144 aa)
Structural and functional homology in first 30 aa.

- Intact hormone (short half life)
- Inactive fragments(longer half life)

Fig. 10.7. Regulation of Secretion of PTH (relation with PTHrP is shown in part B).

- Calcium sensor (receptor)on parathyroid cells, when activated, by calcium ions, activates a G-protein (G_q to activate phospholipase-C, to suppress PTH secretion. Suppression is reduced with low calcium levels.
- PTH receptors (in bone and kidney) are also linked to G-proteins (G_q, which activates phospholipase-C; and G_s, which activates adenylate cyclase)

excretion of nephrogenic cAMP, in a case of hypercalcemia, indicates PTH or PTHrP as the cause of hypercalcemia. Another important action of PTH in kidney is to activate 25 $(OH)D_3$ to 1, 25 $(OH)_2D_3$ (calcitriol). Calcitriol formed in this way promotes absorption of calcium from the intestine.

Vitamin D_3 is present in animal fat and is poorly distributed in food. However, it is also formed in the body from 7-dehydrocholesterol (D_3 formation occurs in skin under the action of UV light). Next, 25 $(OH)D_3$ is formed from D_3 in liver, and activated to calcitriol in kidney (Fig. 10.8). This activation process is triggered by low levels of calcium and phosphate and increased PTH level.

Main action of calcitriol is to promote reabsorption of calcium (and phosphate) from intestine. Low serum calcium is normalized both by PTH and calcitriol. The latter molecule also counteracts phosphate lowering action of PTH. Calcitriol plays the major role in regulation of $Ca^{+2} \times PO_4^{-3}$ ion product; may also play a direct role in the process of bone calcification.

Calcitonin is a polypeptide secreted by C-cells (parafollicular cells of thyroid) in response to the stimulus of hypercalcemia. But its physiological significance is not known since complete removal of thyroid gland does not result in any abnormality of serum calcium. Major known action of calcitonin is to oppose the bone resorptive activity of PTH.

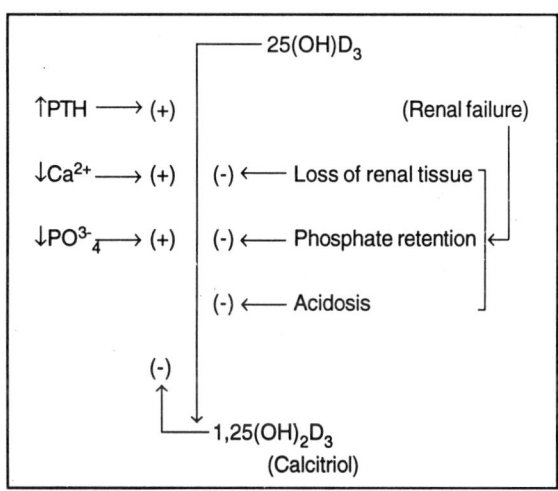

25$(OH)D_3$

↑PTH → (+)   (Renal failure)

↓Ca²⁺ → (+)   (-) ← Loss of renal tissue

↓PO₄³⁻ → (+)   (-) ← Phosphate retention

(-) ← Acidosis

(-)
↑

1,25$(OH)_2D_3$
(Calcitriol)

Fig.10.8. Regulation of formation of calcitriol.

- Enzyme converting 25$(OH)D_3$ to 1, 25$(OH)_2D_3$ is 25(OH)D-1α-hydroxylase.

HYPOCALCEMIA (Table 10.1)

Transient hypocalcemia may be present in acute renal failure, severe burns, sepsis and after extensive transfusions of citrated blood. Some drugs may also produce temporary hypocalcemia. Generally, there are no symptoms and no treatment is required. Chronic hypocalcemia is often symptomatic and needs treatment.

Chronic hypocalcemia may be hereditary when

encountered in a child. Other developmental defects are likely to be present. It may be part of autoimmune polyglandular deficiency and there may be evidence of failure of other endocrine secretions. Acquired hypoparathyroidism may follow neck surgery. In all these (hereditary and acquired cases) there is low serum calcium with high serum phosphate besides unmeasurable or low levels of PTH.

Pseudohypoparathyroidism is also a hereditary disorder in which there is end organ unresponsiveness to PTH. In this condition there may also be developmental abnormalities but PTH levels are elevated. One should remember that the pattern of low calcium with high phosphate in the absence of kidney failure is a key feature pointing to presence of one of the above disorders (hereditary or acquired hypoparathyroidism).

Besides end organ resistance to PTH (mentioned above) there are other causes of PTH ineffectivity resulting in hypocalcemia. These include vitamin D deficiency (absence of exposure to sunlight, malabsorption), defective vitamin D metabolism (anticonvulsant therapy, vitamin D dependant rickets type I, chronic renal disease) and Vitamin D ineffectivity (vitamin-dependant rickets type II). In these conditions PTH is ineffective in the absence of appropriate vitamin D activity and levels of both calcium and phosphate are low with compensatory increase of PTH level. Low serum phosphate is because of continued renal wasting of phosphate since this action of PTH is less dependant on vitamin D activity.

Two other important causes of chronic hypocalcemia are chronic renal failure and magnesium

Table 10.1. Some important causes of chronic hypocalcemia

NEONATAL HYPOCALCEMIA (Chapter 18)

Hereditary causes:

- DiGeorge syndrome (rare) (developmental defect of thymus and parathyroid, associated with special facies and cardiac lesions) $\quad$ ($\downarrow$) PTH
- Autoimmune polyglandular deficiency (autosomal recessive trait; failure of other endocrine secretions; unaffected family members may show presence of autoantibodies) $\quad$ ($\downarrow$) Calcium $\quad$ ($\uparrow$) Phosphate $\quad$ (N) ALP
- Idiopathic hypoparathyroidism (isolated parathyroid failure)

- Pseudohypoparathyroidism (see the Text) $\quad$ (N/$\uparrow$) PTH $\quad$ ($\downarrow$) Calcium $\quad$ ($\uparrow$) Phosphate

Vitamin D deficiency related disorders:

- Nutritional deficiency
- Malabsorption $\quad$ ($\uparrow$, but ineffective) PTH $\quad$ (N/$\downarrow$) Calcium $\quad$ ($\downarrow$) Phosphate
- Anticonvulsant therapy
- Vitamin D dependant rickets type I (1, 25(OH)$_2$D$_3$ $\downarrow$)
- VitaminD dependant rickets type II (1, 25(OH)$_2$D$_3$ $\uparrow$)

Chronic renal failure:

($\downarrow$)Calcium, ($\uparrow$)Phosphate, ($\uparrow$)PTH

Magnesium deficiency[1]:

($\downarrow$)Calcium, ($\downarrow$)Phosphate, ($\downarrow$)PTH

[1] In magnesium deficiency low calcium is due to low PTH and the primary disorder (producing magnesium deficiency); low phosphate is due to primary cause inspite of low PTH.

- The reported value of total serum calcium has to be interpreted in light of unbound calcium. The protein bound calcium is calculated as under:

Protein bound calcium (g/dL) = 0.8 × albumin (g/L) + 0.2 × globulin (g/L) + 3.

This value subtracted from total calcium gives unbound calcium (mg/dL) deficiency, the latter impairs both PTH secretion and PTH response. The laboratory feature of magnesium deficiency are low levels of PTH, calcium and phosphate. In chronic renal failure, low calcium is associated with high phosphate and PTH levels. Causes of hypocalcemia are summarized in Table 10.1.

Acute decrease of calcium (say to <8 mg/dL) may cause paresthesias and tetany (discussed below). Reduced calcium levels when present over a long period may produce cataract/mental retardation. Table 10.2 shows different ways in which patients of hypocalcemia may present.

Tetany

It results from increased neuromuscular irritability because of hypocalcemia (when ionic fraction of calcium is reduced), hypomagnesemia and alkalosis (increases protein binding of calcium, thereby reducing the ionic fraction). In mild form there may be muscular cramps and paresthesia. In more severe form spasms of muscles of hand (carpel spasm) and foot (pedal spasm) occur. In very severe form laryngeal spasm and convulsions may occur. In long standing cases, mental changes and cataract can also develop. In a patient of tetany carpal spasm can be induced by inflating sphygmomanometer cuff around upper arm to mid way between systolic and diastolic pressures (Trousseau's sign). This sign is used to reveal latent tetany.

Tetany may occur in a newborn if mother was suffering from hyperparathyroidism. Neonatal tetany is discussed separately (Chapter 18).

Besides treatment of the cause, the patient may require calcium and vitamin D supplements. In PTH deficiency, activation of vitamin D cannot occur. In such cases active metabolites of vitamin D may be used. Such modes of management need more careful monitoring of serum calcium levels.

Hypoparathyroidism

Most commonly it used to develop in cases of neck surgery when parathyroids were removed, inadvertently. Incidence is much reduced now.

Hereditary hypoparathyroidism may occur in association with thymic aplasia (DiGeorge syndrome) or as part of PGA type I (Chapter 16). Less commonly it may occur in isolation (without any associated endocrine or dermal abnormality) and will be called idiopathic hypoparathyroidism. More commonly these disorders occur in the first decade of life. Hypoparathyroidism should be ruled out in a child presenting with epilepsy, mental/emotional changes, cataracts, poor dentition or changes in skin and nails (moniliasis).

Neonatal hypoparathyroidism may occur in an infant if mother had hyperparathyroidism during pregnancy (suppression of fetal parathyroid glands). Also see Table 10.1.

In hypoparathyroidism serum calcium is reduced with increase of serum phosphate. Serum phosphate however, may not increase if dietary intake of phosphate is reduced.

Hypoparathyroidism may also develop in a person suffering from prolonged deficiency of magnesium. Magnesium is needed both for release as well as for actions of PTH.

Pseudohypoparathyroidism

In this condition serum calcium and phosphate levels are as in hypoparathyroidism (low calcium high phosphate), not because of deficiency of PTH but due to end organ resistance to its actions. After binding to receptors, PTH may fail to generate cAMP or cAMP may be generated but fails to invoke the appropriate response. The two types of end organ resistance in pseudohypoparathyroidism can be differentiated from each other and also from hypoparathyroidism by studying urinary response (effect on excretions of cAMP and phosphate) to administration of exogenous PTH. In normals and patients of hypoparathyroidism PTH administration results in increase of both cAMP and phosphate in urine. In patients of pseudohypoparathyroidism which fail to generate cAMP, there is complete failure of the above response (no increase of cAMP or phosphate in urine); in others there is partial failure of the response (increase of cAMP occurs but not that of phosphate). The patient with complete failure of response often shows other phenotypic abnormalities like short stature, round face, short metacarpals and metatarsals and mental retardation.

Table 10.2. History/clinical presentations in hypocalcemia

Only biochemical hypocalcemia	Find the cause and treat it; long standing hypocalcemia is harmful (see below).
Paresthesias/tetany	• Besides hypocalcemia, increased neuromuscular irritability can also result from hypomagnesemia/alkalosis. • Trousseau's sign is reliable to diagnose latent cases.
Basal ganglia calcification; posterior lens cataract; psychosis; mental deficiency.	Complications of long standing hypocalcemia.
Increased intracranial tension, papilledema	Along with convulsions may mimic a brain tumor.
Presence of developmental defects (round face; short stature, short metacarpals/metatarsals.	Pseudohypoparathyroidism as cause of hypocalcemia.
Associated candidiasis/failure of other endocrines (thyroid, adrenal, gonad).	Idiopathic hypoparathyroidism of autoimmune etiology. (PGA syndromes).
Associated malabsorption; pernicious anemia, vitiligo, alopecia.	Idiopathic hypoparathyroidism of autoimmune etiology. (PGA syndromes).
Malnutrition, malabsorption/chronic renal disease; features of rickets/osteomalacia; history of thyroid surgery	Help to establish cause of hypocalcemia.

This condition is called Albright's hereditary osteodystrophy. Some patients have only phenotype abnormalities without biochemical changes of pseudohypoparathyroidism. This condition is called pseudopseudohypoparathyroidism.

The patients with partial loss of response do not have phenotypic abnormalities. For diagnosis of the latter cases one must rule out vitamin D deficiency since cases of severe vitamind D deficiency also show partial loss of renal response to PTH administration.

Patients of hypoparathyroidism and pseudohypothyroidism are treated with intravenous calcium in acute phase (to relieve spasms of tetany) and then 1α-hydroxy cholecalciferol is given which is converted into calcitriol in liver. During treatment, serum calcium needs to be monitored, every few months.

Vitamin D deficiency can also cause hypocalcemia but not in all cases (read under Rickets and osteomalacia). Hypocalcemia can also occur in chronic renal disease (discussed separately).

Diagnosis of cause of hypocalcemia

Hypocalcemia accompanied with hypoalbuminemia may be asymptomatic (since ionic calcium may be normal) and hypocalcemia of chronic renal disease (serum creatinine raised) will not present with features specific to low ionic calcium. Thus serum calcium should be studied alongwith levels of serum albumin and creatinine.

As already mentioned, commonly estimated calcium is total calcium which includes the bound and free fractions, the latter being clinically significant. If free or ionic calcium is not being measured directly, total calcium can be corrected for variations in serum albumin levels. This is done by adding or substracting 0.8 mg/dL for each g/dL of albumin below or above the normal value (4.7 mg/dL).

If level of unbound calcium is low, the patient should be examined as per information in Table 10.2. In a hypocalcemic neonate it is important to enquire about PTH status of the mother (Chapter 18). If the patient has chronic malabsorption, estimation of serum magnesium should be undertaken. Malabsorption may also produce deficiency of vitamin D. Presence of stigmata of pseudohypoparathyroidism and evidence of calcification of lens and basal ganglion may be useful. Patient may present with evidence of rickets or osteomalacia. Serum phosphate and creatinine levels may also help (Fig. 10.9) in indicating cause of hypocalcemia. Serum phosphate level is low in vitamin D deficiency and high in hypoparathyroidism and pseudohypoparathyroidism and in chronic renal failure. Immunometric estimation of PTH is useful in differentiating

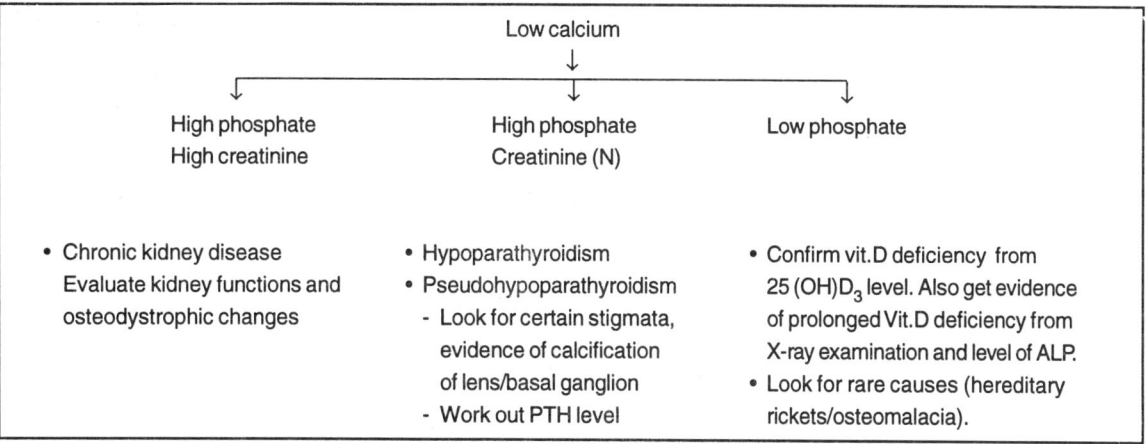

Fig.10.9. Use of serum phosphate level in finding cause of hypocalcemia.

- In the high phosphate, normal creatinine group patients present with features related to neuromuscular irritability (muscle cramps, paresthesia, tetany).
- In the low phosphate group patients present with clinical features related to bone/muscle (bone pains, muscle weakness).

hypoparathyroidism and pseudohypoparathyroidism. Low level of 25 $(OH)D_3$ is the best evidence of vitamin D deficiency.

Rickets and osteomalacia

In these disorders of vitamin D deficiency, there is poor bone mineralization (osteoid formation remains normal). This is due to low serum $Ca^{+2} \times PO^{-3}$ ion product. The product is maintained in the normal range by the effects of vitamin D on intestinal absorption and renal excretion of the two ions. Some other more direct effect of vitamin D on bone mineralization may also be there.

In adults defect is only confined to the remodelling process (as the bones have already grown and the epiphyses already fused). In children besides the remodelling process, bone growth is also occurring and new bone is being laid down in regions of growing epiphyseal cartilage plates. In children both the processes are affected and the condition is called rickets while in adults the disorder is called osteomalacia.

In osteomalacia, in X-ray pictures, bones may present wash out appearance (reduced bone minerals) or pseudofractures (a linear bony rarefaction looking like a fracture). There is also muscular weakness, particularly, confined to the shoulder and hip muscles. Osteomalacia often occurs in women

and manifests during pregnancy when calcium requirement is increased. Bone pains and muscular weakness are common complaints. In children besides bone remodelling, the growing bone ends are affected. These are swollen and show a characteristic appearance on X-ray. These are characteristic rachitic changes. In children general growth and development is also affected, besides bowing of long bones (soft bones bending under pressure).

Vitamin D deficiency may be dietary (growing children and pregnant women) or due to lack of sunshine (elderly and some patients suffering from certain chronic diseases). Malabsorption can also cause deficiency of vitamin D and calcium. In nephrotic syndrome excessive loss of vitamin binding proteins in urine may reduce adequate supply of calcitriol to target tissues. This may also be true in liver disease. Phenytoin and barbitone induce hepatic microsomal enzymes to increase metabolic losses of 25 $(OH)D_3$. Some rare hereditary and acquired disorders which impair normal metabolism of vitamin D or affect some renal function also cause the disorder (Tables 10.1, 10.3).

As already mentioned under hypocalcemia, vitamin D deficiency impairs effects of PTH on calcium metabolism and this causes secondary compensatory hyperparathyroidism, because of which calcium level may be normalized (if vitamin D deficiency is not very severe) or it may remain low (severe vitamin D deficiency). Serum phosphate level is always reduced as an effect of PTH on renal tubules which is less dependant on vitamin D.

Diagnosis

In susceptible groups, patients with bone pains and muscular weakness should be screened for osteomalacia or rickets. Children with poor growth or convulsions should also be investigated for rickets. History of intake of certain drugs and that of malabsorption is also important.

History, clinical features and X-ray examination help diagnosis. Serum phosphate level is reduced while that of calcium may be reduced or normal (see above). Serum alkaline phosphate activity is increased. Reduced level of $25 (OH)D_3$ is the most important evidence of vitamin D deficiency. To establish cause of vitamin D deficiency in less straight forward cases serum creatinine should be estimated and patient evaluated for malabsorption. If the patient does not improve with conventional doses of vitamin D, he may have to be investigated for the following less common diseases (also see Table 10.3).

Vitamin D dependant rickets

There is 1α-hydroxylase deficiency (type I) or target tissue defect (type II). Both are autosomal recessive disorders with hypocalcemia, hypophosphatemia and elevated PTH levels. Serum calcitriol levels (Table 10.1) and associated alopecia in type II differentiate the two. Both respond to large doses of vitamin D (type II need higher doses) or vitamin D metabolites.

Hypophosphatemic rickets (vitamin D resistant rickets)

It includes the characteristic disorder which is X-linked and its variants, autosomal recessive (myopathy associated) hereditary hypophosphatemia with (absorptive) hypercalciuria [(N) Ca, $\downarrow PO_4$)] and autosomal dominant phosphatemic rickets. Other patients may have primary or secondary, more wide spread, tublar reabsorptive defects (phosphate, bicarbonate, glucose, amino acid and uric acid) of Fanconi syndrome. Disorder of vitamin D resistant rickets is more severe than vitamin D dependant rickets and needs treatment with oral phosphate and calcitriol.

Table 10.3. Biochemical profile in different causes of rickets/osteomalacia

Vitamin D deficiency (poor diet, malabsorption, lack of sunshine)	Calcium N/$\downarrow$: Phosphate $\downarrow$: ALP $\uparrow$: PTH $\uparrow$: 25(OH) $D_3 \downarrow$: Aminoaciduria. Investigate for malabsorption.
Chronic renal disease	Calcium N/$\downarrow$: Phosphate $\uparrow$: ALP $\uparrow$: PTH $\uparrow$: 25(OH) D_3– N: 1, 25(OH)$_2$$D_3 \downarrow$; Creatinine $\uparrow$
Renal tubular defects[1] (Vitamin D resistant rickets) • X-linked hypophosphatemia with low 1, 25 (OH)$_2$ D_3^2; autosomal recessive hereditary hypophosphatemic rickets with hypercalciuria, muscle weakness and elevated 1, 25 (OH)$_2$ D_3. Also autosomal dominant. • Fanconi syndrome with low 1, 25(OH)$_2$ D_3 levels.	Calcium N/$\downarrow$; Phosphate$\downarrow\downarrow$; ALP$\uparrow$; PTH N/$\uparrow$; 25 (OH)D_3– N. Conditions are difficult to treat (need active vit.D metabolites for treatment).
Vitamin D dependent rickets (see Table 10.1)	Calcium $\downarrow$: Phosphate $\downarrow$: ALP $\uparrow$: PTH $\uparrow$: Generalized aminoaciduria (unlike vitamin D resistant rickets).
Hypophosphatasia Disease of defective bone mineralization occuring in infants (most severe; autosomal recessive), children and adults. There is deficiency of tissue nonspecific ALP.	Calcium N/$\uparrow$: Phosphate N/$\uparrow$: ALP $\downarrow\downarrow$: Urinary hydroxy proline $\uparrow$; Urinary phosphoryl ethanol amine $\uparrow$. ALP $\downarrow$ in amniotic fluid (prenatal diagnosis)

[1] Rickets/osteomalacia also occurs in RTA - type 1 and RTA - type 2. In these disorders, different factors producing rickets/osteomalacia include, hypophosphatemia, acidosis (altering vitamin D metabolism), acidosis induced loss of bone minerals and low 1,25 (OH)$_2$$D_3$ activity.

[2] Low phosphate fails to stimulate 25 (OH) D-1α-hydroxylase.

Renal tubular acidosis type 1

There is increased urinary excretion of calcium but serum calcium level remains normal because of increased PTH secretion. For the same reason urinary excretion of phosphate is increased leading to low serum phosphate. This causes osteomalacia which is aggravated by acidosis. Rickets/osteomalacia also occurs in RTA type 2.

Hypophosphatasia

In this condition there is severe deficiency of secretion of alkaline phosphatase (ALP) by osteoblasts. Bony lesions, like those of vitamin D deficiency, are produced. Urinary excretions of phosphoryl ethanolamine and pyrophosphate are increased which could be substrates for the enzyme and inhibitory to the calcification process.

Chronic renal failure (Fig. 10.8)

In chronic renal disease calcitriol formation is reduced due to reduced renal tissue, acidosis and hyperphosphatemia. Reduced absorption of calcium from intestine causes hypocalcemia. High serum phosphate level further reduces the ionic fraction of calcium (Fig.10.10). Hypocalcemia causes secondary hyperparathyroidism which tends to normalize serum calcium. Initially the bony changes are osteomalacia type. With substantial PTH response, serum calcium is normalized with healing of osteomalacia but PTH induced bony changes start developing. Also see Fig. 4.5. Only in very advanced renal disease, there is increase of both calcium and phosphate in serum, predisposing to soft tissue calcification. Management requires control of hyperphosphatemia with oral use of calcium or magnesium salts (to prevent absorption of ingested phosphate). Alongwith an active metabolite of vitamin D should be given. All this is meant to prevent hypocalcemia and development of osteomalacia in bones. With treatment of hypocalcemia, development of secondary hyperparathyroidism and consequent bony changes are also prevented.

HYPOPHOSPHATEMIA AND HYPERPHOSPHATEMIA

Clinically significant hypophosphatemia may occur

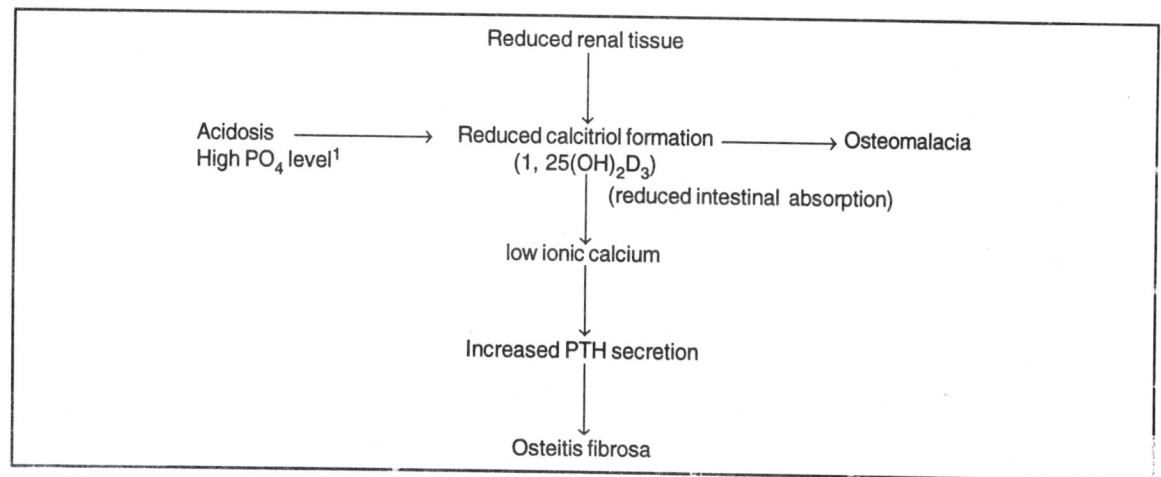

Fig.10.10. Osteodystrophy and serum calcium and phosphate levels with advancing kidney disease.

[1]Hyperphosphatemia inhibits 1-α-hydroxylation of 25(OH)D$_3$. Phosphate may co-precipitate with calcium in soft tissues, thus directly reducing Ca level.

- At a GFR of about 30 mL/min. Ca(N). PO$_4\uparrow$

- With further decrease of GFR, PO$_4$ rises further and Ca is reduced (because of low calcitriol).

- With still more reduction of GFR, there is increase of calcium (high PTH) and of PO$_4$. There is danger of soft tissue calcification.

- Level of PTH goes on increasing with advancing renal disease and can be used to follow osteodystrophic bone changes. These are treated by reducing PO$_4$ intake, increasing Ca intake along with vitamin D.

during restoration of nutrition in alcoholics. These patients are already phosphate depleted and during restoration of nutrition, entry of phosphate into cells worsens hypophosphatemia. In diabetic ketoacidosis hypokalemia associated with acidosis promotes phosphate depletion. Severe hypophosphatemia may develop when phosphate enters cells during treatment with insulin and glucose. Clinically significant hypophosphatemia may also occur during nutritional rehabilitation of starved/malnourished persons (Table 10.4). During intravenous fructose administration, due to unregulated phosphorylation of fructose by fructokinase (unlike regulated phosphorylation of glucose by hexokinase, inhibited by glucose 6-PO_4), severe decrease in serum PO_4 level may occur.

Severe hypophosphatemia may cause ATP depletion in many tissues leading to their dysfunction. There is red cell depletion of 2, 3 BPG and ATP; former reducing O_2 delivery to tissues and latter promoting tendency to hemolysis. There may also be rhabdomyolysis and muscular weakness. Other tissues which may be affected include, CNS (neuroencephalopathy may develop), leukocytes (increased bacterial/fungal infections) and the cardiac muscle (see Table 10.4).

Respiratory alkalosis (considered as the commonest cause of hypophosphatemia of varying severity) accompanies many serious disorders and the associated hypophosphatemia may affect the management of the primary disease. Renal rickets and other vitamin D related disorders produce hypophosphatemia which impairs the calcification process in the bone.

In management of acute hypophosphatemia, intravenous PO_4 should be given carefully, monitoring serum levels of calcium, phosphate, potassium and magnesium during treatment.

Hyperphosphatemia occurs in acute/chronic renal failure (Fig. 10.10) and in conditions associated with massive cell necrosis (acute hemolytic anemia, acute rhabdomyolysis) and when a neoplastic disease (especially hematological) is treated with chemotherapy. In cases of chronic hyperphosphatemia there is risk of metastatic calcification. Hyperphosphatemia in neonates fed on undiluted cow's milk may produce hypocalcemia and tetany (Chapter 18). For significance of increased PO_4 level in hypoparathyroidism and pseudohypoparathyroidism, see Fig. 10.9. Also see Appendix B.

MAGNESIUM (Fig. 10.2)

Total body magnesium is about 21g, of which 67% is present in bone 31% in cells and 1% in ECF. About 39% of dietary magnesium is absorbed and the absorptive process is poorly controlled. Homeostasis is largely maintained by renal excretion. Concentration in intracellular fluid is about 10 times higher than in extracellular fluid.

In cells magnesium is activator of a number of enzymes. These include, those needed in synthesis and hydrolysis of ATP and those involved in synthesis of nucleotides, proteins and lipids. It is also important in stabilization of structures of RNA, DNA and ribosomes. It is involved in transmembrane transport of potassium and calcium, and influences electric properties of membranes. It also influences secretion of PTH and its actions.

30% of serum magnesium is protein bound and most of the rest is in free form. Total serum magnesium is generally measured and has poor correlation with its cellular functions. Low serum magnesium levels correlate poorly with intracellular depletion of magnesium. New methods are becoming available to evaluate magnesium disorders. These include ion selective electrodes for measuring ionic magnesium in blood and microelectrode and NMR based methods for intracellular magnesium.

Magnesium deficiency is more common than hypermagnesemia. In chronic malabsorption there is poor absorption of calcium, phosphate, potassium and magnesium besides other nutrients from the gut. Diuresis (alcohol, osmotic diuresis in diabetes, diuretics) also leads to magnesium depletion. Stresses like trauma, dehydration and even starvation, cause excessive loss of magnesium from cells and excretion in urine. Other causes are chronic dialysis, prolonged lactation, preeclampsia and acute pancreatitis. Magnesium deficiency like calcium deficiency causes increased neuromuscular irritability (magnesium tetany). Seizures and cardiac arrhythmias can also occur.

Three important intracellular elements are potassium, magnesium and phosphate. Deficiency of any

Table 10.4. Important causes of hypophosphatemia and the disturbances produced

Dietary/absorptive deficiencies
- Vitamin D deficiency
- Malabsorption
- Use of antacids along with poor diet

Excessive nutrient utilization causing PO_4 entry into cells
- Hyperalimentation
- Nutritional recovery syndrome
- Recovery from diabetic ketoacidosis (acidosis associated K-depletion promoted PO_4 depletion; during treatment with insulin and glucose, PO_4 enter cells).
- Alcohol withdrawl (alcohol produces acetate which displaces PO_4 from muscle cells to be lost in urine; there is decreased tubular PO_4 reabsorption: During alcohol withdrawl PO_4 enters cells, producing severe hypophosphatemia).

Respiratory alkalosis (the most common cause)
- Sepsis, heat stroke, alcohol withdrawl (intracellular low pCO_2 and high pH stimulate phosphofructokinase to increase glycolysis to increase PO_4 entry into cells)

Increased excretion into urine
- Vitamin D resistant rickets (renal rickets)
- After kidney transplant
- Oncogenic osteomalacia (mesenchymal and other tumors secrete a substance which not only reduces tubular PO_4 reabsorption but also reduces production of $1,25 (OH)_2D_3$

Other causes
- recovery from hypothermia or severe exercise (reactivated metabolism), volume expansion (reduced PO_4 reabsorption), prolonged use of diuretics (loss of PO_4 in urine), severe burns and others

HYPOPHOSPHATEMIA PRODUCED DISTURBANCES

Rhabdomyolysis
- It is produced in severe hypophosphatemia especially if some associated muscle damage is already present.
- It occurs in alcohol withdrawl; during treatment of diabetic ketoacidosis; hyperalimentation and refeeding of severely malnourished

Cardiomyopathy
- It may develop during treatment of septic shock

Respiratory insufficiency
- It is caused by weakness of diaphragm/respiratory muscles, in malnourished individuals receiving I/V nutrients, patients of COPD and others.

Erythrocyte dysfunctions
- It reduces O_2 delivery due to low level of 2,3 BPG in red cell

Nervous system dysfunction
- It reduces O_2 delivery to nervous tissue

Leukocyte dysfunction
- It impairs phagocytosis and opsonization
- It increases susceptibility to bacterial/fungal infections.

Bone demineralization
(hypophosphatemia associated with vitamin D deficiency, impaired activation of $25 (OH)D_3$ etc.)

Metabolic acidosis
- In hypophosphatemia there is impaired H^+ secretion and NH_3 formation but bone provides calcium carbonate to prevent development of acidosis. The compensation is not available in vitamin D deficiency, Mg deficiency and Al poisoning and metabolic acidosis develops.

one promotes deficiency of the other two. Conditions like reduced food intake, malabsorption, cellular atrophy and negative N-balance cause deficiency of all the three elements. In subsequent replenishment, if the nutrient intake is not balanced, there may be synthesis of abnormal protoplasm. For example, if the nutrient mixture used during hyperalimentation is poor in magnesium, ICF may become, undesirably, rich in calcium. This may become important cause of cell injury, by activating proteases and phospholipases.

Other interesting clinical examples also illustrate relationship between magnesium and potassium. About half the patients of selective magnesium deficiency become hypokalemic (magnesium deficiency, may stimulate aldosterone secretion). Further hypokalemia, refractory to potassium supplements, may require correction of magnesium deficiency. Similarly, there is relation between magnesium and calcium. Both hypocalcemia and hypomagnesemia stimulate secretion of PTH (sensitivity for hypocalcemia being much more than for hypomagnesemia). Severe hypomagnesemia, however, produces hypocalcemia which is refractory to calcium supplements alone. In severe hypomagnesemia, both secretion and actions of PTH are impaired.

Important conditions in which serum magnesium should be estimated include hypocalcemia especially when its clinical features do not respond to therapy, non responding hypokalemia, intestinal malabsorption and prolonged diuresis. Cellular magnesium deficiency may exist with serum magnesium in the normal reference range. Thus measurements of ionic serum magnesium or intracellular magnesium may be more useful, when these are easily available. Oral magnesium may result in diarrhea. It can also be given, parenterally. In the presence of renal disease magnesium administration needs careful monitoring of serum levels.

Hypermagnesemia may occur in advanced renal failure, acute diabetic ketoacidosis and after prolonged administration of magnesium containing antacids. It can cause drowsiness, hypotension and paralysis of voluntary muscles. Severe toxicity (renal failure) may result in respiratory paralysis and cardiac arrest. Immediate management may require intravenous calcium infusion followed by dialysis.

OSTEOPOROSIS (Also see Chapter 16)

Osteoporosis is loss of both osteoid and salts from the bone resulting in decrease of bone density. After loss of about 40% of bone material, osteoporotic bone gives a clear glass appearance on X-ray examination (in osteomalacia appearance is ground glass).

In the years of body growth, the bone mass keeps on increasing, as equilibrium, in the remodelling process is in favour of bone formation. Maximum bone mass is attained by about 25 years of age and is determined by genetic make up, physical activity, the level of gonadal hormones and the diet (protein, vitamins D and C). After the age of about 35 years, the equilibrium in bone remodelling process, tilts in favour of bone resorption and there is gradual decline in bone density. This age related osteoporosis is mild, common to both sexes and effects both trabecular (vertebral bodies and distal radius) and cortical (long bones, neck femur) bones. Excessive bone loss predisposes to fractures of vertebral body, distal radius (trabecular bone) and neck femur (cortical bone).

Besides the age related bone mineral loss, there is additional trabecular bone loss due to estrogen deficiency, in females after menopause. Deficiency of calcium, phosphate, vitamins D and C and protein (dietary or due to malabsorption), worsen both primary senile and primary postmenopausal osteoporosis. Immobilization, lack of exercise, smoking and alcohol all tend to add to the process.

Secondary osteoporosis can occur in younger people. Important causes are immobilization, prolonged use of certain drugs (corticosteroids, heparin), excessive alcohol intake, Cushing's syndrome, hyperthyroidism, gonadal failure, diabetes and malabsorption.

Investigations

Serum calcium, phosphate, alkaline phosphatase and PTH levels are within normal limits in senile/postmenopausal osteoporosis. Read objective type question 15 for physical means of diagnosis of bone disorders. During active phase of osteoporosis, increased bone resorption may be indicated by increased urinary excretion of hydroxyproline and calcium, or more specifically, by increased urinary excretion of collagen cross links (pyridinoline and deoxy-pyridinoline).

Serum osteocalcin and alkaline phosphatase are good markers of bone turn over. Also read under "bone formation and bone resorption".

Biochemical investigations are really useful in knowing cause of secondary osteoporosis (See above).

The best way to avoid harmful effects of senile/postmenopausal osteoporosis is to take care of bone formation, during growth period, as discussed above. For decreasing bone resorption treatment

Table 10.5. Some clinical presentations of hyperparathyroidism

- About 50% of patients present with asymptomatic hypercalcemia.
- Patients may present with non-specific features of hypercalcemia (anorexia, nausea, vomiting, constipation, muscle weakness (more of proximal muscles), tiredness) or mental changes (loss of memory, poor concentration, personality changes)[1].
- Renal calculi; more often recurrent calculi. Many patients may present with nephrocalcinosis (X-ray evidence), causing polyuria and polydipsia.
- Features related to bone involvement(bone pains, pathologic fractures). Much more common is X-ray evidence of subperiosteal bone resorption of phalanges and dissolution of phalangeal tufts.
- Hypertension is quite common in hyperparathyroid patients.
- Slit lamp examination (band keratopathy) or ECG (shortened QT interval), may give clue to diagnosis.

[1] In old patients these may be taken as features of dementia.

- Some times patient may present with cardiac arrhythmia, peptic ulcer or pruritis.

Table 10.6. Biochemical profile of certain hypercalcemic disorders

1. Hyperparathyroidism, multiple myeloma, extensive bone metastases and humoral hypercalcemia of malignancy (HHM) (in these cases usually the disorder causing hypercalcemia is not apparent. The biochemical profile of these conditions is presented separately).

2. Granulomatous disorders (sarcoidosis, tuber-culosis): Bilateral hilar enlargement, on X-ray examination; pulmonary opacities; specific disease presentation and specific tests.
   Calcium ↑/N: Phosphate N/↑: ALP ↑/N; PTH↓: Renal functions may be compromised. Urine Ca ↑: 1, 25 $(OH)_2$ D_3↑ in hypercalcemic patients.

3. Vitamin D intoxication[1] (during treatment of renal disease or hypoparathyroidism).
   Calcium ↑; Phosphate N: ALP-↓: PTH↓: Metastatic calcification of soft tissues and renal functions may be compromised. Urine Ca ↑: 25 $(OH)_2D_3$↑.

4. Milk alkali syndrome (self medication by patient of ant-acids for dyspepsia along with increased intake of calcium and bicarbonate. Renal calcinosis may result in renal insufficiency and azotemia.
   Calcium ↑: Phosphate ↑: ALP-N: PTH N/↓: Alkalosis: Renal functions may be compromised. Urine Ca normal..

5. Immobilization (specially in a patient with high rate of bone turnover.
   (In Paget's disease ALP is very high, also there is high level of hydroxy proline in urine).
   Calcium↑/N: Phosphate ↑/N: ALP-N: PTH N/↓:
   - Hypercalciuria in adults.
   - Hypercalcemia in children (effects are severer in presence of some condition causing increased bone turn over).

6. Chronic renal disease (in the terminal stages both calcium and phosphate are high. In early stage phosphate is high but calcium is normal or low). See under differential diagnosis of hypocalcemia.

[1] Besides vitamin D, thiazide diuretics, Li and calcium intakes can also cause hypercalcemia.

- Urine Ca is increased (>400 mg/d on a normal diet, ≥180 mg/d on a low calcium in diet) in PHPT. Excretion of >500 mg/d occurs in malignancy, sarcoidosis, multiple myeloma and hyperthyroidism.
- Low phosphate (<3 mg/dL) occurs in 50% cases of primary hyperparathyroidism (PHPT) and elevated level occurs in non-parathyroid hypercalcemia.
- Urinary cAMP is increased in >90% cases of PHPT and also in cases of HHM. Level is not increased in the presence of osteolytic bony metastases and myelomatosis. Excretion is low in vitamin D intoxication and sarcoidosis.

consists of increasing intake of calcium along with fluoride, protein and vitamin D. Problem with use of vitamin D is that the dose which increases bone deposition is not much lower than the dose that causes bone resorption. Use of a calcitonin analog with calcium has also been used with success. Diphosphonates (which inhibit bone resorption like calcitonin) have also been used.

Paget's disease

This disease is uncommon in our country. It is a disorder of bone remodelling. There is increased osteoclastic activity and increased bone reabsorption. Osteoblastic activity is also increased but the new bone is not laid down properly and is fragile. The disease runs in families. The disease might represent an inflammatory process triggered by a slow virus since inclusion bodies resembling a virus have been found in osteoclasts.

In Paget's disease the newly laid down bone lies in a disorganized way. It may cause pressure on surrounding structures. Bone pain, pathologic fractures and pressure effects on surrounding soft tissue, may be presenting features.

Serum alkaline phosphatase is markedly increased (acid phosphatase may also be increased). Also there is increase in urinary excretion of hydroxyproline, Pyr and D-Pyr (measured by immunoassays or by HPLC). X-ray shows typical punched out lesions of Paget's disease. Calcitonin and biphosphonates have been used in treatment.

HYPERCALCEMIA

Hypercalcemia should be properly confirmed. If the reference range reported by the laboratory lies between 9.0 to 11 mg/dL, mild cases of hypercalcemia may be missed. If samples are free from laboratory contamination the normal reference range lies between 9.0 to 10.5 mg/dL.

In examining the patient early features of hypercalcemia (Table 10.5) should be kept in mind.

Hypercalcemia occurs in two types of situations. In one situation the condition producing hypercalcemia is quite apparent and only alertness is required, to know, as and when it develops (Table 10.6). In the second type (Table 10.7), the condition pro-

ducing increase of serum calcium is not apparent. As diagnosis has to come from clinical features of hypercalcemia, it is quite delayed since clinical features of hypercalcemia are either vague or quite late (Table 10.5). Thus, when a sample is analyzed by a multichannel analyzer and increased calcium is seen as a chance observation, it should never be taken lightly.

Two important causes of hypercalcemia in second category of patients (See above) are malignancy and hyperparathyroidism. The main biochemical features for differential diagnosis are given in Table 10.7. Early features of hypercalcemia are quite vague and patient with unexplained muscular weakness, psychiatric features, hypertension, cardiac arrhythmias or polyuria should be explored for hypercalcemia.

Hyperparathyroidism (primary) (PHPT)

It may be found with frequency of one in one thousand in general population. Condition is commonly due to an adenoma but may be due to diffuse hyperplasia of the gland/s. Most patients have asymptomatic hyercalcemia. Bone pains and renal stones are late features. X-ray evidence of sub-periosteal bone resorption is seen more commonly than other bone lesions. Immunometric assay of intact PTH, using double antibody method will clearly establish diagnosis of hyperparathyroidism. It also helps to differentiate between hyperparathyroidism and idiopathic hypercalciuria in a patient of renal stones. A known case of hyperparathyroidism also needs proper assessment (Table 10.8).

Malignancy

Hypercalcemia is not uncommon in malignancy. The malignant cells present in the bone marrow (leukemia, lymphoma, myeloma) or the malignant cells invading the bone marrow (cancer breast) produce certain cytokines to cause local bone destruction. Some cytokines (IL-1, TNF-α, TNF-β) may be acting by activating osteoclasts and in such cases, osteoblastic reaction also occurs and leads to increase in level of alkaline phosphatase (not seen in multiple myeloma, lymphoma group).

Some tumors (renal/lung) produce parathyroid

Table 10.7. Important causes of hypercalcemia in which the causative disorder may not be evident

Hyperparathyroidism (PHPT): Both bone resorption and formation are increased.	• Family history; renal stones, metabolic bone disease, peptic ulcer disease, endocrine tumors (multiple endocrine neoplasia/familial hyperparathyroidism). • Mother of infant with severe neonatal tetany.	PTH ↑: PO_4↓:Ca↑ ALP ↑/N: Cl↑ (hyperchloremic acidosis): Cl/PO_4 ratio >33: Nephrogenic cAMP excretion ↑/N.
Humoral hypercalcemia of malignancy (HHM) (↑ PTHrP, ↓ PTH): Bone resorption increased but bone formation decreased	Search for primary tumor: Common clinical/metabolic features of malignancy	PTHrP↑; PTH↓ Ca↑↑: ALP-N: PO_4↓ cAMP N/↑ (nephrogenic): Cl ↓ (hypochloremic alkalosis): Cl/PO_4 ratio <30.
Extensive bony metastases/myelomatosis (↓PTH): Both bone resorption and formation increased.	Same as above. Also look for other features of myelomatosis	PTH↓:PO_4↑: ALP[1] N/↑: Ca↑: Nephrogenic cAMP-N:
Familial hypocalciuric hypercalcemia (FHH): • Non progressive harmless hypercalcemia before age of 10 years. • On exploration parathyroids normal and surgical intervention will be of no avail	Look for history of hypercalcemia in family (autosomal dominant inheritance)	Ca mild ↑: Ca excretion ↓ Ca: creatinine clearance ratio usually <0.01 (>0.02 in PHPT): PTH level usually normal: PO_4 variable: ALP-N.

[1]ALP increase > 2 N and increase of LD favour diagnosis of HHM rather than PHPT. ALP remains normal in myelomatosis (because of absence of osteoblastic reaction).

- After ruling out nutritional or medication causes (by history) of hypercalcemia, one has to rule out myeloma and sarcoidosis (ESR, serum proteins, electrophoresis). Then careful differentiation may be required between PHPT and occult cancer. Also one should keep in mind FHH (family history).

hormone related peptide (PTHrP). The PTHrP gene is different from the one encoding PTH but there is marked homology at N-terminal ends of PTH and PTHrP (Fig. 10.7). The latter molecule produced by certain tumors causes humoral hypercalcemia of malignancy (HHM). Immunometric assay of PTHrP is also available. In the presence of PTHrP as a cause of hypercalcemia, level of PTH will be very low (Table 10.7).

Presence of loss of weight, anemia, and raised ESR are common features of malignancy. Increase in level of serum globulin indicates multiple myeloma (also raised in sarcoidosis). In cases of malignancy one should always try to look for the primary tumor (breast, pelvic region and lungs).

Familial hypocalciuric hypercalcemia

It is a rare condition but it is important to know about it, as at times, the recognition may save a patient from unnecessary surgery (for misdiagnosed hyperparathyroidism). In this condition

urinary excretion of calcium is inappropriately low for the serum calcium level. More details are given in Table 10.7.

Differentiating hyperparathyroidism from other causes of hypercalcemia

In hyperparathyroidism, family history of renal stones, metabolic bone disease, peptic ulcer and some other endocrine disorder may be obtained.

Table 10.8. Investigations required for proper evaluation of a case of primary hyperparathyroidism

- For renal stones, nephrocalcinosis and kidney functions.
- For assessment of bone involvement (X-ray of hand/spine).
- Ultrasound of neck region to know about the state of parathyroid glands. Also see the text.

- Treatment may be conservative or partial parathyroidectomy. In conservative treatment increase water intake and ensure sufficient intake of phosphate. Also reduce intake of calcium and oxalate. Drugs increasing urinary excretion of calcium should not be given. For bone lesions controlled exercise and certain drugs may be needed (see under osteoporosis).

With availability of a sensitive immunometric assays for PTH and PTHrP, patients with increased levels of these hormones (in hyperparathyroidism and malignancy) are easily differentiated from other conditions associated with hypercalcemia. In the latter cases (also in malignancy with PTHrP), PTH levels are suppressed. The intact hormone is estimated using two site radio immunometric assay (IRMA), using one Ab against N-terminal region (1-34) as signal Ab and the other against C-terminal (39-84), immunoabsorbed to the solid support.

Reduced level of serum PO_4 favours diagnosis of hyperparathyroidism or HHM. This, however, is only true in the absence of renal disease (Fig. 10.11). Increased level of ALP is more common in cancer cases than hyperparathyroidism. Hypercalcemia of short history, with loss of weight, raised ESR, anemia, and without renal calculi favours diagnosis of malignancy.

Urine examination is important to rule out familial hypocalciuric hypercalcemia.

Urinary excretion of nephrogenic cAMP is increased in hyperparathyroidism and in cases of humoral hypercalcemia of malignancy. This may some times help, if PTH or PTHrP level leaves

some doubt about diagnosis. In a similar situation, the glucocorticoid suppression test may also help. Cortisone or prednisone administration for about 10 days will suppress hypercalcemia of many conditions (vitamin D excess, sarcoidosis, lymphoproliferative disorders and myeloma) but not in cases of hyperparathyroidism and HHM.

To summarize; be sure about presence of hypercalcemia and also whether it is symptomatic or asymptomatic. Take proper dietary history and history of ingestion of vitamins and drugs. Next look for malignancy. Try to locate the tumor if present. Take note of common features of malignancy like weight loss, anemia, muscular weakness, some indication from peripheral blood film and ESR. Bone marrow biopsy and bone scan may be indicated. Also keep in mind familial hypocalciuric hypercalcemia, before recommending the operative treatment.

In a failed surgical excision of hypersecreting parathyroid gland/glands, localization of such a gland for second operation becomes important. This is done with the help of ultrasound, MRI, CT and scanning with [201]Tl (locates parathyroids) and [99m]Tc (locates thyroid). Thyroid angiography and selective

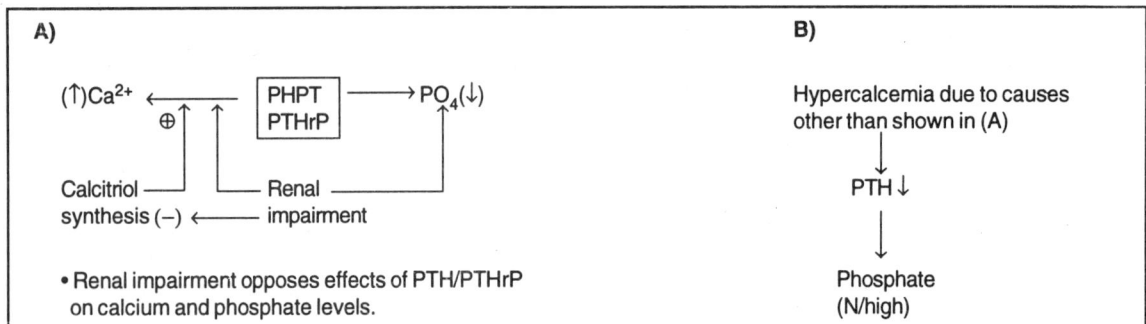

Fig.10.11. Interpretation of phosphate levels in hypercalcemia.

A) Cases of primary hyperparathyroidism or humoral hypercalcemia of malignancy.
- Initially phosphate is low and Ca is high. With rise of serum creatinine level, phosphate is normalized or may rise. This fact needs to be kept in mind while considering diagnosis of PHPT (primary hyperparathyroidism) in a case of renal stones with border line serum calcium.
- Besides renal failure vitamin D deficiency and severe malabsorption also interfere with calcium raising activity of PTH.
- Low serum phosphate of PHPT may become normal in presence of high phosphate intake or azotemia. In about 50% of cases of PHPT, it may be normal without azotemia.
B) Hypercalcemia due to causes other than those shown in A.
- Specificity of phosphate levels of different hypercalcemic disorders is not very good. Phosphate levels are influenced by diet and diurnal variations. Further patients with severe hypercalcemia due to any cause may show low serum phosphate.

venous catheterization, during the operation, for studying PTH levels in veins draining parathyroid glands may also be helpful.

HYPERCALCIURIA AND RENAL STONES

More than 300 mg of calcium excreted daily in urine in a male (and >250 mg in a female) is defined as hypercalciuria. Calcium stones are the most common renal stones (Table 10.9). Most common calcium stones are calcium oxalate stones. Increased urinary excretions of calcium and oxalate predispose to these stones. Magnesium, ammonium phosphate stones are associated with urinary tract infection. Increased uric acid excretion not only predisposes to uric acid stones but also to calcium oxalate stones.

Hypercalciuria occurs in cases of hypercalcemia. In many cases, however, hypercalciuria occurs

Table 10.9. Common types of stones with investigations required in such patients

Calcium stones (75 to 85%):
- Calcium oxalate stones (may have a nidus of uric acid stone).
- Calcium phosphate stones (calcium hydrogen phosphate is easily precipitated in urine of stone formers and may form nidus for both calcium oxalate and phosphate stones)

Triple phosphate stones (10 to 15%):
- Mg ammonium phosphate stones (formed in urine rich in NH_3 formed from urea by bacteria)

Uric acid stones (5 to 8%) **More common in men.**
- In patients with hyperuricosuria, uric acid is precipitated in urinary tract in acid urine; it may also form a nidus for calcium oxalate stones.

Cystine stones (about 1%):

OF CALCIUM STONES:

Idiopathic hypercalciuria (20%):
- The renal leak cases (thiazides reduce hypercalciuria; the drug may be used for diagnosis as well as treatment)
- Absorptive type (intestinal absorption of calcium is increased and is independant of calcitriol; a calcium load increases urinary calcium excretion more than in normals).
- Some cases may turn out as RTA type 1.

Hyperuricemia cases (20%):
- Increased uric acid excretion in urine.

Primary hyperparathyroidism (5%):
- Investigate for the disorder.

Hereditary (rare) **or acquired hyperoxaluria** (less common) **or Hypocitruria** (more common)
- Investigate urine citrate and oxalate levels. Response to pyridoxine administration for cases of hereditary hyperoxaluria.

Idiopathic stone disease (20%)
- Diagnosis by exclusion
- Oral phosphate and fluids to reduce recurrence.

Triple phosphate stones (struvite stones)
- Caused by obstruction and infection in the urinary tract

Investigations
- Investigations in 24h urine sample and blood sample: (calcium, uric acid, creatinine, electrolytes): In only urine (volume, pH, citrate, oxalate).
- Stone analysis will help to establish the cause.
- Investigations to establish presence of a specific cause
- Besides idiopathic hypercalciuria, other causes of hypercalciuria (without hypercalcemia) are hyperthyroidism, Cushing's syndrome, immobilization, malignant tumors, sarcoidosis, rapidly progressive bone disease, renal tubular acidosis, furosemide therapy and Paget's disease.

without hypercalcemia and results in formation of renal stones. These patients may suffer from renal calcium leak (Table 10.9) or unregulated calcium absorption. Hypercalciuria without hypercalcemia also occurs in renal tubular acidosis. In this condition there is hyperchloremic acidosis with high urinary pH (more than 6.8). RTA type 1 is predisposed to renal calculi because of reduced urinary excretion of citrate. Citrate inhibits spontaneous nucleation of calcium oxalate and also prevents crystal growth of both calcium oxalate and calcium phosphate stones. Potassium citrate administration not only inhibits these processes but also corrects hypokalemia produced by RTA type 1.

Hypocitruria occurs (and promotes renal stone formation) in intestinal disorders and with prolonged use of thiazide diuretics. In cases of ileal disease, ulcerative colitis and different forms of gut resections patients suffer from hypocitruria which is proportional to intestinal fluid loss. In addition, in such cases, because of steatorrhea, calcium forms insoluble soaps with fatty acids promoting oxalate absorption from the intestine. Thiazides promote renal tubular reabsorption of calcium. These also cause hypokalemia and intracellular acidosis, which is responsible for hypocitruria. This action of thiazides limits their benefit in calcium nephrolithiasis. Table 10.9 lists important investigations required in cases of renal stones.

A person susceptible to renal stones should eat a diet low in dairy items, without excessive protein but high in phosphate. They should also avoid use of antacids and foods high in oxalate (spinach, beans, brussel sprouts, rhubarb, currants, pine apple, strawberries, tea, cocoa, cashew, almonds). Water intake should be increased, to excrete, atleast 2L urine/d.

CASE HISTORY: 10.1

An old patient presented with complaints of muscular weakness, vague ill health and loss of weight. Serum creatinine level was 3.0 mg/dL. Serum calcium and phosphate levels were 11.2, 6.5 mg/dL respectively. ALP was in the normal range. Kidney X-ray examination did not reveal any calculi or nephrocalcinosis. PTH level was reduced but detectable. PTHrP assay did not reveal evidence of humoral hypercalcemia of malignancy. Secondaries in bones and multiple myeloma were chosen as two important possibilities for diagnosis.

There is no evidence that the renal damage is due to nephrocalcinosis or renal calculi. Direct renal involvement by the tumor can explain increased levels of calcium, phosphate and creatinine. While looking for the primary tumor no evidence was available for cancer prostate and bronchial carcinoma. However, serum globulin level was increased. X-ray examination revealed rounded, punched out lesions in bones. Bence Jones proteinuria was absent (seen in about 50% of patients) but a myeloma band was demonstrated on electrophoresis of serum proteins. In multiple myeloma, bone scan is normal as the myeloma deposits fail to take up bone seeking isotopes.

Renal functions are impaired in about 50% cases of multiple myeloma. Usually there is azotemia and loss of renal concentrating ability. Anemia is out of proportion to azotemia. Occasional cases may present with features of nephrogenic diabetes insipidus or some form of hypophosphatemic rickets. Condition is also discussed in Chapter 5.

CASE HISTORY: 10.2

A 6 year old child presented with short stature and an abnormal round face. His serum calcium was low (7.6 mg/dL), phosphate was raised (9.8 m/dL) and APL was in the normal range. Level of serum creatinine was also in the normal range for the age of the child.

Nutritional rickets was ruled out because of high phosphate level. Main differential diagnosis was between idiopathic hypoparathyroidism and pseudohypoparathyroidism. Short stature and the abnormal face favoured diagnosis of pseudohypoparathyroidism. Child was also mentally retarded.

On X-ray examination of the hand and foot it was shown that fourth and fifth metacarpals and metatarsals were relatively short in length. This established the diagnosis of pseudohypoparathyroidism.

Serum biochemistry of pseudohypoparathyroidism resembles that of hypoparathyroidism but in the former condition plasma PTH level is not reduced. There is end organ resistance to actions of PTH. Either activation of adenyl cyclase is defective (cAMP is not formed after PTH binds to its receptors) or cAMP is normally formed but its response does not occur. In some patients plasma calcium and phosphate levels remain normal but skeletal abnormalities are there. This condition is called pseudopseudohypoparathyroidism.

CASE HISTORY: 10.3

A patient was suffering from chronic diarrhea and presented with skin and mucosal lesions, weight loss, anemia, edema and severe abnormal sensory feelings in fingers and toes. Levels of both serum calcium and phosphate were low. iPTH level was also reduced. The cause of diarrhea could not be ascertained and it continued.

She was also put on rehabilitation diet and her deficiency features started improving except her abnormal sensory feelings in fingers and toes (although she was given vitamin D and calcium supplements). Next she was put on 1α (OH)D$_3$ alongwith a calcium supplement. Still no improvement occurred and it was also shown that she continued with low levels of serum calcium and PTH. At this stage she was given a magnesium supplement and her abnormal sensory feelings disappeared and her serum calcium also improved.

Magnesium deficiency, not only, interferes in secretion of PTH but also in its actions. In the presence of renal function impairment, magnesium administration (especially, parenteral) can become dangerous as it may cause hypermagnesemia. In these situations, serum magnesium level should be monitored during the therapy.

CASE HISTORY: 10.4

A 24 year old female presented in a severe dehydrated condition because of severe vomiting (early pregnancy). She also complained of muscle cramps and tingling sensation in her fingers and toes. Serum calcium was 9.0 mg/dL and serum albumin 4.7 mg/dL. She was in poor state of nutrition. She was administered appropriate fluids and her dehydration was managed but her cramps and tingling sensation did not improve. The two investigations previously done were repeated and her cramps were attributed to hypocalcemia. Trousseu's sign was also demonstrated to be positive.

Serum creatinine was done and was found to be in the normal range. Thus kidney was not responsible for her hypocalcemia. Serum PO$_4$ level was also not increased, ruling out parathyroid related deficiencies as the cause of her low calcium level. She was tentatively diagnosed as a case of nutritional deficiency of vitamin D and it was confirmed by demonstrating low level of 25 (OH)D$_3$ in her plasma.

She was managed by appropriate control of vomiting and supplements of vitamin D and calcium.

CASE HISTORY: 10.5

A 35 year old female was suffering from chronic renal disease. Serum creatinine level was 5.8 mg/dL. Serum calcium and PO$_4$ levels were 8.6 mg/dL, and 10.6 mg/dL, respectively. Plasma level of PTH was just above the normal reference range.

➤ How should she be managed to delay development of osteodystrophic changes?
• In chronic kidney disease activation of 25 (OH)D$_3$ is reduced because of high PO$_4$ level, acidosis

and reduced renal tissue. Calcitriol deficiency produces changes of osteomalacia in bones. In the beginning, with only mild increase in level of PTH (produced by low serum calcium resulting from renal disease) the bony changes are mainly osteomalacia type. But with progressive decrease of GFR and serum calcium, there is further increase of PTH level. As high levels of PTH develop, osteitis fibrosa type of changes also occur. In some cases tertiary hyperparathyroidism (autonomous secretion from parathyroid glands) develops.

The principle of management of renal osteodystrophy is to reduce development of hyperphosphatemia and also to directly treat calcitriol deficiency. This will tend to inhibit the above mentioned sequence ($\uparrow$PO$_4$, $\downarrow$Calcitriol $\rightarrow \downarrow$Ca $\rightarrow \uparrow$PTH $\rightarrow$ bony changes). Thus dietary phosphate is reduced, calcium intake is supplemented and also a phosphate binder is added to diet (administration of calcium carbonate achieves the latter two goals). If the patient is on dialysis, 1α-(OH)D$_3$ is given as it does not need 1α-hydroxylation in kidney for conversion to calcitriol. Treatment of osteodystrophy is preventing its development. Once the bone changes occur, these are resistant to treatment. This is true for both components especially the one produced by PTH excess.

In far advanced renal disease, the excretory functions of kidney can be partly replaced by dialysis but the endocrine and metabolic functions are not replaced and need renal transplant.

OBJECTIVE TYPE QUESTIONS

Pick out incorrect statements

1. Hyperparathyroidism

i) Most common manifestation of hyperparathyroidism is sustained or intermittent hypercalcemia.

ii) In presence of an associated condition which would impair actions of PTH, hyperparathyroidism may present with normocalcemia.

iii) Conditions which impair actions of PTH include, chronic renal failure, severe malabsorption and vitamin D deficiency.

iv) Without presence of conditions listed as item iii), hyperparathyroidism would always present with fasting hypercalcemia.

v) For a given serum calcium level, more calcium is lost in urine in nonparathyroid cases than hyperparathyroidism.

2. Hypercalcemia (asymptomatic)

i) 90% cases of asymptomatic hypercalcemia are due to hyperparathyroidism.

ii) Asymptomatic hypercalcemia of hyperparathyroidism does not require surgical treatment.

iii) Two important causes of hypercalcemia are hyperparathyroidism and malignancy.

iv) If hypercalcemia is of more than one year duration, cause is more likely hyperparathyroidism than malignancy.

v) Lithium therapy causes hypercalcemia by increasing PTH level.

3. Hypercalcemia

i) iPTH may not always be low or undetected, in cases of vitamin D related or high bone turnover cases of hypercalcemia.

ii) 1,25 $(OH)_2D_3$ levels may be increased in many cases of hyperparathyroidism.

iii) History is important in cases of hypercalcemia due to prolonged high intakes of vitamins A and D and thiazides.

iv) In case of a disorder of increased bone turnover, severe hypercalcemia is unusual.

v) 1,25 $(OH)_2D_3$ levels are of real importance in differentiating vitamin D intoxication cases from those of sarcoidosis.

4. PTHrP

i) Different genes produce PTH and PTHrP.

ii) In case of PTHrP multiple fragments are present in blood due to tissue specific cleavages.

iii) PTHrP has roles in both fetal and adult physiology.

iv) In fetus it causes transplacental calcium transfer.

v) In an adult it may have important developmental influence in calcium and bone physiology.

vi) Molecular heterogeneity poses more problems in PTH assay than in PTHrP assay.

vii) PTHrP may cause hypercalcemia of malignancy.

5. Hypercalcemia

i) iPTH levels are high in >90% PTH related cases.

ii) iPTH levels are low or undetected in cases of malignancy.

iii) iPTH levels are undetected or normal in vitamin D related or high bone turnover cases.

iv) Low serum phosphate level in hyperparathyroidism can easily differentiate these cases from non-parathyroid cases (as in item iii) of hypercalcemia.

v) In hyperparathyroidism serum phosphate level is low but may be normal if renal failure starts developing.

6. Malignancy related hypercalcemia

i) More common with overt tumors than with occult ones.

ii) It can occur without bone metastases.

iii) In humoral hypercalcemia of malignancy, a sensitive assay will show decreased level of PTH.

iv) PTH and PTHrP produce similar actions in the body.

v) Features of malignancy like weight loss, muscle weakness, skin rash and anemia may be present in malignancy cases.

vi) Bone scan using technetium labeled biphosphonate can help to detect osteolytic bone lesions.

7. Post operative hypocalcemia (parathyroidectomy)

i) Most common after operation following the first unsuccessful operation.

ii) If serum calcium falls below 8.0 mg/dL, and there is increase in level of phosphate, surgically produced hypoparathyroidism may be there.

iii) It may also be produced by co-existing Mg deficiency.

iv) Presence of bone disease (PTH induced) does not affect post operative hypocalcemia.

v) Most cases of post operative hypocalcemia do not need parenteral calcium therapy.

8. Familial hypocalciuric hypercalcemia (FHH)

i) FHH is an autosomal dominant disorder.

ii) Defect in FHH is in the calcium sensor in parathyroid cells and the renal tubular cells, leading to inappropriate secretion of PTH (increased) by parathyroid cells and excessive reabsorption of calcium by tubules.

iii) FHH involves excessive secretion of PTH and Jansen's disease leads to increased activity of PTH at its receptors.

iv) Both FHH and Jansens disease are treated by parathyroidectomy.

v) FHH presents with hypercalcemia in first ten years of life, whereas in hyperparathyroidism of MEN syndromes, it occurs after the first decade.

vi) For given degree of hypercalcemia iPTH level are higher in hyperparathyroidism than in FHH.

vii) Serum magnesium levels are higher in FHH than in primary hyperparathyroidism.

9. Hypercalcemia in cases of increased bone turnover

i) In hyperthyroidism, hypercalciuria is more common than hypercalcemia.

ii) Immobilization may cause hypercalcemia in children but generally causes hypercalciuria in adults.

iii) Thiazide administration increases serum calcium level in a normal person as long as the drug is continued.

iv) Excess intake of vitamin A causes hypercalcemia by increasing bone resorption.

v) In vitamins A and D intoxications, hyperthyroidism and milk alkali syndrome treatment of the primary disorder leads to normalization of serum calcium.

10. About serum calcium and phosphate level

i) For clinicopathological correlation calcium levels are more useful than phosphate levels.

ii) Prolonged venous occlusion leads to hemoconcentration to affect serum calcium levels.

iii) Changes in serum albumin levels also affects serum calcium levels.

iv) In clinical conditions ionic calcium is often required for proper interpretation.

v) Serum phosphate levels are affected by diet, diurnal variation; samples must be obtained in the morning, in fasting state.

11. Alcohol withdrawl

i) Alcoholics, especially those with associated malabsorption suffer from deficiencies of magnesium, calcium, potassium and phosphate.

ii) Alcohol withdrawl causes accumulation of calcium in smooth muscle cell.

iii) Increased intracellular calcium in vascular smooth muscle increases vascular tone and also potentiates the pressor response to circulating catecholamines.

iv) During alcohol withdrawl there is increased sympathetic nerve activity and increased level of catecholamines.

v) Alcohol withdrawl can result in permanent hypertension in many alcoholics.

12. Effect of magnesium on myocardium

i) Magnesium regulates potassium and calcium movements in myocardial cells.

ii) In magnesium deficiency, ECG changes may resemble those of hypokalemia.

iii) Because of effect on movements of calcium, effects of magnesium therapy may resemble those of calcium channel blockers.

iv) Magnesium deficiency has no independant effect on cardiac rhythm.

v) Deficiency of magnesium or potassium can reduce concentration of myocardial Na, K, Mg - ATPase to increase chances of digitalis toxicity.

13. Bone mineralization

i) Vitamin D metabolites enhance absorption of calcium from the intestine.

ii) $24, 25 \ (OH)_2 \ D_3$ may have a direct role in the mineralization process.

iii) Phosphate depletion can produce osteomalacia.

iv) Chronic acidosis plays a role in development of osteomalacia by altering metabolism of vitamin D or by altering renal handling of calcium/phosphate.

v) Osteomalacia may also occur in hyperchloremic acidosis of ureterocolic anastomosis.

vi) In hypophosphatasia there is deficiency of alkaline phosphatase, low plasma level of phosphate and osteomalatia.

vii) Accumulation of aluminium in bone also produces mineralization defect in the bone.

14. Rickets/osteomalacia

i) Nutritional rickets may affect general body growth and may cause delayed eruption of teeth in children.

ii) In adults, osteomalacia may produce proximal muscle weakness.

iii) Vitamin D dependant rickets may be associated with generalized aminoaciduria and skeletal deformities or epidermal problems.

iv) Vitamin D resistant rickets may present as rickets in an otherwise healthy looking child.

v) All types of rickets/osteomalacia can be treated by vitamin D.

15. Radiological examination

i) In osteoporosis, cortices of long bones may be thin because of endosteal bone resorption but outer margins are sharp unlike sub-periosteal bone resorption of hyperparathyroidism.

ii) Pseudofractures occur only in osteomalacia.

iii) Often it may be impossible to differentiate between osteomalacia and osteoporosis, on radiological ground, only.

iv) Radiologic examination is quite a sensitive indicator of bone density.

v) Bone scan with technetium-labeled bisphosphonate leads to preferential uptake of isotope by lytic lesions of Paget's disease, osteolytic bone secondaries and the fracture sites.

16. Hypercalcemia

i) There is history of hypercalcemia and renal stones in an otherwise asymptomatic person; diagnosis most probably would be hyperparathyroidism.

ii) There is recent symptomatic hypercalcemia; make a thorough search for malignancy.

iii) There is chronic asymptomatic hypercalcemia

and iPTH level is not elevated; malignancy is unlikely, may be occult sarcoidosis.

iv) Serum calcium level of >14.5 is more suggestive of HHM than hyperparathyrodisim.

v) Disorders other than hyperparathyroidism are responsible for about 50% of cases of hypercalcemia.

vi) Repeated analysis should document hypercalcemia (taking into consideration the serum protein level), before declaring it a clinically significant finding.

ANSWERS

1. No.(iv). Condition of normocalcemic hyperparathyroidism, although rare, is known. Patients present with recurrent stone formation without fasting hypercalcemia. Patient may show post prandial hypercalcemia or may be diagnosed by a provocative test using thiazide. Patient will show hypercalcemia throughout the period of drug administration unlike normals who become normocalcemic after some time, during drug therapy.

2. No.(ii). Surgical treatment is recommended in patients below 50 years of age especially: i) if calcium levels is above the upper limit by 1.0 or 1.6 mg/dL; ii) there is history of an episode of severe hypercalcemia resulting from dehydration or some other illness; iii) reduction of creatinine clearance by more than 30% of the normal value for the age of the patient; iv) presence of calcium excretion of more than 400 mg/d; v) when there is considerable decrease of bone mass.

3. No.(v). These are important in establishing diagnosis of sarcoidosis or some B-cell lymphomas as a cause of hypercalcemia.

4. No.(vi). The molecular heterogeneity interferes more in PTHrP assay than in PTH assay.

5. No.(iv). Serum phosphate levels are not low in many cases of hyperparathyroidism. Further even in non-parathyroid cases of severe hypercalcemia serum phosphate may be low.

6. No.(iv). Certain actions of PTH and PTHrP are similar (high calcium, low phosphate and incre-

ased levels of nephrogenic cyclic AMP in urine) while there is difference in other actions (in case of PTH, renal calcium excretion is lower and $1,25 (OH)_2D_3$ level higher than with PTHrP).

7. No.(iv). It causes severe post operative hypocalcemia.

8. No. (iv). Neither of the two disorders are cured by parathyroidectomy.

9. No.(iii). This is true in cases of normocalcemic hyperparathyroidism; in a normal person the initially increased serum calcium level gets normalized, after some days, as the drug is continued.

10. No.(iv). It is often not required. However, effect of high or low serum albumin level should be taken into account before interpreting the significance of serum calcium levels.

11. No.(v). It results only in temporary hypertension.

12. No.(iv). Magnesium deficiency, of its own causes prolongation of QT and predisposes to dangerous arrhythmias.

13. No.(vi). Serum phosphate levels are normal or increased.

14. No.(v). Treatment modality will depend upon the etiology of the disorder. Nutritional rickets is treated with vitamin D; malabsorption cases require higher doses than others with nutritional etiology. Phosphate should not be given as it will lower calcium. Patients of vitamin D resistant rickets need calcitriol along with phosphate supplement. Those associated with chronic acidosis should be given bicarbonate to treat acidosis. Patients of chronic renal failure need active vitamin D metabolite along with restriction of phosphate intake and absorption. There is need to monitor serum calcium and $25(OH)D_3$ levels.

15. No.(iv). It is an insensitive indicator of bone density. The best method is dual-energy X-ray densitometry (DEXA); other methods are single and dual photon absorptiometry, neutron activation analysis of body calcium and quantitative computed tomography.

16. No.(v). Only about 10% of the cases.

CHAPTER 11

Clinical Nutrition – Some Aspects

MALNUTRITION

Malnutrition is an important problem, especially in developing countries. In these countries poverty (including associated environmental factors), ignorance, and cultural practices, all contribute to malnutrition. Malnourished mother produces an under weight baby (intrauterine malnutrition) and as enough food is not available after birth, the catch up growth is not possible. Poor environmental conditions resulting in infections (including diarrheal diseases) aggravate the problem. In adult population, alcoholism aggravates malnutrition produced by poverty. In hospital patients, malnutrition is produced in surgical patients and those suffering from prolonged systemic illnesses due to metabolic changes associated with stress of illness.

In malnutrition, the patient shows evidence of deficiencies of energy, protein, vitamins and minerals. Patient may present with complaints of weight loss (poor growth in a child). There may be increased susceptibility to infection or wound healing may be poor. There may be anemia and poor work capacity.

Evaluation of the patient includes, proper history, clinical examination and certain laboratory tests. In many cases, history will reveal cause of malnutrition. Clinical examination and laboratory tests will indicate its severity. In clinical examination of a malnourished child, record of three parameters is important; the age, the height and the weight. Weight for height is an index of current nutritional status and height for age is an index of past nutrition.

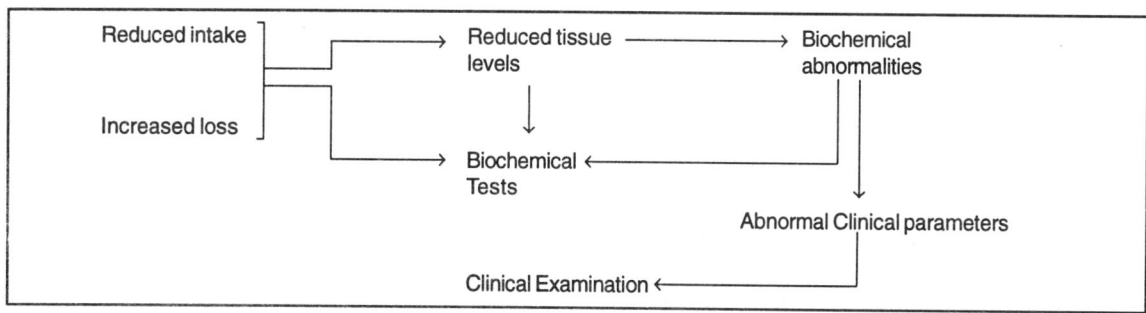

Fig.11.1. Relation between chemical tests and clinical examination in nutrient deficiency disorders.

- Serum levels/urinary excretions of nutrients often represent dietary intakes. For tissue levels/functional status, other tests are available.

Midarm circumference is an index of skeletal muscle mass while skin fold thickness indicates the status of body fat. Proper examination of skin, mucous membrane, hair, nails and teeth may reveal certain specific nutrient deficiencies.

Biochemical tests are also used in diagnosis of different nutrient deficiencies (Appendix 11.1 for vitamin deficiencies). The biochemical tests are supposed to provide evidence of nutrient deficiencies earlier than their clinical evidence (Fig. 11.1). Thus in any situation (malabsorption, reduced intake, intake of alcohol and drugs, infections, trauma, renal and hepatic diseases), where deficiency of a nutrient is expected, a biochemical test will predict need of replacement earlier than the clinical indication. In areas of endemic malnutrition, pre-kwashiorkor can be recognized earlier by measurement of serum albumin than simple clinical examination.

Generally, treatment is based on history and clinical judgement. For single nutrient deficiency, in some situations, however, biochemical tests are relied upon. Thus the biochemical tests may be useful in detecting folic acid deficiency in chronic alcoholics, in pregnancy, in tropical sprue and in patients taking anticonvulsants or oral contraceptives. Similarly pyridoxine deficiency may be detected in patients on antitubercular therapy. Biochemical tests may be needed to differentiate between folic acid and B_{12} deficiencies in megaloblastic anemias. Ascorbate deficiency may need biochemical detection in early infancy and in old age. Vitamin A deficiency may also occur as an isolated deficiency in certain regions. Isolated vitamin D deficiency may occur in liver disease, renal disease, malabsorption syndrome and in certain groups, deprived of sunshine or it may be genetic. Biochemical testing of vitamins A and D may also be required during therapeutic administration of these vitamins to avoid their toxicities.

Role of biochemical tests in monitoring of patients on total parenteral nutrition is discussed separately.

Kwashiorkor and marasmus

Two severe forms of protein energy malnutrition (PEM) are marasmus and kwashiorkor. Marasmus occurs in early infancy by early weaning and putting the infant on a diet poor in both protein and calories. Kwashiorkor occurs in early childhood at about 1.5 years when a child is weaned and put on a diet rich in carbohydrate but poor in protein. Many children have features midway between the two distinct clinical forms.

In marasmus the main features are loss of subcutaneous fat and muscle protein (it is said to be adapted state in stress of PEM). In kwashiorkor, subcutaneous fat and muscle protein are preserved but there is failure of hepatic protein synthesis and edema. Kwashiorkor is said to be the state of PEM in which adaptation has failed. Kwashiorkor is characterized by impaired immune response and also involves free radical injury. Diarrhea and infection play important roles in worsening of PEM.

In developing countries where one encounters cases of marasmus and kwashiorkor, a very large number of children suffer from milder grades of malnutrition. Commonly used parameters in diagnosis of such cases are height/weight for age; weight for height and midarm circumference. Serum levels of albumin or other proteins can help detection of pre-kwashiorkor cases.

IRON METABOLISM

Total body iron is about 4g, of which about 25% is present as storage iron (ferritin and hemosiderin) and about 2.8g in hemoglobin. Besides iron is also present in myoglobin, cytochromes and other enzymes. The recommended iron intake of 10 mg/day for males should be obtained from diet (for females it is 15 mg/day). Normally about 10% of dietary iron is absorbed. It may increase to about 30% in iron deficiency, in pregnancy and during growth. Iron in heme as such and ferritin iron, after solubilization (helped by reducing agents followed by amino acids and sugars, which form complexes) is taken up at receptors in the upper intestine and absorbed by an active process. From inside the cell, it is partly carried to the serosal side (to be handed over to transferrin in the blood) and partly binds to apoferritin to form ferritin and retained in the mucosal cell.

Transferrin carries iron (ferric form) in circula-

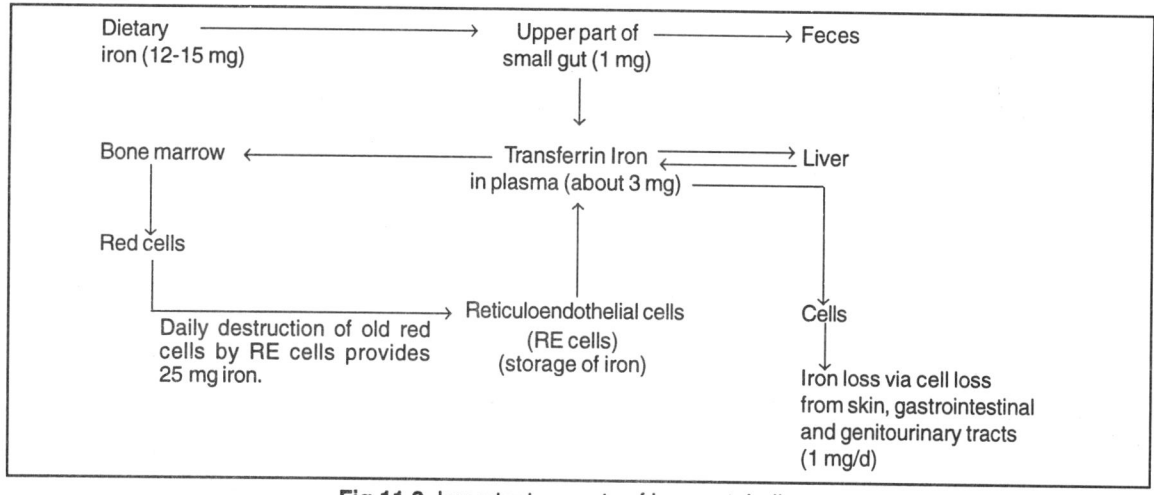

Fig.11.2. Important aspects of iron metabolism.

- Daily iron loss in menstruating females is about 2 mg/d, taking into account iron loss of about 30 mg/month in menstrual blood.
- Iron supply to bone marrow also regulates the proliferative response of marrow to erythropoietin. If iron supply is reduced there is hypoproliferative marrow response and Hb synthesis is also reduced.

tion. Cells take up transferrin with the help of their transferrin receptors (the number of receptors on a cell depends on its need for iron). A very remarkable feature of iron metabolism is the conservation of iron. Iron made available from break down of iron containing compounds is reused for synthesis of iron containing compounds (Fig. 11.2).

Iron deficiency causes microcytic hypochromic anemia. However, effects of iron deficiency are not limited to this anemia. Iron deficiency appears to effect functioning of many tissues (including muscle) which possess iron containing enzymes. Reduced work capacity, in iron deficiency, may partly be independent of anemia. Other independent effects of iron deficiency are behaviour changes and learning problems in children and also impaired thermoregulation.

Iron deficiency anemia

It is the commonest deficiency disorder in our country and results from poor quality of food (cereal based pure vegetarian diet), poor absorption (intestinal malabsorption or achlorhydria) and chronic blood loss (hook worm infection, piles, peptic ulcer). Women in reproductive period of life (increased demand due to menstrual loss and pregnancy) and

growing children (increased demand due to growth) are especially susceptible to this anemia. During iron depletion, body passes through three stages: First of all the stores are depleted and next, probably, the functioning of iron containing or iron activated enzymes is affected along with development of certain compensatory mechanisms (increased synthesis and level of transferrin and decrease in its saturation). Finally, changes in number and morphology of red cells are produced (Table 11.1).

Diagnosis of iron deficiency anemia (IDA)

After examination of the blood film, if there is obvious cause of iron deficiency, no further investigation may be needed. At times, however, differentiation is required from anemia of chronic disease (ACD), sideroblastic anemia and anemia of thalassemia minor. In all these conditions anemia is hypochromic and microcytic as in IDA. Hypochromic normocytic anemia may also be found in hypopituitarism, hypothyroidism and hypogonadism (only in males). The need for differentiation of IDA from these anemias may arise if the patient fails to respond to iron administration. First, a general account of investigations, helpful in differential diagnosis is given below:

Table 11.1. Different stages of iron deficiency

The stage	Biochemical changes / Detection	Remarks
Depletion of store	- No stainable iron[1] in bone marrow smear - Low serum ferritin level (less than 20 µg/L)	No symptoms
Stage of adaptation	- Increased synthesis of transferrin - Reduced transferrin saturation - Increased level of transferrin receptors in serum - Increased level of red cell protoporphyrin	No symptoms
Reduced synthesis of iron containing enzymes	- Transferrin saturation falls to less than 30%	Reduced work capacity. Impaired growth[2]
Stage of anemia	- Reduced number of microcytic hypochromic cells	All features of anemia

[1]There are two storage forms of iron, ferritin (from which iron is readily available for use) and hemosiderin (formed, probably, by degradation of ferritin). The latter is stainable by prussian blue reaction to provide a crude measurement of iron stores in the marrow.

[2]Alongwith cells of growing tissues, cells with short life span (eg; intestinal mucosal cells) are also affected.

Serum iron

There is difficulty in interpretation of serum iron as normal variation of more than 100% can occur in individuals (random variations, circadian variations, monthly variations in women). Serum iron levels in isolation are generally, uninformative (except in cases of iron overload). False increase of serum iron occurs in hemolysed sample and in the presence of iron contaminated glassware. False decrease occurs in lipemic serum.

Serum transferrin or total iron binding capacity (TIBC)

Serum transferrin may be estimated as total iron binding capacity (TIBC) or directly, using a two site enzyme immunoassay, using monoclonal antibodies. See Appendix B for more information. Percent saturation of transferrin (Fe/TIBC × 100) is a better index to differentiate between iron deficiency anemia and anemia of chronic disease.

Serum transferrin level also increases in pregnancy. Its level is reduced in liver disease and malnutrition.

Serum ferritin

Ferritin can be estimated using different methods (RAI, enzyme immuno assay, immuno radiometric assay). It is a good index of iron stores. However, its level rises in infections, inflammatory diseases, chronic liver disease, malignancies, alcoholism and hyperthyroidism as it is an acute phase protein.

Bone marrow iron

It is the most reliable index of iron deficiency. Marrow iron disappears before changes occur in blood film. Only patients with reduced bone marrow iron are likely to benefit from iron therapy.

Free erythrocyte protoporphyrin (FEP)

A rapid micro method is available to estimate FEP in whole blood. FEP is increased in iron deficient erythropoiesis (IDA, ACD) and also lead poisoning, sickle cell disease, eythropoietic porphyria and some cases of sideroblastic anemia but remains normal in thalassemia.

In differential diagnosis between important causes of hypochromic microcytic anemia (see above), bone marrow *storage iron and serum ferritin are decreased in IDA* and normal or elevated in all others (ACD, thalassemia, sideroblastic anemia). *In thalassemia trait the FEP and serum iron are normal and* condition is also present in family members. In β-thalassemia trait the HbA$_2$ and often HbF are increased. HbA$_2$ is often reduced in IDA. *In ACD although serum iron is low (as in IDA), the TIBC is low or normal (Fe/TIBC is more discriminatory).* In sideroblastic anemia (including chronic lead poisoning), serum iron and percent TIBC saturation are increased; also ring sideroblasts are present in the marrow.

Anemia of chronic disorders (ACD)

ACD may be normocytic normochromic but in long standing cases becomes microcytic hypochromic.

Cytokines TNF and IFN-β are mediators produced in bacterial infections and neoplasms and IL-1 and IFN-γ in chronic inflammatory states (e.g., SLE). These cytokines can inhibit proliferative capacity of erythroid precursors, erythropoietin release from kidney and delivery of iron from RE cells. Unlike IDA, in ACD, bone marrow iron stores are increased along with increase of ferritin level, ferritin being an acute phase protein. Further both serum

iron and TIBC are low with normal Fe/TIBC ratio in ACD. ACD require no treatment.

Sideroblastic anemia

Primary disorder is X-linked recessive which results from reduced activity of erythroid form of ALA-synthase leading to ineffective erythropoiesis, causing anemia and weakness in infancy. Secondary causes include alcoholism, lead poisoning, malnutrition and use of antitubercular drugs. Severe cases may respond to vitamin B_6 (forms co-enzyme of ALA-synthase). In peripheral blood film, red cells may show coarse basophilic stippling and bone marrow shows increased iron and cells with peripheral ring of granules (sideroblasts). *Serum iron*

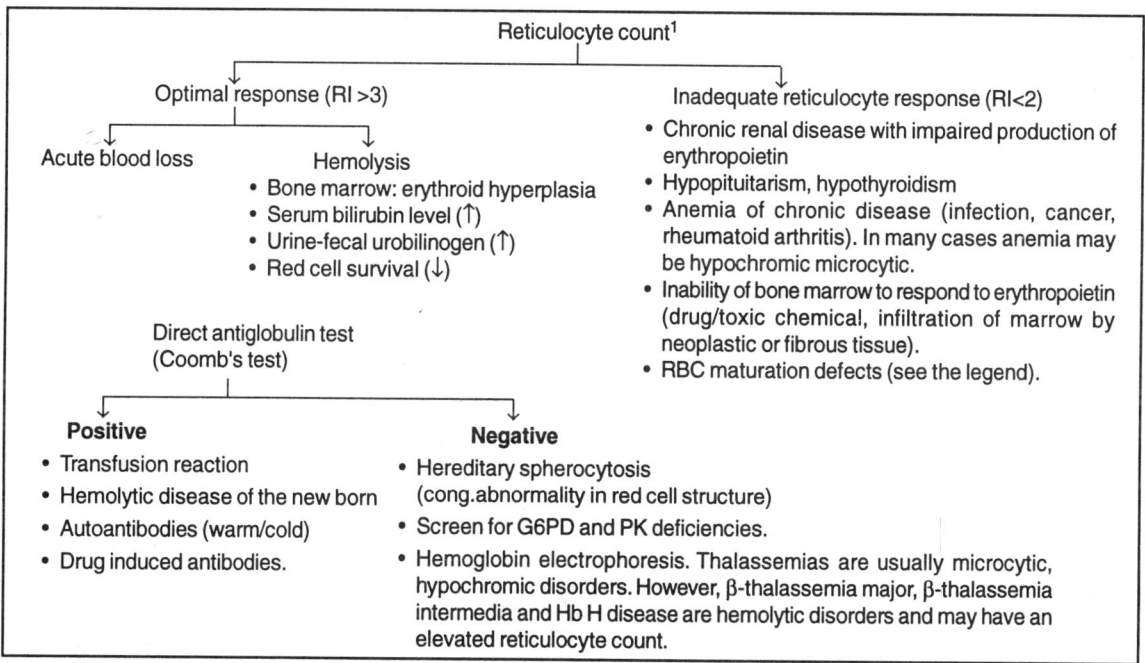

Fig.11.3. Investigating normocytic, normochromic anemia.

---

[1] The reticulocyte count is increased when bone marrow is stimulated due to anemia. This stimulation depends upon hematocrit; lower the hematocrit, more the stimulation. Further it will also be influenced by maturation rate of the precursor cells. If maturation is delayed reticulocytes will stay in circulation for a longer time, tending to cause apparent increase in their number. This delay in maturation is judged by polychromasia of the peripheral blood film. When reticulocyte count is corrected for the above two factors, we get the reticulocyte index (RI) which gives true state of appropriateness of bone marrow response to anemia. RI >3 means appropriate response.

- Index <2 may occur because of hypoproliferative bone marrow (see first four causes under RI <2). In these cases, ratio of erythroid: granulocyte precursors "E:G ratio" in bone marrow is ≤ 1:2. Index <2 may also occur in cases of maturation defect (IDA, thalassemia, folate/B_{12} deficiency) in which E:G ratio is > 1:1.

- Index >3 occurs in hemolytic anemia in which E:G ratio is > 1:1.

and % transferrin saturation are increased (as in thalassemia) but unlike IDA.

Thalassemia minor

It includes heterozygous patients of congenital disorders in which there is defective synthesis of the chains of normal hemoglobin. In β-thalassemia (cases seen in India) defect lies in β-chain synthesis. Hb level is seldom less than 10 g/dL; level of Hb-A_2 is above 3.5% and that of Hb-F is variable.

In α-thalassemia, the heterozygous state is also called Hb-H disease. This condition is more severe and often there is associated splenomegaly. A similar type of anemia also results in presence of Hb-E and the so called Lepore state (functional absence of both δ and β chains of Hb due to presence of δ-β fusion gene)

Important laboratory findings are: i) presence of abnormal hemoglobins; ii) serum and bone marrow iron not reduced and TIBC not increased (unlike IDA); iii) normal level of free erythrocyte porphyrin (FEP) (unlike IDA, ACD and some cases of sideroblastic anemia in which cases FEP levels are increased, an indicator of reduced erythropoiesis).

Type of anemia and its cause

Anemia should be investigated before treatment is started. Also cause of anemia should not be presumed from the presentation of the patient. Preliminary studies include estimations of Hb, hematocrit and erythrocyte count. Blood film should be studied carefully as it may be helpful in pointing to the cause of anemia. Additional help may be provided by the leukocyte, platelet and reticulocyte counts.

Next, the red cell indices are determined to categorize anemia into macrocytic, microcytic hypochromic and normocytic normochromic types.

RDW (red cell distribution width) is a quantitative measure of anisocytosis. It is CV of the distribution of individual red cell volumes. It is derived from central area of the RBC histograms, obtained from use of some newer automated blood cell counting instruments. RDW and MCV taken together have helped to detect early cases of iron, B_{12} and folate deficiency anemias (RDW high and MCV

normal) and also in differential diagnosis of microcytic, hypochromic anemias (see below).

Microcytic hypochromic anemia

In placing a case of anemia in this group, greater reliance is placed on MCV than MCHC which, in many cases, may be in the normal range. RDW and MCV have been used in differentiation of different anemias in this group: RDW (n), MCV (n) in normals and early ACD: RDW (high), MCV (low) in IDA: RDW (low or n), MCV (low) in thalassemia minor. These disorders have already been discussed.

Macrocytic anemias

For anemias of this group, see under deficiencies of folate and B_{12} (Appendix 11.1).

Normochromic normocytic anemia

Sub-classes in this group depend upon the absolute reticulocyte count and the results of the direct antiglobulin test (Coomb's test). See Fig. 11.3.

TRACE ELEMENTS

Besides iron, a number of other metal/non-metal ions are present in human body, in very small amounts. These are called trace elements and include Zn, Cu, Co, Se, Mo, Mn, I, F and Cr. The trace elements form integral components of certain enzymes or some other biomolecules. Generally, there are no special foods rich in specific trace elements. These are present in common foods and their amounts relate to the trace element content of the soil. Trace element deficiencies have been reported in many patients on total parenteral nutrition. (TPN). Excess entry of trace elements into the body may also result in harmful effects. F toxicity is also known in areas where F content of water is high. Plasma levels are used to know trace element deficiencies or excesses. However, the relation of plasma levels to tissue concentrations are not defined properly.

Zinc is present in many enzymes and biomolecules, involved in different biological processes (Table 11.2). Important causes of Zn deficiency due to poor intake are, PEM, malabsorption, chronic alcohol intake and TPN. Stress, infection, and metabolic causes can also result in Zn deficiency. Zn deficiency has been reported in cirrhosis, burns, chronic renal failure acute myocardial infarction, patients on hemodialysis and in other conditions. Achrodermatitis enteropathica is a rare inherited disorder with Zn malabsorption (there is poor wound healing, gonadal dysfunction and immune deficiency). Serum Zn level is reduced. Chronic Zn deficiency has been reported from Middle East countries because of poor cereal based diet resulting in dwarfism and hypogonadism.

Plasma metallothionine levels better correlate with Zn deficiency produced by poor intake while plasma Zn levels are more useful in indicating Zn deficiency due to metabolic and other causes. Atomic absorption spectrophotometry is the method of choice for estimation of plasma Zn. Serum levels are higher than the plasma levels (platelet disintegration releases Zn). Levels are also affected by hemolysis, albumin levels (about 70% of Zn is bound to albumin in plasma) and intake of coticosteroids and oral contraceptives.

Zn deficiency in infants may cause failure to thrive. In children it causes growth failure and delayed sexual development. There is impairment of taste perception and the immune system. In adults it may cause, poor wound healing, alopecia and a skin rash.

In intake deficiency case, Zn therapy is helpful while in cases of deficiency due to metabolic and other causes, its role has not been properly defined.

Cu is component of many enzymes (cytochrome oxidase, tyrosinase, lysyl hydroxylase, dopamine-β-hydroxylase and others). It is involved in synthesis of hemoglobin and in metabolism of connective tissue. Cu deficiency is uncommon except in severe malnutrition and in premature infants in which it causes anemia resembling iron deficiency anemia, which responds, specifically, to copper administration. Menkes' disease is a rare genetic disorder in which there is failure of copper absorption. It affects tissues like connective tissue, bone marrow and myelin. There is failure of hair keratinization, which show kinking.

Free serum copper, total serum copper (free and protein bound) and total blood copper (serum + crythrocyte copper) are all estimated by atomic absorption methods. Metabolically active copper is

---

Table 11.2. Biological significance of zinc

Biomolecules containing Zn:
- Zn is present in different enzymes from all the six classes (eg. cytochrome oxidase, RNA polymerases, alcohol dehydrogenases, carbonic anhydrase, superoxide dismutase, alkaline phosphatase) transcription factors and glucocorticoid receptor.

Functions:
- It has a critical role in spermatogenesis.
- It is needed for normal development of embryo.
- In certain areas of the brain zinc may help neurotransmitters to bind to their receptors.
- Steroid hormone action is zinc dependant.
- It has essential role in formation and function of immune system
- It has a role in sense of taste
- Zn is needed for proper wound healing
- Zn is also important as a free radical scavenger

Zn deficiency[1];
- Zn deficiency may cause failure to thrive in an infant
- In children it may cause somatic and sexual growth failure and impairment of taste perception and immune system
- In an adult it causes poor wound healing, alopecia and a skin rash.
- White cell Zn level indicates bodily status of Zn.

---

[1]Zn deficiency may result from reduced absorption (presence of excess fiber, phytate, calcium in food, malabsorption disorders), hemolytic anemias, catabolic states (trauma, burns, surgery, malignancies, infection) and many other diseases.

better evaluated as RBC superoxide dismutase activity or as leukocyte cytochrome oxidase activity than as serum copper or as ceruloplasmin.

Main interest of Cu in nutrition comes from its involvement in Wilson's disease. It is an inherited disorder of Cu metabolism, in which there is increased absorption of Cu from the intestine and reduced excretion in bile. Plasma ceruloplasmin level is reduced and level of non-ceruloplasmin Cu is increased. There is increased excretion of Cu in urine and Cu is also deposited in tissues (liver, kidney, basal ganglia, cornea). The disease may present in childhood with extensive liver damage or in adulthood with cirrhosis and manifestations of basal ganglia damage (incoordination, rigidity, tremors, choreo-athetotic movements, ataxia). Disease is diagnosed by the corneal ring (green/golden, due to Cu deposition) called the Kayser-Fleischer ring, decreased level of ceruloplasmin in serum and increase of Cu in liver biopsy. Condition is treated with D-penicillamine which chelates Cu to increase its excretion in urine.

SOME INHERITED DISORDERS OF NUTRIENTS

These diseases are not common, still their knowledge is important in differential diagnosis of certain nutritional and other disorders. For example, Wilson's disease and haemochromatosis can produce hepatic cirrhosis in adults. Cystic fibrosis produces pancreatic damage and malabsorption. Some disorders are discussed below.

Inherited disorders causing rickets

These disorders are considered when patient is not responding to ordinary doses of vitamin D, used in treatment of nutritional rickets. See Chapter 10 for more details.

Hemochromatosis

It is an inherited (frequency >3 in 1000 in American Whites) disorder in which excessive iron is absorbed because of failure of regulation of its absorption. Disease is autosomal recessive in which only homozygous individuals are at risk of developing liver damage (see below). Heterozygous individuals are identified from HLA typing and iron

studies. Causes of secondary hemachromatosis include chronic hemolytic disorders, sideroblastic anemia, disorder needing repeated blood transfusions and others.

In the primary cases, with increased iron absorption, as the age advances, more and more iron is deposited in tissues like liver, pancreas, skin and testes. The patient, commonly, presents with hepatomegaly (hepatic cirrhosis with risk of developing carcinoma). Less commonly B-cell damage may cause diabetes mellitus. Disease is more common in males as menstrual blood loss protects women from excess iron accumulation.

Laboratory findings include, raised serum iron, increased % saturation of transferrin, greatly increased serum ferritin and large excess of iron in liver biopsy specimen. The homozygous individuals are treated with desferrioxamine and weekly bleeding to lower systemic iron load.

Wilson's disease

This condition has already been discussed. Also see Chapter 6.

B_{12} related in born errors

A number of inborn errors concerning vitamin B_{12} have been reported. These involve B_{12} absorption (congenital lack of IF; selective B_{12} malabsorption with proteinuria), B_{12} transport (transcobalamin I deficiency; transcobalamin II deficiency) and B_{12} co-enzyme activity (B_{12} responsive methyl malonic aciduria). Megaloblastic anemia of B_{12} deficiency (Appendix 11.1) can result from pernicious anemia (autoimmune damage of gastric mucosa), ileal malabsorption or the above mentioned inborn errors.

B_6 related inborn errors

A number of inborn errors of metabolism are known which involve enzymes requiring B_6 as a co-enzyme. The impaired enzymes include, amino acid decarboxylase (causes convulsions and brain damage), ALA-synthase (causes chronic anemia), kynureninase (causes xanthurenicaciduria), cystathionase (causes cystathioninuria) and cystathionine synthetase (causes homocystinuria). All these metabolic disorders are B_6 responsive.

Menkes' disease, acrodermatitis enteropathica and cystic fibrosis have been discussed separately.

MALABSORPTION SYNDROMES

Malabsorption can be caused by impaired digestion because of reduced secretion or inactivation of pancreatic enzymes. In chronic pancreatitis there is gradual loss of acinar tissue. Cystic fibrosis is a recessively inherited disorder of Cl^- channel. It can present in a new born as meconium ileus because of failure to pass the first feces (made up of bile, mucus and mucosal debris) after birth. Further, in this condition bronchial and pancreatic secretions are thick and block the ducts. Thus a child may present with malabsorption (due to lack of pancreatic secretions) and chronic lung disease.

In obstructive jaundice fat malabsorption occurs as lipase is not activated in the absence of bile salts. In Zollinger-Ellison syndrome (Chapters 6 and 16) pancreatic lipase is inactivated in the presence of low pH of duodenal fluid.

Malabsorption can also be due to intestinal causes like celiac disease, tropical sprue, excessive bacterial growth and giardiasis, PEM, hypogamma-globinemia, cytotoxic drugs. Also it may be associated with extensive inflammation/infiltration of small gut wall (Crohn's, tuberculosis, Whipple's disease and lymphoma). See Appendix 11.2.

Patients of malabsorption present with diarrhea, abdominal pain (distension of inflamed bowel or chronic pancreatitis), weight loss and general malnutrition. The micronutrient deficiencies produce their specific clinical features.

Malabsorption is suspected from history and the clinical examination and established by demonstrating presence of steatorrhea. In X-ray examination, flocculation of barium meal is suggestive of malabsorption. Before demonstrating steatorrhea, simple stool examination (sudan stained), under microscope can indicate excessive fat in stools.

Once malabsorption has been confirmed, different investigations are done to find out the cause. The xylose absorption test is used to distinguish between pancreatic insufficiency and the mucosal disease. Intestinal biopsy may be obtained via an endoscope and it may confirm diagnosis in case of some diseases (Whipple's disease, agammaglobulinemia, a betalipoproteinemia, intestinal lymphoma, amyloidosis, regional enteritis, certain parasitic infestations, intestinal lymphangiectasia). Leakage of protein into intestinal lumen may be indicated by hypoproteinemia and certain specific tests.

Presence of muscle fibers along with excess fat during stool examination, gives indirect evidence of pancreatic insufficiency. Pancreatic insufficiency may be demonstrated by studying pancreatic juice, (by intubation of duodenum), after some stimulation (secretin-pancreozymin test). Pancreatic calcification may be seen by X-ray examination. Pancreatic enlargement may be seen by ultrasound and CT scan. The duct system may be visualized by endoscopic retrograde cholangiopancreatography (ERCP).

Important tests used in diagnosis of malabsorption are listed in Tables 11.3 and 11.4.

Tropical sprue and celiac disease

These two mucosal cell disorders are associated with severe malabsorption. Tropical sprue is common in our country and its cause is not exactly known. It maybe a deficiency disorder (particularly folic acid deficiency), it may be because of a transmissible infection (probably a virus infection) or it may result from some toxins elaborated by some intestinal microorganism.

The celiac disorders (celiac disease in children and celiac sprue in adults) are produced by toxic or immunogenic reaction in ileal mucosa against certain peptides produced from partial hydrolysis of gluten. The problem may fundamentally be related to absence of a specific mucosal peptidase because of which the toxic peptides escape further degradation before absorption. In sera of celiac patients antigliadin, antiendomysial and antireticulin antibodies have been demonstrated and are used for diagnosis and following treatment.

Clinical features include weight loss, muscle wasting and weakness (caused by anorexia and loss of calories and protein). Loss of potassium also contributes to weakness. Microcytic, hypochromic anemia (iron loss) and megaloblastic anemia (folic acid deficiency; B_{12} deficiency if there is

Table 11.3. Important tests in diagnosis of malabsorption and its cause

Estimation of fat in stool: (>6g/24h on fat intake of 100g/d)	Used to confirm steatorrhea
D-Xylose absorption (after 25 g dose, < 4.5 g in urine in next 5h: peak plasma level < 30 mg/dL means reduced absorption)	- Normal in pancreatic insufficiency (PI) - ↓ in mucosal cell disease (MCD)
X-ray examination	- Malabsorption pattern in MCD - No malabsorption pattern in PI but there may be pancreatic calcification.
Breath test using ^{14}C-glycocholate	- Normal in MCD and PI - ↑ $^{14}CO_2$ excretion in bacterial overgrowth and in bile acid malabsorption (ileal diseases)
Serum trypsin like immuno reactivity (TLI)	- ↓ in PI with steatorrhea - Normal in PI without steatorrhea - Normal in any other cause of steatorrhea without PI. - ↑ in acute pancreatitis.
Secretin plus cholecystokinin (pancreozymin) (CCK) test (reduced HCO_3^- secretion occurs early in PI; reduced amylase secretion is also common). Also see Appendix B.	- May even detect occult disease in some cases of PI. (this test is going out of favour because of required intubation and also because of difficulty of sample collections).
Benzoyl-tyrosyl-p-aminobenzoic test (bentiromide test) Chymotrypsin liberates PABA from a synthetic peptide and PABA metabolite estimated in urine)	- Simple and reliable test for demonstrating PI. Estimation of PABA in blood increases sensitivity.
Pancreolauryl test (fluorescein dilaurate is hydrolyzed by pancreatic elastase; fluorescein measured in urine)	- Significance is the same as of the Bentiromide test)
Estimation of chymotrypsin in feces	- Used for diagnosis of cystic fibrosis. Gives 10% false positive and false negative results.
B_{12} malabsorption corrected by administration of pancreatic enzymes.	- Increase in urinary excretion of B_{12} after enzyme administration in PI and cystic fibrosis.
α_1-Antitrypsin clearance by intestine (calculated from levels in plasma and 24h stool sample (g).	- Useful test of detect protein enteropathy. (screening can be done by simply measuring α-antitrypsin in feces)

Table 11.4. Significance of breath tests in malabsorption

- $^{14}CO_2$ is measured in expired air after ingestion of ^{14}C-labeled triglyceride. In pancreatic or intestinal malabsorption there is decrease of radiolabel in expired air (as $^{14}CO_2$).

  To distinguish between pancreatic malabsorption from intestinal malabsorption, the test may be done in two stages. In the second stage radiolabeled triglyceride is given with a dose of pancreatic enzymes. In pancreatic insufficiency, there is relative increase of radiolabeled CO_2 in the second stage.

- Increase of radiolabeled CO_2 in expired air after ingestion of xylose (^{14}C) or glycocolic acid (^{14}C in glycine) indicates bacterial over growth in proximal gut. In the test increase of radiolabeled CO_2 in breath may also occur in ileal disease (Crohn's disease) since unabsorbed bile salts enter large gut and bacterial metabolism of glycine produces radiolabeled CO_2. For the ileal disease, however, the test is not reliable.

- Breath H_2 after ingestion of lactose is used for screening lactose intolerance (there is increase in breath H_2). Breath H_2 after ingestion of lactulose may be used to screen for bacterial over growth in the gut.

involvement of ileum) may be present. Osteomalacia (or rickets) and osteoporosis cause bone pains and skeletal deformities (loss of vitamin D and calcium). Tetany may also occur (loss of calcium and magnesium). Hypoalbuminemia and edema may result from protein losing enteropathy. Other problems may be lactose intolerance (mucosal lactase deficiency) and bleeding tendency (vitamin K loss). Celiac disease, more commonly, occurs in childhood and may present in different ways (Table 11.5).

Both in tropical sprue and celiac disease, X-ray using non-flocculating barium shows dilatation of intestine and some times excessive fluid and gas and suggest malabsorption. There is fat malabsorption and reduced xylose absorption. B_{12} absorption may also be reduced. Intestinal mucosal biopsy changes include villous atrophy which is also found in other causes of malabsorption. In case of celiac disease characteristic endoscopic changes have also been reported. Diagnostic criteria in the two disorders are: evidence of malabsorption, abnormal jejunal biopsy and improvement of clinical, biochemical and biopsy changes on gluten free diet in celiac disease and after treatment with some broad spectrum antibiotic and folic acid in tropical sprue.

Patients of tropical sprue are treated with tetracycline and folate administration while patients of celiac disease require gluten free diet. Patients, otherwise, are give a high protein, high-calorie, low fat diet. Use of medium chain triglycerides reduces steatorrhea. Low residue items are selected in the diet. Micronutrient deficiencies require specific treatment. Severely ill patients of tropical sprue may benefit from administration of corticosteroids.

Cystic fibrosis (CF)

It is quite common in Caucasian populations of North America and much less common in Asian countries.

In cystic fibrosis, there is defect in CF trans-

Table 11.5. Some special presentations of celiac disease

- Failure to thrive in second year of life with fatty diarrhea, abdominal distension, loss of appetite and wasting.
- A child presenting with dwarfism and chronic diarrhea.
- A child presenting with diarrhea, malnutrition and tetany.

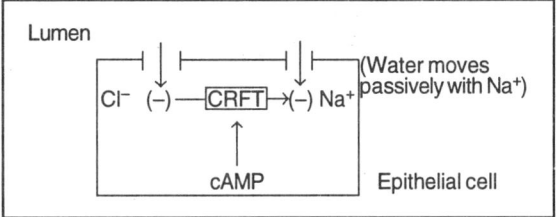

Fig.11.4. Role of defective Cl^- channel in pathogenesis of cystic fibrosis.

- In the respiratory tract epithelial cell cAMP regulated Cl^- channel (CFRT) inhibits close by Cl^- and Na^+ channels (both transport respective ions from lumen into the cell). In cystic fibrosis defective CRFT loses this effect causing increased Na^+ and Cl^- (more of the former) and water loss from respiratory tract mucus, making its thick and poorly cleared. Also PD (lumen -ive) increases from -20 to -50 mv; resistance to infections is reduced.

- Defect of Cl^- channel in pancreatic ductal epithelium limits functioning of an epical membrane Cl^- - HCO_3^- exchanger to secrete HCO_3^- (and passively Na^+) into the duct. Failure to secrete HCO_3^- leads to activation of enzymes in pancreas causing pancreatic damage.

- In ducts of sweat glands absence of functional Cl^- channel limits absorption of NaCl from sweat due to failure of Cl^- absorption from the duct.

membrane regulator (CFTR) which is actually cAMP regulated Cl^- channel, also regulating other ion channels, resulting in disordered ion transport in epithelial cells (Fig. 11.4).

80% of the affected individuals (generally children), present with pulmonary involvement (recurrent respiratory tract infections leading to bronchiectasis) and pancreatic insufficiency. In 15% there is pulmonary involvement without pancreatic insufficiency. All affected males have azospermia. Cytic fibrosis may also present as meconium ileus in a new born.

Diagnosis is established by estimating Cl^- in sweat (collected by pilocarpine induced sweating). In children level should be more than 60 mmol/L for diagnosis (in adults >70 mmol/L). The test limitation lies in proper collection of sweat. In children level of trypsin in stool (digestion of emulsion of X-ray film) has also been used ($\downarrow$ trypsin in stool). Method however, lacks percision and specificity. In neonatal screening, low level of immuno reactive trypsin is demonstrated in blood. Prenatal screening and screening for heterozygotes is possible using DNA techniques. If the mutation is known for the family (and probe is available) the family members can be easily screened for heterozygous state. Also read under diagnosis of inherited disorder by DNA analysis in Chapter 18.

Principles of therapy include control of lung infection and treatment of malabsorption.

METABOLIC RESPONSE TO TRAUMA AND SEPSIS

Severe trauma/infection (sepsis) initiates profound metabolic changes in the body. In case of trauma this response is well characterized into certain stages, starting from time of injury.

The ebb stage

First is the ebb stage; a sort of neurogenic shock coupled with a state of catabolism (increased lipolysis and proteolysis) and reduced O_2 consumption. There is vasodilatation, increased capillary permeability and sequestration of fluid in the interstitial compartment leading to reduced venous return and reduced cardiac out put. The management of this phase includes, careful fluid administration, reducing pain, protecting the patient from extremes of external temperatures and taking care of the injured tissues.

If the patient overcomes the shock phase (about 24h), he enters the flow phase (see details under the specific heading below). This is a state of hypermetabolism (with increased O_2 consumption) while the sequestrated fluid starts entering the vascular compartment and in this way stabilizing the cardiovascular system.

If the patient comes out of this phase also (may take a week or more) he enters the stage of convalescence in which tissue building process starts (the catabolic patten of the flow phase changes into anabolic pattern of metabolism). Complete recovery may take a few months.

The infected patients; those with severe sepsis (septic shock) present with many features of the above mentioned ebb phase while those with more chronic, less severe sepsis show features of the flow phase (hypermetabolic sepsis).

The metabolic response to trauma and sepsis results from associated neuroendocrine response which starts as a sympathoadrenal discharge, followed by changes in levels of a number of other hormones, alongwith increase in levels of many inflammatory cytokines. The neuroendocrine response is produced by pain, fear, anxiety, hypovolemia, infection and hypoxemia.

The flow phase

The essence of metabolic response to trauma and sepsis is the hypermetabolism of the flow phase. Fig. 11.5 shows hormone and cytokine profile of this phase. In this phase there is reduced uptake of glucose in most tissues (to get energy from oxidation of fatty acids and ketones). Hyperglycemia may be produced by this reduced glucose uptake and increased release of glucose by liver (aim is to make plenty of glucose available for use in brain and cells of the immune system). Liver releases glucose, formed by gluconeogenesis from amino acids, released from the muscle, lung and other tissues. In muscle tissue, protein synthesis is inhibited and protein breakdown is increased.

Cortisol plays the most important role in the above changes. Insulin resistance and reduced levels of IGF-l also play a contributory role. Cytokines also augment the action of cortisol. Amino acids released from tissues (see above) are used in liver for gluconeogenesis and synthesis of acute phase proteins (Fig. 11.6). The latter process is also promoted by cytokines. Cytokines also produce features of acute phase response like anorexia, hypotension and fever. Circulating levels of FFA, TAG and cholesterol (C) increase during injury and sepsis. There is increased lipolytic activity in adipose tissue; there is increased synthesis of TAG and apolipoproteins in liver and activity of lipoprotein lipase is reduced. Lipoproteins may bind endotoxins and different viruses.

Interaction between different types of mediators

TNF, IL-l (most potent) and IL-6 stimulate pituitary-adrenal axis to increase release of ACTH and cortisol (Fig. 15.1). TNF may also increase levels of catecholamines, GH and glucagon. TNF and IL-l also reduce levels of T_3 (reduced formation of T_3

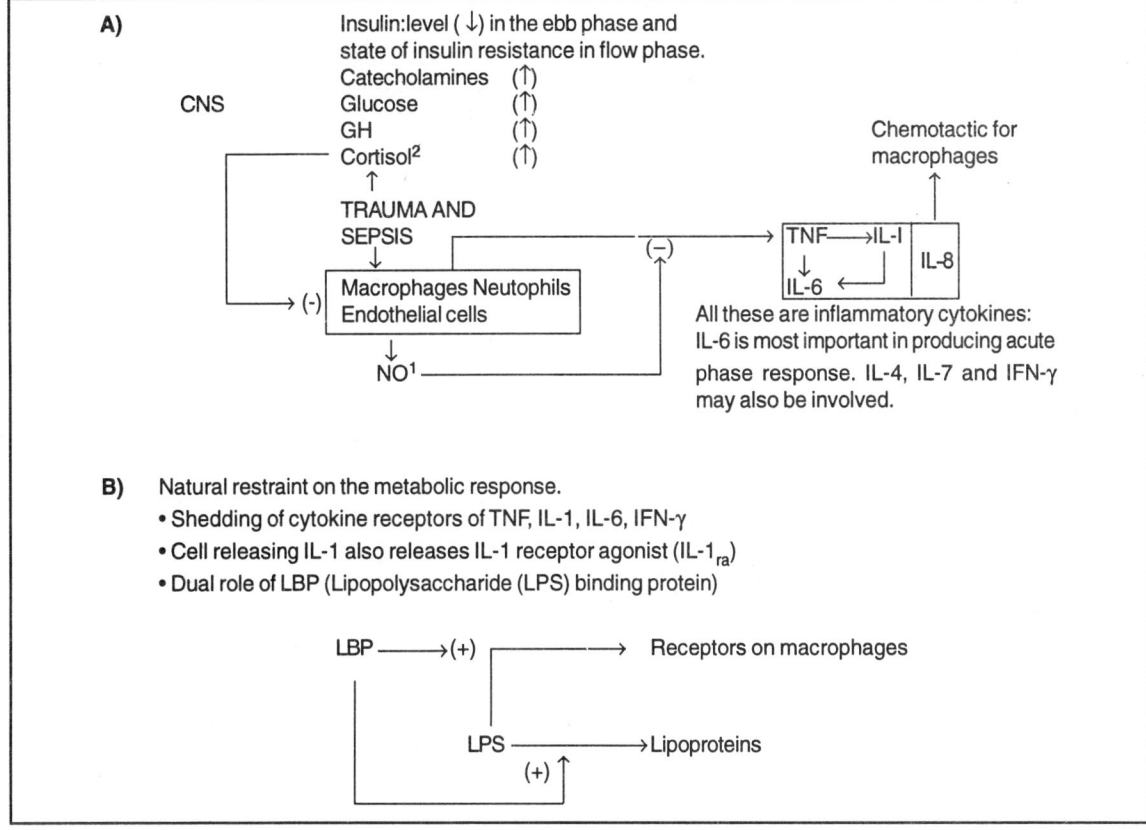

A)

CNS

Insulin:level (↓) in the ebb phase and
state of insulin resistance in flow phase.
Catecholamines (↑)
Glucose (↑)
GH (↑)
Cortisol[2] (↑)
↑
TRAUMA AND
SEPSIS

Chemotactic for
macrophages

→ (-) Macrophages Neutophils
Endothelial cells
↓
NO^1

(−)

TNF——→IL-I
↓
IL-6 ←——
IL-8

All these are inflammatory cytokines:
IL-6 is most important in producing acute
phase response. IL-4, IL-7 and IFN-γ
may also be involved.

B)   Natural restraint on the metabolic response.
• Shedding of cytokine receptors of TNF, IL-1, IL-6, IFN-γ
• Cell releasing IL-1 also releases IL-1 receptor agonist (IL-1$_{ra}$)
• Dual role of LBP (Lipopolysaccharide (LPS) binding protein)

LBP ——→(+)   ——→ Receptors on macrophages

LPS ————————→ Lipoproteins
(+) ↑

Fig. 11.5. Regulation of metabolic response to trauma and sepsis.

[1] NO down regulates endotoxin induced release of cytokines. Cytokines may increase formation of NO (not shown)
[2] Cortisol inhibits release of cytokines and NO. Cytokines stimulate hypothalamus - pituitary - adrenal axis (not shown).
A) Hormone and cytokines producing the metabolic response and their interrelationship.
B) Mechanism to prevent development of excessive response. LBP on one hand facilitates binding of LPS on receptors on
   macrophages and on the other hand helps disposal of LPS into lipoproteins.

from T_4 or increased cellular uptake of T_3, as promoted by catecholamines). Of hormones cortisol modulates production of cytokines and nitric oxide (NO) (Fig. 11.5).

Cytokines appear to be basically, formed in tissues to act in an autocrine or paracrine fashion (originally described to function in immune system but now known to act as regulators of various metabolic processes also). In metabolic stress of trauma and sepsis excessive formation of cytokines in tissues results in their spill over into blood and cause of increased mortality by their systemic effects. Thus therapeutic strategies tending to reduce levels of cytokines may help such patients

(Table 11.6). Cortisol appears to be a natural check on excessive formation of cytokines. Further, the cytokines are produced alongwith their inhibitors (Fig. 11.5). The complex interactions between different types of mediators may be the reason (at least partly) that treatment directed against individual mediators, following trauma/sepsis are not always successful.

Nitric oxide (NO) and septic shock

Nitric oxide is produced by a number of cells when L-arginine is converted to L-citrulline in the presence of O_2. NO degradation results in formation of nitrite (NO_2) and nitrate (NO_3) which are

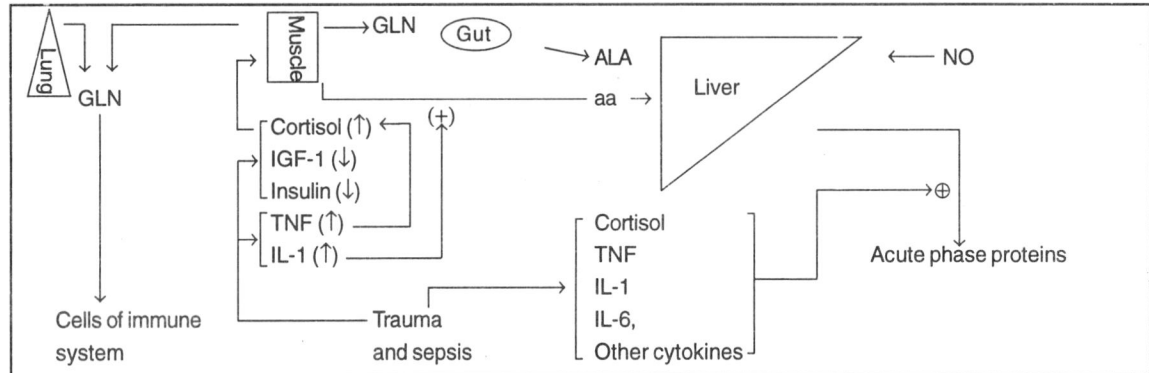

Fig.11.6. Protein metabolism in metabolic response to trauma and sepsis.

---

[1] Note that TNF causes protein breakdown in muscle by increasing cortisol formation while IL-1 acts directly.

- Release of aminoacids from the muscle tissue is increased by protein breakdown (caused by cortisol) and inhibited protein synthesis (caused by insulin resistance and low level of IGF-1). Cytokines (shown) reinforce actions of cortisol. TNF also promotes secretion of cortisol from adrenal cortex

- In the liver cortisol and certain cytokines (shown)increase synthesis of acute phase proteins by increasing gene transcription. NO protects liver from sepsis induced hepatic damage. It may also increase hepatic protein synthesis.

- Liver may also receive amino acids (for gluconeogenesis and for synthesis of acute phase proteins)from gut and lung. The gut, however, is also an important source of cytokines in trauma and sepsis.

- Glutamine is an important source of energy in cells of immune system.

Table 11.6. Therapeutic strategies for improving management of patients passing through metabolic response of trauma or sepsis

---

A) ENTERAL FEEDING:

- Enteral nutrition should be started within hours after trauma. Enteral feeding compared to parenteral feeding results in better survival rate and reduced infective complications. The intestinal mucosal cells remain more fit. Nutrients in the gut lumen (especially, glutamine, short chain fatty acids and nucleotides) support nutrition and integrity of the intestine. Enteral feeding also causes secretion of IgA and EGF, both of which are useful in promoting the barrier function of the gut. As cells remain healthy their damaging contribution in metabolic response to stress/sepsis is reduced. There is reduced formation of cytokines and the hormonal profile is less disturbed.

B) SPECIAL SUPPLEMENTS:

- **Glutamine:** This has been shown to improve N-balance of the patient. Glutamine is used as an energy source by cells of the immune system and intestinal mucosa. Increased cellular levels of this amino acid also inhibit cellular protein breakdown.

- **Arginine:** It may improve immune functions and wound healing. Increased serum level can increase GH release and further, it is substrate for NO biosynthesis.

- **ω-3-polyunsaturated fatty acids[1]:** These are also known to reduce hypermetabolism following trauma and sepsis. These act by promoting eicosanoids of N-3 series and reducing those of N-6 series and certain cytokines.

C) OTHER THERAPIES:

- Insulin administration during parenteral nutrition can improve N-balance but there is danger of hypoglycemia. Administration of IGF-1 holds a promise as this molecule produces anabolic actions of GH.

- Strategies to neutralize or reduce levels of endotoxins (with antibodies), and cytokines like, TNF (with antibodies), IL-6 (with antibodies),IL-1 (with receptor agonist).

- Supplements of branched chain amino acids and nucleotides have also been tried.

---

[1] Short chain fatty acids derived from bacterial breakdown of soluble fibers (pectin) promote cell proliferation and growth of gut mucosa. These form the preferred energy substrate, increase production of enterotropic hormones, pancreatic secretions and intestinal blood flow.

quantitated as an indirect measure of NO. NO acts in a paracrine fashion. For example produced by vascular endothelial cells it acts on vascular smooth muscle. For action, NO activates soluble guanylyl cyclase (SGC) to increase cGMP level to produce smooth muscle cell relaxation.

Production of NO by inducible nitric oxide synthase (iNOS) in macrophages, lymphocytes and neutrophils plays an important role in immune and inflammatory response. Generation of NO by macrophages helps to destroy bacteria, fungi, viruses, parasites and tumor cells. NO appears to be important in non-specific immunity, especially, in the lung and liver. Other functions are given in Table 11.7.

In bacterial sepsis iNOS is induced by endotoxin and cytokines. NO enters general circulation from the septic sites, and accounts for hypotension, myocardial depression and hemorrhagic diathesis (by inhibiting adhesion and aggregation of a platelets) of septic shock. Some other pathophysiological effects are given in Table 11.7.

NEED OF NUTRITIONAL ASSESSMENT IN CLINICAL CASES

Nutritional assessment may be required in different conditions. It may be needed in a child in connection with some growth related problem. It may be needed in a patient who has to undergo a major surgical procedure. A patient may be undergoing treatment for some nutritional problem and may be required to be monitored. A rigorous biochemical monitoring is required in a patient on total parenteral nutrition.

Table 11.7. Biological significance of nitric oxide (NO)

NO produced by vascular endothelial cells (eNOS)[1]:

- Reduces arterial vascular tone in response to flow/agonist mediated calcium accumulated in endothelial cells (which stimulates eNOS).
- Reduced leucocyte adhesion to endothelium (inhibits platelet aggregation and adhesion).
- Inhibits smooth muscle cell migration and proliferation, involved in atherosclerosis. (Hypertension, hyperlipidemia, smoking and diabetes, all predispose to atherosclerosis and are associated with deficiency of vascular endothelial cell NO).

In immune and inflammatory responses:

- See in the text (role of NO in bacterial sepsis and septic shock is also mentioned in text. Inhibition of iNOS[1] has been used in treatment of septic shock). Antimicrobial action of NO is direct, not via cGMP.

Lungs:

- Endogenously produced NO may have a role in producing basal bronchial/pulmonary arterial tone. Inhaled NO selectively, produces pulmonary vasodilatation, as it is inactivated by Hb before entering systemic circulation. This is useful in certain types of pulmonary hypertension. Inhaled NO may also have a role in treatment of sickle cell disease as it increases O_2 affinity of sickle cells.
- Besides lungs, endogenously produced NO is also important in increasing blood flow in the liver and brain.

As a neurotransmitter:

- NO is a likely neurotransmitter of non-adrenergic, non-cholinergic neurons and may have a role in regulating rate/force of heart, bronchial tone, gut motility and penile erection. (Deficiency of NO producing neurons may be responsible for diseases of intestinal motility, Hirschsprung's disease, achalasia).

NO as a cellular protector:

- NO produced by iNOS of hepatocytes protects liver cells from injury from toxins (alcohol, drugs) by reducing liver cell metabolic activity.
- NO can act as cytotoxic or cytoprotective in CNS. In the redox state NO^+, it reacts with N-methyl-D-aspartate receptor to limit excessive Ca^{2+} entry into the cell and protecting from cell toxicity. NO as such promote Ca^{2+} entry and causes cytoxicity.

[1] NO is produced by calcium independant nitric oxide synthase (iNOS) and is involved in inflammatory response and by calcium dependant non inducible enzyme present in neurons (nNOS) and endothelial cells (eNOS).

Table 11.8. Indications of nutritional assessment

- To assess adequacy of growth in a child. (anthropometric parameters and physical examination are commonly sufficient). Also read objective tupe question no. 16.
- To assess a patient for surgical risk. (discussed in text).
- In a chronic illness especially when nutritional compromise is going to effect the course of illness (anthopometric parameters, plasma proteins, lean body mass, N-balance are used). In such cases it is also important to look for an evidence of some marker of metabolic stress and some evidence of inadequate nutrient processing.
- To predict prognosis in a chronically ill patient. (serum albumin level is quite useful in this connection).
- To monitor a dietary intervention. If dietary deficiency is responsible for low serum proteins, increase in serum prealbumin level will give early indication of successful intervention.
- Assessment of a single nutrient deficiency may be required in certain conditions (malabsorption, megaloblastic anemia, alcoholism, antitubercular and other treatments). For vitamin deficiency there should be high degree of suspicion (dietary history and clinical examination). Confirmation is obtained by observing response to treatment to replacement as vitamin levels do not reflect the state of stores except for folate, vitamin D and B_{12}.

  Plasma levels of calcium, phosphorous, magnesium and potassium are used to assess the status of these minerals, although, the levels do not always change in parallel with the body stores. The iron status is discussed separately.

- In child malnutrition, the weight is reduced early and height only in a long standing case. Besides weight for age and height for age, weight/height index is a useful parameter: Weight (kg)/height^2(cm) x 100. Quack stick method is useful in field setting. Triceps skinfold thickness is useful indicator of caloric depletion and mid arm muscle mass and lean body mass for protein depletion (also indicated by low levels of serum albumin/prealbumin).

When nutritional assessment is required as part of growth monitoring in a child, physical examination and anthropometric parameters become the most important items of examination (Table 11.8). The biochemical parameters are often much less used. Nevertheless, a suspected micronutrient deficiency may require biochemical confirmation. The protein nutrition is often assessed by measurement of serum albumin level, although, it is only an insensitive predictor of protein status.

When monitoring is required in a patient receiving a supplement of a micronutrient, a parameter other than, biochemical one, should be chosen. For example, a patient receiving a supplement of B_{12}, should be monitored by examination of his peripheral blood film rather than study of serum levels of B_{12}. If nutritional monitoring is required in a patient who cannot feed himself, properly, because of anorexia or some surgical problem, a record of weight and height (if problem is long extending) is most crucial. Further, depending upon dietary history, one may also investigate for some macro or micro nutrient deficiency.

Malnutrition and its assessment in patients

In patients, malnutrition may be caused by reduced food intake (a type of semistarvation) due to anorexia or some difficulty associated with food intake, digestion or absorption. It may also result from a prevailing catabolic state (post traumatic or sepsis associated). In certain conditions more than one causative factors may be present together. The resulting state of malnutrition also depends upon the rate at which it develops and the relative magnitudes of developing protein and energy depletions. Rapidly developing depletions in which protein depletion is outstanding, result in development of kwashiorkor type of malnutrition in which weight loss is masked by increase of ECF fluid. Slowly developing depletion (and caloric depletion predominating), results in marasmic type of condition. In these conditions, other associated deficiencies of vitamin A, vitamins of B group, folic acid, vitamin C, vitamin K and minerals like iron, zinc and magnesium, may also develop.

Nutritional assessment (presurgical)

Nutritional assessment in a surgical patient is useful to predict outcome of the surgical procedure on the patient. Weight loss should not be more than 15% (or his weight, not less than 80% of the ideal weight for the height). Weight loss becomes more significant under two conditions. Firstly, if it has developed only recently and secondly if it has resulted in some functional impairment. The functional impairment refers to physiological functions of muscular, respiratory, hepatic and renal systems. The weight loss also assumes greater significance if any of the above system dysfunction is already present due to disease of the patient. Hand dynamometry may be used to assess the functional status of the muscle tissue. Muscular function has important relation to respiratory functions of the patient. The protein status of the patient is also important as it may relate to general functioning of different body systems. Deficiency may become clinically apparent if more than 20% of body protein is lost. Serum albumin level of less than 3.0 g/dL may pose a surgical risk. Other serum proteins which have been used for the same purpose are pre-albumin and transferrin. Also are important immunologic and host defence functions including neutrophil functions. Anergy to skin recall antigens by the injection technique may form an important surgical risk. Any history or actual presence of functional impairment is also important.

It is also important in such patients, to know about presence of a catabolic stress. Markers of catabolic stress are:

Increased body temperature (>100°F), increased pulse rate (>100/min) or increased respiratory rate (>30/min), white cell count >12,000 or <3000, positive blood culture or presence of sepsis or trauma. Catabolic index may be calculated by measuring 24h N-intake and excretion of urea over the same period.

Catabolic index = urinary urea N(g) - (dietary N(g)/2 + 3). A value of over 5 indicates severe stress, from 0 to 5, moderate stress and less than 0, no stress.

Knowledge about presence and severity of catabolic stress in such patients is helpful in predicting problems during convalescence and also in assessing their nutritional requirements.

Patients with nutritional and other deficiencies (see above), preoperatively, have increased risk to anaesthesia and surgery. There will also be poor convalescence.

ENTERAL/PARENTERAL NUTRITIONAL SUPPORT

In certain circumstances a patient is not able to obtain necessary amounts of nutrients by ordinary feeding. Patient may be having a catabolic disease and his nutritional state may be very poor. There may be anorexia or impairment of swallowing. A bowel disease may limit oral intake or absorption of nutrients. In these circumstances, if possible, patient should be fed through a nasogastric or naso-duodenal tube or percutaneous gastrostomy/jejunostomy (if intestinal absorptive functions are not disturbed). In case of maldigestion for enteral feeding, an elemental diet is used. Nitrogen is provided as amino acids and very small peptides and carbohydrate as glucose. High osmolality of the elemental diet is likely to cause diarrhea. To avoid this, one may start with half strength diet and increase, gradually, to full strength. Also small feeds should be given, more frequently. Although, enteral nutrition is much more physiological, (Table 11.9), in some circumstances parenteral route has to be used.

Total parenteral nutrition (TPN) is required in inflammatory bowel disease, short bowel syndrome and acute pancreatitis. Supplementation of ordinary feeds may also be required in severe burns, sepsis, crush injuries and other catabolic states. Special formula feeds may also be used, parenterally, in hepatic failure (amino acid solution rich in branched chain amino acids and low in aromatic amino acids delays development of encephalopathy) and in renal failure (a mixture of glucose and amino acids in acute renal failure). Parenteral nutrition may be given through a peripheral vein, in case, it is needed for 1-2 weeks. For longer periods, it should be given through a central venous catheter. Meticulous

Table 11.9. Benefit of enteral feeding over parenteral feeding

- Presence of nutrients in the intestine is important to maintain functional efficiency of mucosal cells. In the absence of nutrients there is atrophy of absorptive cells as well as the goblet cells. There is also loss of brush border enzymes.

- Intestine offers a barriers function against infection (against bacteria, endotoxins, and other antigenic molecules).

- Many of the effects are mediated by enterotrophic gut hormones (which are stimulant to structural and functional aspects of these cells.)

care is needed in insertion and maintenance of catheters to avoid sepsis from the catheter site. Energy and protein requirements of such patients are calculated as described below.

Energy and protein requirements

Total energy expenditure (TEE) of a patient is calculated by adding together, resting metabolic energy (RME), which is 5 to 10% higher than BMR, diet induced thermogenesis (DIT) (calculated by multiplying RME by 0.1), activity energy expenditure (AEE) and the stress factor. Thus:

TEE = RME+DIT+AEE+Stress factor or

TEE = REE+AEE+Stress factor (resting energy expenditure (REE) is sum of RME and DIT).

RME is also calculated using Harris-Benedicts equation:

RME (kcal/d) = 66.5 + 13.8 W + 5 × H - 6.8 × A in males and RME (kcal/d) = 665 + 9.6 W + 1.9 × H - 4.7 × A in females.

W = Weight in kilograms, H is height in cm and A is age in years.

Activity energy expenditure (AEE)

AEE varies from 500 kcal/d (in a sedentary person) to 3000 kcal/d (in a manual labourer). In surgical patients (in ward or in intensive care unit) it is obtained by multiplying REE by 0.3.

Stress Factor

In patients, it is obtained by multiplying REE by a factor, the value of which depends upon the degree of metabolic stress as under: 0.3 for skeletal trauma, 0.1 for post elective surgery, 0.5 for multiple injuries, or serious sepsis and still higher (upto 1.0) for major burns.

In surgical patients, generally, TEE is 35 to 40 kcal/kg/d, except in patients in severe catabolic state (post operative infection).

The protein requirement of a patient is guided by a number of factors. A patient in catabolic phase of metabolism requires adequate calories and dietary protein so that his protein catabolism is not further worsened by lack of calories and dietary essential amino acids. Protein intake of 1.0 to 1.5 (g/kg/d) is generally, enough as higher amounts are not utilized. A patient in anabolic phase can be given more (1.5 to 2.0 g/kg/d). In case the patient is also having some protein loss (protein losing enteropathy) his protein intake may be further increased (2.0 to 2.5 g/kg/d). For each gram of nitrogen (6.5g protein) about 200 kcal energy should be provided as glucose or fat, to ensure efficient nitrogen utilization. Ordinarily (in the absence of fever or other cause of excessive water loss), water requirement is 30 mL/kg body weight. The trace element requirement of an ill patient is more than a normal person.

Table 11.10. Monitoring a patient on total parenternal nutrition and common complications.

- For monitoring hydration, keep record of weight, maintain proper fluid balance chart and keep auscultating lung bases.
- For monitoring adequate caloric intake, keep record of weight and triceps skin fold thickness
- For monitoring adequate protein intake, investigations like N-balance (affected in 24h), serum albumin/ prealbumin levels (affected over days/ weeks), and mid arm muscle mass (to monitor long term effect), are used.
- Other investigated parameters are glucose, urea, creatinine, electrolytes, calcium, magnesium, phosphorous, triglycerides, osmolality, Hb, prothrombin time and total and differential counts.

Complications produced

- Hyperglycemia may be produced because of sepsis/insulin resistance or because of rapid infusion. In the latter case it may cause low serum levels of potassium and phosphate due to their entry into cells with glucose utilization.
- Hypertriglyceridemia because of excessive fat infusion.
- Hypercholremic acidosis because of too rapid infusion of chloride.
- Prerenal azotemia because of too rapid infusion of amino acids.
- In catabolic patients, deficiencies of folate and vitamins C and B_{12} may also be produced. Also trace element deficiencies with long standing use of TPN.

Monitoring of a patient on TPN

A patient of parenteral nutrition can suffer from different complications. These may be mechanical relating to the catheters, infections (also related to catheters and lack of proper asepsis in technique) and metabolic. To avoid metabolic complications proper biochemical monitoring is very essential. (Table 11.10) Glucose overload often causes hyperglycemia. This may stimulate insulin secretion leading to intracellular shift of potassium and phosphorous. These changes may cause arrhythmias, cardiopulmonary dysfunctions and neurological features. Hypokalemia and hypophosphatemia may also reduce glucose utilization. It is also important, in such patients, to monitor their state of hydration. Lung bases should be auscultated for overhydration. It is also important to record urine output and maintain fluid balance charts. Serum sodium level (or osmolality) is used to monitor water excess or deficit and serum creatinine level to indicate prerenal azotemia.

In these patients, adequacy of calories and nitrogen can be judged by record of weight, skin fold thickness (relates to body fat) and mid arm circumference (relate to muscle mass). For more accurate assessment of muscle mass the following relation may be used:

Midarm muscle mass = [Arm circumference - $(\pi \times$ triceps skin fold)]$^2/4\pi$ (all measurements are in cm.).

These patients may also need N balance studies (Table 11.11).

For short term monitoring of protein status during different nutritional support programmes, weekly levels of serum albumin, prealbumin or transferrin may be studied. Best results have been obtained with prealbumin. Recently IGF-1 levels have also been used for the same purpose.

Other complications likely to occur in these patients are acid base disturbances, hypercalcemia, hypomagnesemia and hyperlipidemia. When parenteral nutrition is used over a long period trace elements deficiencies can also occur. Levels of Zn (also Cu and Se in long term treatment) are monitored.

Table 11.11. Some Biochemical parameters related to muscle mass, nitrogen balance and protein status of an individual

Lean body mass
- Lean body mass (kg)=7.138 + 0.02908 x 24h urine creatinine (mg)

Urinary creatinine/Height ratio (mg/24h/height in cm)

N-Balance
- N-Balance (g) = protein intake(g)/ 6.25 - (urine urea-N(g) +2.5) (2.5 g is approximate loss of fecal-N plus non-urea-N in urine).

Serum protein levels
- Serum levels of albumin and other short half life proteins, prealbumin (2-3 d) and transferrin (8-9 d). Half life of serum albumin is 18-20 d. IGF-1 levels have also been used for the same purpose

- The results of first two parameters of body muscle mass are also influenced by kidney functions, exercise, emotional stress, infection, fever and trauma.
- Albumin levels are also influenced by state of hydration, stress (increases albumin catabolism), illness (increase of acute phase proteins reduces hepatic albumin synthesis)

Appendix 11.1. Some vitamin deficiencies and their biochemical diagnosis

Vitamin A (malnutrition due to ignorance and poverty : malabsorption: liver disease: proteinuria: TPN)**:**
- Bitot spots/other ophthalmic features
- Dark adaptation time.
- Rod scotomy; electroretinography
- Serum levels not good indicators of stores
- The therapeutic test

Vitamin K (malabsorption: long term use of antibiotics: new borns with poor hepatic stores. liver disease.)**:**
- Before surgery prothrombin level should not be <70% of normal.
- Plasma level of noncarboxylated prothrombin precursor (↓level along with increased PT means vitamin deficiency and not liver disease).

Vitamin E (Malabsorption especially in children with abetalipoproteinemia or chronic cholestatic liver disease.)**:**
- Ratio of vitamin E level to level of serum lipid.

Vitamin C (Infants on processed milk formula: Elderly because of poor intake of green vegetables and fruits)**:**
- Leucocyte or platelet ascorbate level to know about body status
- Hyperkeratosis of skin
- X-ray changes in bones in infants.
- Plasma ascorbate levels indicate dietary intake
- Therapeutic trial

Thiamine, riboflavin, nicotinamide (thiamine and riboflavin deficiencies occur in alcoholics, during refeeding after starvation, in patients on dialysis and in severe malnutrition)**:** Therapeutic trials will diagnose and abolish deficiencies.
  - For thiamine increase of erythrocyte transketolase activity by > 15% by TPP.
  - Increase of transketolase activity after treatment.
- Niacin deficiency occurs in areas where maize/jawar is staple diet.
- For riboflavin increase of erythrocyte glutathione reductase activity by FAD in the assay procedure.

Pyridoxine (B$_6$) (deficiency is commonly drug induced (isoniazid, cycloserine, penicillamine, oral contraceptives)**:**
- Low level of erythrocyte alanine aminotransaminase, which increases by addition of pyridoxal phosphate (in vitro).
- The loading test (urinary xanthurenic acid after tryptophan load) is less reliable.

Folate/B$_{12}$ deficiencies:
- Establish presence of megaloblastic anemia: MCV is raised (higher than in macrocytosis of liver disease, alcoholism, hypothyroidism and hemolytic disease): Peripheral blood film (oval macrocytosis poikilocytosis, red cell fragmentation and neutrophil hypersegmentation); Hb and reticulocyte count low for degree of anemia: Bone marrow hypercellular with red cell precursors having large nuclei and open chromatin pattern.

Folate deficiency:
- Reduced intake (malnutrition, alcoholism, old age); increased demand (pregnancy, prematurity, chronic hemolysis, malignancy); malabsorption (celiac disease, tropical sprue) and drugs (alcohol, anticonvulsants, oral contraceptives, folate antagonists).
- Red cell folate levels are better index of stores as plasma folate levels relate to intake.
- Elevated homocysteine levels in plasma.
- Therapeutic trial.

B$_{12}$ deficiency:
- Reduced intake (vegetarians, extreme malnutrition), deficient intrinsic factor (pernicious anemia, gastrectomy, rarely transcobalamin II deficiency) and malabsorption (tropical sprue, non-tropical sprue, regional enteritis, intestinal resection, blind loop syndrome).
  - Plasma B$_{12}$ levels correlate better with stores than plasma folate levels (see above).
- Plasma (elevated) levels of methyl malonate and homocysteine are still better indices of stores.

Schilling test[1]:
  - It is used to establish cause of B$_{12}$ deficiency

[1]Patient is given radioactive B$_{12}$ by mouth, immediately followed by an injection of unlabeled B$_{12}$. The excreted radioactivity, in next 24h is an index of absorption. If the test is abnormal, next the patient is given labeled B$_{12}$ bound to IF. If now B$_{12}$ absorption becomes normal, diagnosis is pernicious anemia or some other type of IF deficiency, otherwise it would indicate some other cause (see above).

Appendix 11.2. Important causes of malabsorption

- Celiac disease
- Tropical sprue   } See text
- Cystic fibrosis

Chronic pancreatitis:

- Only extensive damage to pancreas causes steatorrhea.
- It may develop insiduously or it may develop, ultimately, in chronic recurrent pancreatitis
- In chronic pancreatitis there is disparity between abdominal pain and the physical signs (fever, hypotension are mild)
- Deficiencies of fat soluble vitamins and cations (Fe, Zn, Ca, Mg) are rather absent compared to those in mucosal diseases of malabsorption

  - CCK test
  - Xylose absorption and intestinal biopsy normal
  - Bentiromide test.
  - For biliary obstruction, ALP, ultrasound and CT.
  - ERCP to outline bile and pancreatic ducts
  - Pancreatic calcification on X-ray.
  - Malabsorption corrected by pancreatic enzyme supplements.

Contaminated bowel syndrome (causes are blind loops, jejunal diverticulosis, protein energy malnutrition, hypogammaglobulinemia, fistulae, Crohn's)**:**

- Causes moderate steatorrhea.
- Causes macrocytic anemia with megaloblastic bone marrow

  - Xylose absorption and intestinal biopsy usually normal.
  - Breath $^{14}CO_2$ after ^{14}C (xylose) or ^{14}C-labeled bile acids or breath hydrogen after lactulose (screening tests)
  - Impaired B_{12} absorption not corrected by IF.
  - Correction of steatorrhea and impaired B_{12} absorption after antibiotic therapy.
  - Culture of duodenal fluid.

Crohn's disease (with small bowel involvement) Disease occurs with episodes of activity (fever, ↑ESR, ↑CRP and other features) and quiescent periods**:**

- An adult presenting with weight loss and right lower quadrant pain/discomfort.
- Diarrhea often without blood.
- Palpable mass may be there.
- In presentation it may simulate acute appendicitis; may present with malabsorption; may present with obstruction
- Large bowel Crohon's has to be differentiated from ulcerative collitis.

  - Ordinarily easy to diagnose (X-ray shows constriction of some part, the 'string sign'). Difficulty arises if malabsorption is present, and many other possibilities have to be ruled out.

Giardiasis:

- Mild to severe diarrhea in acute or chronic form: malabsorption in severe cases

  - Stool examination

Lymphoma (malabsorption due to mucosal infiltration)[1]**:**

- Commonly occurs in males at about 50 years of age.
- Patient may present with features of celiac sprue, getting incomplete response to gluten free diet and with biopsy features almost those of celiac sprue.
- Abdominal pain and fever also accompany.

  - CT will show abnormal abdominal lymph nodes.
  - Close examination of biopsy.

Contd...

Whipples disease (rare):
- There are dilated lacteals in the intestinal mucosa which cause malabsorption and protein losing enteropathy.
- Malabsorption, fever, enteric loss of serum proteins.
- Associated involvement of other systems, skin, joints, lymph nodes, CNS, heart, eye.
  - Abnormal small bowel X-ray.
  - Confirmation by biopsy study.

After surgical resections:
- Usually, 40 to 50% of small bowel resection is well tolerated, provided proximal duodenum and distal half of the ileum and the ileocecal valve are not lost
- Gastric resection leads to reduced gastric digestion and more rapid transit of food through the gut.
  - Post gastrectomy malabsorption is seldom severe but very often leads to iron deficiency.

---

[1] Other causes of malabsorption due to gut wall infiltration include amyloidosis, intestinal tuberculosis and scleroderma.

- Some endocrinal causes of malabsorption are hyperthyroidism, diabetes mellitus, adrenal insufficiency, carcinoid, Zollinger Ellison syndrome and hypoparathyroidism.

- Two important common intestinal disorders not associated with malabsorption are amoebiasis and irritable bowel syndrome. The latter disorder may result from chronic neurosis. There is no fever, normal ESR and normal mucosal biopsy and X-ray findings. Features are abdominal pain after food intake; relieved by defecation, bloating, stools are in the form of ribbon or pellets with mucous but no blood. There is no organic disease but firm diagnosis is established, only, by ruling out a number of diseases (Crohn's ulcerative collitis, tuberculosis, parasites and cancer colon).

CASE HISTORY: 11.1

A 30 year old female gave history of chronic fatigue and heavy periods. Hb level was 8.0 g/dL, and peripheral blood film showed presence of microcytic hypochromic anemia.

> ➢ Indicate the biochemical investigations required to confirm the type of anemia.
> • In this case low hemoglobin, the typical blood film picture and the apparent cause of blood loss, leave very little doubt about iron deficiency as the cause of anemia. However, if still confirmation is required, the best single test will be estimation of serum ferritin level or study of iron in bone marrow biopsy.

Chronic fatigue of the patient is due to reduced work capacity which, in turn, is related to decreased oxidative metabolism in muscle (probably due to deficiency of iron containing enzymes) and to her anemia. Iron deficiency starts affecting body earlier than it produces iron deficiency anemia. Patients of iron deficiency are treated with iron salts. It takes a few months before iron stores are normalized. Iron salts are gastric irritants and should be taken with food.

Sometimes a person with iron deficiency anemia has no evidence of chronic bleeding and he does not respond to iron therapy. Such a case may has to be investigated and treated as discussed under "diagnosis of iron deficiency anemia".

CASE HISTORY: 11.2

A female patient (age 45 years) was on large doses of non-steroidal analgesics for her active rheumatoid arthritis. Occult blood was present in feces. Peripheral blood film showed microcytic hypochromic picture. Plasma ferritin level was in lower normal range.

> ➢ Discuss significance of plasma ferritin level as indicator of iron stores in this case?
> • Iron deficiency lowers both bone marrow iron as well as plasma ferritin levels whereas chronic inflammation (rheumatoid arthritis) tends to increase ferritin concentration as it is an acute phase protein. Under these circumstances ferritin level no longer remains a good indicator of iron stores. In this case bone marrow should be stained for iron to obtain true status of iron stores. Two other features of ACD are inappropriate reticulocyte response (reticulocyte index <2) and E:G ratio ≤1:2 (Fig. 11.3).

CASE HISTORY: 11.3

A 32 year old female patient gave history of chronic diarrhea following an acute episode. In between the diarrheal episodes, brief quiescent periods were there.

Increased fat intake used to worsen diarrhea. Other complaints were, indigestion, flatulence and abdominal cramps after food intake. She had lost 4 kg weight over the previous 6 months. Her stools were bulky, greasy and foul smelling. The xylose excretion test indicated impaired absorptive function of mucosal cells. A barium meal and follow through revealed dilated intestinal loops and excess of gas.

> ➢ The patient appears to have severe steatorrhea, which may be quantitated by fat absorption study. Describe two important causes of severe steatorrhea, and discuss differential diagnosis between them?
> ➢ How do different nutrient deficiencies present in such cases?
> ➢ How diagnostic is intestinal mucosal biopsy study in malabsorption cases?
> • Tropical sprue and the adult form of celiac (celiac sprue) are two important conditions which could be considered for differential diagnosis, although, celiac sprue is relatively a milder disorder (compared to celiac disease in children and tropical sprue). Tropical sprue is much more common in tropical countries and rare in Western World. The diagnostic criteria of both disorders are evidence of malabsorption and abnormal jejunal mucosa (in biopsy samples). The changes in intestinal mucosa are similar in the two conditions. Further, clinical, biochemical and the biopsy changes improve on gluten free diet in case of celiac sprue and after treatment with antibiotics and folic acid in tropical sprue.
> • Some important nutrient deficiency related clinical presentations are as under:
> - *Loss of weight and weakness:* Caused by loss of calories and nitrogen. Anemia and hypokalemia further add to weakness.
> - *Anemia:* It results from loss of iron, folic acid and B_{12}.
> - *Metabolic bone disease:* There may be X-ray evidence of osteomalacia and osteoporosis. These changes are related to deficiencies of calcium, magnesium and vitamin D.
> - *Edema:* It is due to hypoalbuminemia which in turn results from protein losing enteropathy. Marked protein loss is a special feature of Whipples disease. Other conditions associated with protein losing enteropathy are Crohn's, disease, bacterial overgrowth, infectious enteritis (viral, bacterial, parasitic) and a number of other intestinal diseases. It can be confirmed by finding increased clearance of serum α_1-antitrypsin (protease inhibitor resistant to intestinal proteolysis). The clearance is calculated by multiplying

the ratio of fecal to serum concentration with number of g of feces collected over 24h.

- *Milk intolerance:* This is because of secondary lactase deficiency which occurs very commonly in intestinal disorders.
- *Paresthesia and tetany:* It is because of loss of calcium, magnesium and vitamin D due to malabsorption.
- *Increased bleeding tendency:* Due to malabsorption of vitamin K.
- *Increased incidence of gall stones:* Results from reduced level of bile salts in bile due to their loss in feces.
- *Renal calculi:* Calcium is bound to fatty acids in intestine and that leads to increased absorption of oxalate. Increased oxalate excretion in urine may lead to formation of oxalate stones.
- Peripheral neuropathy (thiamine and B_{12} deficiency) and skin and mucous membrane lesions (vitamin, trace element deficiencies).
- Amenorrhea/decrease of libido may occur due to secondary hypopituitarism because of protein and caloric depletions.
- Azotemia and hypotension may result from water and electrolyte depletions in severe cases.

It may be added that certain presentations from the list discussed above may result from severe nutrient/micronutrient deficiencies in long standing, poorly managed cases of tropical sprue or celiac disease. In most other causes of malabsorption, nutrient/micro-nutrient deficiencies are much less pronounced and many of the clinical presentations listed may be absent. Some patients may present with an isolated deficiency even without apparent steatorrhea. Patient may present with iron deficiency, megaloblastic anemia, abnormal bleeding, bone pain and tenderness or emotional disturbances.

- Jejunal biopsy showing sub-total villous atrophy, is not diagnostic for tropical sprue or celiac disease. This finding occurs in a number of conditions including severe protein energy malnutrition, intestinal infections (bacteria, viruses), milk protein allergy and others. In many other conditions associated with malabsorption, however, biopsy may have diagnostic value. Some examples are Whipple's disease, agammaglobinemia, abetalipoproteinemia, lymphoma, amyloidosis, parasitic infections (giardiasis) and others.

CASE HISTORY: 11.4

A 30 years old patient presented with wasting and the complaint of passing foul smelling bulky stools. There was also history of repeated attacks of abdominal pain accompanied with anorexia and nausea. Patient was known alcoholic. Fat malabsorption was demonstrated by study of fat excretion. Fasting blood glucose level was 120 mg/dL.

➤ What other investigations are needed to arrive at the diagnosis?
➤ Any further investigations which may help to plan management?

- History is suggestive of chronic relapsing pancreatitis. Triad of steatorrhea, pancreatic calcification and diabetes mellitus, is usually enough to establish diagnosis of chronic pancreatitis. Patient is already reported to have steatorrhea and glucose intolerance. X-ray examination should be done to look for pancreatic calcification. One should also investigate the effect of oral administration of pancreatic enzymes on steatorrhea. If steatorrhea is reduced the diagnosis gets established. One must also show that xylose absorption is not reduced. Secretin plus CCK test can detect early cases even without overt steatorrhea while the bentiromide test is commonly useful in patients with established clinical findings.

- There are two important aspects of management in such cases. The first one is to modify diet so as to improve apetite and to reduce malabsorption. Also to increase intake of deficient nutrients. For appropriate supplementation patient should be investigated for nutrient deficiencies. The second aspect of management is to identify some remediable factors in the etiology of the disease. These factors may be chronic cholecystitis, cholelithiasis, stenosis of sphincter of oddi, alcoholism (pancreatic calcification is a good indicator of alcoholic pancreatitis), and hyperparathyroidism.

OBJECTIVE TYPE QUESTIONS

Pick out the wrong statement.

1. Anemia

i) A patient of anemia should be investigated before giving any treatment.
ii) Cause of anemia should not be presumed from clinical presentation of the patient.
iii) Anisocytosis is very prominent in megaloblastic anemias.
iv) Target cells occur in thalassemias.
v) Prominent polychromasia in peripheral smear means early entry of reticulocytes into circulation from bone marrow.

2. Anemia

i) Reticulocyte index <2 means a maturation disorder of red cells.

ii) Reticulocyte index <2 means a hypoproliferative disorder of erythropoiesis.

iii) In maturation disorders, anemia may be microcytic or macrocytic.

iv) Anemia due to chronic disorders is always hypochromic microcytic.

v) Greater importance is attached to MCV than MCHC in diagnosis of microcytic hypochromic anemias.

3. Investigating normocytic normochromic anemia

i) Hemolytic anemias and anemias due to hypoproliferative bone marrow are normochromic, normocytic.

ii) In hemolytic anemias there is optimal reticulocyte response (reticulocyte index >3).

iii) Hemolytic anemias are further categorized depending upon the results of the direct antiglobulin test (Coomb's test).

iv) Coomb's test is positive in hereditary spherocytosis.

v) In cases of anemia due to hypoproliferative bone marrow erythropoiesis, reticulocyte index is <2.

4. Microcytic hypochromic anemia

i) Free erythrocyte protoporphyrin (FEP) level is increased when erythropoiesis is reduced.

ii) FEP is increased in iron deficiency anemia.

iii) FEP is reduced in anemia of chronic disorders.

iv) In iron deficiency anemia serum iron and bone marrow hemosiderin are reduced and total iron binding capacity is increased.

v) In anemia of chronic disorders, serum iron and bone marrow hemosiderin are not reduced and total iron binding capacity is not increased.

5. The reticulocyte response

i) Reticulocyte production index of >3 means appropriate reticulocyte response.

ii) Response is appropriate in hemolytic anemias of autoimmune etiology.

iii) Response is adequate in hemoglobinopathies and red cell membrane and metabolic defects.

iv) Response is inadequate in renal disease as bone marrow is hypoproliferative.

v) Response is adequate in thalassemias.

vi) In cases with adequate reticulocyte response, anemia is normocytic and normochromic. Same is true in cases with hypoproliferative bone marrow.

6. Lactase deficiency

i) Incidence is quite high in Asians and low in Western Whites.

ii) The disorder may not manifest in childhood.

iii) The secondary lactase deficiency occurs only in disorders associated with pathalogic changes in intestinal biopsy.

iv) The breath test using 50g lactose (measuring hydrogen excretion in breath) is both sensitive and specific for diagnosis of lactose intolerance.

v) Excessive milk intake produces abdominal cramps, distension, and diarrhea.

vi) Moderate milk intake may be tolerated.

7. Chronic pancreatitis

i) Serum amylase and lipase levels are not increased, unlike chronic relapsing pancreatitis.

ii) Serum bilirubin and alkaline phosphatase levels may be raised because of accompanying cholestasis.

iii) Pancreatic calcification occurs only in alcohol induced chronic pancreatitis.

iv) Low serum trypsinogen level is suggestive of chronic pancreatitis.

v) Many patients of chronic pancreatitis show glucose intolerance.

8. Chronic pancreatitis

i) Patients of acute pancreatitis and chronic relapsing pancreatitis have often similar etiology as well as presentation.

ii) In Americans, 25% cases of chronic pancreatitis are idiopathic; in the Developing World PEM is an important cause.

iii) Weight loss and excessive fecal fat excretion are common in mucosal cell dysfunction and chronic pancreatitis.

iv) Generally, at presentation, pancreatic damage is much extensive in chronic pancreatitis than in relapsing pancreatitis.

v) Deficiencies of fat soluble vitamins as well as cations like iron, zinc, calcium and magnesium are quite common in pancreatic malabsorption.

9. Small bowel biopsy

i) Upper gastrointestinal endoscope is now commonly used for obtaining biopsy from small intestine.

ii) Intestinal biopsy is normal in pancreatic malabsorption.

iii) Intestinal mucosal biopsy is abnormal in tropical sprue and celiac disease.

iv) Celiac sprue and tropical sprue can be distinguished by study of intestinal biopsy.

v) Biopsy finding are specific for intestinal lymphoma, amyloidosis, regional enteritis and certain parasitic conditions.

10. Chronic pancreatitis

i) Serum trypsin like immunoreactivity (TLI) is decreased in chronic pancreatitis even in the absence of steatorrhea.

ii) The basal, meal stimulated, and CCK stimulated pancreatic polypeptide levels are all decreased in chronic pancreatitis.

iii) Serum pancreatic polypeptide levels have also been used in diagnosis of pancreatic cancer.

iv) Serum level of P-isoenzyme of amylase is more sensitive for diagnosis of acute pancreatitis compared to level of total amylase.

v) Normal C_{am}/C_{cr} ratio is 1 to 4%.

11. Cytokines

i) IL-1, TNF-α, IL-6, IL-8 are inflammatory cytokines.

ii) IL-8 is a potent neutrophil and monocyte chemotactic factor.

iii) IL-6 is considered as prime mediator of acute phase response.

iv) IL-2, IL-4 and TGF-β are involved in growth, differentiation and activation of lymphocytes and monocytes.

v) Pro-inflammatory cytokines also activate immune cells.

vi) Promoting formation of cytokines is helpful in dealing with a septic patient.

12. Protein and caloric requirements of a patient

i) The different components of energy expenditure of a patient are, the resting metabolic rate (RME), diet induced thermogenesis (DIT), the activity energy expenditure (AEE) and the stress factor.

ii) Resting energy expenditure (REE) is calculated by adding DIT to RME.

iii) AEE for a ward patient is calculated by multiplying REE by a factor of 0.3.

iv) The stress factor of energy expenditure component is calculated by multiplying REE by a factor which may vary from 0.1 to 1.0, depending upon the intensity of stress.

v) A patient in catabolic phase of trauma requires high level of protein intake to convert this phase into anabolic phase.

13. Nutritional assessment

i) Anthropometric measurements and physical examination are commonly sufficient to assess adequacy of growth of a child.

ii) Weight loss accompanied by functional impairment needs build up before surgery.

iii) The systems tested for functional impairment before surgery include, cardiac, respiratory, immune, hepatic, renal and muscular.

iv) In a chronic illness, if nutritional compromise will affect course of illness, it becomes important to make nutritional assessment and look for some marker of catabolic stress.

v) In a chronic illness it is also important, to biochemically monitor a patient for vitamin deficiencies.

vi) Monitoring is also important during dietary intervention.

14. Monitoring during total parenteral nutritional

i) For adequacy of calories, monitor weight and triceps skin fold thickness.

ii) For short term adequacy of protein intake serum levels of albumin/prealbumin are useful guides.

iii) For long term adequacy of protein intake the record of mid-arm muscle mass is important.

iv) Trace element estimations should be done on alternate days.

v) For monitoring of patient hydration the record of fluid chart and auscultation of lung bases will be useful.

15. The catabolic stress

i) Catabolic stress is an important risk factor in surgical patients.

ii) Body temperature higher than 100°F is a marker of catabolic stress.

iii) As far as WBC count is concerned only a count >12,000 indicates a catabolic stress.

iv) Pulse rate above 100/min and respiratory rate above 30/min also indicate catabolic stress.

v) The catabolic index can be calculated by recording N-intake and urea excretion over 24h.

16. Height, growth rate and weight assessment

i) Height corrected for mid parental height should not be >2.5 SD below the mean for the age.

ii) Growth rate should not be <5th percentile for the age.

iii) For weight, parameters like body mass index (BMI) (wt. (kg)/(height)^2 (m)) or weight-for-frame size are used.

iv) BMI is a parameter which takes into account the frame size differences.

v) Mid arm muscle mass is used to assess protein malnutritioin.

ANSWERS:

1. No.(iv). Target cells are flat erythrocytes with a central mass of Hb with a pale ring around, These cells appear in peripheral blood film in hemoglobinopathies, liver disease and in the absence of splenic function.

2. No.(iv). Anemia of chronic inflammation may be normocytic normochromic since it is a pure hypoproliferative disorder. In case of long standing disease, however, it becomes hypochromic, microcytic.

3. No.(iv). Coomb's test is negative in hereditary spherocytosis. In this anemia, however, erythrocyte fragility is increased.

4. No.(iii). FEP is increased. Of the three other microcytic hypochromic anemias which do not respond to iron therapy (ACD, thalassemia minor and sideroblastic anemia), only in thalassemia, FEP is normal, in all others it is increased.

5. No.(v). Response is inadequate, as in thalassemias there is erythrocyte maturation defect.

6. No.(iii). 30% patients of irritable bowel syndrome may show lactose intolerance and in this condition there are no intestinal mucosal changes.

7. No.(iii). Although this is the major cause, pancreatic calcification can also occurs in certain other conditions.

8. No.(v). These deficiencies are not common.

9. No.(iv). Intestinal biopsy study cannot distinguish between the two.

10. No.(i). Level of TLI is decreased in chronic pancreatitis with steatorrhea but normal if there is no steatorrhea associated with chronic pancreatitis. Level is also normal in steatorrhea from other causes, in which pancreatic functions remain normal. Level is increased in acute pancreatitis.

11. No.(vi). Cytokines produced locally, in tissues, may be useful locally. Circulating cytokines, represent spill over from tissues when formed in excess. Once in circulation, these produce harmful effects and destabilize circulation. It is believed that reducing formation of cytokines may help such situations.

12. No.(v). The catabolic phase of metabolic response to stress can not be changed into an anabolic phase by any available means. It may, however, be worsened in the absence of adequate amounts of calories and protein intake less than 1.0 to 1.5 g/kg/d. Any amount of protein over and above this level can not be utilized.

13. No.(v). In such cases biochemical monitoring of vitamin deficiencies is not required. Biochemical monitoring of some vitamins may, sometimes, be undertaken when there is high degree of suspicion. In single vitamin deficiency cases confirmation comes from response to the vitamin replacement treatment.

14. No.(iv). It may be required once in a while in catabolic patients on total parenteral nutrition for a very long period.

15. No.(iii). White cell count of less than 3,000 is also an indicator of catabolic stress.

16. No.(v). For the frame size population is divided into three groups depending upon the breadth of epicondyles of humerus. Tables giving appropriate weights for the three groups at different heights are available and are used to know the appropriateness of the weight of the patient.

CHAPTER 12

Chemical Toxicity and Therapeutic Drug Monitoring

CHEMICAL TOXICOLOGY

Chemical toxicology is divided into four areas with different laboratory requirements and management modalities. Acute toxic effects of cyanide, carbon monoxide (CO), alcohols, metal ions, organophosphates and carbamate are well known. The compounds of the last two categories are used as pesticides and herbicides. Next there are air pollutants (benzpyrene and acetyl aminofluorene derivatives) which cause mutations in critical DNA sequences leading to cancer development. The other two areas are concerning drugs of abuse and the therapeutic drugs. Most of the drugs can cause poisoning when taken in overdose and this occurs more commonly in case of drugs with low therapeutic ratio. So diverse are the chemical substances which can produce human toxicity, that a single laboratory cannot cater to its needs. Commonly encountered chemicals in poisoning, in hospital practice, are given in Appendix 12.1.

Screening of urine is often sufficient to confirm poisoning. Quantitative estimation in plasma may only be undertaken, if it helps management. For example it may help to decide about the need of antidote administration. In most of the cases, management is not affected by lack of knowledge of plasma level of the drug. For medicolegal purposes, samples of vomit, gastric wash, urine and plasma (if sample has been taken), from all serious cases of poisoning should be preserved and stored at 4°C.

Management consists of, maintaining the vital functions, removal of the poison by gastric lavage (unless contraindicated) and diuresis in some cases (if poison is not protein bound) and use of the antidote, if available. Antidotes for certain poisons are given in Appendix 12.1. In salicylate poisoning, $NaHCO_3$ administration makes urine alkaline and promotes excretion of salicylate ions. In lithium toxicity intravenous saline promotes urinary excretion of lithium.

In monitoring the case, serum electrolytes, serum creatinine, blood glucose, blood gases and pH and liver function tests are commonly undertaken. Creatinine, electrolytes and blood gases are extremely important in following progress of a patient presenting with dehydration, hypotension and renal impairment. These are also useful in patients undergoing forced diuresis. Liver function tests are especially important in case of hepatotoxic drugs. Blood glucose estimation is important for differential diagnosis, especially in a patient, brought to hospital in coma.

Dialysis may be indicated in many cases (Table 12.1), if the toxin is dialyzable. For a suitable toxin it should be done if: i) lethal dose of the drug has been taken; ii) patient is in deep coma or has complications like severe hypotension, electrolyte and acid base disturbances; iii) patient has associated renal, hepatic, cardiac or pulmonary complication or disease.

During dialysis, the vital signs, central venous

Table 12.1. Toxic substances for which aqueous dialysis is useful for their elimination

Substances for dialysis is effective:
- Alcohols (methanol, ethanol, ethylene glycol)
- Sedative hypnotics like barbiturates
- Non-narcotic analgesics like aspirin, phenacetin, acetaminophen
- Metals like Li, K; and As, Hg, Pb, Fe after use of chelators
- Some other drugs like phenytoin, sulfonamides

Compounds for which dialysis may not be effective:
- Diazepam, digitalis, antihistaminics, atropine, opiates, methaqualone, phenothiazines and tricyclic compounds.

Table 12.2. Some disorders resulting from chronic intake of alcohol.

- Fatty liver and cirrhosis, the latter condition results from actions of hepatic toxins promoted by alcohol. Acute hepatic failure may also occur.
- Acute and chronic pancreatitis.
- Malabsorption due to effect on pancreas.
- Chronic alcohol intake produces nutrient deficiencies by several mechanisms; by reduced intake, by malabsorption, by increasing excretion in urine and by metabolic reasons. Thus deficiencies of thiamine, folate, B_6, riboflavin, Zn and iron may be produced.
- Wernicke's and korsakoff's syndromes, peripheral neuropathy, delirium tremens.
- Cardiomyopathy and myopathy (due to muscle cell damage).
- Peptic ulcer, chronic gastritis.
- Esophageal varices.
- Increase in MCV without anemia and also folic acid deficiency and iron deficiency anemia.
- Changes in WBC functions and immune system may increase incidence of infections and cancer.

pressure, electrolytes and acid base status need careful monitoring.

Some of the important chemical toxicological cases will be discussed as case histories while important features of some others are summarized in Appendix 12.1. Alcohol and lead toxicities are discussed as case histories nos. 12.2 and 12.6. Table 12.2 indicates some disorders resulting from chronic alcohol intake and Fig. 12.1 shows effects of lead interference in heme biosynthesis.

THERAPEUTIC DRUG MONITORING (TDM)

For many drugs clinical indicators help to use the drug in proper therapeutic range. The toxic effects also have their clinical indications. However, these changes are not quantifiable, and more so in complex clinical situations and may be misleading. The next, easiest alternative is to use drug plasma level to optimize its dosage. This is particularly true for drugs for which steady state levels have to be maintained for quite long periods. In such cases treatment is started with a standard dose and after an appropriate period of time (necessary for achievement of steady state concentration; period equal to four half lives of the drug is commonly used), the steady state concentration is compared (sample is collected just before the next administered dose) with the reported therapeutic range. If the plasma concentration (in steady state) of drug lies outside the therapeutic range some dose adjustment will be required. In case of drugs following first order kinetics (Fig. 12.2) the following relation will be of help:

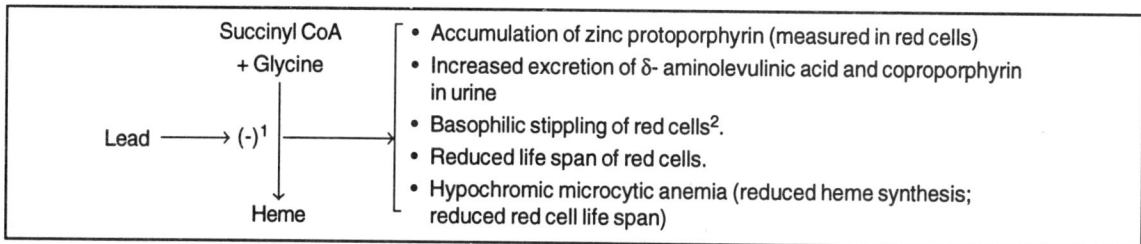

Fig.12.1. Effects of heme synthesis inhibition by lead.

[1] Lead inhibits the enzymes, δ-aminolevulinate dehydratase, ferrochelatase (also probably δ-aminolevulinate synthetase and coproporphyrinogen oxidase (Chapter 8).

[2] Basophilic stippling is aggregation of RNA in red cells. It results from lead inhibiting RNA degradation by inhibiting the enzyme pyrimidine-5-nucleotidase.

- In children the screening test of choice is estimation of lead in blood as estimation of zinc protoporphyrin in red cells lacks sensitivity to detect cases with blood lead level below 25 µg/dL.

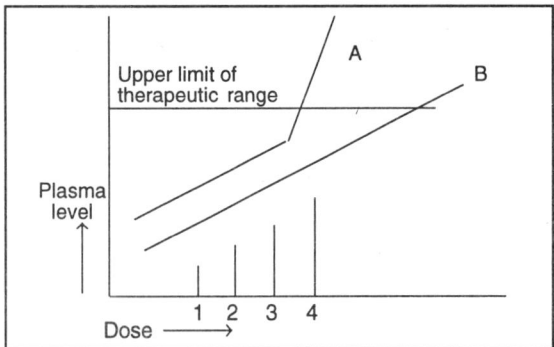

Fig.12.2. Relation between drug dosage and its plasma levels in a drug following first order kinetics and a drug with saturation kinetics.

A) Note sudden increase in plasma level (between doses 3 and 4) when metabolizing enzyme gets saturated (within therapeutic range of the drug)

B) In case of a drug with first order kinetics. There is predictable relationship between dose and plasma level.

$$\frac{\text{Plasma conc. measured (with previous dose)}}{\text{Plasma conc. desired}} = \frac{\text{Dose (previous)}}{\text{Dose (new)}}$$

This relationship cannot be used for drugs having dose dependant kinetics. In such cases dose has to be carefully modified and the whole exercise repeated as change in the plasma level cannot be predicted from change in the dose. Examples of drugs with this type of behaviour are phenytoin and theophylline.

Some drugs are completely eliminated between doses and act only during the early part after the dose. In such a case the sample taken shortly after the dose will be helpful. Further in the presence of renal insufficiency which might cause drug accumulation and toxicity, the sample collected just before the dose will be useful.

Indications for therapeutic drug monitoring are given in Table 12.3. The concept of therapeutic range is explained in Fig. 12.3. Fig. 12.4 mentions different factors which cause difficulties in interpretation of plasma levels during TDM. Corrections for individual factors can be applied with the help of nomograms. For example nomograms are available to help dose modification, when drug accumulation is expected in presence of renal

Table 12.3. Indications for therapeutic drug monitoring.

- Therapeutic effect of the drug is not quantifiable.
- There is poor correlation between dose and the therapeutic effect.
- There is good correlation between plasma level of the drug and the therapeutic effect.
- Drug has low therapeutic ratio.
- Therapeutic drug monitoring is most important when a potentially toxic drug is being given to a seriously ill patient or when the patient has renal or hepatic disease.
- To provide or confirm optimal dosing schedule.
- The drug plasma level is also used to check compliance of drug therapy.
- In a patient showing toxic features of a drug, plasma level of drug can help to confirm drug toxicity.

- Time of sample collection depends upon the purpose for which the plasma sample is desired.

insufficiency. In future computer programmes may be available which may help complicated cases where a number of factors may be involved.

Time of collection of sample has to be carefully selected depending upon the purpose of studying the plasma level of the drug (some examples have already been given). For investigating drug toxicity, any sample may be studied. When it is done for adjustment of the dosage it is best to study the sample just before the next dose. If the drug is almost completely eliminated between doses one should study, one sample, shortly after the dose, to see whether effective concentration is attained and second sample, just before the next dose, to see whether clearance has been, as expected. For starting the maintenance dosage regimen, it should be remembered that the steady state is reached only after four half-lives of the drug.

Toxic reactions of drugs may be pharmacological, pathological or genotoxic. The pharmacological effects are, generally, reversible on stoppage of the drug. The other effects are also repairable, if mild. Patients are also monitored for these effects, when put on prolonged drug therapy.

Examples are discussed below to highlight types of problems that arise during drug monitoring.

Lithium

Lithium is used in psychiatric patients. It has a low therapeutic ratio. The therapeutic range of plasma

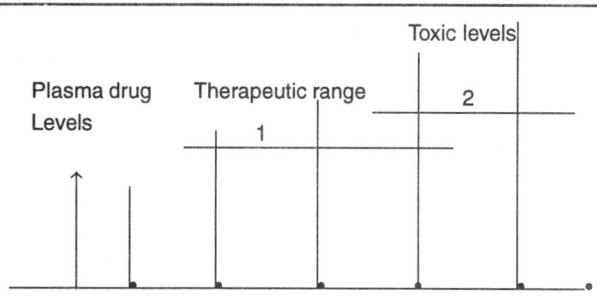

Factors which cause difficulties in correlating the drug dose with plasma level and plasma level with the clinical effect.
- **Plasma level and the drug dose:** Any changes in absorption, distribution, protein binding, metabolism and excretion of the drug; renal and hepatic insufficiencies. Enzyme kinetics of the drug metabolizing enzyme.
- **Plasma level and the drug effect:** Enzyme kinetics of the drug metabolizing enzyme, interaction with other drugs, protein binding.

[1]Therapeutic range = Range of plasma levels which covers 100% patients showing therapeutic response to the drug. Note that some patients show response outside the mentioned therapeutic range of the drug.

[2]Toxic range = Range of plasma levels which covers 100% of the patients showing manifestations of drug toxicity. Note that some patients start showing the drug toxicity at plasma levels within the therapeutic range.

Fig. 12.3. The concept of and uncertainties about therapeutic/toxic levels of a drug.

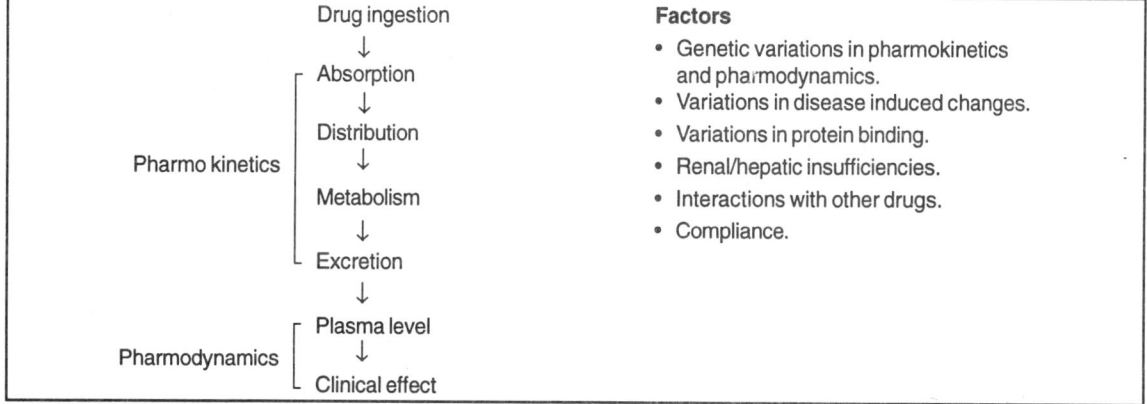

Fig.12.4. Factors which produce uncertainties in correlations between drug dosage and plasma level and between plasma level and the drug effect.

levels is 0.75 to 1.5 mEq/L. Mild to moderate toxicity may be manifested in the range 1.5 to 2.5 mEq/L. Normally a dose of 1.5 g/day (to control the acute attack) should give a plasma level of less than 2.0 mEq/L. However, lithium is eliminated only in urine and a slight renal impairment may raise the plasma level in the toxic range. Luckily, the maintenance dose (after the attack is over) is required to keep plasma concentration of lithium in the range 0.4 to 1.0 mEq/L.

Phenytoin

Phenytoin is used as an anticonvulsant and therapeutic range is 10-20 µg/mL. When this drug is being used in the therapeutic range (say 150 mg/day; plasma level of about 15 µg/mL), the enzymes metabolizing the drug become saturated and if need arises to increase the dose, it is not easy to predict the new plasma level with the increased dose (Fig. 12.2, Curve A). The plasma level will have to be ascertained 1 to 2 weeks after starting the new dose since this much time, the drug will take, to reach the new steady state level.

Digoxin

Digoxin is used in patients of congestive heart failure. Its therapeutic range is 0.5-2 ng/mL. With the usual dose to keep plasma level in therapeutic range, development of slight renal impairment will increase plasma level and may result in toxicity. Even when plasma level is in the therapeutic range, hypokalemia, hypomagnesemia, hypoxia, acidosis and thyroid disease may cause toxicity by enhancing receptor activity.

Theophylline

It is used as a bronchodilator in treatment of asthma. Because of medullary stimulatory action, it is also used for neonatal apnea. This drug is metabolized at different rates in different individuals. The drug response to dosage is quite variable in different patients but response correlates well with plasma level of the drug. If a patient had been on oral drug (especially slow release) and requires intravenous administration, estimation of plasma level (1h after administration) becomes very important. In chronic drug therapy (oral) level in plasma may be ascertained 2h after drug administration, 3 days after start of the drug. In toxic levels, drug may cause severe arrhythmias.

Erythromycin produces interference during theophylline therapy. A patient of asthma, on theophylline therapy may develop lung infection. If erythromycin is given for the infection, plasma level of theophylline may increase and the patient may suffer from toxicity of the drug.

Cyclosporine

This immunosuppressive drug is used to prevent graft rejection in surgery. It is a cyclic polypeptide (11 amino acids), which selectively inhibits T-helper cell function and has no action on augmentation of suppressor T-cell population. It is a nephrotoxic drug and plasma levels are monitored to avoid this toxicity. If evidence of nephrotoxicity appears with drug level in the required range, the cause may be start of graft rejection. Many drugs complicate

cyclosporine therapy, as these are metabolized by the common enzyme system (cytochrome P-450-III-A3.

Table 12.4 shows some other drugs for which TDM is beneficial.

COMA

Coma is defined as complete loss of consciousness. There is no response to any stimulus, however vigorous or painful. Stupor or semicoma is complete loss of consciousness with responses only at reflex level. Depression of ascending reticular system of the brain stem causes coma. Cells of this system lie in the paramedian areas of lower pons and fibers radiate upwards to different areas of the brain.

Coma is an emergency situation in which first priority is the resuscitation measures even before detailed history and clinical examination is undertaken. Patient should be breathing properly. If airway is not clear, intubation may be required. He may even need assisted ventilation. His blood pressure is taken care of. His bleeding should be attended to. In case of trauma, he should not be moved, unnecessarily.

Proper history and physical examination can diagnose majority of cases of coma. History, however, has to be obtained from relatives or friends. One should try to know about any previous history of some physical or mental illness, use of alcohol or drugs and epileptic fits. History about hypertension, kidney, liver, lung and heart diseases should be elicited. Enquire about hysterical attitude of the patient; also about any frustration on part of the patient which could drive him for suicide.

Proper clinical examination is very important. It is important to record depth of coma, not only in the beginning but also from time to time (to monitor progress of the patient). One should also look for focal neurological deficits (say hypotonia) and the state of the pupils. Obtain any evidence of raised intracranial tension (e.g., papilledema, slow irregular breathing). Some other points are stressed in Table 12.5.

Intravenous glucose can always be, safely, given in any patient of coma, where diagnosis is in doubt.

Table 12.4. Drugs for which TDM is considered essential

Digoxin (used in treatment of heart failure):	**Why TDM**
• Therapeutic range (TR) 0.5-2 ng/mL	• Low therapeutic index (TI)
• 20-25% protein bound	• Drug interaction
• Toxic level >2.0 ng/mL (variable)	• Compliance may be poor
	• 50% excreted in urine unchanged
Carbamazapine (anti-convulsant):	
• TR (4-12 µg/mL)	• Low TI
• Toxic level (>9.0 µg/mL)	• Drug interaction
	• Compliance may be poor.
Phenytoin (anticonvulsant):	
• TR (10-20 µg/mL)	• Low TI
• Toxic level (>20 µg/mL)	• Drug interaction
	• Compliance may be poor
	• Saturation kinetics
Phenobarbitone (anticonvulsant):	
• TR (15-30 µg/mL)	• Toxic level >40 µg/mL (however tolerance may develop)
• 40-60% protein bound	
Theophylline (bronchodilator):	
• TR (10-20 µg/mL)	• Low TI
• About 60% protein bound.	• Drug interference
• Toxic level (>20 µg/mL)	• Compliance may be poor
Cyclosporine (used to prevent graft rejection):	
• TR (trough, 12-18h after maintenance dose), 100-300 ng/mL in blood for kidney transplant: renal toxicity[1] ≥ 400 ng/mL.	• Nephrotoxic drug at higher levels • To find cause of elevated creatinine (graft rejection or renal toxicity)

[1] Renal toxicity may occur as delayed graft dysfunction (resolves when drug is withdrawn), acute reversible functional impairment ($\downarrow$ GFR, $\uparrow K^+$, acidosis), responding to decrease of dose, hemolytic uremic syndrome or chronic (irreversible) interstitial fibrosis.
- Low therapeutic levels may result from non-compliance, low dose, malabsorption, increased metabolic clearance.
- High therapeutic levels may result from high dose, increased frequency, improved renal function or impaired hepatic metabolism.
- The four most important drugs for monitoring are digoxin, phenytoin, phenobarbitone and theophyllin.

At the same time samples are submitted for routine investigations (routine urine examination, WBC total and differential counts and for glucose, creatinine and electrolytes).

In acute non-traumatic coma, generally, onset is rapid and there are unilateral signs. CSF examination is important to differentiate between hemorrhage (blood in CSF) and cerebral infarction. In acute infective cases neck rigidity may be present and again CSF examination is required for diagnosis. Bitten tongue and careful history may help diagnosis, of coma due to epilepsy. In space occupying lesions there may be history of days or weeks and there may also be progression of signs (Table 12.5). These may also occur in non-traumatic hemorrhage

or infarction. CT, MRI, EEG and CSF examination are all important in intracranial causes of coma.

In toxic and metabolic causes, evidence of disease or toxic ingestion is generally, available. In these cases there are no features of progressive brain compression. Deep coma may be present without equally severe other clinical signs or vice versa. Pupillary reflexes are preserved in all toxic/ metabolic encephalopathies except when due to hypoxia or due to selected drugs (opiates, tricyclic antidepressants).

Coma in toxic causes takes time to develop and, further, all parts of the body are equally affected. Also read answer to objective type question no. 10. Even when a patient is brought with history of poisoning it is prudent to keep mind open for possibility of some other form of coma (head injury, epilepsy, meningitis, cerebral vascular accident, respiratory failure or metabolic coma).

The following investigations need to be done in all cases of coma unless the cause is quite apparent: i) routine urine examination; ii) routine blood examination for total and differential counts; iii) if there is suspicion of poisoning, analysis of urine/blood/gastric lavage; iv) CSF examination, if there is no contraindication; v) glucose, urea, creatinine, electrolytes in blood/serum samples; vi) X-ray chest, ECG and X-ray skull; vii) CT/MRI, EEG if these are required.

General management includes, care of posture, care of vitals, care of bladder and bowel functions, nutrition of the patient and his fluid balance. In most cases of drug/poison induced coma, the above referred general management is all that is needed till the toxic compound is eliminated by metabolism and excretion. The specific managements for other causes may be looked up in some proper book.

ESTIMATION METHODS FOR DRUG MONITORING OR FOR SCREENING FOR DRUGS OF ABUSE

Drugs are most commonly assayed in serum using immunoassay techniques such as fluorescence polarization immunoassay (FPIA) and enzyme multiplied (or mediated) immunological technique (EMIT). High performance liquid chromatography (HPLC) is also used. TDX-analyzers (Abbot laboratories) and COBAS analyzer (Roche diagnostic laboratories) use immunochemical methods for a wide variety of therapeutic drugs and drugs of abuse. Modalities used are EMIT and FPIA.

Important drugs of abuse are alcohol, opiates, methadone, amphetamine, cocaine and its derivatives, benzodiazepine, barbiturates and other sedative hypnotics, cannabis and lysergic acid diethylamide. Urine samples are used for screening purposes. It is important that the sample is not substituted or adulterated.

For screening of drugs of abuse thin layer chromatography is commonly used. In one method, solvent extraction is used to separate basic (most drugs of abuse fall in this group) and acidic (barbiturates) drugs. Samples are next applied on silica strips for separation of compounds. Different staining reagents are used to identify the compounds. The toxi lab kit (Irvine CA) incorporates the extraction solvent, discrete silicate strips, and colour developing reagents.

As mentioned above, TLC or immunochemical methods are used to detect presence of drug in urine in the screening process. HPLC and gas chromatographic methods may be required in forensic laboratories for confirmation of results of the screening laboratories. These methods, not only estimate the drugs but also their metabolites. Showing the presence of metabolites is, some times, important to be sure that the drug was really taken.

FPIA method

In this fluorescence polarization method, the drug is linked with a fluorescent label (probe) and the linked drug is reacted with its antibody. In the combination, the fluorescent light is polarized into parallel and vertical components. When the sample is added to drug-probe-antibody complex, the drug from the sample displaces probe linked drug from the complex, resulting in diminished fluorescence polarization (Fig. 12.5). Concentration of the displaced molecules will be proportional to the drug molecules in the sample and also to reduced fluorescence polarization.

EMIT

In homogenous immunoassay procedure (or enzyme multiplied immunoassay technique), the enzyme linked drug is reacted with the antibody (this leads to inactivation of the enzyme). On addition of the sample, the free drug molecules in the sample displace the enzyme linked drug molecules from the antibodies. In displaced molecules enzyme becomes active again and its activity is measured. The activity of the displaced enzyme is proportional to the amount of drug in the sample.

Atomic absorption spectroscopy

For Na and K emission technique is better than the absorption one. For others (Li, Ca, Mg, Cu, Fe, Mn,

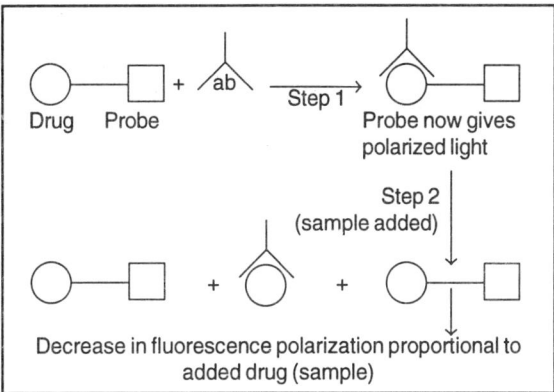

Fig. 12.5. Principle of fluorescence polarization method (FPIA).

Step 1: To the drug-probe (fluorescent) complex, antidrug antibody is added. The new complex gives polarized light.

Step 2: The drug in the added sample shares the antibody, with proportional release of drug-probe complex from the antibody and proportional decrease in fluorescence polarization.

- The instrument optics measure the polarized vertical light. Decrease in this light with addition of the sample drug is proportional to the sample drug concentration.

Cr, CO, Cd, Hg, Pb, Mo, As) the atomic absorption technique is better. In atomic absorption spectroscopy, the analytical principle is just the reverse that of flame photometry (atomic emission spec-

trophotometry) i.e., light absorbed from an incident beam is measured. To maximize sensitivity the incident light is produced by hollow cathode lamp (filled with an inert gas, neon or argon) and its cathode made of the same metal whose ions are to be estimated. The heated metal cathode and the gas atoms emit the spectrum of the incident beam. In the latest models multiple element analysis (upto twelve), from a sample, is possible.

The incident beam is passed through a flame in which ions from the sample are fed and converted into atoms by heat of the flame. These atoms absorb light from the incident beam and this absorbed light is measured.

In the flameless method a graphite furnace is used instead of the flame. A small amount of sample solution is taken in a graphite tube and an electric current is passed through the tube which causes sample vaporization in an inert atmosphere. Result is formation of atoms from the sample ions.

In this procedure spectral interference does not occur since in a single element lamp, one is dealing with only a single wave length. Other types of interferences are encountered (as seen in atomic emission spectrophotometry) when elements are determined without proper processing of the sample.

Table 12.5. Different causes of coma and their important features.

INTRACRANIAL CAUSES

Traumatic:
- Sequence of events between injury and development of unconsciousness and its progression is important to define the brain injury (concussion, laceration, extradural hematoma)
- In laceration focal neurological signs are present.
- X-ray skull for fracture.
- CT/MRI: CT is better for brain hemorrhage (parenchymal/subarachnoid); MRI is better for brain tissue lesions.

Acute non-traumatic:
- In thrombosis there is hemiplegia with previous prodromal episodes(aphasia, dizziness) are likely to be there.
- In embolism hemiplegia develops suddenly. Look for site of origin of embolus.
- In subarachnoid hemorrhage there is sudden onset of symptoms (loss of consciousness, flaccidity of arm/leg muscles along with headache).
- Investigations
  - Lumber puncture should only be done if there is no increase in intracranial pressure as judged from papilloedema, periodic breathing and other evidence: CT/MRI as above.

Acute infective (viral encephalitis/viral or bacterial meningitis):
- These conditions occasionally produce coma.
- Febrile illnesses with accompanying neck rigidity or/and some nervous system problems.
- Investigations
  - CSF examination (Chapter 5); CT, MRI

Coma following epilepsy:
- Examination of patient may show bitten tongue and effect of incontinence.

Contd....

- EEG and others to find cause if any.

Chronic pathologies (abscess, hematoma, tumor):
- History of days/weeks
- Progression of neurological signs (pupil, respiration, eye movement, motor signs) with rostrocaudal progression (in supratentorial pathologies), or as uncal herniation syndrome (in case of laterally placed subdural hematoma, tumor or infarction).

METABOLIC CAUSES OF COMA[1]
(Only important features of presentations are given below; the required investigations will be found in relevant chapters)

Hypoglycemic coma:
- Most common in diabetic patients: also in infants (Chapter 7)
- Epigastric discomfort, sinking sensation: occurs rather rapidly compared to coma of DKA.
- Moist skin and tongue
- Normal blood pressure and bounding pulse.
- Brisk reflexes.

Diabetic ketoacidosis:
- Abdominal pain, anorexia, vomiting
- Dry skin and tongue
- Low blood pressure, feeble pulse
- Laboured breathing
- Diminished reflexes

Uremic coma:
- Patient may be known to have a kidney disease
- Features of chronic renal failure.

Hepatic coma:
- Patient suffering from hepatic disease
- Patient passes through different stages and becomes comatose (altered behaviour; drowsiness; increasing confusion stupor with incoherent speech; liver flap; coma)
- Besides liver function tests other associated metabolic abnormalities are hypoglycemia, metabolic alkalosis (early stages) followed by metabolic acidosis(late stages).
- Evidence of hepatorenal syndrome

Adrenal failure:
- Setting of acute adrenal failure (severe hemorrhage, shock, anticoagulant therapy, overwhelming sepsis eg; meningococcal infection in children)
- A known patient of Addison's disease exposed to severe stress
- Severe electrolyte disturbances:
- Hyponatremia; hyperkalemia

TOXIC AGENTS[1] (alcohol, opiates, barbiturates, tranquilizers, CO):
- Pinpoint pupils in opiate poisoning
- Divergent strabismus in the cyclic antidepressants
- In an alcoholic, coma may be due to head injury, hypothermia or some drug. Coma due to alcohol resolves in 24h unless there is hepatic insufficiency.

Miscellaneous causes:
- Cerebral malaria (results from Falciparum infection[2])
- Hysterical coma (history of hysterical behaviour; inconsistency of physical signs.
- Heat stroke
- Hypothermia (rectal temperature below 35°C)
  (Slowing of circulation; leaking of fluid from capillaries, tissue hypoxia and metabolic acidosis; multiple site thrombosis)
    - Slow pulse and respiration.
    - Commonly there is stupor; coma may occur.

SOME OTHER CAUSES ARE HYPOXIA, CO_2 NARCOSIS AND OTHERS
- If cause of coma is not obvious the following investigations should be undertaken as a routine: X-ray chest, skull; ECG; blood/serum urea, glucose, electrolytes; lumbar puncture (if there is no contraindication); gastric lavage if there is some suspicion of poisoning; routine blood and urine examination.

---

[1] In cases of metabolic/toxic coma there are no features of progressive brain compression. Deep coma may be present without equally severe neurological signs (or vice versa). Pupillary reflexes are preserved in all toxic metabolic encephalopathies when due to anoxia (also see for opiates). All parts of the body are equally affected.

[2] Besides cerebral involvement and coma, the falciparum infection can affect other systems like blood (blackwater fever, DIC), liver (hepatitis), kidney (acute tubular necrosis, pre-renal azotemia), lungs (adult respiratory distress syndrome); hypoglycemia and lactic acidosis.

Appendix 12.1. Some common toxicological agents

Ethyl alcohol (Read case history):

- Disorientation, slurred speech, stupor and coma. Legal intoxication requires level of > 80-100 mg/dL; death may occur at levels between 300-400 mg/dL.
- Investigations: Plasma osmolality (increased), osmolar gap (absence of increased osmolar gap is evidence against increased blood levels of ethanol, methanol or ethylene glycol), acid base status and blood gases (there may be hypochloremic alkalosis, lactic acidosis, alcoholic ketoacidosis), serum electrolytes and LFTs in some cases.
- Alcoholism is associated with increased MCV, increased serum levels of γ-GT, uric acid (about 10% patients), ALT/AST (about 48% patients), ALP (about 16% patients), bilirubin (about 13% patients) and TAG.
- Alcohol ingestion may also cause hypoglycemia and low magnesium levels.
- γ-GT (decrease in its serum level) can be used as a marker of abstinence.
- Hypokalemia during alcohol withdrawl is a useful predictor of delirium tremens.

Methyl alcohol (Read case history):

- Antidote is ethyl alcohol
- It produces severe metabolic acidosis, increased anion gap and increased osmolar gap (as in ethanol poisoning).
- Severe acidosis predisposes to peripheral circulatory failure.
- It causes retrobulbar neuritis and optic atrophy.
- Investigations are as in ethyl alcohol poisoning especially blood gases, pH, electrolytes and kidney functions.
- Patient is treated with alcohol (keep level 100-150 mg/dL), till methanol level is <10 mg/dL, formate level <1.2 mg/dL and anion gap is normalized.
- Hemodialysis at methanol level >50 mg/dL.

Salicylates (Read case history):

- In older children and adults early respiratory alkalosis despite hypermetabolism. Late, in severe cases there is combined primary respiratory alkalosis and primary metabolic acidosis. In infants respiratory alkalosis is overpowered by metabolic acidosis right in the beginning.
- Hyperpyrexia, dehydration, hypotension and renal failure.
- Hypothrombinemia and rarely hemorrhages.
- In older children and adults plasma levels correlate well with severity of toxicity (severe toxicity at about 100 mg/dL); not so in younger children.
- Patients are monitored by studying blood acid base status, glucose (drug causes hypoglycemia) and potassium.

Paracetamol (Read case history):

- Antidote is N-acetylcysteine
- Toxicity depends on dose and is increased by starvation and certain drugs (alcohol) and presence of cirrhosis.
- The most important toxicity is liver damage which can be predicted from the plasma drug level at about 4h after ingestion (not earlier than that).
- Drug level <150 mg/dL at 4h or <30-35 mg/dL at 12h means that no liver damage will occur.
- In first 12-24h no abnormal laboratory results are found and this is the only period when treatment can prevent liver damage. Thus treatment is monitored by drug level.
- In cases in which liver damage occurs, important tests are AST/ALT, PT, bilirubin and blood glucose (as hypoglycemia occurs). Secondary renal failure may also occur.

Lead (Read case history):

- Antidote is penicillamine orally in mild cases and dimercaprol I/V).
- In acute cases abdominal colic, convulsions, hemolytic anemia and kidney damage; in chronic cases encephalopathy and peripheral neuritis.
- Good screening methods for lead poisoning are estimations of red cell ZPP (zinc protoporphyrin estimated by hematofluorometer) and FEP (free erythrocyte protoporphyrin) in blood. These are superior to δ-amino levulinic acid study in urine.
- Lead toxicity is confirmed by level of lead in blood; <20 μg/dL is ignored; >60 μg/dL calls for treatment.
- Basophil stippling of red cells and increased coproporphyrin in urine (increased excretion also occurs in barbiturate and salicylate poisoning) are useful screening tests.

Contd...

Sedatives, hypnotics, antipsychotic and opiates

Barbiturates and benzodiazepines:

- Flumazenil is a useful antidote for benzodiazepines.
- These drugs produce respiratory depression, hypotension, azotemia (especially barbiturates), and CNS depression leading to coma. Features are generally mild with benzodiazepines.
- Investigations should monitor acidosis and azotemia. A patient of barbitruate poisoning should be watched for acute renal failure and pulmonary edema.
- In a patient in coma with barbiturate poisoning, plasma levels is ≥16-20 µg/mL. If level is less, one should look for some other associated cause (head injury, aspiration pneumonia).
- Patient is given gastric lavage with activated charcoal and supportive measures for respiratory failure and hypotension.

Tricyclic compounds:

- Important toxicity features are, retention of urine, absent bowel sounds, cardiac arrhythmias, dilated pupils, divergent strabismus in coma.
- Drugs also cause anxiety, agitation, delirium, convulsions and hypotension.
- Estimation of serum levels of drugs is not useful.
- Gastric lavage and supportive therapy for convulsions, and arrhythmias if these are causing circulatory impairment.

Phenothiazines:

- Important toxicity manifestations are, features like parkinson's disease (muscle rigidity, dyskinesia, tremor), reduced threshold for convulsions, hypotension (adrenergic blockage), hypothermia.
- Drugs may produce cholestatic type of jaundice.
- Estimation of serum levels of drugs is not useful.
- Gastric lavage and supportive therapy for hypotension, convulsions, and extrapyramidal features.

Opiates and related compounds:

- Antidote is naloxone which is given repeatedly for respiratory depression.
- Encountered in opium addicts. Clinical features related to inhibitory effects on brain stem centers. Pulse is slow; there is hypotension, respiration may be slow/periodic, and pupils are constricted and there may be hypothermia. Patient should be watched for acute pancreatitis.
- Gastric lavage with dilute potassium permanganate solution, irrespective of the time of poisoning (drug causes pylorospasm).
- Drug level in plasma is not useful; serum amylase may help.

Carbon monoxide(CO):

- CO poisoning was not uncommon when coal was used for burning in closed rooms for heating purpose. CO is also present in high concentration in exhaust fumes of car engines. When inhaled, it forms carboxyhemoglobin (affinity for Hb is 300 times that of O_2). Carboxyhemoglobin cannot carry O_2 and also interferes in release of O_2 from oxyhemoglobin in tissues. Besides, it also produces histotoxic hypoxia by binding with and inactivating cytochrome a_3. In an atmosphere containing CO (say 1 part per 10,000) an individual will go into coma gradually without warning. Coma (also papilledema) is due to cerebral edema. Myocardial damage and hypotension occurs due to myocardial anoxia.
- Coma can occur at COHb level of >30%.
- Monitor percentage of carboxyhemoglobin with the help of a co-oximeter. For rough estimate, to diluted blood (1 in 10) is added 1ml of 5% sodium hydroxide solution. If solution turns yellow, carboxy Hb is >20% and if it remains red <20%. Give artificial respiration and 90% O_2, 5% CO_2/hyperbaric O_2 (potential danger of hyperbaric O_2 is to produce cerebral vessel spasm and edema).
- Supportive treatment for cerebral edema (IV mannitol) and cardiac damage.
- Patient should be watched for myocardial ischemia or cerebral stroke.

Iron:

- Toxicity occurs in small children who ingest iron tablets taking them as sweets. In fist few hours there is bleeding because of damage to intestinal tract. Subsequently, patient may have encephalopathy, shock, coagulopathy, renal and hepatic damage.
- Diagnosis needs determination of serum iron (≥500 µg/dL in children and ≥840 µg/dL in adults needs treatment).

Contd...

- Desferrioxamine helps to chelate and promote excretion of iron. Supportive measures for shock, acidosis, electrolyte disturbances and blood loss.

Aluminium:

- Aluminium toxicity may occur in a patient using aluminium salts as antacids. It can also occur in patients undergoing renal dialysis employing tap water for dialysis. In both types of cases chronic toxicity occurs leading to renal damage and aluminium osteodystrophy.
- Diagnosis needs estimation of aluminium in serum. Bone biopsy material will show accumulation of aluminium in bone.
- Desferrioxamine can chelate aluminium and promote its excretion.

Arsenic:

- It is used as a rodenticide, herbicide, insecticide and also in paints. In certain parts of the country water content of arsenic is quite high (West Bengal). It produces actions by reacting with SH- groups of biomolecules. Acute ingestion causes profuse vomiting and shock. Chronic ingestion causes diarrhea, dermatitis and polyneuropathy. Cardiovascular and renal damage can also occur.
- In chronic poisoning analysis of urine, hair and nail for arsenic, by ion emission spectroscopy, is useful.
- Chelating agents like N-acetyl penicillamine and dimercaprol are used to promote excretion of arsenic. In severe cases hemodialysis may be needed.

Organophosphates and carbamates:

- These are used as pesticides in agriculture. Toxic manifestations occur because the drugs inhibit acetylcholine esterase (AchE) by binding to its active site. The toxicity features are related to parasympathetic stimulation. It may mimic an abdominal disease (vomiting, diarrhea, abdominal cramps) and a respiratory disease (brochospasm and pulmonary edema due to excessive bronchial secretions). Other features are constricted pupils, excessive salivation and sweating (these features help diagnosis in the absence of proper history), muscle weakness and convulsions.
- Pralidoxime or obidoxime can reactivate the enzyme and can be used as antidotes.
- Diagnosis can be confirmed by showing decrease of erythrocyte acetylcholine esterase (more specific) and plasma pseudocholine esterase.
- Treat respiratory failure (respiratory muscle weakness) with O_2. After correcting cyanosis give atropine to atropinise the patient.

Aluminium phosphide:

- It is commonly used for wheat and other grain preservation by fumigation. The active agent is phosphene gas (PH_3) which is released when the drug comes in contact with moisture. Aluminium phosphide is also a common agent responsible for suicidal/accidental poisoning. After ingestion, contact with HCl of gastric juice causes release of phosphine, which is readily absorbed from stomach and diffuses throughout the body. Precise cause of tissue damage is not known but phosphene is believed to block mitochondrial respiratory chain resulting in severe hypoxia and acidosis. Tissues affected are peripheral vasculature (resulting in wide spread congestion, hemorrhages and fluid leakage from capillaries), heart, lungs and kidney.
- Important clinical features are, severe abdominal pain and profuse vomiting, followed by severe hypotension and shock. After 12 to 24h (if patient survives), respiratory distress develops because of pulmonary edema.
- Impairment of consciousness is late.
- Three tablets (3g each) generally prove fatal.
- Investigations required are, serum electrolytes, blood gases and pH. Serum creatinine helps to follow renal functions. Serum CPK-MB is elevated in almost all cases.
- Cardiac rhythm changes are monitored by ECG.
- Gastric lavage with a dilute solution of $KmnO_4$ followed by a solution of sodium bicarbonate.
- Supportive measures for shock (fluids, dopamine), electrolyte/pH disturbances (KCl, $NaHCO_3$ solutions), rhythm disturbances, and for acute respiratory distress syndrome (O_2 at high flow rate), should be provided.

- In all cases of poisoning, an accurate record of the patient is important, not only for his clinical management but also for legal reasons.
- Any presented medicine, gastric lavage sample, urine and a venous blood sample (heparinised), should be kept for examination.
- It is best to analyze urine for poisoning cases. In case of drugs like phenytoin and theophyllin, plasma levels should be measured to monitor (the patient), till they fall to therapeutic levels.

CASE HISTORY: 12.1

A patient was admitted with complaints of nausea, vomiting, abdominal pain, dizziness and blurred vision. There was history of ingestion of methylated spirit, a few hours back. Blood methanol concentration was reported as 60 mg/dL (for estimation of methanol in blood a GC-MS (gas chromatography - Mass spectroscopy) method is used. A level of >20 mg/dL is considered toxic).

Methanol ingestion (also ethanol ingestion) produce serum hyperosmolality with increased osmolar gap. This may, at times, be helpful in diagnosis. Compared to ethyl alcohol, methanol is less intoxicating but more toxic. Its metabolic clearance is much slower than that of ethyl alcohol. Methanol ingestion produces severe acidosis and that predisposes to peripheral circulatory failure. Plasma level of methanol is used to judge toxicity as well as prognosis (although there is lack of precise correlation). Important laboratory investigations are; level of methanol in blood; acid base status; serum electrolytes and serum creatinine, in case of circulatory failure.

The dreaded toxic effects of methanol is retrobulbar neuritis and optic atrophy which cause diminished vision and even permanent blindness. Methanol is metabolized to formaldehyde and formic acid (by the same enzymes which metabolize ethyl alcohol to acetaldehyde and acetate); formaldehyde has maximum toxic effect on retina. In methanol poisoning, if ethyl alcohol is given intravenously or orally (to maintain plasma level 100-150 mg/dL), it displaces methanol from the enzyme system which produces toxic formaldehyde from methanol, and with time methanol gets excreted in urine. Thus ethyl alcohol is considered an antidote for methanol poisoning. Other aspects of treatment include repeated gastric lavage with 2% sodium bicarbonate (dialysis in severe cases), and maintaining circulation and acid base status. For the latter purpose intravenous sodium bicarbonate is given depending upon acid base status of the patient.

CASE HISTORY: 12.2

A patient was admitted in a state of drowsiness and also had ataxia and disarthria. He was strongly smelling of alcohol.

➤ In this patient what is the importance of analysis of acid base status?

➤ What is the significance of intake of barbiturates/other sedatives by an alcoholic?

➤ After this patient recovers from the present episode, how should he be investigated for effects of chronic alcoholism?

➤ What are different causes of coma which can be expected in an alcoholic.

• In a stuporous/comatose patient smelling of alcohol, presence of acidosis may indicate methyl alcohol or ethylene glycol as the cause of his condition (taken as contaminants of ethyl alcohol).

• When a large bout of alcohol is taken, both cytoplasmic and microsomal enzymes of liver cells (which metabolize alcohol) get saturated. Any intake of a barbiturate or any other sedative (needing same microsomal enzymes for metabolism) may cause severe poisoning. In a chronic alcoholic, on the other hand, activity of microsomal enzymes is increased (induction by alcohol) and these drugs are tolerated in excessive amounts, if taken at separate occasions.

• Chronic use of alcohol along with accompanying malnutrition and B-complex vitamin deficiencies, leads to slowly developing peripheral neuritis (pain, paresthesias and weakness in peripheral parts of the limbs). Other deficiencies and clinical conditions produced are given in Table 12.2. The patient needs to be investigated accordingly. There is no specific and sensitive marker for detection of chronic alcoholism. In a large percentage of chronic alcohol abusers, γ-GT activity is increased in serum. This enzyme however, is also increased in any liver disease and also induced by certain drugs like barbiturates and phenytoin. Other biochemical changes associated with chronic alcohol intake are, hyperuricemia, hypertriglyceridemia, and fasting hypoglycemia. Macrocytosis is also commonly seen as alcohol interferes in folate metabolism. For detecting hepatic involvement serum bilirubin, albumin, ALT and ALP are important parameters.

• It is not necessary, that a person after having taken alcohol may also be suffering from alcoholic coma. Coma may be actually due to some drug taken along with alcohol. It may be that the person after taking alcohol fell down and suffered head injury and went into coma. After a bout of alcohol, the person may get an undue exposure to cold (unable to care for himself) and may suffer from coma due to hypothermia. Coma may result from hypoglycemia produced as a result of alcohol.

For estimation of ethyl alcohol in plasma, enzymatic method (alcohol dehydrogenase converts NAD to NADH which is followed), and methods based on gas chromatography or electro chemical oxidation are used. Arterial and capillary samples give more accurate levels than the venous samples. Legal intoxication requires a level of > 80-100 mg/dL. Ethylene glycol is estimated by HPLC.

CASE HISTORY: 12.3

A patient presented with complaints of nausea and abdominal pain. He admitted having taken 20 tablets of paracetamol (acetaminophen) which, previously he had been using during attacks of common cold. There was also tenderness on deep palpation in right upper quadrant but liver and spleen were not palpable.

> ➤ What is the importance of estimation of drug in serum in this case?
> ➤ What other investigations will be helpful?
> ➤ What is the mechanism of hepatic damage with this drug?
> ➤ What supportive treatment will be needed?

• It is important to estimate serum level of this drug since an antidote (N-acetyl cysteine) is available for its toxicity and has to be used depending upon the serum level of the drug and the time after ingestion. Antidote treatment is needed if plasma level is above 200 mg/L at 4h and above 50 mg/L at 12h after the drug ingestion. In the absence of knowledge of plasma level of the drug, the antidote can still be given (upto 24h after the ingestion of the drug), if a potentially toxic dose had been taken. It is not required after 24h, if no evidence of liver or kidney damage appears.

• These are the investigations evaluating liver damage (prothrombin time, serum bilirubin, AST), acid base status (danger of acidosis) and blood glucose (danger of hypoglycemia). Tendency to liver damage increases in the elderly and malnourished. Patient should be watched for liver damage from second to fifth day.

• Major metabolites of the drug are excreted as glucuronate/sulphate conjugates and are harmless. A small amount of highly reactive metabolite N-acetyl-p-benzoquinonimine (which binds to many hepatic cell enzymes) is formed by mixed function oxidase enzyme system of microsomes. It is detoxified by glutathione. With depletion of glutathione, the metabolite causes liver cell damage (the compound is also nephrotoxic). With ingestion of a toxic dose of paracetamol this metabolite is formed in large amounts. If the patient had been taking some enzyme inducing drug (carbamazepine, phenytoin, alcohol, barbiturate), larger amounts of the toxic metabolite of paracetamol will be formed and chances of liver damage will increase. In such a case antidote treatment has to be started at lower plasma drug levels (see above).

• Gastric lavage is useful only within a few hours after ingestion of the drug (not of use, after 4h of drug ingestion). If hepatic damage is expected, medical treatment, in that connection should be started, in anticipation.

CASE HISTORY: 12.4

A student (age 24 years), was brought in a state of drowsiness. He had been in the habit of using barbiturates for sleep. The previous night he had a large dose because of his tension. He had Cheyne-Stokes respiration. Blood pressure was 90/50. Pupils were constricted and there were no reflexes. Apparently, he was suffering from barbiturate poisoning.

> ➤ How do important clinical features of barbiturate poisoning arise?
> ➤ What are the investigations required in this case?
> ➤ How are drugs eliminated by alkaline diuresis? How safe is the procedure?
> ➤ What supportive measures are required in treatment of the case.

• Barbiturates cause depression of cerebral and brain stem functions. The brain stem depression results in respiratory failure, hypotension, venous pooling and reduced cardiac out put. Impaired circulation leads to renal failure. Drowsiness and coma are produced because of cerebral depression.

• Barbiturates are detected in urine to confirm barbiturate poisoning by thin layer chromatography. Immunoassay is used to study serum level. The serum levels is used to know the severity of poisoning. After alkaline diuresis serum levels are helpful in following the progress of treatment. Other investigations required in this case are analysis of acid base status and serum creatinine.

• Forced alkaline diuresis helps to increase urinary excretion of weak organic acids from the body. It is used in cases of barbiturate poisoning and aspirin poisoning. These drugs are organic acids and are passively secreted into the tubular fluid, undissociated, at the pH of the tubular cells. Undissociated, these can easily cross the plasma membrane to enter tubular fluid. In case the tubular fluid is alkaline, dissociation occurs and organic acid anions are formed and get trapped and excreted since ions cannot cross back into the tubular cells easily. The procedure, however, is not very safe. It should only be undertaken in adults with normal renal and cardiac functions. Also, blood pH and serum potassium levels should be, carefully, monitored during the procedure.

• Gastric lavage, and supportive measures for respiratory failure, hypothermia and hypotension are required. Dialysis may be needed if the patient is already suffering from hepatic or renal disease.

CASE HISTORY: 12.5

A 12 year old school student was brought to hospital with history of having ingested a large number of aspirin tablets in frustration before his examination. The boy was in a confused state, hyperventilating and sweating. He also complained of tinnitis and blurred vision. There was smell of ketones in his breath. His pulse was 110/min and blood pressure was 90/65. The boy was also running high temperature.

➢ What important investigations are required in this case?

➢ Explain causes of dehydration, ketosis and hyperpyrexia, often encountered, in such cases.

➢ What are common toxic presenting features of an adult getting toxicity from his therapeutic intake of aspirin?

➢ What is the importance of studying serum aspirin level in this case?

➢ What is the importance of urine examination in this case?

➢ What supportive measures are required in management of this case?

➢ Why are salicylates not recommended in children suffering from chicken pox or influenza?

• Besides serum salicylate level, serum potassium, blood acid base status and prothrombin time should be studied. Serum creatinine level is used to monitor azotemia because of dehydration. Blood glucose level is also estimated, as in severe cases, in children, hypoglycemia can occur leading to convulsions and coma.

• Hyperventilation, sweating and vomiting (gastric irritation) cause dehydration. Inhibition of citric acid cycle enzymes causes reduced aerobic metabolism and acidosis. This also increases lipolysis resulting in ketosis. In salicylate poisoning, initially there is alkalosis due to hyperventilation (more commonly seen in adults) and this is followed by acidosis (more severe in children). Severe acidosis can result in pulmonary edema and cardiac arrest.

• These are patients in which there is no history of drug overdose, although, they have been taking the drug over a long period. These patients show acid base disturbances, unexplained ketosis and prolonged prothrombin time. These patients are likely to show pulmonary edema (non-cardiogenic) and certain neurological manifestations.

• In a patient suffering from some drug toxicity plasma level of the drug is studied, only, if it is useful in management since the diagnosis is, generally, established from history. Plasma salicylate levels are used to indicate severity of toxicity (level more than 100 mg/dL indicates severe

toxicity and need for alkaline diuresis). For estimation of salicylate in plasma, a simple colorimetric method is used based on reaction of Fe^{+++} with phenol group of salicylic acid.

• Because of presence of salicylate metabolites in urine, it becomes false positive for glucose and ketones. Actual ketones, however, can also be present in urine because of salicylate toxicity. Ferric chloride test, for urinary ketones can be used, to diagnose salicylate toxicity.

• The supportive measures include gastric lavage, intravenous fluids (also potassium) to correct dehydration and hyperthermia and alkaline diuresis (if drug level is more than 100 mg/dL). Vitamin K (IM) is given if prothrombin time is prolonged. In very severe cases dialysis may be needed. Patient should be watched for hyperthermia and acute renal failure.

• Reye's syndrome may develop if salicylates are given in these virus infections. Salicylates and these virus infections have additive effect in producing mitochondrial damage.

CASE HISTORY: 12.6

A 4 year old child presented with anorexia, abdominal colic and convulsions. Her mother reported that child had been often seen licking paint material on her toys and elsewhere. In view of the history, the child was considered to be suffering from acute lead poisoning. Other features of acute lead poisoning not seen in this child are evidence of hemolytic anemia, black colour of stools (due to presence of lead sulphide) and evidence of kidney damage. Treatment involves use of chelator, dimercaprol (given parenterally). Milder cases can be treated with oral penicillamine.

In chronic lead poisoning, there is involvement of gastrointestinal system (constipation and severe colic), hemopoietic system (anemia and basophilic stippling of red cells), encephalopathy (more common in children), peripheral neuropathy (involvement of motor nerves) and a blue line (due to lead sulphide) developing on gums. In children growth, intellectual development and hearing may be affected. History is very important in diagnosis of cases of lead poisoning. In the absence of history encephalopathic features will be attributed to various degenerative disorders in adults. Similarly abdominal colic will be attributed to other abdominal disorders.

In environment lead fumes are released from exhaust of automobiles and near lead smelters where discarded battery cases are burnt. Food, beverages and wines may be contaminated with lead when stored in lead soldered cans. Water from lead pipes and lead tanks is also contaminated.

Fig. 12.1 indicates certain tests useful in diagnosis of patients of lead poisoning.

OBJECTIVE TYPE QUESTIONS

Pick out the wrong statement.

1. Diagnosis of drug toxicities

i) In lead poisoning red cells zinc protoporphyrin and serum lead are estimated.

ii) Serum iron level is useful to diagnose poisoning by iron salts in children.

iii) Liver function tests are important in diagnosis of paracetamol poisoning.

iv) In CO poisoning, blood carboxyhemoglobin level will indicate diagnosis.

v) Plasma levels of all drugs play a very useful role in treatment of their toxicities.

2. Drug toxicity

i) Methyl alcohol has lower metabolic clearance compared to ethanol.

ii) The main toxic metabolite of acetaminophen, N-acetyl-p-benzoquinonimine is toxic to liver.

iii) Prolonged prothrombin time is the best marker of hepatic toxicity of acetaminophen (paracetamol).

iv) Plasma level of N-acetyl-p-benzoquinonimine is routinely estimated to know prognosis of the patient.

v) Plasma level of paracetamol is important to decide, whether or not to give the antidote N-acetyl cysteine.

3. Alcohol

i) Worsens porphyria, pancreatitis and epilepsy.

ii) Should not be used with sedatives, hypnotics and tranquillizers.

iii) Affects normal functioning of many systems except the pulmonary system.

iv) May produce fatty liver or cirrhosis.

v) May produce lactic acidosis, hypoglycemia, hypomagnesemia and hyperlipidemia.

vi) May produce coma.

4. Binding of drugs by plasma proteins

i) Hypoalbuminemia decreases binding of basic drugs.

ii) Malnutrition, chronic liver disease and nephrotic syndrome may produce hypoalbuminemia.

iii) α_1-Acid glycoprotein (an acute phase reactant) is elevated in blood in myocardial infarction, surgery, neoplastic disease, burns and rheumatoid arthritis.

iv) Lidocaine binding to α_1-acid glycoprotein can cause drug accumulation, when used to control arrhythmias during acute phase of myocardial infarction.

v) Altered levels of plasma proteins modify effectivity of those drugs which are more than 90% bound.

5. Drug toxicity

i) Patients of organophosphate pesticide and strychnine poisoning may present with convulsions and need I/V diazepam for treatment.

ii) Patients with corrosive poisoning may present with severe epigastric pain and require I/V morphine for that.

iii) In aluminium phosphide poisoning cellular damage occurs most prominently in the brain tissue.

iv) In opiate poisoning patient may present with acute pancreatitis.

v) In barbiturate poisoning patient may present with acute respiratory failure needing assisted ventilation.

vi) In barbiturate poisoning patient may present with peripheral circulatory failure needing I/V fluids and dopamine.

6. Forced alkaline diuresis

i) Patient is given 500 mL of glucose saline every 1 to 2h and 300 mL of 20% mannitol every 6 to 12h.

ii) Urine pH is maintained near 8.5 with infusion of 7.5% sodium bicarbonate.

iii) Alkalemia by itself increases rate of urine flow.

iv) Urine out put should increase to over 8L/d.

v) This method of drug excretion is useful in different types of drug poisonings which do not lead to kidney damage.

7. Acute alcoholic toxicity

i) Patient may present in coma.

ii) If alcoholic coma persists for more than 24h, some superadded cause of coma is likely to be present.

iii) Alcoholic toxicity can appear with superadded acute hepatic failure.

iv) Alcoholics tolerate barbiturates better than normals.

v) Alcoholic toxicity is reduced if barbiturates are taken along with alcohol.

vi) An alcoholic may present with gastrointestinal bleeding.

8. Drug toxicity

i) In salicylate poisoning severity of poisoning can be judged from serum level of the drug.

ii) In barbiturate poisoning blood levels are useful in management but do not faithfully predict chances of survival of the patient.

iii) CO poisoning leads to severe tissue hypoxia.

iv) CO poisoning in the elderly may lead to myocardial infarction or cerebral stroke.

v) Deep coma is characteristic of aluminium phosphide poisoning.

vi) Hepatic toxicity of paracetamol is increased by alcohol.

9. Alcohol poisoning

i) Methanol is metabolized to formic acid and ethylene glycol to oxalic acid.

ii) Both at item i) produce acidosis.

iii) Ethylene glycol poisoning produces hypocalcemia.

iv) Ethyl alcohol and benzodiazepines taken together may prove lethal.

v) Ethyl alcohol and ethylene glycol taken together produce severe toxicity.

10. Coma (diagnosing the cause)

i) Cause may be obvious, such as trauma, stroke, hypoxia, diabetes, liver disease or kidney disease.

ii) Acute adrenal failure may be the cause in the presence of an overwhelming sepsis.

iii) Common toxic agents causing coma are, alcohol, opiates, barbiturates, carbon monoxide and tranquillizers.

iv) In case the cause in obvious, that becomes the point of focus

v) In case the cause is not obvious cerebral stroke is the first possibility to be excluded.

vi) In case of cerebral stroke, different signs and symptoms may help to localize the damaged area.

11. Therapeutic drug monitoring (TDM)

i) Dosage of antihypertensives can be easily adjusted depending upon the changes produced in blood pressure.

ii) Laboratory markers can be used in adjusting dosage of lipid lowering and hypoglycemic drugs.

iii) TDM is important in case of drugs like antidepressants or antiseizure drugs which are used over long periods.

iv) TDM is essential for all drugs whose response is not easily measurable by any clinical or biochemical parameter.

iv) It may also be used to confirm that the toxic features of the patient are due to drug toxicity.

v) It is also required for checking the drug compliance.

12. Amino glycosides (about gentamycin)

i) Gentamycin is largely excreted through kidney and is also nephrotoxic.

ii) Simultaneous use of diuretics, further increase toxicity.

iii) Drug plasma level, relevant to its bactericidal action may be determined, just before dose administration, after 4 half lives.

iv) K^+ depletion increases toxicity of the drug.

v) Pre-renal failure increases the drug toxicity.

vi) Likelihood of toxicity also increases in old age and in the presence of hepatic insufficiency.

13. Phenytoin

i) May produce abnormal results in thyroid function tests.

ii) Moderate increase in serum enzymes related to liver functions, is an indication to withdraw the drug.

iii) Altered metabolism of vitamin D may produce osteomalacia.

iv) Hyperglycemia may be produced by inhibition of insulin secretion.

v) May alter metabolism of folic acid to produce megaloblastic anemia.

14. Oral contraceptives

i) May exacerbate porphyria.

ii) May increase cholesterol level in bile to promote cholelithiasis.

iii) These should not be used by women with acute or chronic liver disease.

iv) May produce increase in VLDL and TAG levels and decrease in HDL level.

v) Impaired glucose tolerance is a very common and harmless effect.

vi) Cholestatic jaundice in those predisposed to recurrent jaundice of pregnancy.

15. Diuretics

i) Both thiazides and loop diuretics increase LDL-C.

ii) Both thiazides and loop diuretics produce hypomagnesemia and hypocalcemia.

iii) Thiazides impair diabetic control.

iv) Thiazides produce hyperuricemia.

v) Both thiazides and loopdiuretics produce hypokalemia.

ANSWERS

1. No.(v). Diagnosis of poisoning is commonly made clinically. However, information about presence of the drug in the body fluids of the patient may

help. Generally, qualitative analysis of the drug (urine is more useful than plasma) is enough. Urine, blood and stomach contents may be submitted for analysis. Plasma levels are used in some cases especially when antidote has to be given.

2. No.(iv). The major pathway of metabolism of paracetamol is formation of glucuronate and sulphate conjugates (and these are not toxic). Only when the major pathway is saturated, hepatotoxic metabolite N-acetyl-p-benzoquinonimine is formed. Plasma level of this toxic metabolite, however, is not routinely estimated for lack of a suitable method.

3. No.(iii). Lung volumes, airway resistance and the gas exchanges are all adversely affected.

4. No.(i). Albumin binds acidic and neutral drugs.

5. No.(iii). Cellular damage most prominantly occurs in heart, lung and kidney. Important features are severe hypotension and respiratory distress syndrome. Consciousness is not lost

6. No.(v). Drugs which are weak acids are trapped in alkaline urine. Examples are phenobarbitone and other long acting barbiturates, salicylates, sulfonamides and methotrexate. Saline diuresis increases excretion of calcium, lithium and alcohols. Acid diuresis increases renal loss of basic drugs like amphetamine, cocaine, quinidine, quinine, tricyclic antidepressants and strychnine.

7. No.(v). Ethyl alcohol and barbiturates both are metabolized by cytochrome P450 microsomal enzyme system. Thus in chronic alccholics tolerance to barbiturates increases. When alcohol and barbiturates are taken together barbiturates delay metabolism of ethyl alcohol and increase its effects.

8. No.(v). See answer to question no.5.

9. No.(v). Ethyl alcohol is used as an antidote to ethylene glycol and methanol poisonings.

10. No.(v). Hypoglycemia is first ruled out. The order of actions, in case the cause of coma is not obvious is as follows: i) after taking care of vitals and making a brief assessment of pupils, depth of coma, heart and lungs and collecting blood and urine samples for analysis, glucose is administered to rule out hypoglycemia as the cause; ii) hypoglycemia ruled out, next is the turn of detailed history and examination for trauma and drug toxicity; iii) after ruling out the above possibilities focus shifts to diabetic ketoacidosis, followed by meningitis, sub-arachnoid hæmorrhage, epilepsy, cerebrovascular accident and hysteria, in that order.

11. No.(iii). It may not be required in all such drugs; for example it may not be required if margin of safety between desirable and toxic concentration is quite wide. Important criteria for useful TDM are: i) poor correlation between dose and effect (because of inter-individual variations in pharmokinetics of the drug); ii) there is low margin of safety between desirable and toxic concentrations; iii) plasma levels correlate well with the effect.

12. No.(iii). Bactericidal action of the drug is related to the peak drug concentration (found shortly after the dose) and toxicity is related to trough concentration of the drug (found just before next dose). If a small dose can give adequate peak concentration, the drug should be given in this small amount, more frequently.

13. No.(ii). Increase in enzyme levels is transitory and not an indication to withdraw the drug.

14. No.(v). It is not very common but if it occurs an alternative method of contraception should be used. Lipid changes produced by oral contraceptives are not atherogenic, ordinarily. However, if the woman is a heavy smoker oral contraceptives induced changes become strongly atherogenic.

15. No.(ii). Thiazides may produce hypercalcemia and not hypocalcemia.

CHAPTER 13

Pituitary Functions and Disorders

PITUITARY GLAND

It weighs about 0.5g in an adult and lies in a bony cavity (sella turcica) in the sphenoid bone at the base of skull. It is related above to the optic chiasma, laterally to the cavernous venous sinuses (passage for third, fourth and sixth cranial nerves) and below and anteriorly to sphenoid air sinus. The gland is connected to hypothalamus by a stalk. The stalk carries nerve fibres, originating in supraoptic nucleus (SON) and paraventricular nucleus (PVN) of either side and ending in posterior pituitary. It also contains the vessels of hypophyseal portal plexus, which receives blood from superior and inferior hypophyseal arteries and drains into the sinusoids of anterior pituitary. The stalk and posterior pituitary develop from the floor of third ventricle while anterior pituitary develops from Rathke's pouch, an upward extension from embryonic oral ectoderm.

Paired supraoptic and paraventricular nuclei lie in anterior part of hypothalamus and form antidiuretic hormone (ADH), now called arginine vasopressin or AVP and oxytocin, respectively. The two hormones are stored in and secreted from posterior pituitary. Some fibres carrying AVP also terminate in median eminence.

The peptidergic neurons producing hypophyseotropic hormones lie in the lateral wall of the third ventricle. Their nerve terminals converge on median eminence and release their neurosecretions or hypophyseotropic hormones. These hormones enter hypophyseal portal plexus and reach anterior pituitary to regulate secretion of pituitary hormones from different groups of anterior pituitary cells (Fig. 13.1). Autonomous activity of these peptidergic neurones is able to maintain basal level of secretion of pituitary hormones. However, these peptidergic neurones receive numerous inputs from both within hypothalamus and outside hypothalamus (anterior thalamus, amygdala, pyriform cortex, septum hippocampus and midbrain). Neurotransmitters/neuromodulators at these inputs include noradrenaline, adrenaline, dopamine 5-HT, acetyl choline, GABA, opioids, IL-1 and somatostatin. Fig. 13.2 shows general plan of regulation of secretion of anterior pituitary hormones.

Hypothalamic neurohormones are released in a pulsatile manner and this is important to their actions on anterior pituitary cells. The frequency as well as the amplitude of pulses may have additional regulatory influence on the pituitary cells. The anterior pituitary hormones are also secreted in a pulsatile fashion. All the pituitary hormones also exhibit circadian rhythms in their secretion (See later under general remarks on pituitary hormone studies). Most of the pituitary hormones are influenced by stress, obesity, depression and malnutrition.

Growth hormone

This 191 amino acid protein is secreted in sporadic bursts (each lasting for 1-2h), mainly during sleep.

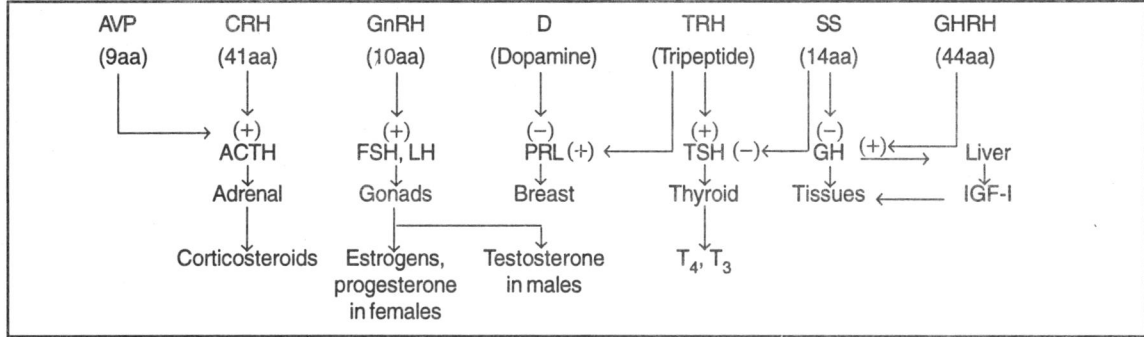

Fig. 13.1. Role of hypothalamic neurohormones in regulating secetion of pituitary hormones.

- AVP (arginine vasopressin or ADH), CRH (corticotropin - releasing hormone), GnRH (gonadotropin releasing hormone), D (dopamine), TRH (thyrotropin releasing hormone).
- GH (growth hormone, 191aa, Mol.wt. 22,000).
- PRL (prolactin, 198aa, Mol.wt. 23,000).
- ACTH (adrenocorticotropin, 39aa, Mol.wt. 4500).
- TSH (thyroid stimulating hormone, α-chain 89aa, β-chain 112aa, Mol.wt. 29,000).
- LH (luteinizing hormone, α-chain 89aa, β-chain 112aa, Mol.wt.29,000).
- FSH (follicle stimulating hormone, α-chain 89aa, β-chain 112aa Mol.wt. 29,000).
- TSH, LH and FSH have different β-chains which carry specificity but the α-chains of all these hormones are identical. Human chorionic gonadotropin (hCG) has α-chain (92aa) almost identical to α-chains of TSH, FSH and LH, β-chain (145aa) has 67% homology with β-chain of LH.
- Besides, GH and TSH, SS can inhibit secretion of a number of other hormones. Its long acting analog, octreotide is used for treatment of carcinoid tumors, glucagonoma, VIPomas and acromegaly.
- Besides TSH, TRH can stimulate secretion of other hormones (PRL, GH, gonadotropins). This is the basis of provocative tests used in diagnosis of PRL deficiency, in predicting recurrence of a GH secreting tumor after surgery and in diagnosis of gonadotropin secreting tumors.

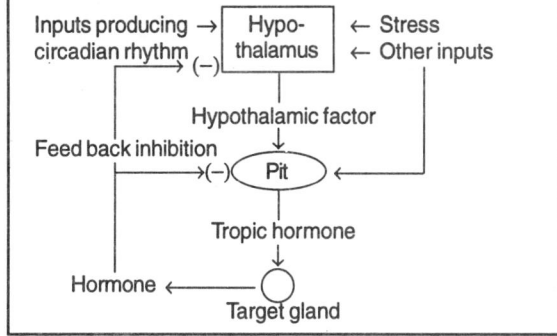

Fig. 13.2. The general plan of hypothalamic-pituitary-target gland axis.

- There are two negative feedback effects; the effect of pituitary hormone at hypothalamus (short loop) and the effect of target gland hormone at both pituitary and hypothalamus (long loop).
- For prolactin secretion there is only short loop inhibitory effect and in case of GH, IGF-1 produces the long loop inhibitory effect.
- Feedback effect of thyroid hormones at pituitary level plays a major role in precise regulation of TSH.
- Pituitary hormones are secreted in a pulsatile fashion and also show circadian rhythms.

Secretion is more in children and adolescents than adults and there is very little secretion after the age of 40 years. Release of growth hormone (GH) is under control of two hypothalamic factors, growth hormone releasing hormone (GHRH) and somatostatin (SS), latter being inhibitory. Stresses like exercise, trauma, excitement, increase GH secretion. Increased secretion also occurs during sleep. Certain metabolites in blood also affect GH secretion (hypoglycemia increases the secretion). Increased levels of certain amino acids (especially arginine) increase the secretion while free fatty acids reduce the release. Certain hormones also modify secretion of GH. Presence of T_3 on its nuclear receptors, in somatotrophs, increases transcription of GH gene. Some other factors are shown in Fig. 13.3.

GH actions

GH produces two types of actions in the body, the growth promoting and the metabolic actions. The metabolic actions are direct actions of GH. The

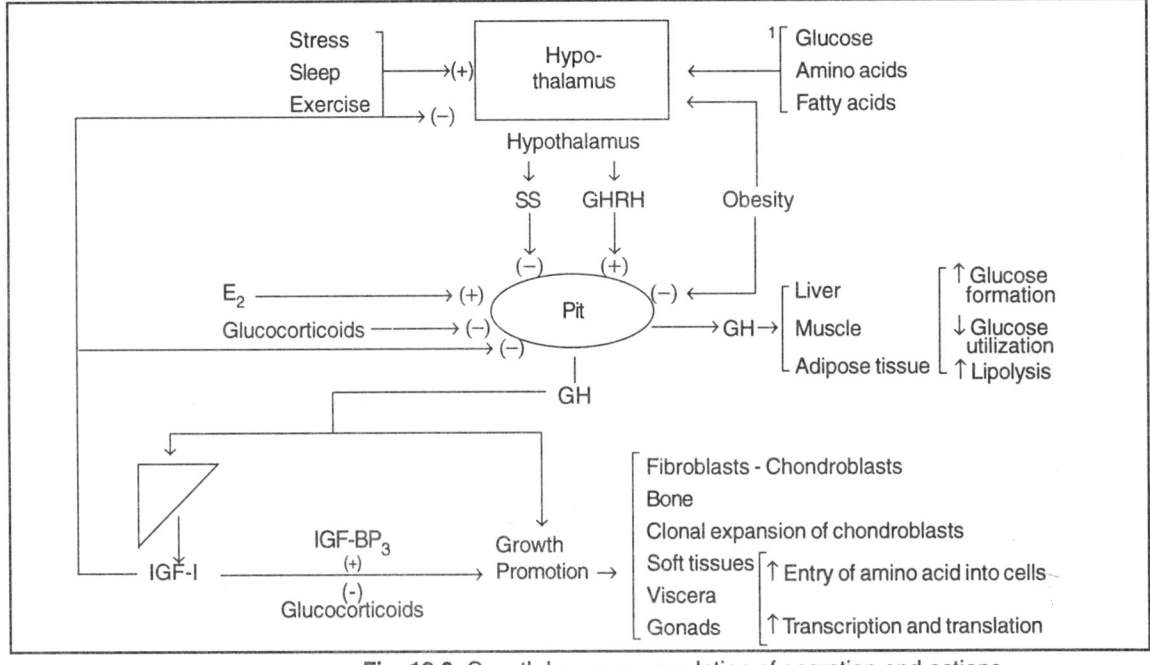

Fig. 13.3. Growth hormone; regulation of secretion and actions.

[1] Hypoglycemia, hyperaminoacidemia increase GH secretion; elevated fatty acid level and obesity reduces GH secretion.

- Clonidine (α-2 adrenergic agonist) and levodopa (dopaminergic agonist) stimulate formation of GHRH.

- Arginine inhibits SS secretion.

- Emotional stress (psychosocial deprivation) ↓ GH secretion.

- IGF-II level is low in hypopituitarism but not increased is acromegaly (unlike IGF-I).

growth promoting actions are produced indirectly, through insulin like growth factor 1 (IGF-I) which is released from liver, under the action of GH (Fig. 13.3). Unlike GH, level of IGF-I does not fluctuate in plasma. A very significant effect of growth promoting activity of GH (and IGF-I) is to increase proliferation of the cartilage cells of the epiphyseal plates of the long bones. Role of binding proteins for GH and IGF-I in plasma is not understood. GH binding proteins have structural homology with GH receptor and may tend to increase half life of GH in plasma, which ordinarily, is only about 30 minutes.

The role of IGF-I in regulation and actions of GH is well known (see above). IGF-II has 70% structural homology with IGF-I (both IGF-I and IGF-II have 50% homology with insulin), but its regulation by GH and the physiological roles are not well understood. GH is involved in regulation of IGF-II as its level is low (like IGF-I) in hypopituitarism but level is not increased in acromegaly (unlike IGF-I). Although role of IGF-II in growth, is not properly known (it may be more important in fetal growth), it is believed to be the cause of hypoglycemia produced by many tumors (large fibroma, sarcoma and adrenal cancer).

GH receptor is a single chain glycoprotein. GH first binds to a receptor in the plasma membrane. The second GH receptor is then associated. As the receptor dimer is formed, a membrane based tyrosine kinase is then associated with the receptor dimer. In this way modes of action of GH and insulin resemble, in a general way. IGF-I receptor resembles the insulin receptor which is a dimer composed of two glycoprotein subunits. Both have tyrosine kinase activities in their cytoplasmic domains. IGF-II receptor however, is a single chain structure. It has been postulated that IGF-II receptor someway, only indirectly helps IGF-II which actually acts through the IGF-I receptors to produce its actions.

Prolactin

It has 199 amino acids and is secreted by lactotrophs. Its secretion, from otherwise autonomously secreting lactotrophs (Fig. 13.4) is under inhibitory control of dopamine (from hypothalamus). TRH and AVP increase secretion from lactotrophs. Prolactin secretion also occurs in bursts (although peaks are less discrete), but half life of the hormone is sufficiently long and therefore a single fasting sample is good enough for studying the hormone levels. Prolactin secretion is also higher during sleep but is not associated with any sleep phase. In pregnancy prolactin secretion increases with progress of pregnancy and the high levels attained at term are maintained by suckling during lactation. Breast feeding sustains increased level of prolactin for about 3 months after delivery. Stress (as with most other pituitary hormones), increases release of prolactin. In primary hypothyroidism prolactin

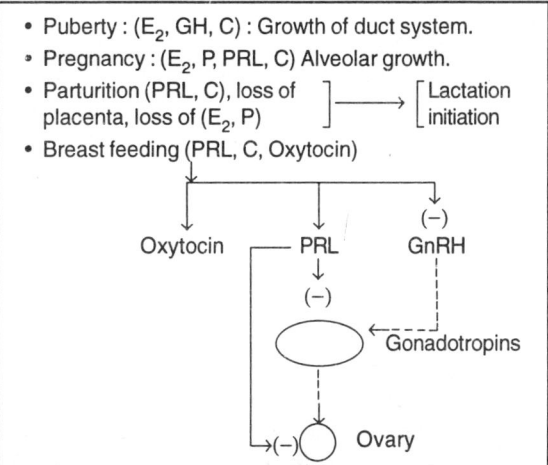

Fig. 13.5. Breast development, lactation and lactational amenorrhea.

- Additionally, insulin and thyroid hormones are also important in both breast development and lactation.
- C=Cortisol, E_2=Estrogens, P=Progesterone, PRL-Prolactin
- Note inhibitory action of breast feeding on ovary (lactation amenorrhea).

secretion is increased because of raised levels of TRH. Many drugs increase secretion of prolactin (see the Appendix A).

Fig. 13.5 explains role of prolactin in lactation and lactational amenorrhea.

Adrenocorticotropic hormone (ACTH)

It is a 39 amino acid polypeptide derived from a much larger precursor pro-opiomelanocortin (POMC). Before release, POMC is cleaved into different fragments including ACTH and β-lipotropin or β-LPH (the latter molecule contains sequences of β–MSH and β-endorphin in its structure). Three important controls of ACTH secretion are, stress, the CNS inputs, producing circadian rhythm and the feed back effect of cortisol. In humans, secretions of ACTH, and β-lipotropin (and β-endorphin) occur in parallel and there is no separate MSH hormone. Elevated levels of ACTH produce pigmentation since it contains the sequence of α-MSH (Fig. 13.6). The significance of secretion of β-endorphin is not properly understood. It belongs to a group of peptides (opioids) having morphine like properties (besides pituitary, these peptides have been

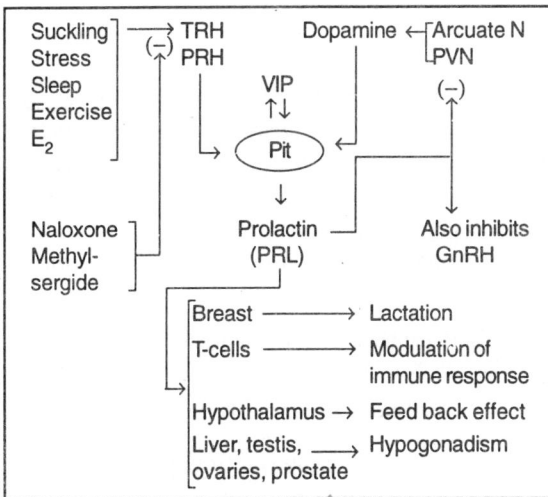

Fig. 13.4. Factors in regulation of PRL.

- VIP secreted by lactotrops acts in an autocrine fashion to regulate secretion of PRL by these cells. Basal level of secretion of PRL is controlled by a short loop formed by dopamine and PRL as shown.
- Suckling stress and other factors increase PRL secretion by release of some stimulatory factor from hypothalamus (TRH or PRH). Opioid and serotonin neurons may be involved in the stimulatory path.

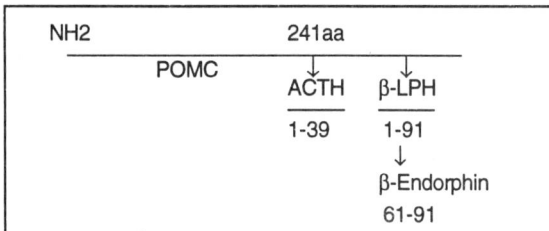

Fig. 13.6. Fragments of POMC secreted by anterior pituitary.

- POMC is cleaved differently in different tissues; in hypothalamus POMC serves as a precursor of β-endorphin (not ACTH).
- Tumor producing ACTH process POMC incompletely, leading to higher ratio of β-LPH to ACTH (pituitary cells release ACTH and β-LPH in equimolar amounts).
- 1-13 sequence in ACTH is that of α-MSH.

found in many other tissues including brain). These may have a role in inhibiting signals to brain, arising from severe stress or pain.

ACTH activates steroidogenesis in adrenal cortex and also exerts a trophic action, increasing the size of the cortical portion of the adrenal gland. As its extra adrenal actions, ACTH promotes lipolysis in adipose tissue and pigmentation of skin and mucous membrane. Also read about ACTH in Chapter 15.

Thyroid stimulating hormone (TSH)

It is a glycoprotein hormone composed of one α and one β subunit. Gonadotropins (FSH and LH) and hCG are also similarly composed of α and β subunits. In all the above hormones, α-subunits have quite similar structures but the β-subunits are unique for the different hormones. Basal level of TSH depends upon tonic release of TRH from hypothalamus. The most important control of TSH lies in feed back inhibitory influence of T_3 (and T_4) on pituitary and hypothalamus. Also see Chapter 14. TSH stimulates a number of metabolic reactions in thyroid follicular cells including synthesis and release of T_4 and T_3. Through its trophic action, it increases size and vascularity of the gland.

Gonadotropins

One hypothalamic factor, GnRH (Gonadotropin releasing hormone) is responsible for release of both FSH and LH from the same pituitary cells. Selective release of LH or FSH depends on pulse frequency of GnRH and selective feed back effects of gonadal factors. Before puberty, secretion of GnRH from hypothalamus is inhibited by small amounts of steroid hormones produced by the gonads. Puberty is brought about by reduced sensitivity of hypothalamic cells secreting GnRH, to the gonadal steroids. This starts pulsatile secretion of GnRH causing pulsatile secretion of FSH and LH. First, the pulsatile secretions occur during sleep and then during day also. The pulsatile release of FSH and LH occurs, both in males and females. The LH pulses are higher than FSH pulses (main reason being the much longer half life of FSH than that of LH). The FSH and LH pulses occur every 1.5 to 2.0h in males and every 1.0 to 5.0h in females. In men FSH and LH secretions are fairly parallel. In females, however, in reproductive period of life, it is not so. This is because of complex interaction of FSH and LH (regulating ovarian changes of menstrual cycle) with steroid and peptide ovarian factors (producing cyclic changes in endometrium), required in the normal menstrual cycle. The FSH and LH patterns in menstrual cycle are briefly:

- Both FSH and LH are higher in preovulatory than the luteal phase.
- There is apparent fall in FSH (LH level does not change much) as follicular phase progresses.
- At mid-cycle there is a larger LH surge and a smaller FSH surge.

After menopause gonadotropins continue to be secreted in pulsatile fashion. FSH levels, however, become higher than those seen earlier (due to lack of inhibin production by ovary). Because of continued availability of estradiol (from adrenals) the LH levels after menopause are not much changed. In men, in sixth decade, there is gradual increase in levels of FSH and LH.

Some general remarks regarding hormone studies in pituitary disorders

Laboratory plays a very important role in diagnosis of pituitary disorders. However, for proper inter-

Table 13.1. About modes of secretion of pituitary hormones and their use in diagnosis

Growth hormone:

Discontinuous secretory bursts; one or two major bursts at night shortly after going to sleep.

- Three blood samples collected at 20 minute intervals should be pooled for one assay (half life of hormone 20-50 minutes)
- In cases of GH excess, estimation of IGF-I (level is more uniform) provides a better method. For confirmation one should demonstrate reduced suppression (compared to normal) by hyperglycemia.
- In GH deficiency cases loss of secretory capacity should be demonstrated by at least two provocative stimuli since some patients with normal GH secretory capacity are not able to respond to any one stimulus at a given time.

Prolactin:

Compared to GH, secretory bursts of PRL occur more regularly and half life of PRL is also longer (> 50 minutes). Thus a single sample estimation maybe enough; although many workers prefer pooling of three samples as for GH.

- In clinical setting hyperprolactinemia is much more common than PRL deficiency; increased levels can be demonstrated in a single/pooled sample (as above). Deficiency (Sheehan's syndrome: pituitary infarction due to postpartum hemorrhage) may be revealed by PRL stimulation test using TRH or chlorpromazine (rise of < 200% suggests deficiency).

ACTH:

Secretion is pulsatile and there is peak before awakening and decline as the day passes (circadian rhythm). Half life of ACTH is ~ 5 minutes.

- Both primary and secondary adrenal insufficiencies are first revealed by cortisol levels and need confirmation by the stimulation test.
- Sample for cortisol estimation is collected in the morning (ACTH and cortisol levels are higher in the morning than evening); further confirmation of adrenal insufficiency requires study of cortisol following stimulation (ACTH stimulation test) and hyperfunctioning (Cushing's syndrome) is diagnosed by studying dexamethasone inhibition of cortisol.
- ACTH levels are studied in finding cause of Cushing's syndrome.

TSH:

Thyroid hormone levels have a sensitive feedback effect in regulation of TSH and unlike ACTH, stress and other factors acting via hypothalamus are relatively less effective. It is for this reason that primary hypothyroidism as well as primary hyperthyroidism are best evaluated in terms of TSH levels.

- The new immunoradiometric assay of TSH can differentiate between lower normal limit and the low TSH levels produced in primary hyperthyroidism.

LH/FSH:

In early puberty there is, mostly, nocturnal pulsatile secretion of these hormones, subsequently pulses of similar magnitude occur in sleep and waking hours. In the male FSH and LH releases are fairly concordant but their secretory pattern is more complex in the female as per stages of the menstrual cycle.

- Unlike other hormones, clinical assessments of gonadotropins and gonadal hormones are commonly used instead of their plasma levels. Thus regular predictable events in menstrual cycle imply normal pituitary gonadotropins as well as ovarian hormones. LH, FSH levels (and also testosterone levels in the male) are used to differentiate primary causes (gonadal) from secondary causes of hypogonadism. Prolactin levels are also important since this hormone influences both secretion and actions of gonadotropins.
- Pooled samples (as incase of GH) should be used for estimations of FSH and LH.

pretation of results one must be familiar with certain peculiarities of secretion of these hormones. Because of pulsatile nature, circadian rhythms (Table 13.1) and short half lives of pituitary hormones, single sample analysis, generally, does not give clinically useful information. For that reason, in certain cases (see under individual hormones), a number of samples collected at regular intervals are pooled for analysis. Alternatively, urinary excretion of the hormone (if available) may be studied as it does not show any pulsatile variations and gives a more representative level of bodily status of the hormone. In view of the circadian rhythms seen in secretion of these hormones the time of sample collection for any particular hormone has to be carefully selected and should be the same in all laboratories. Deficiencies of those pituitary hormones which act on their target endocrine glands, can be more easily recognized from plasma levels of the target gland secretions, than their own levels (Tables 13.1 and 13.2). The problems created by uncertainties of the plasma levels of pituitary hormones may also be overcome by the use of provocative tests (in deficiency states) and the suppression tests (in hypersecretion states). It should also be borne in mind that stress, obesity, depression, starvation, malnutrition and disorders like uremia and diabetes mellitus, all affect secretions of different pituitary hormones.

HYPOPITUITARISM

It is relatively a rare condition. It may be produced by tumors, granulomatous diseases (sarcoidosis, tuberculosis), trauma (surgery, head injury, radiation injury), infiltrative disorders (hemochromatosis, amyloidosis), vascular disorders (Sheehan's postpartum necrosis, due to severe postpartum hemorrhage accompanied by spasm of hypophyseal vessels) and as an autoimmune disorder. Single hormone deficiency cases are more often due to genetic failure of hypothalamic factors. Functional hypopituitarism is common. Anorexia nervosa, any severe stress or stress of any severe diseases may result in temporary GnRH deficiency. Psychosocial dwarfism is also an example of stress induced GH deficiency. A severe illness may be associated with euthyroid sick syndrome (deficiencies of T_4 or TSH and T_4).

Clinical features

In panhypopituitarism, the most common features in children relate to GH deficiency and in adults to lack of gonadotropins and ACTH. TSH deficiency and related symptoms are less common. In adults GH deficiency occurs but produces changes like decreased muscle mass, increased subcutaneous fat and wrinkling of face, as well as sleep and personality disorders. There may be increased mortality from cardiovascular disease in GH deficient adults. GnRH deficiency may produce amenorrhea and infertility in women and decreased libido in men,

due to low testosterone level. ACTH deficiency produces cortisol deficiency, which in turn causes, weight loss, fatigue, anorexia and abnormal response to stress (acute adrenal failure may be produced).

In many cases of pituitary deficiency, prolactin may be increased and contributes to hypogonadal features. However, in postpartum pituitary necrosis there is prolactin deficiency resulting in failure of lactation.

Hypothalamic pituitary axis is very sensitive to radiation damage and GH secretion is particularly affected. Metastatic cancer, sarcoidosis and non-anterior pituitary local tumors commonly cause diabetes inspidus along with damage to anterior pituitary secretory cells. Also see Table 13.2 in which some presentations of pituitary failure cases are given. A careful history is very important in such cases.

Investigations (Table 13.2)

The straight forward use of pituitary hormones in diagnosis of hypopituitarism has problems and more reliance is placed on levels of the target gland secretions. The dynamic tests also try to overcome these uncertainties associated with the plasma levels of pituitary hormones.

In children, growth failure is a common feature and requires evaluation of plasma GH level. The basal GH and IGF-I levels are less reliable in diagnosis of GH deficiency since, in a normal individual, plasma GH levels are undetectable during much of the time, during the day and for IGF-I, there is lot of overlap of plasma levels between normals and GH deficiency cases. The insulin stimulation test is most reliable in younger patients without heart disease or history of seizures (Table 13.3).

Prolactin should be estimated if hypogonadism is suspected. In most patients of hypopituitarism due to tumor (which may distort the stalk) or some disorders (sarcoidosis, cancer secondaries) which specifically, damage the stalk, prolactin levels will be raised. However, in panhypopituitarism resulting from pituitary infarction in peripartum period prolactin levels are reduced. Detection of increased levels offers no problem (see under hyperprolacti-

Table 13.2. Common endocrinal changes, presentation and diagnosis of hypopituitarism

GH deficiency:

- Growth failure is a common presenting complaint in children. It may be the earliest feature in case of an enlarging non-functional pituitary tumor or may be congenital. Isolated congenital deficiencies of only GH and gonadotropins are common.
- Mutation of a pituitary specific transcription factor (Pit-1) may, however, cause combined deficiency of GH, prolactin and TSH.
- A diabetic becoming GH deficient may present with increased insulin sensitivity.
- A child with emotional stress may present with functional GH deficiency (psychosocial dwarfism)

Gonadotropin deficiency:

- An adult woman may present with amenorrhea and infertility and an adult man with decreased libido as well as beard and body hair loss.
- A child may present with delay in puberty. Next to loss of GH, loss of gonadotropins occurs in case of an enlarging non-functional tumor.
- Severe stress, a major illness and anorexia nervosa are often associated with reversible gonadotropin deficiency.

Other presentations:

- An enlarging non-functional tumor of pituitary region produces late deficiency of ACTH followed by TSH deficiency.
- With primary defect in hypothalamus or high in pituitary stalk (secondaries from some tumor) diabetes insipidus is always present along with mild hyperprolactinemia and anterior pituitary deficiency
- Person may present with increased fatigue, decreased appetite, weight loss, fasting hypoglycemia and reduced resistance to stress (ACTH deficiency).
- Person may present with fatigue cold intolerance and puffy skin without goitre (TSH deficiency)
- In hypothalamic and stalk lesions patient may present with polyuria and increased thrist (AVP deficiency)
- An acromegalic may present with developing features of hypo-pituitarism.
- Patient may present with mass effects of the enlarging tumor (loss of partial or complete vision, headache, behaviour changes, sleep and appetite disturbances).
- Patient may fail to lactate postpartum (Sheehan's post partum necrosis).

Diagnosis:

Gonadotropin deficiency: In the presence of normal menstrual cycles in females, no hormone testing is required; in postmenopausal ladies normal gonadotropin levels suggest a deficiency state. In men if testosterone levels and spermatogenes are normal there is no need to measure gonadotropin levels. In suspicious cases, low estrogen (in women) and low testosterone (in men), without elevated gonadotropins imply hypopituitarism.

GH deficiency: Simple GH (levels are undetectable for most part of the day) and IFG-1 (there is overlap with normal range) alone are not of much use. The insulin stimulation test can be performed in the absence of heart disease or seizures. Alternatively, provocative tests using arginine or clonidine may be used.

ACTH deficiency: In chronic deficiency cases (>3 months old) the rapid ACTH stimulation test is a convenient and safe screening test and in pituitary/hyothalamic deficiency states of shorter duration use the insulin stimulation test (it can be used for both GH and ACTH deficiencies). If primary adrenal insufficiency can be ruled out, metyrapone test can also be used. In the presence of primary adrenal insufficiency it can precipitate acute adrenal crisis. The CRH test can also be used (at present there is limited experience with this test).

TSH deficiency: First measure T_4 (or free T_4 index). If the levels are low (and not if the levels are in mid normal range), TSH should be estimated. In central hypothyroidism TSH level should not be increased.

nemia) but most methods will not distinguish between normal and low levels. TRH or chlorpromazine stimulation test may be used.

To screen for ACTH deficiency produced by pituitary/hypothalamus disease, basal cortisol levels are often not helpful since basal cortisol secretion is not affected even in presence of extensive pituitary damage and the rapid ACTH stimulation test is used. Also read in Chapter 15.

The biochemical tests to evaluate status of gonadotropins are only undertaken if there is some evidence of hypogonadism. Thus gonadotropin levels are taken as normal in women with normal menses. In men if spermatogenesis and plasma testosterone levels are normal other investigations are not undertaken. Also read in Chapter 16 for more details.

To investigate TSH secretory deficiency of pituitary/hypothalamic disease, serum T_4 and free T_4 index are estimated. If these levels are in mid-normal range, TSH will be most likely normal. If these levels are low, serum TSH level is estimated for proper diagnosis. For further details see Chapter 14.

The dynamic tests useful in hypopituitarism

Because of pulsatile nature of pituitary hormone secretions the interpretation of a single hormone estimation often carries an element of uncertainty. Thus the dynamic tests are needed to confirm the diagnosis. Besides, these tests may reveal the degree of dysfunction/endocrine reserve and the level of disease (hypothalamus or pituitary). An appropriate stimulation test is used for specific deficiency. Thus for gonadotropin deficiency, GnRH or clomiphene stimulation test is used, for GH deficiency or for ACTH deficiency, insulin stimulation test is used (insulin acts by producing hypoglycemia). TRH stimulation test is used in diagnosis of thyroid disorders. Interpretation of different tests is discussed at different places in this and other chapters.

For total hypopituitarism the combined anterior pituitary function test can be done. In this test, first, the base line levels of glucose, GH, cortisol (or ACTH), LH (FSH may also be included), TSH and testosterone are established. Next, TRH, GnRH and insulin are given by a single injection. This is followed by estimation of levels of glucose, cortisol (or ACTH), TSH, LH (FSH), GH. Glucose level is estimated to know that adequate hypoglycemia has been produced.

Hypopituitary patient needs to be given replacement therapy throughout life, of corticosteroids, thyroid hormone and sex steroids. In a patient of adrenal insufficiency, thyroid hormone should only be given after glucocorticoid therapy has already been started, as patients of adrenal failure are extremely sensitive to thyroid hormone. In some, GH therapy is also recommended.

PITUITARY DWARFISM

GH deficiency is an uncommon cause of retarted growth. It may occur as part of pan-hypopituitarism or due to isolated deficiency of GH. The isolated GH deficiency is generally caused by hypothalamic genetic defect. Children with emotional deprivation have also hypothalamic cause of GH deficiency. In some cases there is only insensitivity to GH because of hepatic receptor defect with reduced formation of IGF-I (although there is no deficiency of GH). Before discussing diagnosis of growth retardation due to GH deficiency a brief account of normal growth process will be presented.

NORMAL GROWTH

Prenatal growth rate depends upon uterine blood flow, maternal height and other maternal influences. Correlation between body length at birth and the adult height is quite weak. Postnatal growth depends upon genetic, nutritional and hormonal factors. Height is a polygenic trait and there is a correlation between mean height of the parents and that of their child. Nutrition is the next important factor which affects growth of a child. Overall subnormal nutrition and selective deficiencies of vitamins and minerals impair growth.

A number of hormones are also intimately involved in growth. GH has a central role in growth from birth upto end of puberty. In total absence of growth hormone linear body growth rate is reduced to about less than half the normal growth rate. GH may act, directly, as well as through IGF-I and IGFBPs (especially IGFBP-3). Both IGF-I and IGFBP-3 are formed under the action of GH. IGFBP-3 binds IGF-I and increases its half life. Insulin also has growth promoting actions. These actions include promoting protein synthesis and cell division. Insulin has structural resemblance with IGF group of growth factors and some growth promoting actions of insulin may be because that it can attach to IGF-I receptors. Thyroid hormone is another hormone having very significant effect on growth. Effect of thyroid hormone on growth starts earlier than that of GH (it starts influencing growth even earlier than birth, in third trimester of pregnancy) and the effect is stronger than that of GH. Thyroid hormone has direct effect on cell metabolism; its deficiency also reduces secretion of GH in

Table 13.3. About GH estimation

Single blood sample:
• Random sample not useful; sample collected during night through an indwelling catheter may be useful in acromegalics.
Multiple samples pooled for analysis:
• Cumbersome; overlap between deficient and normals; more useful in acromegalics than cases of deficiency.
GH estimation in urine sample (needs a more sensitive method)**:**
• Gives better idea of the average plasma level; more useful in acromegalics. Sensitivity and specificity for deficiency cases can be increased by repeated testing.
IGF-1 level in plasma:
• No variations in plasma levels as seen for GH. Useful for screening purpose (especially acromegalics) if age related normal values are used and a reliable kit is available.
• IGF-1 and IGFBP-3 together used to screen GH deficient children as in most patients of GH deficiency these levels are also low.
Stimulation test using exercise of about 15 minutes (making the child breathless) (Normal: increase of >5 ng/mL)**:**
• It is often used as a screening test in deficiency states.
Stimulation test using insulin induced hypoglycemia (Normal: increase of >10 ng/mL)**:**
• It is a very good test but carries risk (of dangerous hypoglycemia) in children, heart patients and epileptics.
• Useful in diagnosis of deficiency states.
The clonidine stimulation test (Normal as for hypoglycemia)**:**
• An alternative to the insulin stimulation test.
The suppression test (estimation of GH during glucose tolerance test)**:**
• Not as good as the stimulation tests in deficiency states.
• Useful in diagnosis of acromegaly.

- All laboratories should have their own cut off values in these cases since different kits using different antibodies (monoclonal or polyclonal) and GH standards (pituitary derived or recombinant) will give different results.
- Simple GH estimation should be done after an overnight fast (except for estimation during sleep) since carbohydrate intake reduces GH secretion.
- False positives and false negatives are common in these tests
- Loran dwarfism cases have low IGF-1 and GHBP levels and elevated GH levels.

response to stimulation and further some effects of IGF-I require presence of thyroid hormone (eg; action of IGF-I on cartilage cells).

Androgens and estrogens are important for stimulation of growth at puberty. Much of growth spurt at puberty is because of these hormones. Androgens cause positive N-balance and have a direct role in growth of muscle, cartilage and growth and maturation of bone. Estrogens stimulate growth at low levels and inhibit growth at higher levels. Both estrogens and androgens cause closure of epiphyses, stopping the linear growth.

A number of other growth factors are known to participate in growth and repair of certain specific tissues. These include, nerve growth factor (NGF), epidermal growth factor (EGF), platelet derived growth factor (PDGF) and others. The exact physiological role of these growth factors in general process of growth remains to be found out.

When to investigate a child for growth retardation

If height of the child is three standard deviations (SD) below the mean height for age, he/she should be immediately investigated for the cause of retarded growth (for finding SD below the mean height, the mid parental height should be taken into account). If it is only 2 SD below the mean value, his growth rate should be determined. A growth rate consistently below normal also needs to be investigated.

DIAGNOSING A GROWTH DISORDER

Table 13.4 presents important causes of growth

retardation. Most common cause is constitutional delay in growth. Diagnosis of this condition is by exclusion.

Important points in history are, weight and gestational age at birth and development during early infancy. One should look for presence of some systemic disease. Family history of growth, stature and puberty of parents and first and second degree relatives should also be obtained. In physical examination body proportions should be determined. If limbs are short relative to the trunk, it may suggest long standing hypothyroidism or one of the chondrodystrophies. Examine height to weight ratio. If height is low and child is also underweight for height, the cause may be malnutrition or some systemic disease. A child who is short but overweight might be suffering from Cushing's syndrome, hypothyroidism or GH deficiency. If bone age is delayed the child should be investigated for constitutional delayed development, GH and thyroid hormone deficiencies. One should also look for certain special physical features which may suggest the cause (Table 13.4). It is also very important to have an idea of psychosocial environment of the child. Important investigations are also listed in Table 13.4.

Assessment of GH secretion

Because of pulsatile secretion of GH along with its very short half life and also because secretion is less during the day, analysis of a single sample collected during the day has very little clinical significance. Result of a single sample collected during the night, 1h after going to sleep, is more useful, particularly, a high level pointing against the deficiency of GH. For other alternatives, see Table 13.4. When a stimulation test is required, in most of the cases, rise of GH after an exercise of 15 minutes is enough. A proper provocative test is only occasionally required. The best stimulation test uses insulin induced hypoglycemia. However, because of the dangers of the test some centres use clonidine induced stimulation.

Incidence of GH deficiency may be 1 in 10,000 children and in about half, the deficiency is idiopathic (due to hypothalamic defect) and in the other half secondary to tumors and other causes. Recombinant GH is used for treatment. Children with deficiencies of IGF-I, IGFBP-3 and GHBR (without GH deficiency) also benefit from the treatment. Treatment also helps children with short stature due to chronic renal disease and gonadal dysgenesis.

Disease of hypothalamus

Tumors are the most common cause of hypothalamic disorders. Craniopharyngiomas arise from remnants of Rathke's pouch. Most of these are suprasellar (about 15% are intrasellar). Other tumors are glioma of optic nerve, germinoma, pinealoma (may be a germinoma), teratoma, meningioma, hamartoma (a fetal rest growth), a pituitary tumor (may grow into hypothalamus) and metastatic cancer. Common inflammatory diseases are tuberculosis and encephalitis. Granulomas, sarcoidosis and histiocytosis X also occur. Trauma to base of skull also can cause hypothalamic dysfunction. Genetic or idiopathic deficiencies of releasing hormones also occur. Hypothalamic disorders cause sexual abnormalities (precocious puberty, hypogonadism) most frequently and also may produce DI or SIADH and hypopituitarism (partial or complete). Pineal tumors may produce sexual precocity in boys and delayed puberty in girls.

PITUITARY TUMORS (Appendix 13.1)

These may be functional (secrete hormones) or non-functional. Most common tumor in adults is prolactin secreting adenoma and in children, craniopharyngioma (arising from remnants of pouch of Rathke). Tumors producing GH and ACTH also occur but other functional tumors are very rare. Tumors may be small (microadenoma) or large (macroadenoma). Macroadenomas may destroy the surrounding normal glandular tissue and produce deficiency of some pituitary hormones. The large tumors may produce pressure feature by pressing on surrounding structures. If a tumor happens to destroy/distort the pituitary stalk, it may produce disconnection hyperprolactinemia by interfering with transport of dopamine from hypothalamus to pituitary. In this way, besides adenomas of lactotrophs (prolactinomas), many other tumors of

Table 13.4. Important causes of retarded/delayed growth

Hormonal disorders:
- GH deficiency (short stature obvious at 1-2 years of age, obesity, high pitched voice); infant normal at birth; nutrition for height normal; bone age reduced. Partial GH deficiency is responsible for some forms of constitutional short stature with delayed onset of adolescence.
- Thyroid hormone deficiency (dry skin, coarse hair, large tongue peculiar facies); constipation; delayed mile stones; epiphysial dysgenesis.
- Cushing's syndrome (central obesity, striae, hypertension)
- Pseudohypoparathyroidism (moon facies, obesity, short metacarpals, mental retardation)

Genetic short stature:
- Genetic cause; height comes closer to mean after correction for mid parental height.
- Family history about growth.

Primordial dwarfism (small for age babies due to proportionate intrauterine growth retardation):
- There is no family history
- History of baby weight at birth.
- Bone age, age at onset of puberty and yearly growth rate are normal.
  (Read under SGA infants in chapter 18).

Constitutional delayed development[1]:
- The most common cause
- Delayed growth and delayed onset of puberty; bone age is also correspondingly delayed.
- Final attained growth is normal (although delayed); in a subgroup final height is moderately reduced (constitutional short stature).
- A similar history in parents

Psychosocial deprivation
Malnutrition/malabsorption/chronic diseases:
- Protein energy malnutrition
- Celiac disease and other malabsorption disorders including cystic fibrosis and inflammatory bowel disease.
- Chronic renal disease (anorexia, uremic toxins and secondary hormonal changes may impair growth).
- Chronic cardiac/respiratory diseases (hypoxemia may be the cause of impaired growth).
- Hematological disorders including sickle cell disease and thalassemia (hypoxemia may be the cause of impaired growth)
- Diabetes mellitus (being a catabolic state)

Conditions in which impaired growth is not the main concern:
- Bone cartilage dysplasia (abnormal proportions, macrocephaly)
- Mucopolysaccharidosis(organomegaly, corneal clouding, joint/bone problems).
- Chromosomal disorders (unexplained short stature in a female with features of gonadal dysgenesis along with webbed neck, sheild chest)

Other rare cause
- Renal tubular acidosis, vitamin D resistant rickets, many in born errors.

---

[1] Incidence of delayed puberty in these patients is highly variable in different countries because of great variations of other factors which independently influence age of onset of puberty.
- History and family history is important in delayed development and constitutional growth delay.
- Enquiry about psychosocial enviornment is important.
- Nutritional history, history of diarrheal and infective episodes.
- Knowledge about baby at birth.
- The bone age (if delayed, investigate for constitutional delayed development, GH and thyroid hormone deficiencies).
- Special physical features including body proportions.
- *Investigations:* Hb and blood count (malnutrition, hematological disorders), blood urea, kidney ability to acidify urine (chronic renal disease, RTA), ESR (chronic infections, inflammatory bowel syndrome, connective tissue disease), serum calcium, phosphate and alkaline phosphatase (pseudohypoparathyroidism, vitamin D resistant rickets), X-ray examination of hand/wrist bones for skeletal maturity and of pituitary fossa, chromosomal karyotyping (gonadal dysgenesis or other disorders).
- Specialized investigations for GH deficiency/GH insensitivity, hypothyroidism, Cushing's syndrome and pseudohypoparathyroidism.

hypothalamus/pituitary area can produce hyper-prolactinemia.

If posterior pituitary is involved (generally, a site of tumor secondaries), there will be AVP deficiency. However, damage confined to posterior pituitary alone may not produce DI; the suprasellar extension of the tumor must be able to destroy the AVP producing cells (as some fibres end in anterior pituitary). Further AVP deficiency in the presence of ACTH deficiency does not produce DI since cortisol is needed for proper formation of GFR and urine. If a patient has deficiencies of both AVP and ACTH, DI will only develop when glucocorticoid replacement therapy is started.

Pressure features produced by large tumors are visual disturbances, by pressure on optic chiasma/optic tract; headache, by pressure on dura and nerve palsies due to involvement of nerves in cavernous sinus. If the tumor extends into hypothalamus, disturbances of sleep, thirst, appetite and temperature regulation may appear.

Diagnosis

Diagnosis is based on clinical presentation, biochemical and other investigations. Lateral X-ray of skull reveals the size of sella. CT-scan or MRI defines structures in and around sella (MRI is better). In case of a functional tumor, increased level of a particular hormone in serum can be demonstrated. Deficiencies of certain pituitary hormones may be produced in case of macroadenomas or other large tumors/secondary deposits.

Empty sella syndrome

Radiological evidence of an enlarged sella may be produced by a pituitary growth or empty sella syndrome. In the latter condition shape of the sella is not distorted as happens in case of a tumor (CT/MRI may be done to rule out tumor in any case of enlarged sella). Empty sella syndrome is produced by herniation of suprasellar subarachnoid space into sella, which gets uniformly enlarged. It is more common in middle aged, obese women with hypertension and headache. Some patients have associated hyperprolactinemia with associated problems for which surveillance may be needed.

HYPERSECRETION OF PITUITARY HORMONES

Patients of increased secretions of prolactin or growth hormone occur more commonly than those of other pituitary hormones (Appendix 13.1). Cushing's disease (hypersecretion of ACTH) is discussed in the Chapter 15.

Hyperprolactinemia

Increased serum prolactin levels can be caused by a prolactinoma (micro or macro adenoma of lactotrophs) or a large non-functional pituitary tumor interfering in delivery of dopamine from hypothalamus to anterior pituitary (disconnection hyperprolcatinemia). Relatively smaller increase in prolactin levels is produced by a number of drugs or physiological states like pregnancy, lactation and others (Table 13.5). High levels of prolactin result in menstrual disorders and infertility in females and infertility (and loss of libido) in males. Galactorrhea can also occur, more commonly, in females.

Prolactin secretion occurs in bursts (like other pituitary hormones), but half life of the hormone is sufficiently long. Thus a single sample is good enough for studying the hormone level. The sample should be taken without undue stress to the patient. In interpretation of the reported value, it should be kept in mind that a number of drugs, pregnancy (high estrogen level), lactation, sleep, exercise, stress, hypoglycemia and dietary protein, increase prolactin secretion. In hypothyroidism increased prolactin secretion is mediated through increased level of TRH.

Two other groups of investigations become important in case a tumor is responsible for high level of prolactin. Firstly, the investigations to establish deficiency of other pituitary hormones (discussed under hypopituitarism); secondly, the investigations to define the exact location of the tumor (Table 13.6). Bromocriptine is used to treat hyperprolactinemia. In adenomas, it not only reduces secretion of prolactin but also causes shrinkage of tumor, for easy resection, if required.

Excess GH secretion

It is, mostly, caused by a pituitary tumor secreting

Table 13.5. Important conditions increasing prolactin secretion

Physiological causes:

- Pregnancy leads to 8-20 times increase in PRL secretion by delivery which returns to normal in 2-4 weeks post partum.
- Sukling also increases PRL secretion to sustain lactation in postpartum period.
- PRL levels are also high in neonates.
- Sharp increase occurs during sleep; levels are higher in the morning than in the afternoon.
- Some increase (<30 ng/mL) is produced by stress (hypoglycemia, exercise)

Tumors and hypothalamic causes:

- Large tumors (not secreting PRL) cause hyperprolactinemia (up to 50-100 ng/mL) by stalk distortion. A similar increase may also be produced by hypothalamic disorders (interfere in dopamine formation). These disorders include sarcoidosis, eosinophilic granuloma, tuberculosis, glioma, craniopharyngioma and others. Prolactinomas (PRL secreting pituitary tumors) secrete PRL according to their size (>100 ng/mL; commonly >150 ng/mL). In diagnosis of prolactinomas elevated PRL level should be demonstrated in repeated samples collected at the same time every day.
- Idiopathic cases of hyperprolactinemia probably represent early cases of microadenomas nor detected by CT.

Endocrine causes:

- Hypothyroidism (and drugs) often cause increase PRL levels in the same range as produced by stalk distortion. *Hypothyroidism is an important cause of elevated PRL levels (mediated by elevated TRH levels).*

Drugs:

- A large number of drugs (neuroleptics, dopamine antagonists, opiates, oral contraceptives, isoniazid and others) increase serum PRL levels. Thus drugs should be discontinued for about 2 weeks prior to collection of a sample for PRL estimation.

Other causes:

- These include liver disease (reduced clearance), chronic renal failure, neurogenic causes (spinal cord and chest wall lesions, seizures)

- Important causes of hyperprolactinemia resulting in clinical syndromes include tumors, hypothyroidism, hypothalamic disorders and drugs. Rest of the causes are important to take note of while investigating clinical disorders produced by hyperprolactinemia.

Table 13.6. Imaging and other investigations in hyperprolactinemia and other pituitary hormone hypersecretions

- Patients with unexplained hyperprolactinemia should undergo X-ray study.
- If there is some abnormality ($\uparrow$ in size of sella, wall erosion, calcification in sellar region), CT or MRI is done (MRI has better tissue contrast to define relation to surrounding structures; CT is better for detecting bone erosion, calcification).
- Macroadenomas and most microadenomas are well delineated on MRI. Also suprasellar tumors are differentiated from intrasellar ones.
- However 20% of normal persons show pituitary abnormalities (microadenomas, cysts, infarcts) on MRI/ contrast enhanced CT.
- In cases with modest elevation of PRL (20-100 ng/mL) the main aim of MRI is to exclude large clinically significant lesions, actual detection of a microadenoma (PRL secreting) is less important as management is non-surgical.
- In case of Cushing's disease localization of adenoma (to decide surgical approach) is done by estimating ACTH in samples collected by catheterization of inferior petrosal sinus on both sides.
- In case of acromegaly enlarged paranasal sinuses (on X-ray) and other bony changes supplement diagnosis.

- An enlarging tumor can produce clinical effects by pressure on surrounding structures; optic tract/chiasma (defects in visual fields), meninges (headache), hypothalamus (appetite/sleep disturbances), and cranial nerves (III, IV, V, VI).

GH. If it develops in childhood, before closure of epiphyses, there will be excessive linear growth of long bones resulting in excessive height and the condition is called gigantism. If the condition develops after the fusion of epiphyses, increase in height is not possible. The condition is called acromegaly. Features common to the two conditions are listed in Table 13.7. As the tumor enlarges, features may develop from deficiency of other pituitary hormones and also from pressure on surrounding structures.

There may also be increased secretion of prolactin, if tumor is large. Also in cases of MEN 1 syndrome study of other hormones (insulin, PTH) may become relevant.

Table 13.7. Some clinical and biochemical manifestations of acromegaly.

- Increased cortical thickening of bones of hands and feet (along with added soft tissue overgrowth produces large hands and feet), also there is increased growth of facial bones and vertebral bodies. Often these may not be the presenting complaints.
- Neurological and musculoskeletal symptoms (muscle weakness, paresthesias, osteoarthritis).
- Low renin, aldosterone, hypertension (due to expanded plasma volume), cardiac enlargement may be important in reducing life expectancy.
- Increased tissue tags may increase risk for carcinoma of colon.
- Goitre occurs in about 40% of patients (IGF-1 stimulated growth of thyroid cells).
- Glucose tolerance is impaired in most patients; mild diabetes (insulin resistance) is found in about 15% patients.
- Hyperprolactinemia occurs in about 50% of patients and may produce hypogonadism (in these patients, the tumor cells produce both GH and PRL).
- Patient feels weak and tired with increased BMR and excessive sweating.
- Women may show adrenal virilism with increased excretion of 17-ketosteroids in urine.
- There is increased α-1-hydroxylase activity which causes hyperphosphatemia, hypercalciuria and renal stones.
- Less commonly other endocrinopathies may also coexist (as part of MEN-syndromes).

- Acromegaly may result from increased GH levels due to pituitary adenoma, hyperplasia or carcinoma. There may be ectopic pituitary tissue in sphenoid or parapharyngeal sinus or there may be ectopic formation of GH (tumors of pancreas, lung, ovary, breast).
- The disorder can also result from excess production of GHRH (hamartoma, ganglioneuroma) or from an ectopic source (carcinoids, pancreatic islet cell tumor, small cell carcinoma of lung, pheochromocytoma, adrenal adenoma).

Table 13.8. The different molecular forms of GR and prolactin.

Growth hormone:

191 aa single peptide (22,000 mol. wt.)	The main form in circulation
Dimeric and polymeric forms 20,000 mol.wt. form	- These forms are less active and less immunogenic.
GH circulating with GH binding protein (GHBP)	- Different Abs. used in different kits react differently with different forms.
	- Binding of GH with GHBP increases its half life.

Prolactin:

198 aa (23,000 mol. wt.)	The main form in circulation
Dimer, polymer and protein bound forms	- Normally present in small amount.
	- Larger amounts present in adenomas.
	- These forms have reduced activity and immunogenicity.

- Normal GHBP has structure like that of GH receptor and increases half life of GH in circulation. In a GH resistant dwarfism abnormal protein (and receptor) is present.

Diagnosis

Rough face and large hands are important suggestive features, provided it can be ascertained that these have developed only, recently. Lateral X-ray skull often (in 90% of acromegalics) shows enlargement of pituitary fossa. Other tests may also be helpful (Table 13.3). If level of GH is not appropriately high in a single sample (see under "pituitary dwarfism"), estimation of IGF1, if available, should be done. Alternatively, estimation of GH in a urine sample may help to solve the problem.

Trans-sphenoidal surgery is done to remove a small adenoma and leads to cure. In case of a large tumor, partial resection is done to remove the pressure effects. This is followed by radiotherapy. Medical treatment using a long acting analog of somatostatin is also used.

GH estimation

There are several molecular forms of GH in circulation 22 kD (190 aa), 20 kDa and other monomers, the oligomeric and protein bound forms (Table 13.8). The 22 kDa form has most biological properties of GH and is the main hormone form in circulation (although not always). The immunological methods use antibodies against 22 kDa form. These methods measure total hormone (22 kDa monomer, oligomers and protein bound). About 45% is protein bound. Although, GH antibodies have much greater affinity for GH than growth hormone binding proteins (GHBPs), in some assay procedures GHBPs produce interference. The sandwich technique (has greater sensitivity and specificity) is used, these days, in the estimation procedure.

POSTERIOR PITUITARY HORMONES

AVP and oxytocin are synthesized in hypothalamus and released in posterior pituitary. Both are nona-peptides with quite similar structures. AVP is mostly synthesized in supraoptic nuclei and oxytocin, mostly, in paraventricular nuclei. Each hormone is secreted as a large precursor molecule

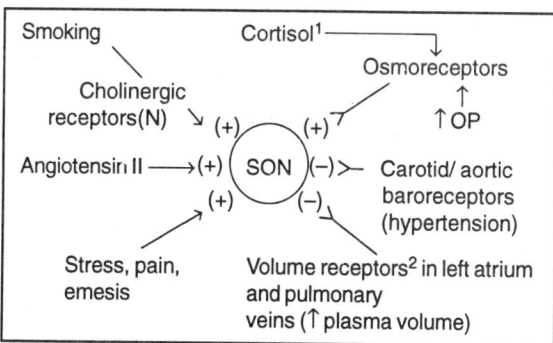

Fig. 13.7. Regulation of AVP release.

---

[1] Cortisol increases osmotic threshold for AVP release and also acts directly on renal tubules to decrease water permeability.

[2] This effect could also be mediated by release of atrial natriuretic peptide (ANP) released from atrial myocytes when there is increased atrial pressure.

- Osmotic factors ordinarily predominate and maintain plasma osmolality within a narrow range. Large changes in volume (in hemorrhage) may first blunt and then overpower osmotic influence (when the two have opposite effect on AVP release).

which contains both the hormone and its carrier protein (neurophysin). The granules containing the large precursor molecules are released in posterior pituitary after proteolytic cleavage resulting in release of separated hormones. Physiological action of AVP is antidiuresis (reduced urine formation) although, in pharmacological amounts it has vasopressor action on peripheral vessels. The regulatory signals for AVP arise from changes in plasma volume and osmotic pressure (Fig. 13.7).

Oxytocin causes contraction of myoepithelial cells around milk ducts. But its name is derived from its action of hastening the process of labour by causing myometrial contraction. Oxytocin appears to have a role in final expulsion of fetus and placenta. The stimulatory impulses for oxytocin arise from suckling and stretching of the birth canal.

SIADH (syndrome of inappropriate antidiuretic hormone secretion)

Disturbances of water metabolism in disorders of AVP excess and deficiency, clinically, present as SIADH and diabetes insipidus, respectively. SIADH is most commonly caused by ectopic formation of AVP from certain malignant tumors especially small cell carcinoma of the lung. Other causes are pulmonary disorders (tuberculosis, empyema), central nervous system disorders (trauma, cerebrovascular accidents, infections) and certain drugs (see the Appendix A).

There is hyponatremia and urine is concentrated (osmolality >300 mmol/kg). Clinical features of hyponatremia are mentioned in chapter 2. SIADH should be suspected in a patient with hyponatremia, passing concentrated urine (in the presence of appropriate clinical findings and history of the case), in the absence of edema, orthostatic hypotension and features of dehydration. It is one of the causes in differential diagnosis of hyponatremia with near normal volumes (see Chapter 2). Often diagnosis is not difficult. Table 13.10 outline a useful approach in less clear cases.

Treatment of SIADH lies in treatment of the cause. However, symptomatic hyponatremia is treated with water restriction (800 to 1000 mL/d).

In more severe cases hypertonic NaCl (3%) may be infused in small amount (200 mL) to gradually increase plasma sodium level. For avoiding fluid overload a loop diuretic may be used along with. For long term management demelocycline can be used as it produces a reversible type of DI. AVP antagonists are under development.

Table 13.9. The random studies in diagnosis of diabetes insipidus

- If daily excretion of urine is more than 6L and osmolality is less than 200 (sp.gr. of about 1.005), the patient is quite likely to be suffering from DI.
- In DI there is water intake following water loss, therefore plasma osmolality is increased (>295 mosmol/kg); there is hypernatremia. In psychogenic water intake, water loss follows water intake and therefore, there is hyponatremia and serum osmolality is reduced (<280 mosmol/kg).
- Large volume of dilute urine with plasma osmolality low normal or slightly reduced means psychogenic polydypsia; but with plasma osmolality increased means DI.

Table 13.10. Diagnosing SIADH as a cause of hyponatremia

- There are no hypovolemic features (orthostatic hypotension, tachycardia, prerenal azotemia), no history of recent diuretic therapy and it is not a case of edema or ascites.
- There is no hyperlipidemia, plasma osmolality is not increased (to rule out pseudohyponatremia) and urine osmolality is not less than 200 mosmol/kg (to rule out psychogenic polydipsia).
- Thyroid/adrenal insufficiencies ruled out.
- No cause of mildly increased AVP secretion (pain, stress, nausea, hypotension, drugs).
- Sick cell syndrome ruled out.
- Water excretion test: Patient is given water (20 mL/kg body wt.) to drink in 10 to 20 min. In SIADH <80% of the water load is excreted in urine in next 5h. Also the lowest urine osmolality attained is >100 mosmol/kg.
  - This test should not be done unless serum Na$^+$ is >125 mmol/L.
  - Main aim of the test is to differentiate cases of low set osmoreceptor threshold, who excrete water load like normals.

- Two basic features of SIADH patients are hyponatremia and urine osmolality >300 mmol/kg.
- AVP estimation is seldom required in diagnosis of SIADH. However, AVP is often unmeasurable in hyponatremic states except in SIADH in which it remains detectable even after water load.

Diabetes insipidus (DI)

In diabetes insipidus (DI), there is reduced formation of AVP (neurogenic DI) or there is impaired renal response to AVP (nephrogenic DI). Neurogenic DI is caused (compare with causes of SIADH) by hypothalamic/pituitary neoplasms including metastatic tumors, infiltrative and granulomatous (sarcoidosis) disorders. Neurogenic DI may also result from severe head trauma or surgery in this region. Other causes are cerebrovascular accidents and infections. Some drugs also reduce AVP secretion by the AVP secreting cells (see the Appendix A).

Idiopathic DI (when no cause is found) usually starts in childhood and in majority of cases, it is not accompanied by features of pituitary deficiency. Inherited cases are rare (autosomal recessive disorder with DI, diabetes mellitus, optic atrophy and deafness). DI may appear during pregnancy and last upto a few days after delivery; or it may appear as a part of Sheehan's syndrome after parturition. It may manifest only after start of cortisol therapy.

Some children suffering from nocturnal enuresis may have AVP deficiency and benefit from AVP supplementation. In these children the first morning urine sample shows a specific gravity of less than 1.015.

Nephrogenic DI may be congenital and familial or acquired. The acquired cases may result from renal disorders (severe chronic renal disease, after obstructive uropathy, unilateral renal artery stenosis, after renal transplantation and after acute tubular necrosis) and from certain systemic disorders (multiple myeloma, amyloidosis, sickle cell disease, Sjogren syndrome). Nephrogenic DI may also be drug induced (see the Appendix A) or caused by chronic hypercalcemia and hypokalemia.

Clinical features and diagnosis

Patient suffers from polyuria, severe thirst and polydipsia. There is preference for cold water. Generally, 24h urine volume is more than 6L and specific gravity less than 1.006. Restriction of fluids causes features of severe dehydration, fever, psychic disturbances, hypotension, prostration and death.

The first aim in diagnosis of DI is to rule out

causes of non-hypotonic diuresis (diabetes mellitus, chronic renal disease, including chronic pyelonephritis and diuretic induced diuresis). In all these cases polyuria is not hypotonic (urine osmolality is >300 mmol/kg). Next one should find out whether or not hypotonic polyuria is because of nephrogenic DI. There is not much difficulty in acquired cases. History may help certain cases. Examples are obstructive uropathy, acute tubular necrosis. Certain simple tests will recognize cases like hypokalemia, hypercalcemia, multiple myeloma and sickle cell disease. Some chronic kidney diseases also produce hypotonic polyuria (others cause polyuria because of salt wasting). Serum creatinine levels will recognize chronic renal failure cases.

Problem may arise in diagnosis of primary and some secondary cases of nephrogenic DI. Certain special tests may be required in differentiating certain cases of nephrogenic DI from neurogenic DI and psychogenic polydipsia (see below).

Finally, if diagnosis is neurogenic DI, its cause should be established (diagnosis of idiopathic neurogenic DI is by exclusion). Search should be made for some lesion (tumor, infiltration, vascular lesion) in the region of hypothalamus and pituitary. Presence of clinical or radiological of evidence hyperprolactinemia/hypopituitarism should further stimulate to pin point the cause.

For differentiating between neurogenic DI, nephrogenic DI and psychogenic polydipsia consult Tables 13.9 and 13.11. A simple approach in a difficult case is as under:

i) Test AVP response in a hydrated patient with 5U AVP. No change in urine osmolality indicates nephrogenic DI while doubling of urine osmolality occurs in central DI and psychogenic polydipsia.

ii) Water deprivation test should be done as per procedure outlined in Table 13.11. It should however, be remembered that many disorders interfere in interpretation of this test eg; kidney/urinary disorders, adrenal insufficiency, diabetes mellitus and thyroid disorders. Many patients of partial DI and those of psychogenic polydipsia of long duration may not be easily differentiated as the water

Table 13.11. The dehydration test[1] in diagnosis of DI.

- No fluids and hourly urine collection, till urine osmolality rise is stable (<30 mmol/kg/h) for 3 consecutive hours.
- Draw blood sample to confirm that serum osmolality is >288 mmol/kg (prerequisite for the next step).
- Administer 5 units aqueous AVP subcutaneously.
- Collect urine and measure osmolality after 1h of AVP dose.
- Interpretation
  - In normals urinary osmolality does not rise more than 9% after AVP injection, whatever, the maximum urinary osmolality achieved (it is > that of plasma) during the earlier period of dehydration.
  - In central DI, after AVP administration rise is >100% (at least >9%) in complete DI and >9-67% (at least >9%) in partial cases. Earlier dehydration may be completely ineffective (complete DI) or partially effective in increasing urine osmolality.
  - In nephrogenic DI, or those having polyuria due to renal disease or hypokalemia, there is very little increase of osmolality during dehydration and no further rise (or <9% after AVP injection.
  - In psychogenic polydipsia cases often the required osmolality of >288 mosmol/kg is reached after a prolonged (> usual 6-12h) period of dehydration and AVP injection increases urine osmolality >9% (unlike nephrogenic DI). These cases may be difficult to differentiate from partial cases of DI unless retested after a period of high salt and low water intake.

[1] For this test patient should not be already dehydrated (plasma osmolality should be <295 mosmol/kg). During the test, to avoid severe hypotension from excessive dehydration the test is terminated if weight loss exceeds 3 kg. Before AVP injection plasma osmolality should be >288 mosmol/kg as only then nephrogenic DI needs to be considered for diagnosis (AVP secretion occurs only above plasma osmolality of 285 mosmol/kg).
- In an alternative test to distinguish between partial central DI and psychogenic polydipsia, instead of water deprivation, saline infusion is used to increase plasma osmolality. If correctly performed and tolerated by the patient, is superior to the water deprivation test. It is, however, seldom used for patients. Study of relationship between plasma and urine osmolalities in nomograms in dehydration/saline infusion test is more useful in diagnosing partial cases of DI.
- ADH levels are rarely required in differential diagnosis. Study of relationship between plasma osmolality and ADH levels during dehydration/saline infusion test (in a nomogram) can however be used for the purpose.

deprivation test may give intermediate values in both disorders (the polydipsia cases poorly respond to the test, due to suppression of AVP release by chronic water intake and washing out of medullary gradient due to chronic polyuria). Such patients should be retested after a period of high sodium and low water intake to normalize medullary hypertonicity.

Patients of DI are treated with desmopressin which can be used intranasaly, subcutaneously or intravenously. For treatment of nephrogenic DI, thiazide diuretics may be used along with salt restriction. The regimen produces sodium depletion leading to low GFR and increased fluid reabsorption in proximal tubules resulting in reduced delivery of Na^+ to the later nephron segments, thereby reducing capacity to dilute urine. In psychogenic polydipsia (or primary polydipsia) the causative factor should be treated. Also read Case history 13.4.

Appendix 13.1. Pituitary tumors and their clinical presentations

Classification is based on specific immunochemical staining characteristics of cells; terms chromophils/chromophobes have been avoided.

Prolactinomas:

- These tumors constitute about 30% of all pituitary tumors (pituitary tumors make up about 10% of all intracranial tumors). Microadenomas (size <10 mm) are more common than macroadenoma (size >10 mm); microadenomas occur, predominantly in women and macroadenomas in men.
- These tumors secrete PRL according to their size and those presenting in women with irregular menses, amenorrhea and galactorrhea are easily diagnosed, early.
- Amenorrhea caused by hyperprolactinemia is most commonly associated with low or absent estrogen but some times it may be associated with chronic anovulation with estrogen present.
- Increased PRL may be associated with low LH and FSH (in both sexes) producing hypogonadotropic hypogonadism.
- Although sexual dysfunction occurs in most men with prolactinomas but only in 15% of these it occurs as the presenting complaint.

Tumors producing GH:

These tumors are generally macroadenomas and produce acromegaly.

Tumors producing glycoprotein hormones/their fragments:

Most of these tumors are non-functional, although these show positive reaction in immunochemical staining; being non-functional the tumors often attain a large size producing mass effects.

- TSH functional tumors are very rare.
- Functional FSH/LH secreting tumors may be diagnosed in men with reduced libido, low testosterone, normal or elevated PRL, variable FSH and low or normal LH (LH may be inactive).
- Occuring in females the gonadotropic tumors produce hormonal profile and clinical presentation of a post menopausal woman.[1]

ACTH producing tumors:

These functional tumors are generally microadenomas (more than 90% cases) and produce Cushing's disease. These are referred in Chapter 15.

Null cell tumors:

Cells of these tumors do not take up any stain; commonly seen as macroadenomas and produce mass effects.

Craniopharyngiomas (form 3% of all intracranial tumors):

These tumors arise from remnants of Rathke's pouch and occur more commonly in children. The tumor gets calcified and this helps radiological diagnosis.

- Hormone related presentations include, short stature, delayed sexual development, hyperprolactinemia and diabetes insipidus.
- Patient may present with increased intracranial tension/visual defects.
- As the tumor is cystic it may rupture and produce aseptic meningitis.
- In a few cases it may produce panhypopituitarism.

The germ cell tumors:

These are common ovarian and testicular tumors but also occur in pineal gland. The germ cell tumors produce hCG and AFP and/or only hCG and these tumor markers help diagnosis, determining prognosis and in management. Also read in Chapter 5.

- hCG produced by these tumors does not cause female precocity since hCG (or LH) without FSH, does not cause increased secretion of estrogen. However, in the male it increases secretion of testosterone and or estrogen and hence patient can present with pseudoprecocity or gynecomastia.

The secondary tumors (from breast, bronchus):

These tumors produce diabetes insipidus, hyperprolactinemia along with some deficiencies of anterior pituitary hormones. Secondaries are located in hypothalamus/upper stalk.

---

[1] FSH response to TRH occurs in 40% patients with gonadotropin secreting tumors but not in normals or hypogonadal men or postmenopausal women.

CASE HISTORY: 13.1

A 40 year old male presented with complaints of weight loss, gradually increasing visual impairment, loss of libido, and also loss of axillary and pubic hair. He also had features of postural hypotension (he felt dizzy on suddenly getting up from lying down position).

These are typical features of hypopituitarism caused by a tumor. The visual impairment is due to pressure on optic nerve pathway. Loss of libido and loss of axillary and pubic hair could be explained by gonadotropin deficiency. Postural hypotension could be explained by ACTH deficiency leading to cortisol deficiency. Testosterone level was below the normal reference range while cortisol level was in the lower part of normal reference range. Serum Na^+ level was 120 mmol/L. Lateral X-ray skull revealed enlarged sella.

The patient should be investigated for different anterior pituitary hormone deficiencies. This is also essential to decide about management. In presence of both secondary hypothyroidism and secondary adrenal deficiency, cortisol replacement should be started first and followed by thyroxine replacement. In case of gonadotropin deficiency, sex hormone replacement is important not only to restore sexual functions but also to prevent osteoporosis.

Hyponatremia is because of reduced free water elimination due to reduced amount of urine formation due to glucocorticoid deficiency. It will be corrected by cortisol administration.

CASE HISTORY: 13.2

Romesh was brought for consultation because of smaller height than his age mates. The family physician noted that his height was 3SD below the average height at his age. The lag in increase in height had been noted, only, during past 6-8 months. Romesh was otherwise smart, active and well nourished for his height. Also he had normal body proportions and his parents were of normal height and without any history of abnormality in their growth progress.

➤ Should this child be investigated for his short stature?

➤ What investigations are needed?

• As the height of the child is 3SD below the average height for his age, he needs to be investigated. First of all the common causes should be ruled out (Table 13.4, App. B). In this smart child, height retardation has been noted in third year. His bone age should be found out and if delayed, he should be investigated for GH deficiency.

• Purpose of investigations is three fold. Firstly, to arrive at the diagnosis. Urinary excretion of GH should be used as a screening test. Confirmation

should be obtained from the stimulation test using insulin hypoglycemia as the stimulant. The second purpose of investigation is to find out the cause of GH deficiency, especially, to investigate for presence of a tumor in pituitary-hypothalamic region. For this, the lateral X-ray of skull is taken to know the size of sella. CT-scan or MRI define structures in and around the sella (MRI is better). Thirdly, if tumor is found, secretion of other hormones should be investigated. Treatment will depend upon the cause. For GH deficiency, human GH is available from recombinant DNA technology. Therapeutic potential of GH-releasing peptide (GHRP), a synthetic hexapeptide which stimulates GH release but does not interact with GHRH or opiate receptors is under investigation.

CASE HISTORY: 13.3

A 35 year old woman had prolonged and difficult labour and her much desired child could not be saved. She lost her appetite and started losing weight. About 6 months after her delivery, she presented with severe cachexia and malnutrition. She had also amenorrhea.

➤ How should she be investigated?

• The patient might have developed pituitary failure following severe post partum hemorrhage, or she might have developed anorexia nervosa because of her emotional upset after losing her much wanted child. In anorexia nervosa there is aversion to food and severe weight loss. In this condition, however, loss of pubic and axillary hair (seen in pituitary deficiency), does not occur. Plasma levels of thyroid hormones, cortisol and GH should be determined. Levels of these hormones (likely to be reduced in pituitary failure) are not reduced in anorexia nervosa.

In anorexia nervosa the hormonal changes are secondary to nutrient deficiencies but are not specific. These include increase in basal GH level with normal response to provocative tests; LH/FSH may be low with impaired response to LHRH. There is no adrenal insufficiency but there may be loss of circadian rhythm, incomplete suppression with dexamethazone and increased respone to ACTH. TSH is normal, T_3/T_4 normal or low. In anorexia nervosa anemia and vitamin deficiencies are uncommon. There may be prerenal azotemia. Diagnosis of anorexia nervosa remains clinical.

CASE HISTORY: 13.4

A known patient of lung cancer presented with complaints of increased thirst and of passing large volumes of urine. Urine osmolality was tested, a number of times and was found around 200 mosmol/kg.

This patient, most likely, has DI due to secondaries in the pituitary region. He should be evaluated as per information in Table 13.9, 13.11 and also for pituitary hormones. This will help his management also. The patient, however, does not appear to have adrenal insufficiency at present. In a patient of DI, with loss of ACTH (and cortisol) secretion, polyuria disappears.

Neurogenic DI is managed by DDAVP (1-desamino -D- arginine vasopressin) given intranasally. The amount required should be adequate to keep the patient in water balance. Chlorpropamide given orally enhances renal effectivity of ADH but there is danger of hypoglycemia. Carbamazepine has a similar action. For nephrogenic DI, thiazide diuretics are used, and K^+ carefully monitored.

OBJECTIVE TYPE QUESTIONS

Pick out the wrong statement.

1. Growth hormone (regulation of secretion)

   i) Hypothalamic factors GHRH (stimulatory) and somatostatin (inhibitory) regulate GH secretion from pituitary.
   ii) IGF-I produces feedback effect by increasing secretion of somatostatin and by producing inhibitory action at pituitary.
   iii) Obesity and major depression reduce basal and stimulated secretions of GH.
   iv) Malnourished individuals and patients of anorexia nervosa have increased plasma GH levels.
   v) The correlation between plasma levels of IGF-I and GH is better at higher levels of GH than at its lower levels.

2. GH and growth

   i) Levels peak during adolescence and start decreasing after 50 years of age.
   ii) Most of the secretion occurs during sleep (especially, during third and fourth stages).
   iii) Thyroid hormone is important in growth because of its direct effect on cell metabolism, its requirement in GH secretion and its involvement in certain actions of IGF-I on cells.
   iv) Anabolic actions of insulin include those for protein synthesis and cell division.
   v) Much of the growth spurt at puberty is due to GH again.
   vi) Estrogens stimulate growth at low levels and inhibit growth at high levels.
   vii) Androgens directly stimulate growth and maturation of bone, cartilage and muscle.

3. IGF-I

   i) It is a basic protein and structurally similar to proinsulin, and exerts some insulin like actions.
   ii) IGF-I circulates bound to a number of IGF binding proteins (IGF-BPs) which increase half life of IGF-I.
   iii) IGF-BPs also modulate actions of IGF-I at cellular level.
   iv) IGF-BP3 is the major IGF binding protein and is itself GH dependant.
   v) Estrogen increases levels of both GH and IGF-I.

4. GH secreting tumor

   i) MRI is required for proper defining of the tumor size and relation to surrounding structures.
   ii) X-ray examination may show enlarged air sinuses.
   iii) X-ray examination may show tufting of distal phalanges of hand and feet.
   iv) Level of prolactin may be increased due to co-secretion of prolactin or due to compression of pituitary stalk.
   v) It is very easy for the family physician to make diagnosis of acromegaly due to peculiar facial features.
   vi) A large tumor may produce visual field defects, III or VI cranial nerve lesions or hypothalamic pressure effects.
   vii) There may be increased associated secretions of PTH and insulin.

5. Acromegaly

   i) GH excess may cause increase in BMR and increased sweating.
   ii) GH excess may cause hypertension.
   iii) Increased levels of IGF-I may cause goitre.
   iv) GH excess is associated with insulin resistance.
   v) In acromegaly both hypercalcemia and hyperphosphatemia result from renal tubular effects of excess GH.

6. Hyperprolactinemia - presentation

   i) Men may present with decreased libido, impotence or infertility.
   ii) Women developing galactorrhea on oral contraceptives.
   iii) Women developing amenorrhea on withdrawl of contraceptives.
   iv) Patient may present with primary amenorrhea.
   v) Macroprolactinomas are more common in women than men.

vi) Enlargement of macroadenoma during pregnancy may cause headache and visual disturbances.

7. Prolactinomas

i) Microprolactinomas are more common than macroprolactinomas.

ii) Macroprolactinomas produce more prolactin than microprolactinomas.

iii) A large pituitary tumor with only modest increase in prolactin level is not a true prolactinoma.

iv) Some times a microadenoma producing a small pituitary lesion (on MRI) may present with hypopituitarism and hyperprolactinemia.

v) Pituitary macroadenomas and most microadenomas are easily visualized by MRI scan.

vi) In macroadenomas or patients with hypothalamic lesions, evaluation of visual fields and pituitary functions should be done.

8. Interpreting hyperprolactinemia

i) Rule out pregnancy.

ii) Rule out cirrhosis.

iii) Rule out postpartum period.

iv) Rule out medication.

v) Rule out renal insufficiency and hypothyroidism.

vi) Serum prolactin level of >100 mg/L is diagnostic of prolactinoma.

9. Prolactinoma

i) Size correlates with hormone secretion by the tumor.

ii) Microprolactinoma may produce hypogonadism.

iii) Macroadneoma may produce features of panhypopituitarism.

iv) Dopamine receptors antagonists produce modest hyperprolactinemia.

v) TRH stimulation test is very useful to differentiate between different causes of hyperprolactinemia.

10. Prolactinomas

i) These can cause amenorrhea.

ii) These can cause amenorrhea and galactorrhea.

iii) These can cause irregular menses.

iv) These can cause infertility despite regular menses.

v) The regular menstrual period becomes infertile because of absent LH surge.

11. Gonadotropin deficiency

i) It may produce infertility and amenorrhea in females.

ii) It may produce loss of beard, body hair and libido in males.

iii) Gonadotropin measurements are not required if a woman has regular menses.

iv) In post menopausal women, gonadotropin levels are lower than premenopausal women.

v) Increased gonadotropin levels and low gonadal hormone levels can occur together.

12. Growth disorders

i) A height below 3SD from mean for age should be immediately investigated for the cause.

ii) A growth rate consistently below normal for the age, also needs to be investigated.

iii) A height less than mean but difference less than 2SD, means that the child is likely to be normal depending upon his growth rate.

iv) Simple biochemical parameters can easily diagnose constitutional delay of growth.

v) Three important causes of growth retardation requiring intervention are hypothyroidism, GH deficiency and some common systemic diseases.

13. Growth retardation

i) Short limbs relative to skeleton, indicates long standing hypothyroidism or one of the chondrodystrophies.

ii) A child who is short and also underweight for height could have malnutrition or some systemic disease.

iii) A child who is short but overweight for height could have an endocrine disorder.

iv) A normal looking child at birth could be hypothyroid or GH deficient.

v) Central obesity, hypertension and striae indicate Cushing's syndrome.

vi) Webbed neck and multiple pigmented nevi indicate gonadal dysgenesis.

14. Growth retardation

i) Serum TSH and T_4 levels help diagnosis of hypothyroidism.

ii) Random measurement of GH in serum is quite adequate for diagnosing GH deficiency.

iii) Serum GHBR levels help diagnosis of GH ineffectivity syndromes.

iv) Serum phosphate levels may help diagnosis of vitamin D resistant rickets.

v) Serum bicarbonate levels may help diagnosis of RTA.

15. Tests using hypothalamic releasing hormones

i) GnRH stimulation test can be used to test capacity of gonadotrophs to secrete LH and FSH.

ii) Failure of LH response to clomiphene means hypothalamic disease.

iii) Clomiphene is also used for treatment of anovulatory women which show progesterone withdrawl bleeding.

iv) The main use of TRH test is to confirm diagnosis of hyperthyroidism.

v) Persistent GH response to TRH after resection of a GH secreting tumor means that recurrence may occur.

vi) In a postmenopausal woman gonadotropin elevation is due to a microadenoma (not simply because of menopause) if LH level increases in response to TRH.

vii) If confirmation of Sheehan's syndrome needs demonstration of low prolactin level, reduced response to TRH is useful, as many prolactin assays do not distinguish between low and normal levels, as such.

16. Thirst and AVP release

i) With increasing plasma osmolality ADH release occurs earlier than perception of thirst.

ii) Angiotensin II increases AVP release and thirst under conditions of volume depletion.

iii) In DI patient prefers to take cold drinks.

iv) Adipsia is a common finding in idiopathic DI.

v) In DI accompanied by adipsia patient develops severe dehydration causing weakness, fever, psychic disturbances, hypotension tachycardia, prostration and death.

17. Diabetes insipidus

i) In complete form there is no evidence of AVP release.

ii) In one form of DI saline infusion does not lead to release of AVP at any stage but increasing dehydration causes AVP release at a certain stage of plasma osmolality.

iii) In another form of DI there is elevated osmotic threshold for AVP release.

iv) In fourth type there is subnormal release of AVP, although it occurs at proper plasma osmolality.

v) AVP response to nausea, smoking and certain drugs is maintained in all forms of DI.

18. AVP release

i) There is osmoregulation, volume regulation and baroreceptor regulation of AVP release.

ii) Hypotension increases AVP release through activation of aortic/carotid baroreceptors.

iii) The volume regulation mechanism is involved in decrease of AVP release during lack of gravitational force (space travel), negative pressure breathing and exposure to cold.

iv) Hypotension or volume contraction act through the volume regulation mechanism (which involves stretch receptors in left atrium and perhaps in pulmonary veins) to increase AVP release.

v) Osmoregulation of AVP release is always more powerful than volume regulation of AVP.

vi) Stress, emesis and pain are antidiuretic.

19. AVP release

i) Cortisol elevates the osmotic threshold for AVP release caused by hypertonic saline infusion in a water loaded normal person.

ii) AVP binds to its receptor (V_2) on basolateral surface of the principal cell of medullary collecting duct.

iii) Receptor stimulation by AVP leads to insertion of water channels into apical membrane of the cell (via cAMP mediated process).

iv) AVP also stimulates prostaglandin E_2 production which potentiates action of AVP to reabsorb water.

v) Presence of calcium and lithium and potassium depletion interfere in the above activation process of AVP.

20. Polyuric syndromes

i) Polyuria is hypotonic (osmolality <300 mmol/kg) in DI and psychogenic polydipsia.

ii) In osmotic diuresis, polyuria is not hypotonic.

iii) Thiazide diuretics cause excretion of hypotonic urine, and with loop diuretics, urine may not be hypotonic.

iv) Some chronic kidney diseases produce nephrogenic DI and some cause osmotic diuresis.

v) In water deprivation test urine osmolality always increases normally (with increase in plasma osmolality) in psychogenic polydipsia and subnormally in DI, making differentiation between the two quite easy.

ANSWERS

1. No.(v). In patients of acromegaly, with increased GH levels, there is parallel increase in plasma IGF-I levels upto a GH level of about 20 μg/L. After this there is platueing of IGF-I levels on further increase of GH levels.

2. No.(v). Much of the growth spurt at puberty is due to testosterone in the male and estrogens in the female.

3. No.(v). Estrogens increase production of GH but

inhibit its actions by blocking production of IGF-I. Because of the estrogen effect, most GH stimulants produce higher GH levels in women than men.

4. No.(v). The family physician may fail to detect the characteristic changes if these have been developing, gradually. A new physcian may note the features more easily.

5. No.(v). GH increases tubular reabsorption of phosphate to increase serum phosphate level. There is increased formation of calcitriol in acromegaly which often results in hypercalciuria. In MEN 1 syndrome, along with excess of GH there may also be increased formation of parathyroid hormone which may cause hypercalcemia.

6. No.(v). Macroadenomas are more common in males as detection is delayed because of vague clinical effects.

7. No.(iv). Microadenomas do not produce hypopituitarism (except hypogonadism). A small lesion in the stalk (detected by MRI) produced by sarcoidosis or some other pathology (however, not an adenoma), can result in both hyperprolactinemia and hyperpituitarism.

8. No.(v). A level >150 ng/mL generally indicates a prolactinoma. some microprolactinomas produce lower levels (<100 ng/mL) and cause diagnostic problems.

9. No.(v). In prolactinoma, there is no increase in prolactin secretion after TRH and only modest increase occurs in most other causes of hyperprolactinemia. Increase is quite sharp in normals. However, results are variable and the test is not much used.

10. No.(v). It is because of short luteal phase.

11. No.(iv). The gonadotropin levels are higher (especially that of FSH).

12. No.(iv). Diagnosis of constitutional delay is by exclusion.

13. No.(iv). It is true for GH deficient child but not for the hypothyroid child.

14. No.(ii). If age related standards are used, IGF-I and IGFFBP-3 provide a useful screen. For GH some stimulation test is needed.

15. No.(iv). This was the main use when sensitive TSH assay was not available. It may be useful in some cases of euthyroid hyperthyroidism and some times in diagnosis of primary hypothyroidism although with sensitive TSH assays the test is generally not required. TRH test is also not useful in diagnosis of secondary hypothyroidism or for distinguishing between hypothalamic and pituitary cause of hypothyroidism.

16. No.(iv). It does not occur in idiopathic cases. It occurs if some lesion causing DI extends to involve the hypothalamic thirst centre.

17. No.(v). Except in complete form.

18. No.(v). In dehydration both mechanisms tend to increase AVP release and osmoregulatory mechanism is more sensitive than the volume regulatory one. However, when volume changes are large as in hemorrhage the volume regulatory mechanism becomes more powerful and may over come the osmoregulatory influences if working in opposite direction.

19. No.(iv). Prostaglandin E_2 produces feedback inhibition by inhibiting cAMP formation in response to V_2 receptor stimulation.

20. No.(v). It may not be always so. In many cases due to chronic ingestion of water may suppress release of AVP and chronic polyuria may cause washing out of medullary gradient. These changes would lead to subnormal increase of urine osmolality on water deprivation.

CHAPTER 14

Thyroid Hormones and Disorders

It is the largest endocrine gland releasing two related hormones, tetraiodothyronine (T_4) and triiodothyronine (T_3), from the acinar cells and the third hormone, calcitonin (unrelated to the first two hormones) from the parafollicular cells (C-cells). Calcitonin has a role in calcium metabolism and is discussed in Chapter 10. Thyroid hormones are required for growth and development. They produce certain well known metabolic effects including increase of BMR. These also potentiate cardiovascular and central nervous system effects of catecholamines. Thyroid hormones act through their nuclear receptors and modify transcriptional activities of cells. In pharmacological amounts, thyroid hormones promote overall catabolic activities of cells.

BIOSYNTHESIS OF THYROID HORMONES

Thyroid hormone synthesis involves iodination of tyrosine residues on a protein called thyroglobulin. The acinar cells take up I^- from blood by an active process. This is oxidized and incorporated into tyrosine residues of thyroglobulin. This reaction is called organification. This reaction and also the subsequent ones leading to synthesis of T_3 and T_4 take place while the substrate and the products of reaction remain attached in the structure of thyroglobulin molecule. The reactions take place at apical borders of the acinar cells, where thyroglobulin is undergoing exocytosis into the acinar lumen (Fig. 14.1). Thus thyroglobulin present in the acinus is charged with T_3/T_4 and the intermediate products, monoiodotyrosine (MIT) and diiodotyrosine (DIT). All the reactions of T_3/T_4 synthesis and also secretion of these hormones, are stimulated by TSH. Synthesis of thyroglobulin (TGB) is also increased. Prolonged presence of excess of TSH also causes acinar cell hyperplasia and hypertrophy.

Release of T_4 and T_3

Thyroglobulin is present in colloid of thyroid acini. A small amount of colloid is taken into follicular cell by endocytosis. A lysosome fuses with the endocytic vesicle. The lysosomal endopeptidases degrade thyroglobulin and release T_3, T_4, MIT and DIT in free form. T_3 and T_4 are released into circulation. From MIT and DIT, I^- is released by the enzyme deiodinase and added to I^- pool of the cell. This contribution of I^- is quite significant since deiodinase deficiency can result in iodine deficiency goitre (MIT and DIT enter circulation and are excreted in urine along with their iodine).

Normal thyroid secretes about 10 times more T_4 than T_3. Some of the secreted T_3 also arises from conversion of T_4 to T_3 during the process of secretion. This conversion increases in Graves' disease. However, 80% of T_3 in circulation arises from deiodination of T_4 in peripheral tissues.

THYROID HORMONES IN CIRCULATION

Most of T_4 and T_3 circulating in plasma are bound

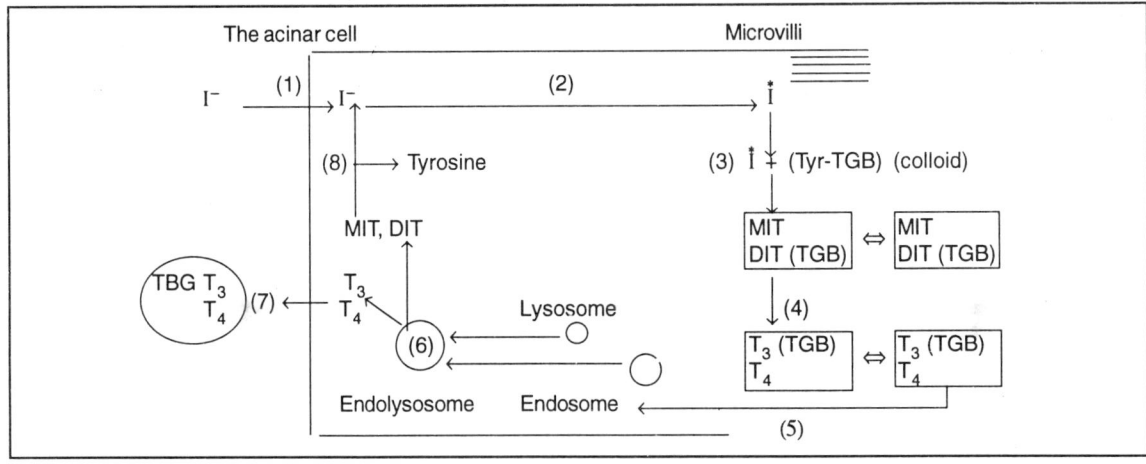

Fig. 14.1. Biosynthesis of thyroid hormones.

1. Iodine trapping   2. Oxidation of $I^- \rightarrow \overset{*}{I}$ 3. Iodination of tyrosine (in thyroglobulin)   4. Formation of T_3 and T_4
5. Endocytosis of colloid into follicular cell   6. Hydrolytic cleavage of TGB and release of T_3, T_4, MIT and DIT
7. Release of T_3 and T_4 into circulation binding to TBG   8. Deiodination of MIT and DIT
- Steps 2, 3 and 4 are mediated by the same enzyme. Inborn errors related to steps 2, 3 and 8 are known.

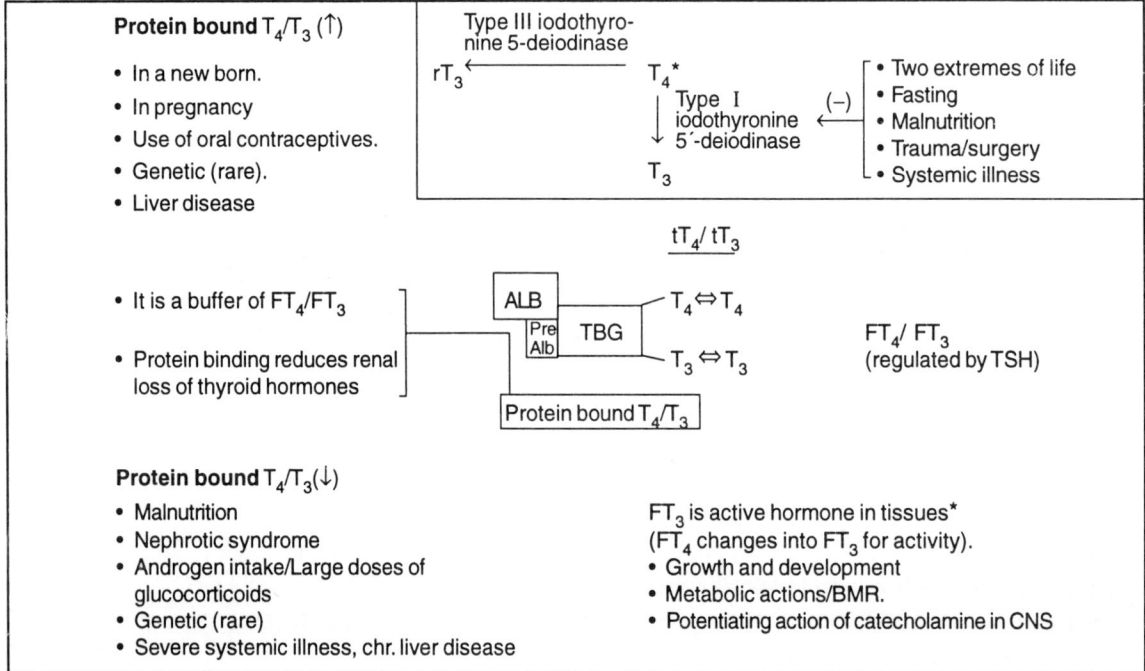

Fig. 14.2. Thyroid hormones in circulation and their main actions in tissues.

- Increase/decrease of TBG affects levels of total hormones but the free hormone levels remain unchanged since these are regulated by TSH.
- The inset of the figure shows conditioins which favour formation of inactive rT_3.

to thyroxine binding globulin (TBG), thyroxine binding prealbumin (transthyretin) and albumin and only small fractions circulate in free form. T_3 is the active form and T_4 (prohormone) is converted into T_3 in tissues for producing actions.

Total T_4 (tT_4 or T_4) or total T_3 (tT_3 or T_3) are easily measured in plasma. In these measurements both free and protein bound hormones are included. However, the thyroid status of an individual is only determined by levels of free T_4 (FT_4) and free T_3 (FT_3). Further, hypothalamic - pituitary axis is also regulated by free hormone levels. Changes in plasma levels of thyroid hormone binding proteins (Fig. 14.2) would alter T_4 and T_3 levels in plasma, without affecting FT_4 and FT_3 and thyroid status of the person.

METABOLISM (also see page 286)

Besides conversion of T_4 to active T_3 in tissues, some T_4 is also converted into rT_3 (reverse T_3) (Fig. 14.2), which is totally inactive. In some conditions (surgical stress, starvation, chronic malnutrition) more T_4 is converted into rT_3 than normal.

Like iron, there is reuse of I^- liberated during metabolism of T_4 and T_3. Daily about 60 μg of I^- is used for synthesis of T_4 and T_3 and 40 to 50 μg of I^- is liberated during daily catabolism of T_4 and T_3. Thus only 10 to 20 μg of I^- is lost when iodinated metabolites of T_4 and T_3 are lost in bile. For 10 to 20 μg of I^-, as daily physiological requirement, dietary requirement is about 150 μg (with almost 100% absorption), probably, to maintain adequate plasma level of I^- for sufficient uptake by the thyroid gland.

REGULATION OF SECRETION OF THYROID HORMONES

Thyroid hormones exert feed back inhibitory effect at pituitary and hypothalamus and this is the main regulatory influence controlling secretion of TSH. It is because of this relationship that TSH levels acts as a sensitive indicator of thyroid activity in primary thyroid disorders (Fig. 14.3). Hypothalamic factors, TRH (stimulatory) and probably somatostatin (inhibitory), modify activity of thyrotrophs secreting TSH. Day to day temperature variations do not appear to have any significant effect in modulating

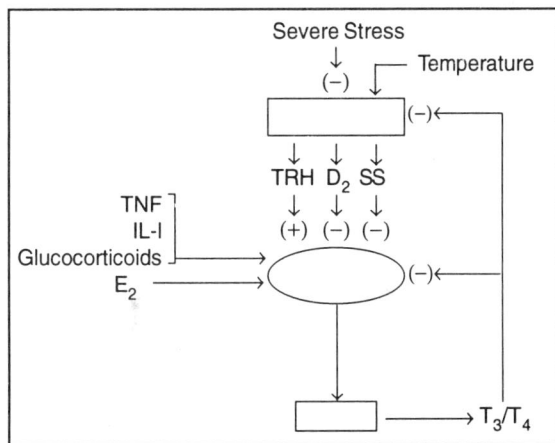

Fig.14.3. Hypothalamic-pituitary-thyroid axis.

- Effect of cold in increasing TSH secretion has been demonstrated in humans only at birth. Direct effect of stress has also not been clearly demonstrated; the effect may be an indirect one.
- Both dopamine (D_2) and somatostatin (SS) appear to be physiological inhibitors of TSH secretion.
- Estrogens enhance pituitary responsiveness to TRH; glucocorticoids reduce it. Inhibitory effect of cytokines may explain sick euthyroid syndrome.
- Because of sharp sensing of thyroid hormones by pituitary, TSH has become the most important test for thyroid disorders. It is an indirect faithful measure of free thyroid hormones.
- Although at the level of pituitary, the inhibitory effect is produced by T_3 (T_4 is converted into T_3 inside thyrotropes for producing the effect), serum T_4 levels are more effective for feed back inhibition than serum T_3. T_4, probably, enters thyrotropes more readily than T_3.

secretion of TSH. However, extremes of temperature do affect pituitary TSH secretion. Severe stress, depresses hypothalamic-pituitary-thyroid axis. Tumor necrosis factor (TNF) and IL-1, inhibit TSH secretion by acting at pituitary level. This may have a role in sick euthyroid syndrome.

TSH acting through cell surface receptors (and via cAMP) increases metabolic activity of thyroid cells including synthesis and secretion of thyroid hormones and also synthesis of thyroglobulin. With prolonged administration, there is thyroid cell hypertrophy and hyperplasia. Vascularity of the gland also increases.

Autoregulation

Thyroid gland has capacity to autoregulate its

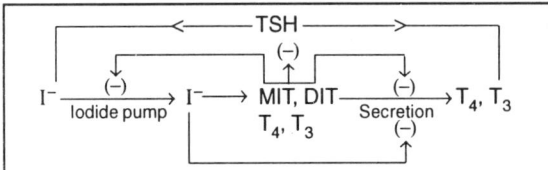

Fig. 14.4. Autoregulation of secretion of thyroid hormones.

- With increase of plasma I⁻ level, organic iodide level in thyroid cells increases and prevents excessive formation and secretion of thyroid hormones by reducing thyroid responsiveness to TSH and by inhibiting iodide trapping. Accumulated I⁻ reduces secretion of the hormones. In this way, generally, the secretion of thyroid hormones is not allowed to increase, with increase in plasma I⁻ level.

- Reverse happens with decrease of plasma I⁻ level. This helps to maintain normal thyroid status in iodine deficiency goitre. In cases of too much decrease of plasma I⁻ levels, however, secretion of thyroid hormones does decrease and hypothyroidism occurs.

activity and maintain normal secretions of thyroid hormones, under variable intakes of dietary I⁻ (Fig. 14.4). Thus in iodine deficiency goitre, hypothyroidism occurs only rarely when I⁻ intake is very poor.

TESTS FOR ASSESSMENT OF THYROID FUNCTIONS

TSH

With availability of a very reliable and ultra sensitive method for TSH, it has become the single most important investigation in diagnosis of thyroid diseases. Method uses two monoclonal antibodies against TSH. One is fixed to a solid support and is used to fix TSH from the serum sample. The second monoclonal antibody against a separate epitope on TSH (this antibody carries the label) is used to quantitate TSH bound to the support.

These days TSH is one single investigation on which maximum reliance is placed in diagnosis of thyroid disorders. At the secondary level diagnostic support is obtained from levels of total or free T_4/T_3.

Total T_4 (T_4) and total T_3 (T_3)

T_4 and T_3 are estimated by immunoassay procedures using specific antisera. In most of the cases of thyroid disorders T_4/T_3 is good enough to sup-

Table 14.1. Calculation of adjusted FT_4I and FT_3I values in resin T_4 uptake (RT_3U)

- The reaction mixture consists of the sample, known amount of radiolabeled T_3 or T_4 (more often T_3) and the resin in excess (to take up radiolabeled T_3/T_4 beyond the capacity of the binding sites on TBG).

- Find out the percentage of labeled hormone taken up by the resin. It is called RT_3U (resin T_3 uptake).

- RT_3U multiplied by total serum T_4 and total serum T_3 will, respectively, yield FT_4I (free T_4 index) and FT_3I.

- In an improved version of the method, one finds out the ratio of the counts on the resin and the counts remaining in the reaction mixture. This ratio is called THBR (thyroid hormone binding ratio). Patient's THBR is normalized by dividing it by THBR of the reference serum of the laboratory.

- Normalized THBR multiplied by total serum T_4 and total serum T_3 will, respectively, yield adjusted FT_4I and adjusted FT_3I. These values are less likely to differ from method to method or laboratory to laboratory than FT_4I and FT_3I.

- FT_4 estimate (FT_4E) refers to free T_4 fraction determined by equilibrium dialysis or the indirect (using RT_3U) method.

---

port TSH for diagnosis. Problem with T_4 and T_3, however, is that levels are affected by changes in levels or binding capacity of TBG. From this angle, estimations of free T_4 and free T_3 offer a distinct advantage, since levels of these parameters relate more faithfully to the thyroid status of the patient.

Free T_4 and free T_3

Free T_4 and free T_3 are often estimated, indirectly, by calculating free T_4 index (FT_4I) and FT_3I, after estimating T_4 or T_3 and then estimating radiolabeled hormone uptake by resin (RT_3U). In this test (which is an estimate of free binding sites on TBG), one may use radiolabeled T_4 or T_3 (T_3 is preferred). Adjusted FT_4I and FT_3I are calculated as shown in Table 14.1.

Direct methods are also available for estimation of FT_4 and FT_3. Principle of one such method is illustrated in Fig. 14.5.

TRH test

In this test, plasma TSH is assayed before and after TRH administration. With availability of a very sensitive assay procedure for TSH, the TRH test may

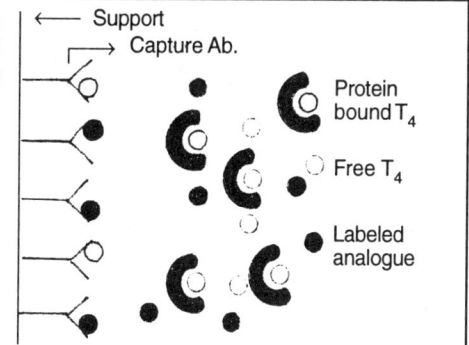

- A capture antibody held on a solid support is used. The antibody can react with free T_4 in the sample as well as a labeled T_4 analogue (label may be as an enzyme, a radio isotope or a chemilumiscent substance).

- The known amount of the analogue and serum sample are incubated with the capture antibody.

- The two uptakes are proportional to the respective concentrations.

- The analogue uptake being known (from a known amount), FT_4 of sample can be calculated..

- As only 1 to 5% of free T_4 is taken up by the capture antibody; free pool is not increased by release of T_4 from TBG bound T_4.

Fig. 14.5. Principle of single step immuno extraction method for estimation of free T_4.

- With improvement in assay techniques FT_4 is preferred over T_4 or FT_4I. However the highly sensitive assay of TSH is the most sensitive test of thyroid function.
- Relatively a fewer protein bound T_4 molecules are shown in the figure for convenience.

only be required in some borderline cases of primary hyperthyroidism and primary hypothyroidism. It may also help to distinguish between pituitary and hypothalamic cause of hypothyroidism. In the former, the response is reduced while in the latter, response is delayed.

Thyroglobulin

It is measured by double antibody radioimmunoassay. However, the endogenous antibodies interfere, in the assay procedure. This has been used in the follow up of thyroid cancer cases after surgery or ^{131}I therapy. If levels are not sufficiently reduced or increase following undetectable values, it indicates inadequate surgery/radioablation and/or metastases. Besides differentiated thyroid cancer, many other thyroid disorders cause release of thyroglobulin from the gland. The levels in serum depend upon the size of the gland (raised levels in large goitres), the gland activity (raised in hyperthyroid states) and leakage from the gland due to chronic inflammation (sub-acute thyroiditis). Appendix 14.1 gives a summary of investigative requirements in thyroid disorders.

Thyroid radioactive iodine uptake (RAIU)

[123]I is preferred because it exposes the patient to lesser radiation dose compared to [131]I. As normal 24h RAIU may be in the range of 20 to 30% of the test dose, the test will not be of much use in diagnosis of hypothyroidism (associated with reduced RAIU), since the lower limit of uptake is quite low even in normal cases. In thyrotoxicosis associated with hyperactive gland (hyperthyroidism) RAIU is increased. In certain cases of thyrotoxicosis the gland is not hyperactive and RAIU is not increased (Table 14.2). It is in such cases that RAIU is useful for diagnosis. This test is not done in pregnancy because of harmful effect of radiations on fetal development.

RAIU is also used as part of thyroid suppression test. RAIU is studied before and after liothyronine administration (serum T_4 levels may also be studied). Liothyronine suppresses TSH and thereby the thyroid gland. Normal suppression would exclude hyperthyroidism (hyperactive thyroid gland). However, this test is not used because of harmful effects of exogenous thyroid hormone especially in the elderly and those with cardiovascular disease and also because of availability of sensitive TSH assay.

USE OF THYROID INVESTIGATIONS IN DIAGNOSIS

History and clinical examination often detect cases of thyroid dysfunction. The detection rate of clinically inapparent cases, in adults, by thyroid related investigations is quite low. Thus investigations should be requested judiciously, to confirm a good clinical suspicion, in adults. In the elderly,

Table 14.2. Throtoxicosis without increase of RAIU

Iodine induced thyrotoxicosis:

- In iodine deficiency areas, during iodine supplementation some individuals may develop thyrotoxicosis. More commonly, in patients of non-toxic multinodular goitre. Some area of the gland is provoked to become autonomous; but as the gland is loaded with iodine RAIU does not increase.

Factitious hyperthyroidism:

- Thyroid hormone intake by a malingerer or inadvertently; thyrotoxicosis is due to the ingested hormone, which in turn inhibits TSH secretion from pituitary to decrease RAIU.
- Sub-normal serum thyroglobulin levels
- Thyroid gland is not palpable.

Thyroiditis patients:

- Thyrotoxicosis is produced by thyroid hormones leaked out of the thyroid gland and not because of its hyperactivity.
- Gland may be tender.

Functional ectopic thyroid tissue:

- In wide spread metastases of thyroid carcinoma, and struma ovarii.
- The thyroid gland is suppressed because of low TSH levels (pituitary is suppressed by ectopic thyroid hormones).
- The ectopic thyroid tissue may be located by scintillation scanning.
- Increased serum thyroglobulin levels
- Thyroid gland is not palpable.

- In trophoblastic tumors hCG causes stimulation of thyroid gland to increase total and free levels of both T_3 and T_4. Relation to pregnancy and high blood/urine levels of hCG help diagnosis. In this case however, RAIU is increased.

however, the clinical presentation may be atypical or may be masked by some other problem and the thyroid related tests may play a more significant role in diagnosis.

TSH level (by a sensitive assay) in the normal range excludes thyroid dysfunction. But TSH level outside the normal limits may not always indicate thyroid disease. If TSH is high, low T_4 indicates primary hypothyroidism; T_4 may be normal indicating euthyroid status or subclinical primary hypothyroidism. If TSH is undetectable, high T_4 (or T_3) indicates primary hyperthyroidism; T_4 (T_3) may be normal, indicating euthyroid status or subclinical primary hyperthyroidism (in most such euthyroid cases and some subclinical primary hyperthyroid

patients TSH is detectable although low). The TRH test may help diagnosis of subclinical cases.

Hypothalamic/pituitary hypothyroid patients present with detectable low TSH and low T_4. Hypothalamic/pituitary hyperthyroid patients are rare and present with elevated TSH and T_4/T_3. Thyroid hormone resistance cases are mentioned under euthyroid hyperthyroxinemia.

Many drugs alter parameters used in assessment of thyroid status of patients (Table 14.3). These drugs should be withheld for a few weeks (if possible) before the investigations are undertaken.

Many non-thyroidal disorders (infection, systemic illness, malignancy, malnutrition, surgery, myocardial infarction) also alter thyroid related biochemical parameters (Fig. 14.2) and the parameters may fail to convey the correct information regarding the thyroid status. One should wait for the illness to subside, before, undertaking the tests.

When newborns are screened for hypothyroidism, their TSH is estimated and if the level is high, T_4 is estimated for confirmation. However, in a premature or in a highly stressed infant, TSH level may be spuriously increased. Some other cases may be missed as rise of TSH may be delayed because of some subtle problem at the hypothalamus-pituitary axis. In some cases low T_4 may be due to TBG deficiency. In doubtful cases a second blood sample 2 to 6 weeks postpartum may be analyzed.

Table 14.3. Effect of some drugs on thyroid functions

- A drug may increase (clofibrate, phenothiazines, progestins, estrogens, fluorouracil) or decrease (anabolic steroids, aspirin in large doses, chlorpropamide, prednisone, sulfonamides) TBG concentration.
- A drug may increase or decrease TBG binding. (heparin causes release of FFA which reduce binding).
- A drug may block conversion of T_4 to T_3. (glucocorticoids, amiodarone)[1]
- A drug may reduce secretion of TSH. (glucocorticoids, dopamine, phenytoin)
- A drug may increase hepatic metabolism of T_4 specifically but not of T_3. (Rifampicin, antiepileptic drugs)

[1] β-Adrenergic drugs and oral cholecystographic agents also lead to formation of rT_3 from T_4. Other factors which block conversion of T_4 to T_3 are, low caloric intake, hepatic disease, major systemic illness and fetal life.

Determination of bone age may also help such cases.

Because of TSH surge at delivery, it is best to delay evaluation of neonatal hypothyroidism for about a week after delivery.

SICK EUTHYROID SYNDROME

Severe illness, physical stress and psychological trauma can alter various aspects of thyroid hormone metabolism. Such changes are more common than changes in metabolism of thyroid hormone by real thyroid disorders. Important factors producing the said changes are; reduced levels of TBG and transthyretin; increased formation of $rT3$ from T_4; inappropriate secretion of TSH in response to low T_4 and T_3 (due to effects of somatostatin and cytokines like TNF and IL-1). Commonly, only T_3 is reduced and as illness becomes more serious along with low T_3, T_4 and TSH are also reduced. Less commonly T_4 is elevated with normal T_3 (Fig. 14.6). In all these cases, thyroid status remains normal. One may have to differentiate such cases from a case of true thyroid disorder with superimposed non-thyroid illness.

EUTHYROID HYPERTHYROXINEMIA

Serum T_4 is increased but metabolic state of the patient is normal. This may result from increased T_4 binding. Examples are conditions of elevated TBG levels, familial dysalbuminemia (inherited as

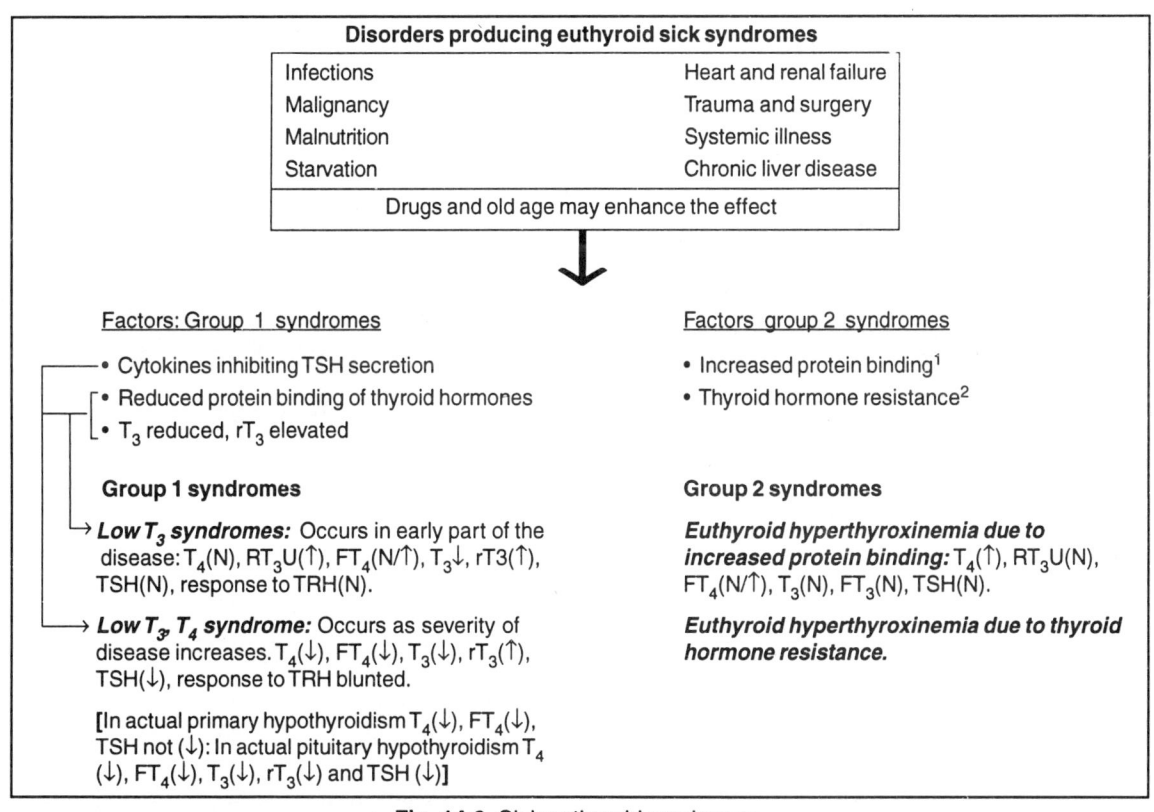

Fig. 14.6. Sick euthyroid syndromes.

[1] Illness commonly increases prealbumin which has higher affinity for T_4 than T_3.

[2] Resistance to thyroid hormone may occur rarely as part of sick thyroid syndrome or as a genetic disorder. In generalized resistance (pituitary and peripheral tissues) cases there is variable increase in TSH, T_4 and FT_4 with or without hypothyroidism. In genetic cases an adult may present with goitre and a child with growth and mental retardation. In cases of isolated resistance at pituitary there is variable increase of T_4 without suppression of TSH.

autosomal dominant trait in which a variant of albumin is present with very high affinity for T_4 but not for T_3), increased T_4 binding by transthyretin (prealbumin) and presence of anti-T_4 antibodies. In all these conditions FT_4 is normal, FT_4I may be increased. In cases of T_4-antibodies and dysalbuminemia the abnormal proteins have affinity, only for T_4 and not for T_3 (prealbumin has some affinity for T_3, although the affinity is more for T_4) and therefore, the fraction obtained as RT_3U is not reduced since it is obtained using T_3 (for which the increased protein has no increased affinity). This results in increased values of FT_4I (obtained by multiplying T_4 by RT_3U). FT_3I, if calculated will have normal value since T_3 is normal. In cases of increased TBG levels, FT_4I and FT_3I remain normal and both T_3 and T_4 are increased since TBG has almost same affinity for both T_4 and T_3. Some drugs also increase TBG affinity for T_4 (for T_3 the effect is variable) (see Table 14.3).

TSH, T_4 and FT_4I are increased (without altering metabolic status) in cases of pituitary plus peripheral, thyroid hormone resistance or only peripheral, thyroid hormone resistance (if there is only pituitary level resistance, hyperthyroidism will occur) (Fig. 14.3). Temporary hormone resistance of this type is seen in acute psychiatric illness and hyperemesis gravidarum. It may also be seen, rarely, in cases of sick thyroid syndrome.

IODINE DEFICIENCY AND THYROID DISORDERS

Fig. 14.7 shows dynamics of iodine balance and Fig. 14.4 presents the process of autoregulation of secretion of thyroid gland.

Iodine deficiency is the commonest cause of thyroid disorders in our country. Simple endemic goitre is common in iodine deficiency areas. Dietary or water borne goitrogens, dyshormogenesis and stimulants like epidermal growth factor and certain immunoglobulins may also play roles in development of simple goitre. Only, if iodine deficiency is severe, hypothyroidism is associated with goitre. In areas of endemic iodine deficiency, the size and prevalence of goitre and frequency of cretinism has been reduced by use of iodized salt or periodic injections of iodized oil.

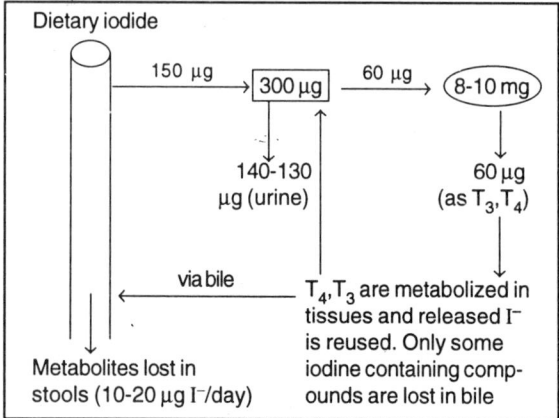

Fig. 14.7. Iodide equilibrium of a healthy adult. In areas of endemic goitre iodide intake may be less than 20 μg/day.

- All figures are per 24h.

Table 14.4. Iodine induced hypothyroidism and hyperthyroidism

Patients susceptible to Goitre/Hypothyroidism (Wolff-Chaikoff effect)
- Hashimoto's disease
- Euthyroid patients of Graves' disease (radioiodine or surgically treated cases)
- Normal fetus (fetus is susceptible to develop hypothyroidism in response to excess iodide received from mother. Goitrogens received via placenta also produce similar effect)

Patients susceptible to Hyperthyroidism (Jodbasedow effect)
- Multinodular goitre
- Elderly persons in iodine deficiency areas exposed to excess iodine
- Ill individuals (T_4 toxicosis)

- Iodine excess may produce goitre with or without hypothyroidism. The sensitivity of the thyroid glands to develop goitre/ hypothyroidism may be due to organic iodide binding defect present in the sensitive glands.
- In iodine depleted thyroids exposure to excess iodine may promote autonomous secretion of hormone by the thyroid tissue.

Under certain circumstances excessive iodine intake may produce hypothyroidism or hyperthyroidism (Table 14.4).

THYROID DISORDERS

The most common thyroid disorder is, diffuse or nodular swelling of the gland (goitre). The metaboli syndrome produced by increased production of thyroid hormone is called thyrotoxicosis; while hyperactivity (and increased secretion) of the gland is called hyperthyroidism. Thyrotoxicosis generally, results from hyperthyroidism but it may also occur without hyperthyroidism, for example when excess thyroxine is being produced from an ectopic site. In this case, in fact, thyroid gland activity is reduced. Reduced production of thyroid hormone is called hypothyroidism and this may also be used to indicate the resulting metabolic syndrome, although the term myxedema has also been used for that. But all cases of hypothyroidism are not associated with myxedema.

In ill patients many aspects of thyroid hormone metabolism are changed (see above). Although, in these ill patients, thyroid hormone status does not change and no thyroid hormone treatment is required, but difficulties arise in assessment of actual thyroid disorder which may, simultaneously be present.

Thyroid tumors may arise from follicular cells (adenoma, papillary/follicular/anaplastic carcinoma), from parafollicular cells (medullary carcinoma) or from lymphocytes (lymphoma). Medullary carcinoma may secrete calcitonin along with serotonin and various peptides of the tachykinin family, ACTH and prostaglandins. Medullary carcinoma may also occur as part of the familial multiple endocrine neoplasia (MEN) syndromes.

Goitre

Goitre is the most common disorder of the thyroid gland. It implies a swelling of the thyroid gland. Goitre is simple or non-toxic if there is euthyroid state. If associated with thyrotoxicosis (and hyperthyroidism) it is called toxic goitre. Goitre may also be associated with the hypothyroidism. An inflammatory or malignant process of thyroid gland may also produce a goitre.

Simple goitre

The term implies thyroid enlargement, not due to inflammation or neoplastic process and initially associated with euthyroid state of the body. Simple goitre of iodine deficiency is common in our country.

As thyroid gland is depleted of iodine, its sensitivity to TSH increases, resulting in increased gland mass. The person remains euthyroid as thyroid hormone production (even with low plasma iodine level) remains normal due to increased gland sensitivity to TSH. With more severe iodine deficiency hormone production may fall and the patient may become hypothyroid. In this case TSH level will increase due to low thyroid hormone level. Presence of goitrogens in diet or water intensifies the effect of iodine deficiency. Certain biosynthetic defects of thyroid hormones (legend to Fig. 14.1) may also result in goitre and increase chances of hypothyroidism in iodine deficiency goitre.

In developed countries, goitre occurs, most commonly, due to Hashimoto's disease (see later). This disease, however, is an autoimmune disorder and the patient may be euthyroid, hyperthyroid or hypothyroid, depending upon the stage of the disease.

In case of iodine deficiency or hormone dysgenesis, the gland is initially, uniformly swollen but over years (etiological factors continuing), multinodular goitre is formed. One or more nodules of the multinodular goitre may later become autonomous resulting in formation of multinodular toxic goitre.

Besides producing disfigurement, goitre, if large, may produce pressure effects on surrounding structures. This is especially true for large retrosternal goitres.

Diagnosis

Diagnosis is easy in a simple diffuse goitre. In case of nodular goitre, it is important to carefully rule out presence of a toxic or a malignant nodule. In simple goitre (diffuse or multinodular) the patient is euthyroid and has serum T_4 and T_3 levels in the normal range. At an early stage of development of toxic multinodular goitre, serum T_4 and T_3 levels are only in the upper part of the normal range. In the multinodular goitre, the best way to confirm euthyroid state is to show TSH level in the normal range. In simple goitre, RAIU is usually normal but may be increased in the presence of iodine deficiency or the biosynthetic defect.

Absence or presence of a hot nodule (secreting

excessive thyroid hormone) may be shown with isotopic scanning (Appendix 14.1). Also there is absence of detectable basal TSH by a sensitive assay in the presence of an autonomous or hot nodule.

The single nodule, may have to be differentiated from a neoplasm by fine needle biopsy (neoplastic nodule will also be cold). Growth of nodule is followed by ultrasound.

The Hashimoto's thyroiditis cases are differentiated by study of autoantibodies in serum or by fine needle biopsy.

The simple goitre cases need L-thyroxine (in some cases, especially in iodine deficiency areas small doses of iodide may prove effective). It suppresses TSH to reduce the size of the thyroid gland. Minimum possible dose of the drug should be used, as there is risk of excessive bone loss (particularly in post menopausal women). The therapeutic dose is titrated to serum TSH levels or RAIU. For good suppression of TSH, RAIU should decrease to less than 5% of the administered dose at 24h.

Before starting L-thyroxine treatment in multinodular goitre, one should carefully rule out presence of an autonomous nodule (see above). Such cases should be treated with the help of radioiodine. Surgical removal of simple or toxic multinodular goitre is not favoured.

Hypothyroidism (Table 14.5)

In areas of severe iodine deficiency goitre may be associated with varying degree of hypothyroidism. Cretinism both goitrous and non-goitrous is common in children of goitrous parents in these areas. In United States most common cause of goitrous hypothyroidism is Hashimoto's thyroiditis. Quite frequently, in this condition, there is abnormal organic binding of iodide and secretion of abnormal iodoproteins. Excessive iodine intake in certain types of thyroid gland may induce hypothyroidism (Table 14.4).

Non-goitrous (thyroprivic) hypothyroidism may be because of use of radioiodine or surgery for some thyroid diseases. It may also occur as primary idiopathic disorder which is, usually, due to an autoimmune etiology (there may be co-existing diabetes mellitus, pernicious anemia, SLE and other

similar disorders), and circulating antibodies against thyroid antigens may be present. It could also result as part of PGA syndromes. All these diseases appear to be associated with specific HLA haplotypes. Thyroprivic case could also result from a developmental defect of the thyroid gland.

Early clinical features in adults (features in children and cretinism will be discussed later), are vague and start insidiously. Features include fatigue, sluggishness (in movements, speech, thought process and reflexes), cold intolerance, constipation, hoarseness, scant eyebrows and other (Fig. 14.8). An elderly patient may appear as a patient of depression, Alzheimer disease or even Parkinson's disease. Heart is enlarged due to dilatation and pericardial effusion. Heart may be small in pituitary hypothyroidism (because of associated deficiency of ACTH) or if there is coexisting primary adrenal insufficiency (PGA syndromes). In severe cases there is accumulation of hydrophilic mucopolysaccharides in dermis and other tissues. This condition is called myxedema. A severe long standing case, exposed to cold, trauma, infection or with the use of some central nervous system depressant may become stuporous, hypothermic and may develop respiratory depression (myxedema coma).

Diagnosis

Diagnosis is based on clinical presentation and estimations of TSH and T_4. In primary hypothyroidism TSH in high and T_4 low (TSH levels carry greater significance than T_4 levels). Presence of thyroid antibodies would suggest the autoimmune cause. In secondary hypothyroidism T_4 level is low and TSH level is also low and there may be deficiency of other pituitary hormones also. However, even in primary hypothyroidism, status of other hormones may not be quite normal since thyroid hormones are needed for other glandular functions.

Other laboratory parameters of hypothyroid state are, increased serum cholesterol (only primary hypothyroidism), and increased serum levels of certain enzymes (CK, AST, LDH). Echocardiography may show increased preejection period and there may be specific ECG changes.

Nephrotic syndrome may present many features similar to those of hypothyroidism. These include,

Table 14.5. Causes of goitre, hypothyroidism and hyperthyroidism

Site of disorder	Goitre	Hypothyroidism	Hyperthyroidism
Hypothalamus/ pituitary	-	Pituitary failure (secondary hypothyroidism)	-
Thyroid: Diet and drugs	Goitre due to I⁻ deficiency or goitrogens. Enlargement is diffuse in the beginning and becomes multinodular with time.	Goitrous hypothyroidism: Endemic cretinism (with goitre): Wolff-Chaikoff effect	• Toxic multinodular goitre • Jodbasedow effect
Heritable/ Autoimmune	see below under goitrous hypothyroidism	See below under atrophic hypothyroidism (autoimmune including Hashimoto's, developmental defects and others)	• Graves' disease. • Hashimoto's disease with hyperthyroidism
Infection	Viral thyroiditis	Later stage of viral thyroiditis	Initial stages of viral thyroiditis

Important casues of hypothyroidism

Causes in thyroid (goitrous)
• Iodine deficiency, intake of goitrogens
• Heritable defects (dyshormogenesis)
• Maternally transmitted iodine, goitrogens
• Goitrous cretinism
• Hashimoto's thyroiditis

Causes in thyroid (atrophic)
• Primary iodiopathic including those with autoimmune etiology
• Part of polyglandular endocrine deficiency
• Congenital developmental defects
• Result of surgical, radioiodine damage
• Damage due to malignancy

Causes in pituitary/ hypothalamus
• Secondary hypothyroidism

Important causes of hyperthyroidism

Causes in thyroid (goitrous)
• Excessive stimulation in Graves' disease
• Excessive stimulation in trophoblastic tumor
• Autonomous thyroid tissue (adenoma, toxic multinodular goitre)
• Thyroiditis (autoimmune, viral)

Causes due to ectopic functional thyroid tissue
(thyroid gland not palpable)
• Thyroid carcinoma with metastases
• Struma ovarii
• Factitious causes (see Table 14.3)

Cause in pituitary
• Rare

facial pallor and puffiness, anemia, high serum cholesterol level, anasarca, low T_4 (because of loss of TBG in urine), and often low T_3 (reduced conversion of T_4 to T_3 in tissues). However, TSH and FT_4 are normal, in nephrotic syndrome.

In mild subclinical cases, serum T_4 and T_3 levels may be normal but TSH and TSH response to TRH are both increased. With further increase of TSH, with advance of the disease, serum T_4 level falls but T_3 remains normal (because of TSH induced hypersecretion of T_3 relative to T_4).

Hypothyroid patients are put on T_4 replacement therapy. In an old patient, treatment is started with a smaller dose which is gradually increased to

stabilize the patient. This avoids risk of myocardial ischemia or even myocardial infarction, during the treatment. Biochemical monitoring of patients of replacement therapy is discussed in case history 14.2. In secondary hypothyroidism, T_4 replacement therapy is given along with cortisol, otherwise, increase in metabolic rate of the patient may produce acute adrenal failure.

Cretinism (read objective type Question 16)

This condition is caused by inadequacy of thyroid hormones during fetal and neonatal development. There may be agenesis or improper development of fetal thyroid (in sporadic case). These cases

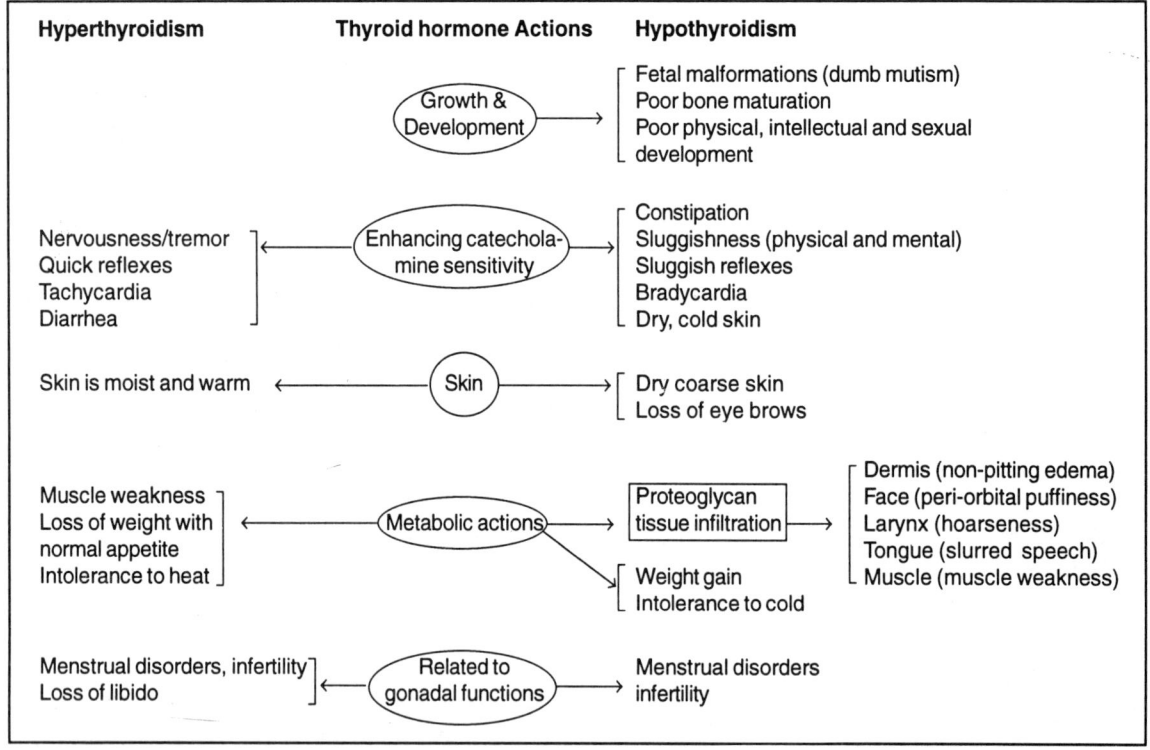

Fig.14.8. Features of hyperthyroidism and hypothyroidism based on actions of thyroid hormones.

- In hypothyroidism (myxedema) proteoglycan degradation is reduced.
- Thyroid hormones induce LDL receptors on liver cells. Thus serum cholesterol level is reduced in hyperthyroidism and increased in hypothyroidism.
- Stare, because of upper lid retraction, is very common in hyperthyroidism because of contraction of a smooth muscle (innervated by sympathetic fibers) in the upper lid. Real eye ball protrusion, however, occurs in Graves' disease in which autoantibodies produce inflammatory reaction in orbital muscles. This condition is called exophthalmos.
- In primary hypothyroidism, pituitary gland may enlarge with increased secretions of TSH and prolactin. There may be misdiagnosis of prolactinoma. However, pituitary size decreases with treatment.
- In severe primary hypothyroidism there may be reduced secretions of GH and ACTH and increased secretion of FSH and ovarian estrogens. True precocious puberty may occur in girls.

occur because of embryonic defect. Endemic cases are seen in areas of iodine deficiency (as mentioned earlier).

The condition may manifest at birth or in early infancy. The affected newborn may have persistence of physiological jaundice, hoarse cry, respiratory difficulty and poor feeding. As infant grows, there is delay in his milestones of development. The characteristic features of cretinism appear which include, short stature, coarse skin with sparse hair, protruding tongue, protuberant abdomen and umbilical hernia. There is also impaired mental develop-

ment, retarded bone age, epiphyseal dysgenesis and delayed dentition.

Hypothyroidism in children presents with retarded growth, reduced IQ and poor performance at school. Puberty is delayed. In these infants and children living in endemic iodine deficiency areas, iodide excretion in urine is reduced along with increased TSH and low T_4. Principles of treatment are the same as mentioned under simple goitre.

Screening for hypothyroid disorders

Incidence of neonatal hypothyroidism is estimated

as 1 in 3500 to 4000 live births in developed countries. In iodine deficiency regions of the World, the incidence is much higher. Besides the confirmed hypothyroid cases, in these areas, there are many milder cases who can also benefit from early treatment with thyroxine. For screening, blood may be collected at 6 to 8 days of life. According to one plan TSH is first studied and if raised T_4 is also studied. Either investigation, in isolation, will have inadequacy (see under investigations for thyroid disorders). X-ray will show evidence of delay in bone age in these cases. This parameter may be required, some times.

In a pregnant mother with Hashimoto's thyroiditis TSH receptor blocking antibodies can cross to fetus and produce transitory hypothyroidism after birth. In Graves' disease receptor stimulatory and receptor inhibitory antibodies crossing to fetus may produce transitory hyperthyroidism and hypothyroidism, respectively, in the new born. These antibodies could be studied in maternal plasma in last months of pregnancy.

Hashimoto's thyroiditis

It is the most common cause of goitrous hypothyroidism in developed countries. It is an autoimmune disorder. In the initial stages there is slight hyperthyroidism because of increased release of thyroid hormones from thyroid cells due to inflammatory process. However, with continued destruction of thyroid tissue hypothyroidism supervenes. In final stages the thyroid gland may, no longer, remain swollen. At this stage TSH level is increased and T_4 is normal or low. For diagnosis of etiology, serum is investigated for high levels of autoantibodies (thyroglobulin antibodies or thyroid peroxidase antibodies) (Appendix 14.1). Fine needle biopsy can also be used for the same purpose.

In viral subacute thyroiditis the inflammatory process has a limited course of some weeks during which the gland functions are disturbed (increased release of hormone followed by reduced release of hormone).

Hyperthyroidism

Most commonly it is caused by Graves' disease which is an autoimmune disorder with familial tendency (Table 14.5). It occurs, more commonly, in females in the age group of 20 to 40 years. Important features are weakness, sweating, weight loss (with normal apetite), nervousness and diarrhea. Skin is moist and warm (Fig. 14.8). Hands may show fine tremor. Pulse is rapid and bounding. There is slight enlargement of thyroid gland. In Graves' disease, autoantibodies are synthesized against TSH receptors which stimulate the receptors and increase formation of thyroid hormones. The thyroid cell antigen, (against which autoantibodies are formed) is common with certain antigens of orbital muscles. The sensitized T-cells, in the presence of cytotoxic autoantibodies, produce orbital inflammatory changes leading to thyroid ophthalmopathy. This is seen in about 50% of cases of Graves' disease and less common in older patients in whom myopathic findings (severe muscle weakness) are more common.

Besides Graves' disease, hyperthyroidism may occur in a case of long standing nodular goitre (Table 14.5) when some nodules start hypersecreting, autonomously. In multinodular goitre hyperthyroidism may be precipitated by iodine administration (Table 14.4). Besides, multinodular goitre, a benign adenoma of thyroid gland, may some times, start hypersecreting, autonomously, T_4 and T_3, to cause hyperthyroidism. The hypersecreting nodules (of a multinodular goiter) or hypersecreting adenoma can be recognized as hot nodules on 99m Tc pertechnetate and ^{123}I scans (Appendix 14.1). These occur in older individuals compared to the age group of patients of Graves' disease. In these patients, ophthalmic features are rare. Further features like weakness, nervousness, tremor, excessive sweating are mild. In older patients, of multinodular goitre and over 60 years, generally, features of atrial fibrillation and cardiac failure, predominate (Table 14.6). In toxic adenoma in about 50% cases there is increase in only T_3 level in serum.

Diagnosis

Hyperthyroidism is mostly primary and reduced level of TSH is the most important indicator of the disease. Along with low TSH, both T_4 and T_3 are increased in most cases but there is greater increase in T_3 than T_4. In a few patients, T_3 is elevated but

Table 14.6. Some unusual presentations of a thyrotoxicosis patient

Severe weakness and wasting	- Patient may require differentiation from some mypopathy.
Severe weakness, wasting and anorexia	- Presentation in some cases of toxic multinodular goitre - May require differentiation from malignancy.
Atrial fibrillation and depression in a patient of about 60 years[1]	- Seen in toxic multinodular cases - Severe depression as such is not uncommon in old age; atrial fibrillation could arise from some other cause.
Patient presenting with ophthalmic features without catecholamine hyperactivity features	- In such a case one may find low TSH as the only finding. If so one should keep patient under observation; other features may develop subsequently. - Rule out intraorbital/intracranial cause of unilateral ophthalmopathy
Features of thyrotoxicosis without ophthalmopathy and without symmetric diffuse thyroid enlargement	- Pituitary hyperthyroidism due to adenoma or due to resistance to TSH suppression. Thyroid gland may be palpable but not goitrous. - Trophoblastic tumor (hydatidiform mole, choriocarcinoma) producing hCG which is a stimulator of thyroid. - Excess hormone secretion from ectopic thyroid tissue (struma ovarii) or widespread secondaries of thyroid carcinoma. Thyroid gland is not palpable. - Thyrotoxicosis (clinical features) without hyperthyroidism can also occur by inadvertent ingestion of large amounts of thyroid hormone (thyrotoxicosis factitia).
A young woman may present with amenorrhea and infertility or osteoporosis.	

[1] In old patients difficulty of diagnosis arises from three reasons: Firstly it may be mild T_3 toxicosis and patient may also have non-thyroid illness. Secondly, in old patients raised levels of thyroid hormones may not suppress TSH or TSH may be normally suppressed. Thirdly, the patient may be taking some drugs which might interfere with thyroid hormone physiology.
- In trophoblastic tumors there is increase of T_4, T_3, and $F T_4$. There is no ophthalmopathy and high levels of β-hCG are present in serum and urine.
- In thyrotoxicosis factitia there is thyrotoxicosis without hyperthyroidism. There is reduced RAIU. TSH is reduced. Increase of T_4 or T_3 depends upon the ingested drug.

T_4 remains in the normal range (T_3 thyrotoxicosis). Levels of T_4 and T_3, however, vary with varying levels of TBG, independent of the thyroid status of the patient. From this angle estimations of FT_4 or FT_4I and FT_3 or FT_3I offer a distinct advantage.

Many features of thyrotoxicosis and anxiety neurosis are similar (tachycardia, tremor, irritability, weakness). Some of these features and other symptoms like sweating, heat intolerance, and hypermetabolic state, are common between thyrotoxicosis and pheochromocytoma. In anxiety neurosis there is anorexia and peripheral skin may be cold while in thyrotoxicosis, apetite is generally increased and peripheral skin is warm and moist. Laboratory tests may be, some times, needed to differentiate between these disorders.

Table 14.6 mentions certain unusual features found in certain patients of thyrotoxicosis especially elderly persons suffering from toxic nodular goitre. These features also present problems of differential diagnosis. Also read carefully objective type questions related to thyrotoxicosis.

Young patients are usually treated with antithyroid drugs (carbimazole), which has to be given for many years. This treatment effectively reduces thyroid hormone production but is ineffective in reducing thyroid receptor antibodies (TRAbs). The latter is the limiting factor in deciding duration of this treatment in Graves' disease. Relapse is more common in younger patients than older ones.

Treatment is monitored by estimations of T_4/T_3 or TSH (read in case history 14.1). Treatment with an antithyroid agent will correct the suppressed

TSH but it may be delayed because of previous prolonged suppression. Excessive rise may mean over treatment. This rise of overtreatment may also be delayed. Other modes of treatment are sub-total thyroidectomy (if goitre is large or if there had been recurrent relapses) or the radioiodine therapy (in old patients or if there is recurrence after surgery).

Diagnosis of toxic multinodular goitre

It is a disease of the elderly since it occurs when a person has been suffering from long standing simple goitre. Some times iodine administration in a patient of multinodular goitre results in development of toxicity. Problems in diagnosis of hyperthyroidism are as under:

i) Clinical features are different from those of Graves' disease as already mentioned.

ii) Serum T_4, T_3, FT_4I or FT_4 may be only slightly increased as the patients are elderly and even normal values for these parameters decrease with age.

iii) TSH response to TRH, in a normal elderly patient, may be subnormal.

Toxic multinodular goitre is confirmed if basal TSH level is undetectable and TSH response to TRH is subnormal. In many elderly persons, even normally, TSH is suppressed.

In diagnosis of toxic multinodular goitre, one should also be able to palpate nodularity of the gland or get evidence of structural heterogeneity from scintiscan. If diagnosis is in doubt, therapeutic trial with an antithyroid drug may be tried. It is important that patients in which the toxic state is suspected should never be treated with thyroxine (for simple multinodular goitre). Table 14.2 shows some less common causes of thyrotoxicosis.

THYROID NODULES

Palpable thyroid nodules are found in about 5% of female patients. A solitary nodule may be a cyst, a colloid nodule or a neoplasm. A solitary nodule may be malignant, if there is previous history of irridiation of the neck region or if it has appeared in an elderly person or if rapid increase in size has been noted. A cystic nodule may also show sudden increase in size with the nodule becoming painful (because of hemorrhage, into the cyst).

Fine needle biopsy, followed by cytological examination is very useful for diagnosis; a benign (80%) nodule may be distinguished from a malignant nodule (20%). However, results may be inconclusive in highly cellular nodules. Radionuclide scan may also help as cold nodules are likely to be malignant. Ultrasound will differentiate a solid nodule from a cystic one. Ultrasound may also be used to follow the increase in size of the nodule. If it is a colloid nodule, it is important to know whether or not it is autonomous. This requires estimations of TSH, T_4 and T_3 levels. Undetectable TSH indicates that the nodule is autonomous. It may be confirmed by isotopic scanning. This nodule is almost always benign and is treated by surgery or radioiodine.

Appendix 14.1. Use of thyroid function tests in diagnosis

Hyperthyroidism/postpartum thyroiditis:

- Graves' disease, toxic nodular goitre (See text)
- Subclinical exophthalmic Graves' disease, multinodular goitre
  - TSH is suppressed and T_4 is in upper part of normal reference range.
- Post partum thyroiditis: (A variant of chronic thyroiditis with transient thyrotoxicosis, CT/TT[1]).
  - Mild autoimmune disorder suppressed by pregnancy and manifesting after delivery (for about 6 months).
  - Radioiodine uptake will be low.
- Factitious hyperthyroidism: (intake of T_4 for some extra therapeutic purpose)
  - High T_4/T_3 ratio, poor radioiodine uptake, low thyroglobulin level. Also see the text.

Non-thyroidal illness (Patients are generally euthyroid): See the text.

Psychiatric non-thyroid illness:

- $T_4 \uparrow., FT_4 \uparrow, T_3 \downarrow$

Following a patient of Graves' disease:

- TSH, T_4 or T_3 have all been used in following a case of hyperthyroidism during treatment. T_3 is better than T_4; it decreases faster than T4 and also predicts a relapse better than T_4.
- Measurements of TSH receptor antibodies have been used to predict the outcome of drug therapy in a patient treated with antithyroid drugs (detectable after therapy, predicts relapse).
- Monitoring TB II (blocking antibodies called thyrotropin-binding inhibitor immunoglobulin) and TSH can be used to prevent over treatment with antithyroid drugs.
- TSH receptor antibodies have been used to predict thyroid dysfunction in newborns of mothers with Graves' disease.

Screening a population of new borns for neonatal hypothyroidism: See the text.

Hashimoto's thyroiditis

- Antibodies to thyroid peroxidase (TPO) is a laboratory marker of this autoimmune disorder. An ELISA procedure is available for measurement of antibody level
- Antibodies to TPO and TgAb (thyroglobulin antibodies) are used to identify patients of endogenous depression associated with sub-clinical autoimmune thyroiditis.

Thyroid nodule

- Scintiscanning using radioiodine or sodium ^{99m}Tc pertechnetate are used to locate cold, warm and hot nodules depending upon accumulation of radionuclide in the nodule and/or the surrounding tissue.
- Ultrasound differentiates solid from cystic nodules.

---

[1] It is a condition of unknown pathophysiology in which an episode of transient thyrotoxicosis (2 to 5 months) is followed by transient hypothyroidism. Patient may recover or have recurrent episodes. As increase of T_4/T_3 is due to leakage of the hormones, TSH is suppressed and RAIU low.

- BMR, once an important test, is rarely used. Increased serum cholesterol is commonly seen in primary hypothyroidism. Systolic time indices (say pre ejection period) are prolonged in hypothyroidism and reduced in hyperthyroidism. The last investigation may be used in monitoring thyroid replacement therapy in elders or patients of heart disease.

CASE HISTORY: 14.1

A 30 year old female presented with complaints of nervousness, palpitation, excessive sweating, fine tremor of hands and loss of weight. She also felt that her eyes had become more prominent. On examination pulse was 92/min. Her thyroid gland was modestly enlarged. To rule out anxiety neurosis TSH and T_4 were estimated. Diagnosis of hyperthyroidism was confirmed as TSH was low and T_4 raised. She was put on carbimazole treatment.

> ➤ How to monitor her treatment with the help of biochemical tests?
> ➤ What could be other investigative profiles in hyperthyroidism?
> ➤ Mention some other presentations of patients of thyrotoxicosis?
> • Treatment is monitored by periodic estimation of T_3, T_4 or TSH and from her clinical condition. Treatment with an antithyroid agent generally, results in decrease of T_4 and increase of TSH. In many cases, however, TSH may remain suppressed. In case of a relapse there is increase in T_4 and decrease in TSH. Spurious increase in T_4 produced by some drug being taken by the patient, should, however, be kept in mind. In some cases apparent decrease in TSH may not occur during a relapse. Also see Appendix 14.1.
> • Besides, increase of both T_4 and T_3 with low TSH, there may be increase only in T_3 with low or normal TSH in some cases of hyperthyroidism. This is often seen in case of an autonomous nodule in a multinodular goitre, in an elderly patient. Suppressed TSH level, generally, indicates hyperthyroidism even with normal levels of thyroid hormones expect in individuals over 60 years of age in which this hormone profile is often associated with euthyroid status. Secondary hyperthyroidism (raised TSH and raised levels of thyroid hormones) is very rare.
> • For unusual presentations see Table 14.6.

CASE HISTORY: 14.2

A 60 year old male presented with effort angina and gradually increasing hoarseness. History and examination revealed mental sluggishness, scanty eye brows, puffiness around eyes, intolerance to cold and bradycardia. Knee jerk was sluggish. In this case there was strong suspicion of hypothyroidism and it was confirmed by elevated serum TSH and low T_4 levels.

> ➤ What is a better indicator of hypothyroidism, elevated TSH and T_4 in lower part of the normal range or TSH in upper part of normal range and low T_4?
> ➤ What are consequences of infiltration of different tissues by proteoglycans in hypothyroidism?
> ➤ How is T_4 replacement therapy guided by the investigations?
> ➤ Could the patient have autoimmune etiology?
> • TSH has greater diagnostic significance than T_4, and therefore elevated TSH and T_4 in the lower normal range is better indicator of primary hypothyroidism than the other alternative. Clinical features of the patient are also given lot of significance in diagnosis of hypothyroidism. In cases in which both clinical presentation as well as results of investigations, are subtle, greater reliance is placed on the clinical features. In the present case the clinical features are quite suggestive of hypothyroidism.
> • In the present case, hoarseness is caused by proteoglycan infiltration of larynx. Other tissues which may be infiltrated are tongue (slurred speech), wrist (compression of median nerve), dermis (non-pitting edema or myxedema), face (periorbital puffiness), pleura/pericardium (effusions).
> • For adjustment of the replacement therapy, it is best to keep TSH in the normal range and also to keep a watch on the clinical picture. Elevated TSH means that the treatment dose is insufficient. If desired, the metabolic status be monitored from T_4 or T_3 (former is better) levels. Elevated T_4 would mean that the dose is excessive. It may be added that after starting the therapy, the desired steady state of the hormones may not be attained rapidly. It may take a few weeks or even more. In central hypothyroidism the replacement therapy should be guided by T_4 and not by TSH levels.
> • Primary idiopathic hypothyroidism, hypothyroidism as part of PGA syndromes and hypothyroidism resulting from Hashimoto's thyroiditis have autoimmune etiology. Hashimoto's thyroiditis is diagnosed by study of autoantibodies and biopsy. Also in these hypothyroid patients presence of certain associated disorders (see the text) and study of HLA haplotype will help diagnosis of autoimmune etiology.

CASE HISTORY: 14.3

A 4 year old child was quite small compared to his age mates. Growth faltering had been noted, almost, since birth. Mile stones were delayed and dental development was poor. Thyroid gland was not palpable. Radiological examination of hand revealed poor maturation of the epiphyseal centres. His elder brother and parents were normal. The family never lived in an iodine deficient area. Level of TSH was high and that of T_4 low.

It is a typical case of sporadic neonatal hypothyroidism.

> What about size of thyroid gland in sporadic and endemic neonatal hypothyroidism?
> How do hypothyroid cases present at birth in endemic iodine deficiency areas? How does hypothyroidism in pregnancy affect fetus/neonate?
> How will T_4 replacement therapy help the child under reference.

- In endemic neonatal hypothyroidism, the thyroid gland is normal, atrophied, or goitrous. In sporadic cases the gland is generally absent or rudimentary. Only in a case of dyshormogenesis, the gland may be enlarged.
- It may be seen in a new born and is called cretinism. At birth there may be respiratory difficulty, jaundice, hoarse cry, poor feeding. The new born, later may turn out to be a deaf mute. Relation between maternal hypothyroidism and fetal thyroid status is quite poor. Hypothyroid mothers frequently deliver newborns with normal thyroid status. However, chances of hypothyroid mothers of delivering cretins is much more in areas of iodine deficiency. In such a case mother should be treated with T_4 as well as with iodine.

In a mother with Hashimoto's thyroiditis, transfer of TSH-R Ab (block) to fetus may result in agenesis of thyroid gland in the fetus or transitory neonatal hypothyroidism.

- In the present child, treatment will promote his physical growth and later his sexual growth but much intellectual development cannot be expected. If treatment is delayed by about 3 months, only 75% will achieve RQ of 90% or more. Monitoring is done by assessment of growth, bone age, physical appearance and thyroid function tests.

OBJECTIVE TYPE QUESTIONS

Pick out the wrong statement.

1. The TRH test

i) There may be blunted TRH response in euthyroid cases of Graves' disease or toxic adenoma.
ii) TRH response is often reduced in normal elderly males.
iii) TRH test is commonly used to confirm clinical hyperthyroidism.
iv) TRH test may help to establish, an adenoma as a cause of increased gonadotropin levels in a postmenopausal woman.
v) TRH test may help to establish mild deficiency of prolactin in cases of pituitary disease.

2. Sick euthyroid syndrome

i) There may be nT_4 and low T_3 with normal TSH and TSH response to TRH.
ii) The pattern at i) is easy to differentiate from hypothyroidism as T_3 is not used in diagnosis of hypothyroidism.
iii) Findings in more severe cases are low T_4, low T_3, low TSH and blunted TRH response.
iv) The pattern at iii) makes it impossible to distinguish the patient from that of pituitary hypothyroidism.
v) In a patient of primary hypothyroidism with associated illness, TSH level remains increased, although less than in a case of primary hypothyroidism without illness.
vi) Rarely levels of T_4 and FT_4I are both increased in risk euthyroid syndrome.

3. Goitre (multinodular)

i) In elderly, euthyroid state may be difficult to confirm as manifestations of thyrotoxicosis are vague or atypical.
ii) T_4 and T_3 may only be near the upper limit of the normal range in toxic nodular goitre.
iii) T_3 is reduced in normal elderly.
iv) The best index of euthyroid state is measurable serum TSH level by a sensitive assay procedure.
v) Multinodularity is more common in Hashimoto's disease than the multinodular goitre.
vi) If a prominent single nodule is present, carcinoma thyroid will have to be excluded.

4. Central hypothyroidism

i) At the first level serum T_4, and free T_4 (or free T_4 index) must be at least low normal.
ii) The test profile at i) in the presence of clinical features of hypothyroidism and some other evidence of pituitary deficiency is an adequate evidence of hypothyroidism.
iii) With evidence at ii), further support may be provided by showing that TSH level is not increased, although, in some cases (hypothalamic defect) slight increase of TSH (bioinactive) may be there.
iv) In the syndrome of TBG deficiency, there is low T_4, elevated RT_3U, low to low normal free T_4 index and normal TSH.
v) In euthyroid sick syndrome, there is low T_4, low free T_4 index and increased TSH.

5. Hypothyroidism

i) Hypothyroidism in a neonate may manifest as

persistence of physiological jaundice, a hoarse cry, constipation and delayed mile stones.

ii) In the elderly, early symptoms are vague (fatigue, cold intolerance, constipation, stiffness, menorrhagia, slowing of motor and intellectual activity and increase of weight), and could be attributed to ageing, Parkinson's disease, depression or Alzheimer's disease.

iii) Plasma TSH is single most important test useful in diagnosis of hypothyroidism.

iv) In the primary cases, T_4 is decreased more than T_3, since increased TSH causes relatively, more secretion of T_3 than T_4.

v) In primary hypothyroidism reduced ^{123}I uptake by thyroid may also be used for diagnosis.

vi) In subclinical hypothyroidism, T_3 and T_4 levels are normal and serum TSH and its response to TRH is increased.

vii) Subclinical hypothyroidism is most commonly seen in patients of Hashimoto's disease and patients of Graves' disease treated with ^{131}I or surgery.

6. Goitre

i) Iodine deficiency, ingestion of goitrogens or some defect in biosynthesis of thyroid hormones may cause their deficiency as per tissue needs.

ii) Because of reduced thyroid hormones, TSH level increases to increase functional thyroid mass.

iii) With increase in thyroid cell mass (goitre) the thyroid hormone output becomes adequate and patient remains euthyroid.

iv) In severe cases inspite of increased TSH and presence of goitre, there is hypothyroidism.

v) In elderly patients with multinodular goitre, treatment is given only if basal TSH level is normal.

7. Hypothyroidism

i) In all forms of hypothyroidism there is decrease of T_4 and FT_4.

ii) In both primary (thyroid disease) and secondary (pituitary disease) hypothyroidism serum T_3 remains normal or is only slightly reduced.

iii) Serum cholesterol level is increased only in primary cases.

iv) RAIU is low to high in goitrous cases but uniformly low in thyroprivic cases.

v) In primary thyroprivic cases pernicious anemia occurs in some patients.

8. Iodine and thyroid

i) Excess iodine ingested by mother may produce goitrous hypothyroidism in fetus due to iodine

sensitivity of fetal thyroid.

ii) Acute excessive iodine administration in a normal person may produce transitory or long lasting hypothyroidism with or without goitre.

iii) Many patients of Graves' disease especially after surgery or radioiodine treatment also become sensitive to inhibitory effect of iodine and develop hypothyroidism.

iv) However, in iodine deficient areas excess iodine produces no harmful effect.

v) Incidence of Hashimoto's thyroiditis, has increased in United States probably by increased iodine ingestion.

9. Hyperthyroidism

i) In Graves' disease antibodies are produced which stimulate TSH receptors (thyroid stimulating immunoglobulins; TSIs also called thyroid stimulating antibodies, (TSAbs).

ii) In Graves' disease blocking antibodies may also be produced which inhibit binding of TSH to TSH receptors called TSH binding inhibitory immunoglobulins (TBIIs).

iii) Patient may be euthyroid if there is dominance of TBIIs over TSAbs.

iv) Hormonal profiles in hyperthyroidism are only two; elevated T_3 and T_4 and elevated T_3 with normal T_4.

v) In Graves' disease, prolonged remission is likely if there is reversion of TRH stimulation test, reduction of gland size, normalization of T_3 and disappearance of above antibodies from serum (together called TSH receptor antibodies, TRAbs).

10. Toxic multinodular goitre

i) It is a disease of the elderly.

ii) Ophthalmopathy is rare.

iii) Patient may present with congestive heart failure or arrhythmia.

iv) Patient may present with features of myopathy.

v) Often T_4 and FT_4I are only slightly above normal.

vi) Subnormal response to TRH confirms thyrotoxicosis while normal response does not exclude it.

11. Thyrotoxicosis

i) Tachycardia, tremor, irritability, fatigue (features of thyrotoxicosis), can also occur in anxiety states.

ii) In anxiety states weight loss occurs with anorexia.

iii) Hypermetabolism, tachycardia, sweating occur both in thyrotoxicosis as well as pheochromocytoma.

iv) Skin is warm and moist in thyrotoxicosis and cold and clammy in anxiety states.

v) Thyrotoxicosis may require differentiation from myopathic disorders.

vi) All patients with unexplained cardiac failure or atrial arrythmias should be investigated for thyrotoxicosis.

vii) Spastic type of ophthalmopathy may be seen in diabetes, myopathies and mysasthenia gravis.

viii) Ophthalmopathy with proptosis (exophthalmos) occurs only in thyrotoxicosis.

12. Thyrotoxicosis

i) A diffuse symmetric goitre of small or moderate size suggests diagnosis of Graves' disease.

ii) Hydatidiform mole or choriocarcinoma of uterus or testis can also cause diffuse symmetric enlargement of thyroid gland.

iii) Increased ^{123}I uptake may help diagnosis of thyrotoxicosis due to ectopic thyroid tissue.

iv) Thyrotoxicosis and hyperthyroidism carry the same meaning.

v) Serum levels of thyroglobulin are increased in Graves' disease and thyroiditis; reduced in factitious hyperthyroidism.

13. Thyroid adenoma

i) Unifocal follicular adenoma is most common.

ii) It grows slowly over years.

iii) Initially, its basal secretion is independant of TSH, although, it is stimulated by TSH.

iv) Initially, on scintiscan, it appears as a warm nodule (accumulates radioiodine more than the surrounding thyroid tissue).

v) With growth and increased activity of the nodule, TSH is suppressed, producing hot nodule associated with chemical thyrotoxicosis.

vi) Terms warm nodule and hot nodule are used interchangeably.

vii) Finally, toxic adenoma results producing clinical thyrotoxicosis.

14. Thyroid nodule

i) A solitary nodule is more likely to be malignant than one nodule among many.

ii) A hot nodule is less likely to be malignant.

iii) A cystic lesion is less likely to be malignant.

iv) Elevated level of serum thyroglobulin is specific for thyroid carcinoma.

v) Benign nodules are more common in women.

vi) History of radiation exposure to neck (years back) makes malignancy more likely.

15. Thyroid nodule

i) FNC requires presence of an experienced cytologist.

ii) FNC may show that the lesion is malignant.

iii) FNC may show that the lesion is benign

iv) FNC may show that the lesion is follicular.

v) Follicular lesions are considered as malignant and removed.

vi) Results of FNC may be inconclusive.

vii) In inconclusive cases keep a check on size of the nodule.

16. Neonatal hypothyroidism

i) Primary causes (aplasia, ectopic gland, inborn errors, iodine deficiency) are mostly responsible (about 86%).

ii) In endemic areas of iodine deficiency neonatal hypothyroidism incidence is much higher.

iii) Secondary causes (pituitary/hypothalamic disorder, TBG deficiency) are much less common.

iv) Transient hypothyroidism (premature, SGA, placental transfer of drugs/antibodies) (about 10%).

v) 2-4% of cases are missed in neonatal screening.

vi) Prenatal diagnosis is not required.

ANSWERS

1. No.(iii). Because of availability of sensitive TSH assay, the test is not commonly used. However, it can be used in borderline cases, keeping in mind that it may give false positive results in some elderly persons and also that it may diagnose some clinically euthyroid cases of Graves' disease/toxic adenoma (see nos. i&ii). The test also cannot reliably separate pituitary hypothyroidism from hypothalamic hypothyroidism.

2. No.(iv). In sick euthyroid syndrome rT_3 is increased whereas its level is reduced in pituitary hypothyroidism. One should avoid thyroid function tests during an illness since difficulties arise in their interpretation.

3. No.(v). Multinodularity is more a feature of nontoxic multinodular goitre than Hashimoto's disease. In the latter condition presence of high titres of certain antibodies (anti-microsomal, also called antiperoxidase and antithyroglobulin) may help diagnosis.

4. No.(v). TSH should be low or normal. TBG deficiency and euthyroid syndrome become significant in differential diagnosis in isolated deficiencies of TSH than in panhypopituitarism when some additional evidence of pituitary hormone deficiency may be present.

5. No.(v). It is not a useful test. In thyroprivic cases

^{123}I uptake is reduced but it is difficult to distinguish it from the lower normal limit, which itself is quite low. In goitrous cases ^{123}I uptake is low to increased.

6. No.(ii). In early stages TSH level is normal. However, as gland is hormone depleted, its responsiveness to normal TSH increases leading to increase in functional mass of the gland.

7. No.(ii). It occurs only in primary cases since compensatory hypersecretion of TSH promotes increased relative secretion of T_3.

8. No.(iv). It may produce hyperthyroidism due to excessive hormone production from autonomous areas of the gland.

9. No.(iv). In T_4 toxicosis, T_4 level is elevated while T_3 is normal. It is likely to occur in an old/ill patient, previously exposed to high doses of iodine.

10. No.(vi). It is the other way round. A normal response excludes thyrotoxicosis but subnormal response does not, always confirm thyrotoxicosis. Many euthyroid patients with multinodular goitre show a subnormal response. Response is reduced with age as well as presence of multinodular goitre. Toxic multinodular goitre is confirmed if at its basal secretion, TSH is undetectable and level is subnormal in TRH test.

11. No.(viii). It can occur in a number of disorders including, retrobulbar tumors, cavernous sinus thrombosis, uremia, accelerated hypertension, chronic obstructive pulmonary disease, Cushing's syndrome, chronic alcoholism and others.

12. No.(iv). Thyrotoxiocosis (metabolic state produced by elevated level of thyroid hormones) can occur in the absence of hyperthyroidism (increased hormone synthesis by thyroid gland). It may occur in subacute thyroiditis or chronic thyroiditis (due to leakage of hormones during gland degradation) or thyrotoxicosis factitia. In all these conditions ^{123}I uptake by the thyroid gland is suppressed. Same is also true when ectopic thyroid tissue is cause of thyrotoxicosis.

13. No.(vi). The term hot nodule means when radioiodine is taken up by adenoma only and not the surrounding thyroid tissue (relative atrophy due to suppressed TSH). Hot nodule may produce only suppression of TSH (chemical thyrotoxicosis) or overt disease.

14. No.(iv). Elevation of thyroglobulin is not specific for differentiating thyroid carcinoma, as it is also associated with benign adenoma, simple goitre and Graves' disease. However elevated serum calcitonin is a good tumor marker for medullary thyroid carcinoma.

15. No.(v). Such lesions are subjected to radionuclide scan. The cold lesions are removed and the hot ones are evaluated for hyperthyroidism.

16. No.(vi). If discovered by study of amniotic fluid iodothyronines, weekly intraamniotic injections of T_4 may take care of some aspects of development.

CHAPTER 15

Functions and Disorders
of the Adrenal Gland

THE ADRENAL GLAND

There are two adrenal glands, one on either side, on the upper pole of the kidney. Each gland has two distinct parts, each with different histology and embryonic origin. The outer cortex comprises about 90% of the gland and almost surrounds (except at hilum) the centrally located medulla. Medulla is a part of sympathetic nervous system and releases adrenaline (80%) and nor adrenaline (20%). Approximate secretions (mg/24h) of major hormones of adrenal cortex are; glucocorticoids (cortisol 10, corticosterone 2.5), mineralocorticoids (aldosterone 0.15) and androgens (dehydroepiandrosterone 2.0). Adrenal cortex has three histologic zones, zona glomerulosa (the outermost), zona fasciculata (the middle zone) and zona reticularis (the inner most zone). Aldosterone is produced by zona glomerulosa and its secretion is regulated by renin-angiotensin mechanism. The other two zones produce glucocorticoids and androgens regulated by hypothalamic-pituitary - adrenal axis. Hormones of both the parts of the adrenal gland help the body to adapt to different types of stresses. Life is, however, possible without medulla but not without cortex.

Regulation of secretion of cortisol

Cortisol is produced under the action of CRH and ACTH (Fig. 15.1). Stresses like fever, infection, trauma, exercise, hypoglycemia, and anxiety, exert influence at hypothalamus to increase secretion of CRH. There is circadian rhythm in secretion of CRH, ACTH and cortisol (peak secretion occurs in early morning and goes on declining with the lowest level at about midnight. Fig. 15.1 also shows relation between hypothalamic-pituitary - adrenal axis and the immune system. Cortisol exercises negative feed back effect at hypothalamus and pituitary to regulate secretion of CRH and ACTH. The following are based on this feed back effect:

i) Dexamethasone (acts like cortisol) administration inhibits ACTH formation from pituitary but not from an ectopic source. This is the principle of high dose dexamethasone suppression test.

ii) On reduction of cortisol formation, increased formation of ACTH occurs. This explains increased ACTH production in primary adrenal failure. Further removal of hypertrophic and hypersecreting adrenal gland increases secretion of CRH, stimulating ACTH production and causing pigmentation (Nelson's syndrome).

iii) Use of therapeutic amounts of cortisol or some similar steroid, in patients, tends to suppress ACTH production. If administration is continued for a long time and then suddenly stopped, reduced endogenous secretion of cortisol will result. Thus the steroid administration should not be stopped suddenly after a prolonged therapy.

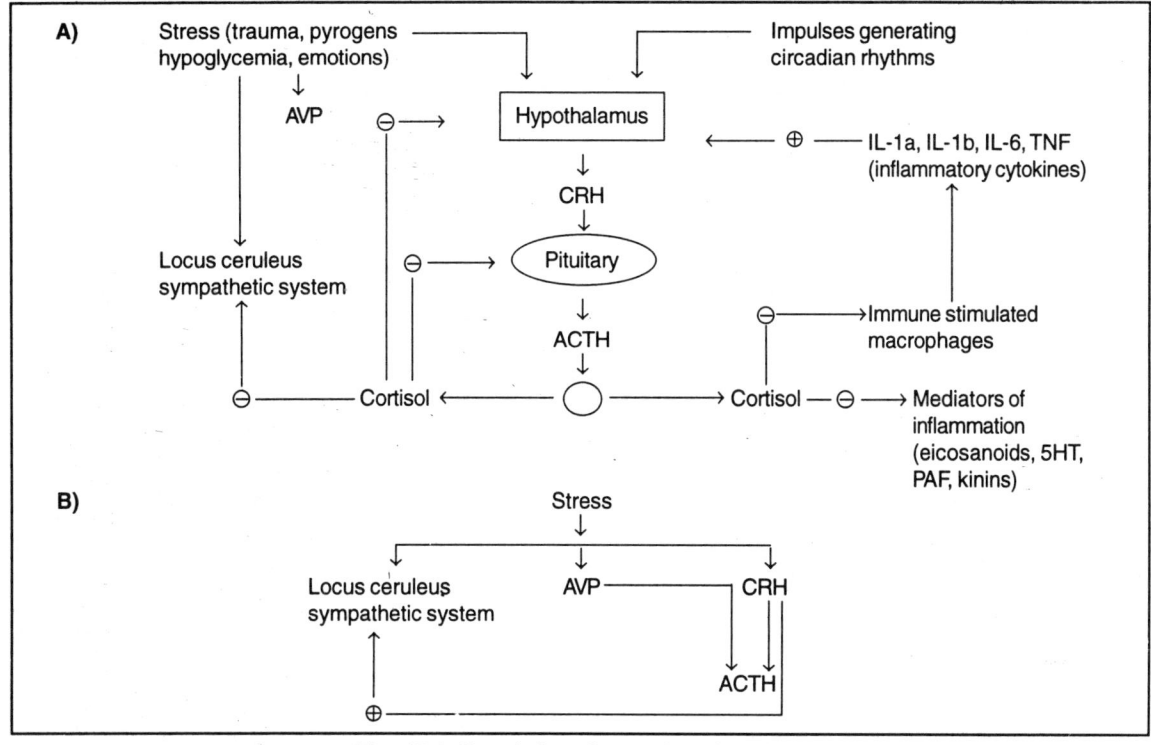

Fig. 15.1. Regulation of secretion of cortisol.

- Note effect of stress on release of CRH, AVP and stimulation of sympathetic system; the immune adrenal relationship and feed back effect of cortisol.
B) AVP enhances effect of CRH on secretion of ACTH; CRH also activates sympathetic system
- Endogenous opioids and exogenous opiates block secretion of ACTH by corticotrophs (also inhibit release of TSH and gonadotropins); on the other hand increase secretion of GH and PRL. Amenorrhea is common in narcotic addicts.

Regulation of aldosterone secretion (Fig. 15.2)

Juxta glomerular apparatus consists of the renin secreting cells of the afferent arteriole entering glomerulus and part of distal convoluted tubule (macula densa) closely applied to the secretory region of the afferent arteriole. This structure is involved in secretion of renin under three influences: i) when reduced amount of blood flows through the afferent arteriole (in malignant hypertension, hypovolemia or renal artery stenosis); ii) with reduced sodium delivery to distal tubules (reduced GFR and sodium depletion; iii) with increased sympathetic activity. Also read objective type question no.11 in Chapter 2.

Renin has a specific proteolytic action on a protein, angiotensinogen produced by liver generating a decapeptide called angiotensin I. Angiotensin I is converted into angiotensin II by angiotensin converting enzyme (ACE) located on luminal surface of vascular endothelium, most abundantly, in lungs. Angiotensin II stimulates secretion of aldosterone by cells of zona glomerulosa. Raised serum K^+ level is a direct stimulus for aldosterone secretion.

Biosynthesis of adrenal hormones

The pathways for synthesis of cortisol, aldosterone and adrenal androgens are shown in Fig. 15.3. Cholesterol is obtained from circulating LDL as well as by biosynthesis in the cortical cells. The side-chain cleavage enzyme (converting cholesterol into pregnenolone) is the key enzyme and is stimulated by ACTH.

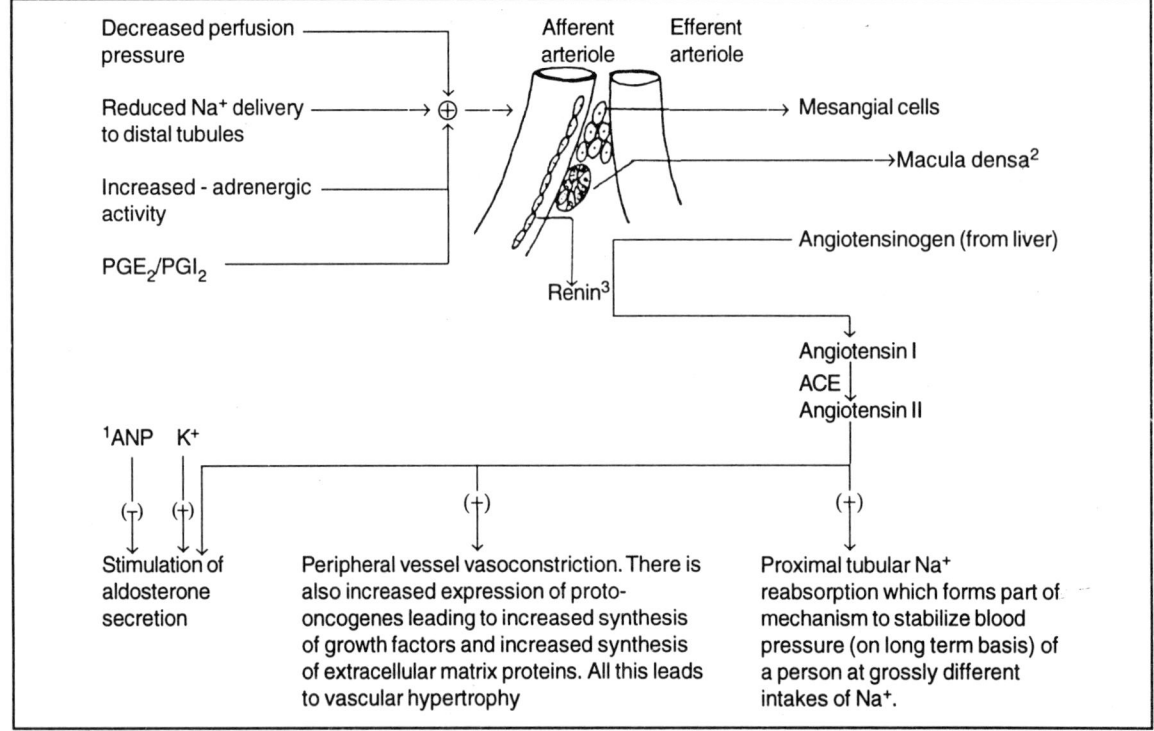

Fig. 15.2. Stimulation of JG apparatus and actions of angiotensin II.

[1] Atrial distension or Na^+ load causes release of atrial natriuretic peptide (ANP) from atrial myocytes. It promotes sodium excretion by: i) increasing GFR; ii) inhibiting Na^+ reabsorption in proximal tribules; iii) inhibiting release of aldosterone. ANP also causes arteriolar and venous dilatation by opposing effects of angiotensin II and sympathetic stimulation.

[2] Senses Na^+ delivery to distal tubules and alters GFR via renin release (local A-II constricting afferent arteriole).

[3] The initiating enzyme in the renin angiotensin system (RAS) is cleaved from prorenin in several tissues, although, the major site is JG apparatus. Thus two renin angiotensin systems (functionally similar and perhaps interrelated) are there. Besides regulation of aldosterone RAS is related to coronary artery disease (CAD) and essential hypertension, for the latter local angiotensin II (A-II) produces growth factors (causing vascular hypertrophy) and local vascular regulators (producing vasoconstriction) including endothelni and prostaglandins.

- Angiotensin II reduces Na^+ excretion by modifying renal hemodynamics, by causing secretion of aldosterone and by increasing proximal tubular Na^+ reabsorption.

- Aldosterone releasing effect of angiotensin II is enhanced by hyponatremia or hyperkalemia.

- Na^+ retention is self limited under aldosterone excess due to aldosterone escape caused by increased GFR and by release of natriuretic peptides. K^+ excretion is not limited however.

Functions of adrenal cortex

Adrenal cortex plays an important role in bodily reactions to different types of stresses. Cortisol helps to provide fuel molecules (glucose, amino acids, fatty acids) and molecules needed for anabolic processes (amino acids, nucleotides) in tissues needing repair (during stress), by its actions on intermediary metabolism. Glucose uptake is reduced in a number of tissues like muscle, skin,

connective tissue, adipose tissue, bone and lymphoid tissue. This leads to increase in level of glucose in plasma. Lipolysis is promoted in adipose tissue to increase plasma fatty acid level. Similarly, levels of amino acids and nucleotides are increased in plasma by actions of cortisol on metabolism of proteins and nucleic acids in most of the above mentioned tissues.

Through a number of effects, cortisol helps to

maintain cardiovascular system during a stress. Besides retention of Na^+ (to increase plasma volume) by weak binding of cortisol to aldosterone receptors, cortisol increases synthesis of angiotensinogen and also sensitivity of tissues to angiotensin II. Further, the hormone also enhances vasopressor actions of catecholamines.

Again in relation to stress, cortisol might also be involved in modulating secretions/actions of many other hormones.

Regulatory effects of cortisol in reducing formation of prostaglandins, leukotrienes, kinins and proteases in tissues is also physiologically significant. These compounds are produced for local functions, in tissues, in certain stresses and if produced in excessive amounts, may leak into circulation and cause circulatory decompensation.

Two other physiological actions of cortisol also need mention. First, the feedback effect at hypothalamus/pituitary and second, of promoting water

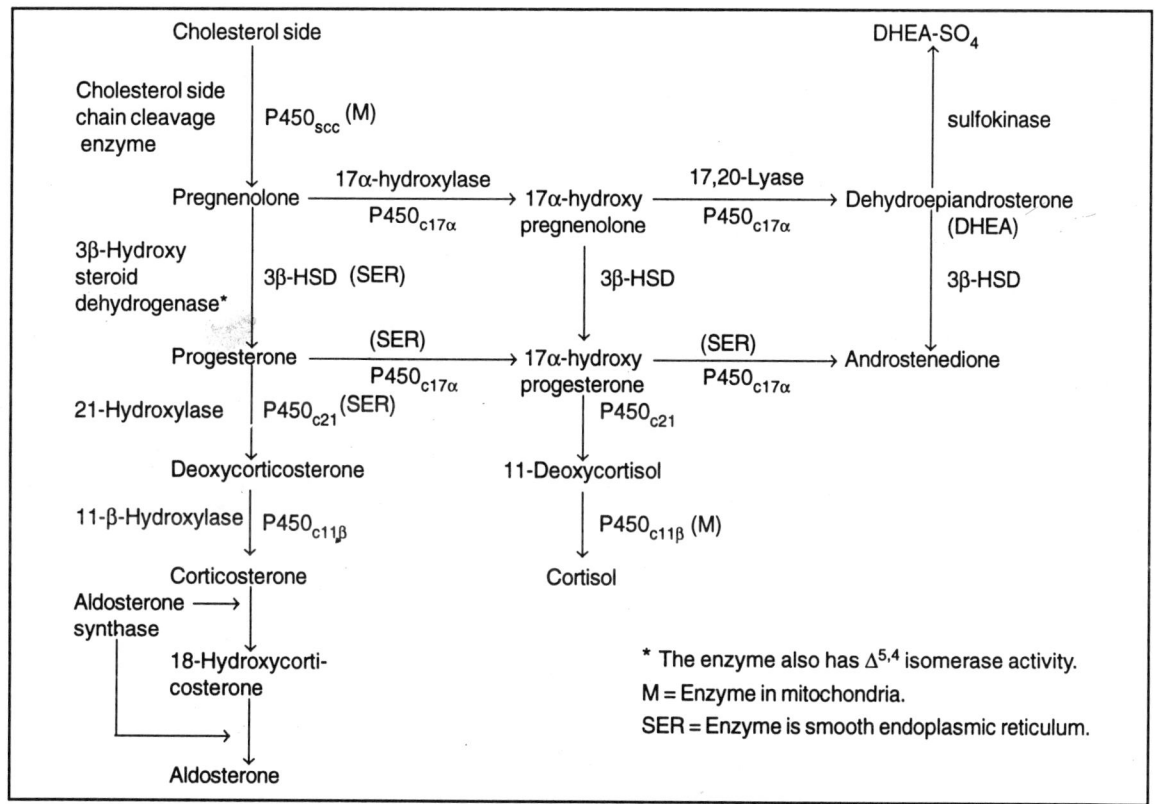

Fig. 15.3. Biosynthesis of adrenal steroids.

- The pathway shown is operative in zona fasciculata and zona reticularis. In zona glomerulosa corticosterone is formed by the same enzymes as shown; followed by formation of aldosterone by the enzyme aldosterone synthase P450$_{AS}$) only present in zona glomerulosa. Zona glomerulosa lacks P450$_{c17\alpha}$ activity.
- Major adrenal androgen is DHEA (and its sulphate); there is minimal secretion of androstenedione. But qualitatively the latter is more important as it is peripherally converted into testosterone.
- In zona fasciculata/ reticularis the main pathway is via 17-OH pregnenolone with formation of cortisol or DHEA. Pregnenolone ⟶ 17-OH pregnenolone ⟶ DHEA is called Δ^5 pathway. Pregnenolone ⟶ progesterone ⟶ androstenedione is called Δ^4 pathway. The latter pathway is important in testes and ovaries.
- 21-Hydroxylase and 11-β-hydroxylase are absent from gonads.
- In case of P450$_{c17\alpha}$, deficiency of 17, 20 lyase activity may occur independent of deficiency of 17-α hydroxylase activity (see Chapter 17).

excretion by the kidney probably by having a role in maintaining GFR and other effects (Fig. 13.7).

Therapeutic use of cortisol and cortisol like synthetic corticosteroids

Glucocorticoids block the inflammatory process by inhibiting generation of different mediators of inflammation like prostaglandins, leukotrienes (by inhibiting phospholipase A_2) and kinins (by inhibiting plasminogen activator). The antiallergic actions of glucocorticoids are because these compounds block stimulation of mast cells by antigen-IgE complexes. Glucocorticoids are also used to prevent rejection of transplanted organs by affecting the T-cell response. These are also useful in treatment of autoimmune disorders which are caused by an imbalance between different sub-types of T cells. In congenital adrenal hyperplasia, because of cortisol deficiency, the aberrant steroidogenesis is stimulated (absence of feedback by cortisol). Cortisol administration reduces synthesis of abnormal steroids, when given as replacement therapy.

Problems associated with therapeutic use of steroids

During therapeutic use of glucocorticoids, certain clinical conditions may get worsened, because of metabolic and other actions of these drugs. Patient should be screened for a number of clinical disorders, before starting steroid therapy. These disorders include, any chronic infection (especially tuberculosis), osteoporosis, diabetes mellitus, gastritis (or gastrointestinal ulcers), hypertension or some cardiovascular disease and psychological disorders. Patient should also be monitored for development of any of these disorders. During therapeutic use of steroids, patient's own hypothalamic-pituitary-adrenal axis is suppressed. Therefore, for any stressful period during steroid therapy, the dose of the drug should be increased.

When glucocorticoids are used for some therapeutic purpose, for a long time, some features of Cushing's syndrome are produced which are reversed on withdrawl of the drug. Further, glucocorticoids should never be withdrawn suddenly after prolonged therapy as it may result in acute adrenal insufficiency.

Actions of aldosterone

Aldosterone stimulates reabsorption of Na^+ by distal convoluted tubules and collecting ducts in the kidney and in exchange, promotes secretions of K^+ and H^+. In this way, aldosterone has a very important role in maintaining Na^+ and K^+ homeostasis and ECF/plasma volume. Stimulated renin-angiotensin system increases blood pressure by increasing plasma volume (via increased aldosterone secretion) and by vasopressor action of angiotensin-II.

Adrenal androgens

Dehydroepiandrosterone (DHAE), its sulfated form (DHAE sulfate) and androstenedione are weak androgens. The latter is partly converted into testosterone in adipose tissue and elsewhere (Fig. 17.3). In females adrenal cortex is an important source of androgens. These help prepubertal general body growth and growth of axillary and pubic hair in females, at puberty.

Renin angiotensin system (RAS) and coronary artery disease (CAD) and hypertention

Besides regulating aldosterone secretion A-II has other actions related to CAD and essential hypertension (Fig. 15.2). Certain polymorphic mutations in ACE (Chapter 18), angiotensin II type receptor and angiotensinogen predispose to the disorders.

LABORATORY EVALUATION OF DISORDERS OF ADRENAL CORTEX

Plasma ACTH, cortisol and 24h urinary cortisol excretion

ACTH is measured using a sensitive immunometric assay. ACTH, however, is very labile and the samples should be estimated without delay and contact with glass should be avoided. The method has poor sensitivity and percision at low concentrations. Further any stress, greatly affects the plasma level. Immunoassay of cortisol has better specificity than the fluorimetric assay (maximum interference comes from corticosterone) and the protein binding assay (cortisone, 11-deoxy cortisol, progesterone, all interfere). In immunoassay, the specificity depends upon the antibody used (its cross reactivity with other steroids). Conjugated metabolite (which may accumulate in serum in renal failure), also binds like cortisol. The HPLC method, however, is very sensitive and there is possibility of simultaneous estimation of some other steroids. The HPLC method is capable of automatization.

In severe adrenal insufficiency, both plasma level and urinary excretion of cortisol are markedly reduced. The latter test is preferred as it better correlates with free plasma cortisol level. With estimations of plasma cortisol and free cortisol, in urine, estimation of 17-hydroxycorticosteroids has become obsolete. It is important to keep a check on proper collection of urine (urine creatinine may be estimated, simultaneously). In mild deficiency, plasma and urine cortisol levels overlap with the normal ranges and therefore diagnosis of both primary and secondary adrenal insufficiencies should be established, only with ACTH stimulation test (see below). Plasma ACTH level, in isolation is not used for diagnosis of primary or secondary adrenal insufficiency because of overlap with normal values. This estimation, however, is helpful in differentiating between primary and secondary adrenal insufficiencies. Plasma ACTH and β-lipoprotein levels are elevated in primary adrenal insufficiency and plasma ACTH level is low or low normal in secondary insufficiency. Many times clinical features alone help this differentiation.

For Cushing's syndrome, also, because of circadian rhythm, plasma cortisol or ACTH, in isolation are not much helpful for diagnosis. Lack of evening fall of cortisol level in Cushing's syndrome, may however, be useful. ACTH estimation may be helpful in finding cause of Cushing's syndrome.

The dynamic tests

The rapid ACTH stimulation test is used to screen patients for both primary and secondary adrenal insufficiency. The test explores the adrenal reserve. In the test 0.25 mg of cosyntropin is given intramuscularly or intravenously and plasma cortisol levels are measured before and half an hour and one hour, after drug administration. Compared to normals the cortisol response is reduced in adrenal insufficiency. Reduction of response is more in primary cases than secondary ones. The reason for reduced response in secondary cases is atrophy of adrenal cortex (as zona glomerulosa is not atrophied, aldosterone secretion is not affected), in ACTH deficiency. It however, takes about 3 months for adrenal cortex to atrophy in the absence of ACTH. If the test is performed before this period the expected response may not occur. Further in partial cases of secondary adrenal insufficiency, this test remains normal and tests evaluating pituitary reserve (see below) are needed.

The rapid ACTH test, does not provide maximal stimulation. For that prolonged ACTH infusion (for 24h or longer) is needed. This test helps to discover patients of primary adrenal insufficiency with only mild loss of adrenal reserve (not evident in rapid ACTH stimulation test). Patients of only mild loss of pituitary reserve (secondary adrenal insufficiency) are not expected to lose adrenal reserve.

Testing of pituitary-adrenal axis or pituitary reserve

The ACTH stimulation test is used to diagnose adrenal reserve. The stimulation tests using insulin induced hypoglycemia, the CRH test and the metyrapone test, evaluate pituitary reserve. Metyrapone inhibits 11-hydroxylase enzyme, inhibiting formation of cortisol from 11-deoxycortisol, tending to increase ACTH (removal from feedback inhibitory effect). Patients with poor pituitary reserve may fail to increase ACTH and suffer from severe cortisol deficiency since drug has already reduced cortisol level. Thus the test is suitable only in cases of mild loss of pituitary reserve without loss of adrenal reserve.

The metyrapone test is more useful for differential diagnosis of Cushing's syndrome (as overnight metyrapone test) and may be superior to the high dose dexamethasone suppression test for the same purpose (see below).

The dexamethasone suppression test

The drug dexamethasone inhibits pituitary (like cortisol) to reduce ACTH secretion. Urinary excretion of cortisol or 17-OH corticosteroids is estimated, both before and after drug intake to know presence or absence of suppression. In the low dose, the test is used to diagnose presence of Cushing's syndrome and in high dose, to find cause of the disorder (see under Cushing's syndrome).

DISORDERS OF ADRENAL CORTEX

In Addison's disease there is failure of function of adrenal cortex and in Cushing's syndrome there is hyperactivity of adrenal cortex (except of zona glomerulosa). In aldosteronism there is increased secretion of, only aldosterone. Congenital, specific enzymatic deficiencies in the pathway of adrenal steroidogenesis are also known.

Addison's disease

Important causes of adrenal insufficiency are autoimmune atrophy, infection (tuberculosis, viral) and metastatic invasion. Secondary insufficiency due to exogenous or endogenous steroids is also common (Table 15.1). In about half the patients, there is evidence of autoimmune damage and in some of these cases, there may be associated evidence of damage to some other endocrine gland and/or presence of pernicious anemia and/or vitiligo (polyglandular autoimmune syndromes I and II). Panhypopituitarism is less common a cause of adrenal insufficiency. In AIDS patients, there may be evidence of reduced adrenal reserve. Some drugs like rifampin, phenytoin, ketoconazole and opiates also increase chances of development of adrenal insufficiency. Adrenal insufficiency may occur in chronic (gradual damage) or acute form. In chronic cases, exposure to some severe stress (trauma, infection, surgery) may produce acute adrenal insufficiency. Important causes are given in Table 15.1.

Cortisol deficiency causes hypoglycemia and muscle weakness. Aldosterone deficiency leads to electrolyte abnormalities (low Na^+, raised K^+), and acidosis which produce gastrointestinal manifestations like anorexia, nausea and vomiting and also contribute to muscular weakness. Due to Na^+ deficiency there is hypovolemia which leads to low blood pressure, shock and azotemia (Fig. 15.4). Increased body pigmentation occurs, only, in primary cases of adrenal failure.

Cortisol deficiency also leads to poor tolerance to stress. Such patients when exposed to stress (infection, trauma) are likely to go into acute adrenal failure with severe shock and hypotension, fever, intractable gastrointestinal manifestations leading to severe dehydration, hyponatremia and hyperkalemia.

Diagnosis

In chronic form early features are asthenia, anorexia and weight loss; pigmentation if present, will be quite suggestive of the disorder. In early cases postural hypotension is more common than actual hypotension. In severe cases dehydration, hyponatremia, hyperkalemia, eosinophilia and relative lymphocytosis may be present.

X-ray examination (adrenal calcification in tuberculosis) and CT-scan also help. The latter investigation may show an enlarged gland (infection, granuloma, hemorrhage or malignancy) or atrophic gland.

In many cases of Addison's disease, plasma and urinary cortisol levels are only in the lower part of the normal range as only adrenal reserve is reduced.

Table 15.1. Primary and secondary causes of chronic adrenal insufficiency

Primary insufficiency:	Secondary insufficiency:
• Autoimmune	• Therapeutic use of steroids.
- Polyglandular deficiencies type I and II	• Cortisol deficiency in congenital adrenal hyperplasia.
- Sporadic	• Panhypopituitarism
• Tubercular/due to other infection	
• Metastatic tumor	
• Amyloidosis	
- Less common	- More common
- Total cortex is destroyed; there is deficiency of cortisol as well as aldosterone.	- There is no deficiency of aldosterone.
- Pigmentation due to increased ACTH levels.	- No pigmentation as ACTH level is low.

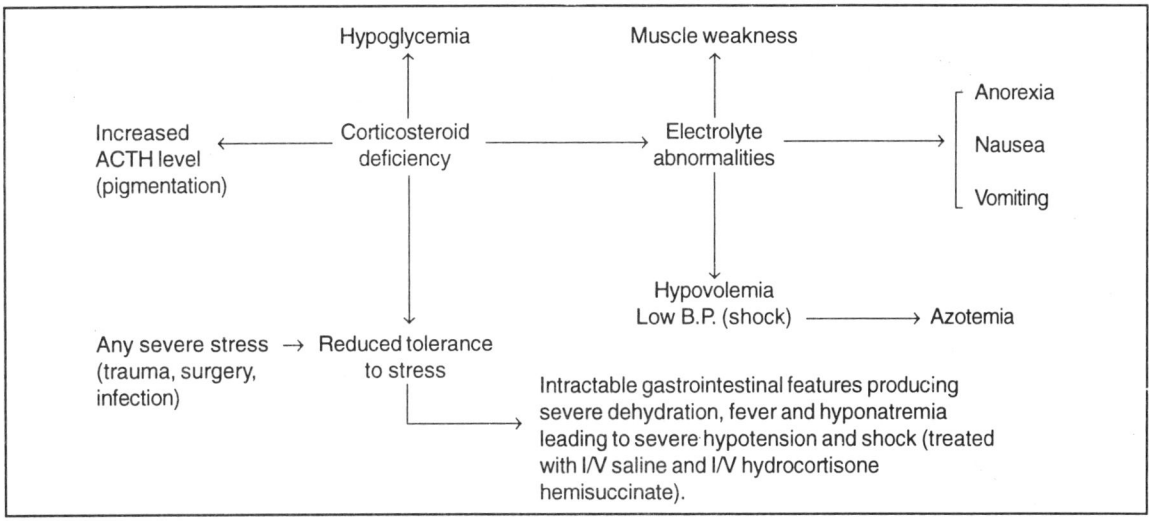

Fig. 15.4. Important features of Addison's disease.

- Five common features of chronic adrenal insufficiency are asthenia, weight loss, anorexia (with or without nausea and vomiting), recently increased pigmentations and hypotension (especially postural hypotension).
- Severe dehydration, hyponatremia and hyperkalemia are characteristics of primary insufficiency cases. Pigmentation, also, is not a feature of secondary adrenal insufficiency.

In such cases the rapid ACTH stimulation test is helpful. If the rapid ACTH test indicates adrenal deficiency and there is also other strong suggestive evidence of the disorder, no further confirmation is required. Otherwise, the long synacthen test is done to confirm the diagnosis. To differentiate between primary and secondary adrenal failure, estimation of plasma ACTH is very useful. In primary cases ACTH is raised due to absence of negative feed back effect of cortisol. In the secondary cases, ACTH is low, there is near normal level of plasma aldosterone and there may be evidence of deficiency of some other pituitary hormone. It may also be recalled that in secondary cases, there is no pigmentation and dehydration and hyponatremia are only mild.

The hypothalamic-pituitary-adrenal axis is suppressed in long term steroid therapy. There is reduced release of ACTH and also failure of adrenal response to ACTH. The baseline levels of cortisol and ACTH are low. The rapid ACTH stimulation test is often adequate to assess the suppression and also (after drug withdrawl) recovery from suppression (which may take days to months). Other stimulation tests (insulin hypoglycemia or metyrapone stimulation test) are less often, required.

Patients of Addison's disease need life long therapy with cortisol and 9α-fluorocortisol (some patients may become symptom free with cortisol and high salt intake). Adequacy of drugs is best judged by clinical assessment of the patient. Excessive cortisol may cause weight gain and features resembling Cushing's syndrome. Excessive intake of 9α-fluorocortisol will cause hypokalemia and hypertension. Patient should be aware that any stress (trauma, surgery, infection) will increase his requirement of the drug. Acute adrenal failure is a medical emergency and treated with normal saline and 5% dextrose (for hypoglycemia). Hydrocortisone hemisuccinate is added to the fluids. Once vomiting is controlled, oral therapy is started.

Cushing's syndrome (Fig. 15.5)

This condition is produced by increased secretion of cortisol. It is, most commonly caused by bilateral adrenal hyperplasia, resulting from increased secretion of ACTH, resulting from some hypothalamic

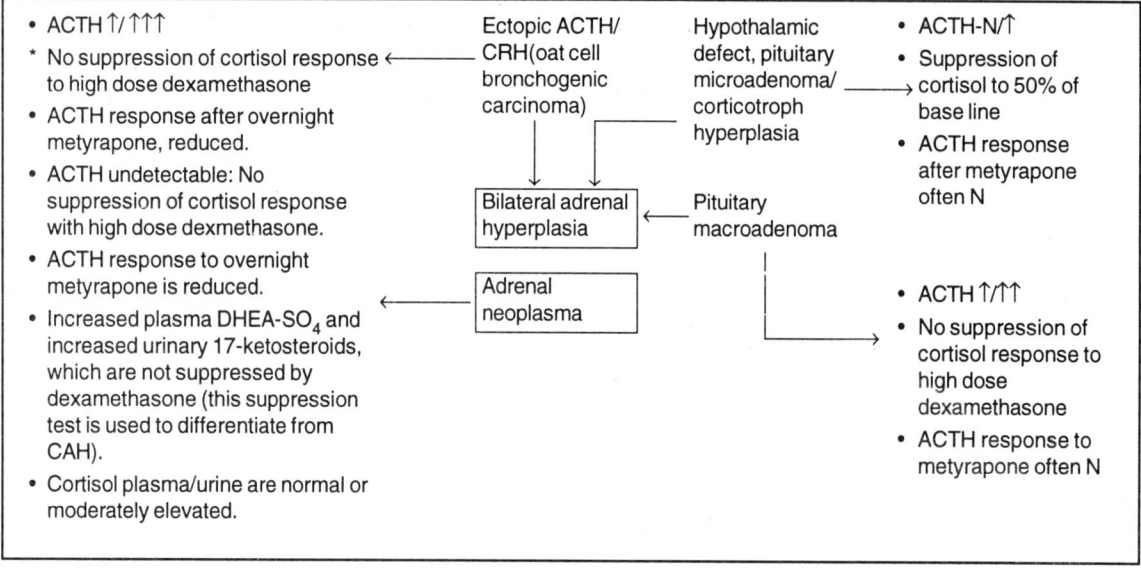

Fig. 15.5. Important causes of Cushings syndrome with diagnostic feature (investigative).

- Besides metyrapone stimulation test, CRH stimulation test is also used. In the CRH test no response is obtained in the ectopic cases and adrenal neoplasm.
- Frequency of different causes of Cushing's syndrome: Cushing's disease 50-80%; ectopic ACTH cases 15%; ectopic CRH <1%; adrenal adenoma 9%; carcinoma 8% and nodular hyperplasia <2%.

defect (in many cases there may be basophil cell microadenoma formation due to CRH excess, in others there may be hyperplasia of corticotropic cells).

There are also other causes of bilateral adrenal hyperplasia but the cases of the above etiology are most common and their incidence is three times more in women than in men, in the age group of 30 to 40 years. Other less common causes of bilateral adrenal hyperplasia are primary pituitary macroadenoma, and ectopic formation of ACTH or CRH. Common cause of ectopic ACTH formation is oat cell bronchogenic carcinoma (Table 16.1). Less commonly, it may be produced by carcinoids or pheochromocytomas. About 20 to 25% patients of Cushing's syndrome are caused by adrenal neoplasms. These adrenal tumors are usually unilateral and about 50% are malignant.

A small group of bilateral adrenal hyperplasia patients appear to have autonomous cortisol secretion (like adrenal tumors) but with variable increase in ACTH levels (Cushing's syndrome related nodular hyperplasia). About 50% of these patients show

autosomal dominant inheritance. Test profile of these cases lies inbetween those of Cushing's disease (the term Cushing's disease is used if cause lies in hypothalamus/pituitary; Cushing's syndrome is a general term covering all types of cases) and adrenal tumor. These cases are treated by bilateral adrenalectomy.

Prolonged therapeutic administration of glucocorticoids produces features of Cushing's syndrome. These iatrogenic cases are infact, the commonest cause of Cushing's syndrome. Tendency to develop the disorder varies in patients. Drug intake in the evening is more likely to produce the disorder.

Diagnosis

Suspicion is based on clinical features (Table 15.2). Other associated findings are eosinopenia and lymphopenia, glucose intolerance (post prandial hyperglycemia) hypokalemia and alkalosis. Obesity in association with features like, diabetes mellitus, hirsutism, amenorrhea and muscle wasting should raise suspicion. Similarly, elderly women with osteoporosis, diabetes and mild hirsutism should also be

Table 15.2. Clinical features of Cushing's syndrome

Five most common features:
- Obesity with centripetal distribution of fat.
- Increased body weight.
- Fatiguability and muscle weakness, with greater involvement of proximal muscles.
- Hypertension
- Hirsutism

Three more specific features:
- Bruising and striae (caused by breakdown of collagen and thinning of skin).
- Muscle weakness with greater involvement of proximal muscles.
- Hirsutism and menstrual problems in females and impotence in males.

Other features include osteoporosis, psychiatric problems in adults, steroid diabetes and pigmentation in ectopic cases.

About 70% cases are due to pituitary adenoma (Cushing's disease). Disease is more common in females and shows slow progression over years. Hypokalemia, alkalosis and pigmentation are rare.

About 15% patients have ectopic ACTH production (most commonly due to small cell carcinoma of bronchus). It is more common in males and important features are hypertension, hypokalemia, alkalosis (there is increased secretion of deoxycorticosterone (DOC) and androgens along with cortisol) and glucose intolerance (impaired insulin release due to hypokalemia). Hypokalemia also causes severe muscle weakness. In slow growing tumors (carcinoids) there is also time to produce central obesity, pigmentation and hirsutism.

Adrenal carcinoma produces large amounts of androgens, DOC, 11-deoxycortisol and even aldosterone and estrogens, besides cortisol. Important features are hirsutism, masculinization and menstrual disturbances along with hypertension and hypokalemia.

Table 15.3. Patients with the following presenting features may or may not be suffering from Cushing's syndrome
- Obesity associated with diabetes and mild hirsutism.
- Patient with amenorrhea (or oligomenorrhea), hirsutism and some other features of masculinization.
- An elderly woman with diabetes, osteoporosis and hirsutism.
- An obese woman with severe muscle weakness.
- Pseudocushing's (alcoholics, psychotics). In these individuals small dose dexamethasone test may be abnormal.

- In a patient presenting with features of Cushing's syndromes one must take history of steroid administration.
- Patients with above presentations should be thoroughly investigated for Cushing's syndrome.

investigated for Cushing's syndrome. An alcoholic may present with features resembling those of Cushing's syndrome (pseudo-Cushing's) but may not be suffering from the disease (Table 15.3).

Investigations

ACTH and cortisol estimations, in isolation, generally, do not help. These levels are affected by any mild stress and so many other factors (Table 15.4). However, determination of cortisol in the sample collected at night, without stress may be useful, as increased cortisol level in this sample will reveal loss of circadian variation. Alternatively, estimation of 24h urinary excretion of free cortisol is a useful test. In this test, the main problem is collection of proper urine sample (study of sample creatinine may be used to be sure about that). Some people use overnight urine sample and express results in terms of creatinine excretion.

It is however, best to screen the patient using overnight dexamethasone suppression test. A small dose of the drug (1 mg) is given at 11P.M. and plasma cortisol is estimated at 8A.M. Cortisol level of <5 µg/dL in the 8A.M. sample suggests normal suppression (whatever the baseline value). This may be followed by the low dose dexamethasone test. In this test cortisol response is tested on the second day after oral administration of 0.5 mg of the drug, given 6 hourly.

For determining etiology (Fig. 15.5, Table 15.5) the different tests have low specificity. Two commonly used tests are plasma ACTH estimation and

Table 15.4. Conditions mimicking test profile seen in Cushing's syndrome

Obesity (Cushingoid features):
- Urinary and plasma cortisol levels and diurnal pattern usually normal; some patients however, show abnormalities. In about 13% even overnight dexamethasone test may show abnormality.

Chronic alcoholism (Cushingoid features):
- Modest changes in blood and urine steroid levels along with loss of diurnal pattern.
- Resistance to overnight dexamethasone suppression.
- Normal response to insulin induced hypoglycemia.

Depression:
- As for chronic alcoholism but there are no cushingoid features.

Severely ill patients (as in intensive care unit): **Septic shock**
- Elevated cortisol level.
- No suppression by dexamethasone.

- Many drugs (phenobarbitone, phenytoin, methyldopa, meprobamate, reserpine, spironolactone) interfere in interpretation of adrenal function tests.
- Diseases including cardiac failure, uncontrolled diabetes mellitus, fever, pulmonary disease and anorexia also interfere in interpretation of adrenal function tests.

Table 15.5. Tests used to determine etiology of Cushing's syndrome.

	Plasma ACTH	High dose dexamethasone (% of cases responding with suppression)	CRH test (% cases with positive ACTH response)
Hypothalamic dysfunction/ primary pituitary microadenoma	N to ↑	>95	>90
Pituitary macroadenoma	↑ to ↑↑	<10	>90
Ectopic ACTH/ CRH production	↑ to ↑↑↑	<10	<10
Adrenal tumor	↓	<10	<10

- In difficult cases response of ACTH or cortisol secretion to CRH (test not widely available) or metyrapone is studied. In ectopic etiology cases and adrenal tumors response is reduced as pituitary is suppressed (CRH test is similar to TRH test for hyperthyroidism).
- High dose dexamethasone has high specificity for confirmation of cases of category 1.
- In many patients of the first three categories ACTH levels may be similar; if CT of pituitary gland is normal (rules out category 2), CRH/metyrapone tests may be required to distinguish between categories 1 and 3.

the high dose dexamethasone test. In the latter test, 2 mg dexamethasone is given 6 hourly and percentage decrease in plasma cortisol level is studied on the second day. In difficult cases the stimulation tests (the CRH test and the metyrapone test) may be used (Table 15.5). CRH test has however, not been extensively used due to limited availability of CRH but may become a useful test in future. In the ectopic cases special clinical features (Table 15.2) may also help. This may be especially so in cases of carcinoids and pheochromocytomas (features like flush, diarrhea and episodic hypertension). The imaging studies may be required to define pituitary adenomas. In case of negative results of imaging studies, some times, selective venous sampling for ACTH/CRH may be used. History of drug intake may help detecting iatrogenic cases. In these patients the basal cortisol level is low due to suppression of pituitary.

Principles of treatment are given in case history 15.2.

Congenital adrenal hyperplasia (CAH) (Table 15.6)

It represents a group of disorders with inborn errors of enzymes of adrenal steroid biosynthesis. Clinical picture depends upon, the enzyme involved, whether deficiency is partial or complete and sex of the patient. However, the common changes in common forms are, deficiency of cortisol and increased formation of androgens. Cortisol deficiency results in increased formation of ACTH (lack of negative feedback effect) resulting in adrenal hyperplasia and stimulation of the aberrant pathway. The three common disorders are, 21-hydroxylase deficiency, 3-β hydroxy steroid dehydrogenase deficiency and 11-β-hydroxylase deficiency. The estimated frequency of the first one is about half that of phenylketonuria and neonatal diagnosis can be made by testing of the same blood as is collected for screening of phenylketonuria. 11-β-hydroxylase deficiency, more often, is partial.

In case of 21-hydroxylase ($P450_{c21}$) deficiency, in addition to cortisol deficiency, aldosterone secretion is also reduced in about one third of the patients, accounting for salt losing tendency in these patients. 11-β-Hydroxylase ($P450_{c11\beta}$) deficiency, there is impaired convertion of 11-deoxycorticosterone to corticosterone, resulting in accumulation of 11-deoxycorticosterone, a potent mineralocorticoid. This accounts for hypertension in these patients. Deficiencies of these two enzymes in the female may produce female pseudohermaphroditism (in a newborn), virilization (in a female child). A male newborn/child may present with isosexual pseudoprecocity. In cases of partial enzyme deficiency, the adult female patients present with hirsutism, amenorrhea, male type voice and other signs of virilization (late onset adrenal hyperplasia). Adult female patients with features of virilization may also result from adrenal cancer or ovarian causes of increased androgen production. These causes will be discussed in Chapter 17.

In deficiency of 3-β-hydroxy steroid dehydrogenase (3-β-HSD), there is block in synthesis of both cortisol and aldosterone, with increased synthesis of adrenal adrogens via 17-hydroxypregnenolone and DHEA. Deficiency is also present in gonads. For male fetus DHEA is a weak androgen and therefore male fetus is incompletely virilized (male pseudohermaphroditism). In female fetus there is partial virilization. $P450_{c17\alpha}$ deficiency (rare) is also present both in adrenals and gonads. There is hypogonadism (primary amenorrhea and lack of development of secondary sex characters in females; and in males, ambiguous genitalia or female phenotype (male pseudohermaphroditism), hypokalemia and hypertension (also see in Chapter 17).

Diagnosis and basis of treatment

Because of inappropriate androgenic steroids produced in congenital adrenal hyperplasia, this condition becomes an important disorder in differential diagnosis of many clinical conditions like hirsutism, virilizing syndrome, female pseudohermaphroditism, in females and in incomplete isosexual precocity (precocious pseudopuberty) in the male. Important adrenal specific tests which are often used in these disorders are as follows: i) urinary 17-ketosteroids; ii) plasma DHEA-sulfate; iii) dexamethasone suppression test; 17-ketosteroids and DHEA-sulfate levels falling to normal in response to dexamethasone suppression (0.5 mg, orally, every 6h for 2 days) in CAH and not in case of adrenal tumor or any other androgen secreting tumor; iv) cortisol precursor levels (17-hydroxy progesterone, 11-deoxycortisol and 17-hydroxy pregnenolone in plasma) both basal and after ACTH infusion (increased levels which further increase with ACTH, only in CAH); v) plasma cortisol, basal and after dexamethasone suppression. For diagnostic features of individual enzyme deficiencies. Also see Table 15.6.

The patients are treated with daily administration of glucocorticoids, not only to compensate for deficiency of cortisol but also to suppress excessive synthesis of ACTH. Dose is adjusted in relation to repetitive analysis of urinary 17-ketosteroids, plasma DHEA-sulfate and/or precursors of cortisol. Overtreatment in children can, retard linear growth; therefore skeletal growth and maturation should also be monitored.

Table 15.6. Important features of different forms of congenital adrenal hyperplasia (CAH)

This is an autosomal recessive disorder caused by different enzyme defects in biosynthesis of cortisol; 21-hydroxylase deficiency accounting for 95% of total cases.

ENZYMATIC DEFECTS ASSOCIATED WITH FEMALE PSEUDOHERMAPHRODITISM/ MALE VIRILIZATION:

21-hydroxylase deficiency:

- In less severe cases adrenal hyperplasia (increased ACTH due to reduced feedback control) maintains cortisol and aldosterone levels in normal range but increased androgens produce external genital changes.
- In severe form, the salt losing form is produced with low levels of cortisol and aldosterone.
- Besides the external genital changes patient may present with hyponatremia or episodes of acute adrenal insufficiency (hyponatremia, hyperkalemia, vomiting and dehydration).
  - Increased urinary 17-ketosteroids and plasma DHEA-SO$_4$ levels which are suppressed by dexamethasone.
  - Increased precursor molecules (17-hydroxyprogesterone and 11-deoxycortisol in plasma and pregnanetriol in urine), basal and after stimulation with ACTH.
  - Normal or decreased cortisol levels which are suppressed by dexamethasone.
  - Prenatal diagnosis is established by demonstrating elevated levels of 17-OH progesterone in amniotic fluid at 14 to 16 weeks of gestation.
  - HLA typing, amniotic fluid 17-hydroxy progesterone and by DNA study (linkage analysis) can be used to diagnose affected fetuses and carriers in some families.

11-β-hydroxylase deficiency:

- Adrenal virilization associated with salt retension and hypertension.
  - Most characteristic are increased plasma levels of 11-deoxycortisol and 11-deoxycorticosterone (and urinary excretion of tetrahydro 11-deoxycortisol).
  - Levels of 17-ketosteroids and 17-OH progesterone are also increased.

Late onset adrenal hyperplasia

  - Presents as virilization of females; there is no defect in external genitalia at birth (no pseudohermaphroditism).
  - Caused by partial deficiencies of 21-hydroxylase (P450$_{c21}$), 11-hydroxylase (P450$_{c11β}$), and 3β-hydroxysteroid dehydrogenase/ isomerase (3β-HSD).
  - Moderate metabolite changes depending upon the enzyme involved; most common is 21-hydroxylase deficiency as already pointed out.

ENZYMATIC DEFECTS ASSOCIATED WITH MALE PSEUDOHERMAPHRODITISM:

3β-hydroxysteroid dehydrogenase deficiency:

- Male pseudohermaphroditism is produced because of lack of testosterone synthesis in testes in male fetuses. Female fetus is not much affected as the accumulated adrenal androgen (DHEA) is weak for affecting fetal differentiation[1].
- Synthesis of cortisol, 17-OH progesterone and aldosterone is blocked (plasma levels very low).
  - Increased levels of DHEA and 17-ketosteroids (DHEA is the only source).
  - Levels of cortisol, aldosterone and their precursors are very low.

17α-hydroxylase deficiency: 17-20 lyase deficiency:

- As 17-hydroxysteroids are precursors of androgens as well as cortisol (also estrogens are derived from androgens); there is male pseudohermaphroditism and sexual infantilism in female (lack of secondary sex characters and amenorrhea).
- There is increased synthesis of corticosterone and deoxycorticosterone (DOC); the latter is a mineralocorticoid and increases plasma volume to suppress renin-angiotensin system and aldosterone. No adrenal deficiency due to presence of corticosterone. Main urinary steroids are DOC and corticosterone; ↓ 17-ketosteroids; ↑ urinary gonadotropins: ↓ plasma cortisol, aldosterone.
- Hypertension and hypokalemic alkalosis (due to DOC).
- In isolated 17-20 lyase deficiency there is normal function of adernal cortex (no hypertension, alkolosis): Male pseudohermaphroditism, female infantilism. Low levels of androgens and estrogens and urinary 17-ketosteroids.

[1] Some female newborns may present with female pseudohermaphroditism.

Primary aldosteronism (Conn's syndrome)

Table 15.7 records characterizing features of this condition. 40% of these patients also have proteinuria.

Diagnosis

In a patient of diastolic hypertension, if there is hypokalemia, one should rule out use of diuretics or drugs like licorice and carbenoxolone. If there is no such history, patient is given KCl supplement for ten days. If hypokalemia persists, it confirms presence of excess of aldosterone or some other mineralocorticoid. Next, plasma aldosterone and plasma renin activity (PRA) are measured to differentiate between three possibilities: i) Secondary aldosteronism (both levels high); one should look for renal artery stenosis or a renin producing tumor; ii) adrenal tumor/CAH (both levels low); one should do other investigations for firm diagnosis; iii) primary aldosteronism (low renin activity and high aldosterone level. Some times when results are not clear cut (especially when hypokalemia is also doubtful), increased aldosterone, renin ratio may be helpful, to differentiate primary aldosteronism from essential hypertension. In essential hypertension, about 25% patients may present with low renin and increased aldosterone levels. Table 15.8 lists some conditions with hypertension and low renin and aldosterone levels.

Some centres measure urinary excretions (24h) of potassium and aldosterone to confirm primary aldosteronism, after the condition is indicated by

Table 15.7. Characterizing features of primary aldosteronism

- Systolic and diastolic hypertension.
- High aldosterone to renin ratio (>50).
- Potassium wastage.
- Sodium retention.
- 40% patients have proteinuria.

- Low salt diet, upright posture and diuretics all increase plasma aldosterone level in normals (and classic hyperplasia cases but there is no effect in classic adenoma cases (which are autonomous). Similarly, saline infusion expands ECF and reduces aldosterone secretion in normals (and low renin essential hypertension cases) but fails to suppress plasma aldosterone into the normal range in cases of adenoma or hyperplasia.

Table 15.8. Low renin hypertension

- Mineralocorticoid excess in congenital adrenal hyperplasia, adrenal carcinoma and some cases of Cushing's syndrome.
- Liddle syndrome (renal tubular defect causing increased sodium reabsorption and hypertension, hypokalemia and expanded ECF).
- Glycyrrhizinic acid (tobacco chewing, licorice) inhibiting 11-hydroxysteroid dehydrogenase promoting formation of adrenal mineralocorticoids (other than aldosterone) at the cost of reduced formation of adrenal glucocorticoids.
- Some patients of diabetes mellitus, renal disease and long standing hypertension. Also read under hypoaldosteronism.

- In first three cases, there is Na^+ retention due to a cause other than aldosterone excess, with expansion of ECF leading to suppression of renin and aldosterone. Na^+ retention causes hypertension.
- In the fourth category, cases are called hyporeninemic hypoaldosteronism. In these patients: i) hyperkalemia and metabolic acidosis are out of proportion to decrease in GFR; ii) plasma renin fails to increase following sodium restriction and postural changes; iii) hypertension, increased volume and increased potassium are present; iv) cause may be a renal tubular defect.

plasma aldosterone and PRA. Patient should be on unrestricted salt intake during these studies.

Once diagnosis of primary aldosteronism is established, it is important to differentiate between, adenoma (most common), bilateral nodular hyperplasia (idiopathic hyperaldosteronism) and rare glucocorticoid remediable aldosteronism (GRA), since the treatment modalities are different. Important differentiating features and investigations are listed in Table 15.9. The adenoma cases (compared to hyperplasia patients) have higher blood pressure, more severe hypokalemia and may be treated by surgical excision of adenoma. CT scan or adrenal vein sampling may be used to demonstrate whether or not the disease is confined to one adrenal gland. In bilateral nodular hyperplasia, surgery (bilateral adrenalectomy) is indicated only if hypokalemia cannot be controlled by medical treatment. Medical treatment consists of dietary salt restriction and administration of spironolactone. This may be able to control both hypertension and hypokalemia. In fact the bilateral hyperplasia cases who are likely to benefit from subtotal or total adrenalectomy behave more like adenoma cases (in suppressive

Table 15.9. Disorders producing hypertension and hypokalemia.

Primary aldosteronism (adenoma):
- Usually unilateral
- Low renin activity; high aldosterone level
- No aldosterone suppression
- Adenoma localization by CT scan
- Unilateral adrenal vein sample showing high aldosterone level
- Elevated plasma 18-hydroxycorticosterone level.
- Lowering of plasma aldosterone or no change in erect posture

Primary aldosteronism (bilateral cortical nodular hyperplasia; idiopathic hyperaldosteronism):
- All investigative features as above, although these patients have less severe hypokalemia and less severe changes in renin and aldosterone levels, further, CT/MRI and the unilateral vein sample studies do not reveal adenoma.
- Plasma 18-hydroxycorticosterone not high.
- About 30% increase of aldosterone over basal level in erect posture.

Deoxycorticosterone (DOC) secreting adrenal tumor:
- Reduced renin activity
- Aldosterone level normal or reduced.

Glucocorticoid remediable aldosteronism (GRA) with chimeric gene for aldosterone:
- Elevated cortisol precursors in plasma or urine
- Direct demonstration of genetic defect
- Aldosterone level not suppressed by saline infusion but suppressed by dexamethasone (2mg/d for 2 weeks)

Liddle syndrome (autosomal dominant defective epithelial sodium channel):
- Both aldosterone and renin activities are low (continuous sodium reabsorption)
- Increased sodium reabsorption (promotes potassium secretion) is responsible for both hypertension and hypokalemia.

11-β-hydroxysteroid dehydrogenase deficiency[1]:
- Increased ratio of cortisol to cortisone in urine
- Genetic analysis

Chewing tobacco containing licorice:
- Licorice is inhibitor of 11-β-hydroxydehydrogenase
- Proper history will be useful

[1.] Cortisol cannot be converted into cortisone and hence binds to glucocorticoid type 1 (mineralocorticoid) receptors.
- Hypertension and hypokalemia may also be produced in some varities of CAH.
- Common feature in all these disorders is hypertension with associated hypokalemia.
- In the last three causes, hypervolemia and hypertension (added associated hypokalemia) is not produced by aldosterone. Rather hypervolemia results in low renin and aldosterone activities.
- Saline infusion fails to suppress aldosterone level in the normal range in aldosterone secreting adenoma or idiopathic hyperaldosteronism but prompt suppression occurs in essential hypertension.

and stimulatory manoeuvres) than more common idiopathic hyperaldosteronism cases. This subgroup is named as primary adrenal hyperplasia. In GRA cases (a very small group of nodular hyperplasia cases), small doses of glucocorticoids are used for treatment. One should watch for development of iatrogenic Cushing's syndrome. Alternatively, medical treatment mentioned above may be used.

Besides aldosteronism, low renin activity is also found in patients with increased secretion of adrenal mineralocorticoids other than aldosterone (Table 15.8) and in some other conditions, as already pointed out.

Secondary aldosteronism

Renin-angiotensin-aldosterone system is stimulated by reduced effective circulatory volume leading to reduced perfusion of afferent arterioles in the kidney. This explains secondary aldosteronism of congestive heart failure and in edematous states (cirrhosis, nephrotic syndrome). The renin-angio-tensin-aldosterone system can also be stimulated by narrowing of major renal arterial vessels, on one or both sides by artherosclerosis or fibromuscular hyperplasia, with profound renal vasoconstriction (accelerated phase of hypertension), and severe arteriolar nephrosclerosis (malignant hypertension). Secondary aldosteronism is associated with hypokalemic alkalosis, moderate to severe increase in plasma renin activity and marked increase in aldosterone level. Often aldosterone production in secondary aldosteronism is more than in primary aldosteronism. In rare, renin producing tumors of juxtaglomerular cells, there will be normal renal vasculature but presence of a space occupying lesion in the kidney (Chapter 4).

In the above account, many intrarenal causes of secondary aldosteronism are associated with hypertension, which in some instances, is remediable by removal of the local lesion. Secondary aldosteronism can occur without edema or hypertension as in Bartter's syndrome. In this condition, there is defect in renal Na/Cl conservations. Resulting hypovolemia produces secondary aldosteronism which produces hypokalemia. Hypokalemia can stimulate renal prostaglandin production which in turn increases stimulation of JG-cells (juxta glomerular cells) for renin secretion. Excessive prostaglandin production may be the primary event stimulating JG-cells (but preventing development of hypertension because of vasodilatory effect of renal prostaglandins).

Hypoaldosteronism

Most patients of isolated hypoaldosteronism result from deficiency of renin production (hyporeninemic hypoaldosteronism). Renin production to usual stimuli is impaired in chronic tubulointerstitial diseases, diabetic neuropathy and during use of certain drugs (ACE-inhibitors, NSAIDs, heparin). Presence of mild renal insufficiency is the usual accompniment of hyporeninemic hypoaldosteronism and potentiates the effect of these drugs. In hyporeninemic hypoaldosteronism there is tendency to develop hyperchloremic acidosis and hyperkalemia, out of proportion to impairment of GFR. Hyperchloremic acidosis is also

a feature of early chronic renal failure before metabolic acidosis with increased anion gap develops.

Patients with tubular resistance to aldosterone, present with clinical features as those of hyporeninemic hypoaldosteronism. Resistance to aldosterone occurs in tubulointerstitial disease, obstructive uropathy and sickle cell disease. In fact both the mechanisms may be operative (aldosterone resistance as well as impaired production of renin) in these disorders. Pseudohypoaldosteronism is a rare familial disorder with end organ resistance to aldosterone (more complete than for conditions mentioned above) and there is acidosis, hyperkalemia along with renal sodium wasting. Resistance may also develop in SLE, drug induced interstitial nephritis, cyclosporin therapy and kidney transplant rejection.

In a rare disorder there is electroneutral reabsorption of sodium (with chloride), interfering with H^+ and K^+ secretory effects of aldosterone (Gordon's syndrome). The patients are commonly volume expanded, acidotic (metabolic acidosis) and hyperkalemic.

A combination of high renin and low aldosterone level implies primary adrenal damage or a biosynthetic defect for aldosterone synthesis. In case of the former cortisol response to ACTH will be impaired. In diagnosis of hyporeninemic hypoaldosteronism, there is normal cortisol response to ACTH but renin-aldosterone response to sodium restriction or posture is impaired.

RTA type 4 is associated with either insufficient aldosterone production or intrinsic renal disease causing aldosterone resistance.

ADRENAL MEDULLA

It is composed of chromaffin cells (so called, as these cells stain with potassium dichromate), and lies enclosed in cortical portion of adrenal gland. Blood passing through medulla is rich in corticosteroid hormones. This increases synthesis of catecholamines (especially epinephrine) during stress. Epinephrine and norepinephrine are stored in vesicles before release. The adrenal medullary cells are innervated by cholinergic preganglionic autonomic fibers (these cells are therefore like cells of

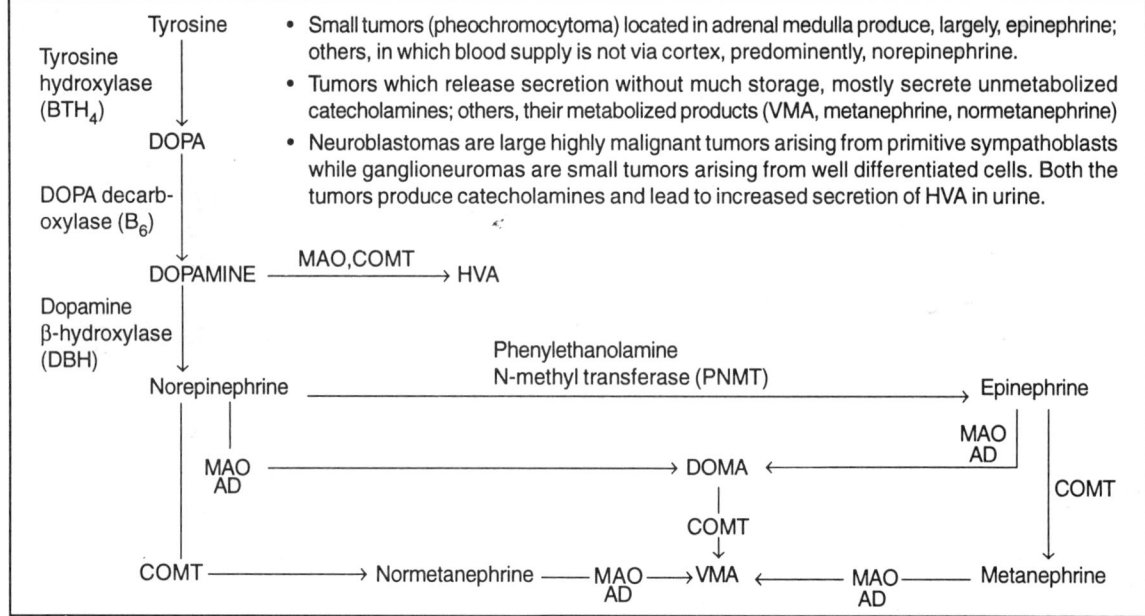

Fig. 15.6. Biosynthesis and catabolism of catecholamines.

- Tyrosine hydroxylase is the regulatory enzyme activated by the nerve stimulation and inhibited (feedback inhibition) by catecholamines. There is no innervation of the tumor tissue in pheochromocytoma and mechanism of hormone secretion is not known.
- In the pathway shown, both epinephrine and norepinephrine are metabolized to VMA with the help of enzymes MAO, AD and COMT.
- In an alternative pathway MHPG (3-methoxy 4-hydroxy phenyl ethylene glycol) is formed with the help of enzymes MAO, AR and COMT. MHPG and VMA (and also 5-HIAA) levels increase in CSF in depressive illness.

MAO=Mono amino oxidase COMT=Catechol-O-methyltransferase AD=Aldehyde dehydrogenase AR=Aldehyde reductase VMA=3-methoxy 4-hydroxy mandelic acid HVA=Homovanillic acid DOMA=3,4 dihydroxy mandelic acid: BTH_4: Terahydrobiopterin.

sympathetic ganglia). Cell depolarization by acetylcholine causes entry of calcium into the chromaffin cells which leads to release of catecolamines by causing exocytosis of vesicles storing catecholamines. Although, 80% of catecholamines present in adrenal medulla is epinephrine, the proportion of the two hormones differs with the type of stress. In anger more of norepinephrine is released while in fear more of epinephrine is secreted. Fig. 15.6. shows the pathway of biosynthesis of catecholamines.

For terminating the actions of the two hormones there is no local availability of a catecholamine degrading enzyme, at the site of action (unlike acetylcholine). The hormone action is terminated, firstly, by its uptake into post ganglionic sympathatic fiber terminals (for entry into storage vesicles or degra-

dation by MAO present on mitochondrial surface) and secondly, by diffusion from site of action, to get degraded in non-neuronal tissues (especially, liver and kidney) by COMT which is a cytoplasmic enzyme. The first pathway of disposal is more important for norepinephrine, released at the nerve terminals and the second one for the hormones of adrenal medulla. The metabolic transformation of catecholamines is outlined in Fig. 15.6. 5% of catecholamines are excreted in urine, unchanged and 95% as metabolites.

Role in stress

Important actions of catecholamines and the receptors involved are shown in Table 15.10. Catecholamines are hormones of stress and their actions help survival of the animal during stress. In the initial

Table 15.10. Catecholamine actions and function

Smooth muscle contraction:
- Vascular smooth muscle (in skin, kidney, mucous membranes), tending increased peripheral vascular resistance and diastolic blood pressure (by activating α_1 receptors).
- Smooth muscle of sphincters (gut, urinary bladder), leading to closure of sphincters (α_1 receptors).

Smooth muscle relaxation:
- Vascular smooth muscle of skeletal vessels (β_2 receptors). Smooth muscle in bronchial walls (β_2 receptors).
- Through activation of inhibitory β receptors on smooth muscle of intestine and through inhibitory α-receptors on parasympathetic ganglion cells of auerbach's plexus, there is relaxation of the gut wall.

Skeletal muscle:
- Increased contractility, glycogenolysis and K^+ uptake (β_2 receptors)

Liver:
- Increased glycogenolysis and gluconeogenesis (α_1, β_2 receptors)

Adipose tissue:
- Increased lipolysis, thermogenesis (α_2, β_1(β_3) receptors)

Sweat glands:
- Increased secretion (α_1-receptors).

Cardiac tissue activation:
- Stimulation of SA node, atria, AV node and ventricles (β_1 receptors)

Stimulation of secretion of glucagon, renin, thyroxine, gastrin and some other hormones (β-receptors) and inhibition of insulin secretion (α_2 receptors)

Modulation of neurotransmitter release by binding to presynaptic receptors:
- There is increased synaptic release of norepinephrine (β receptors) and inhibition of release of acetyl choline at postganglionic parasympathetic fibers (α_2 receptors)

CNS
- Stimulation of medullary respiratory centre cells to stimulate respiration and cells of reticular activating system to produce alertness and anxiety.
- As a part of sympathetic nervous system, adrenal medullary hormones play important role in response to stresses like exposure to cold, hypoglycemia (and starvation), exercise, trauma, hypoxia and circulatory failure through the above listed effects.

---

period, the actions on cardiovascular system tend to increase blood flow to more essential organs at the cost of relatively less important ones. Thus blood is diverted from skin and splanchnic areas to brain, heart and lungs. Subsequently, the metabolic actions are meant to provide fuel and other metabolites for quick tissue repair in damaged tissues.

Pheochromocytoma

It is a tumor of adrenal medullary cells but may also arise from extra adrenal chromaffin cell rests. There is no innervation of the tumor tissue and mechanism of hormone secretion is not known. Small tumors located in adrenal medulla produce, predominantly, epinephrine while others and large ones, which do not depend upon blood supply coming

via cortex, produced, largely norepinephrine. Further, those tumors which release their secretion without much storage, secrete, mostly, unmetabolized catecholamines and produce clinical features early while those tumors which excessively store their hormones, secrete, mostly the metabolites and produce clinical features quite late.

Incidence of pheochromocytoma is about 0.1% of the hypertensive patients. Tumors are, generally, benign and only 10% are malignant. 90% of tumors are found in adrenal medulla. The tumor also occurs as part of multiple endocrine hyperplasia (MEN) syndromes. Related tumors, ganglioneuromas (small well differentiated tumors arising from ganglion cells) and neuroblastomas (highly malignant tumors arising from primitive sympathoblastic cells) produce dopamine as the major catecholamine metabolizing to homovanillic acid (HVA) which appears in urine.

Diagnosis

About 40% patients may present with paroxysms of hypertension, (with headache, visual blurring, tremor, anxiety, sweating and raised blood glucose). In about 60% cases, headache, hypertension and features of hypermetabolism are sustained. Some cases present with postural hypotension, tachycardia and cardiac enlargement.

Postural hypotension results from reduced plasma volume and blunted sympathetic reflexes (also release of adrenomedullin from the tumor).

A hypertensive should be investigated for pheochromocytoma when: i) there are paroxysmal clinical features; ii) patient is a child; iii) an adult with severe hypertension, not responding to therapy; iv) the paroxysmal features are evoked by exercise, emotional disturbances, change or posture or certain drugs; v) blood pressure is quite labile; vi) mild stress or a simple surgical procedure induces shock. Also in hypertensives with some associated abnormality (neurofibromatosis, retinal and cerebellar hemangioblastomas, medullary carcinoma of thyroid as part of MEN 2). Some times it may be familial.

Two conditions which need careful differentiation from pheochromocytoma are hypertension with adrenergic features (tachycardia, sweating) and a severe attack of anxiety.

Investigations (Table 15.11)

For diagnosis of pheochromocytoma, urinary excretions of vanillyl mandelic acid (VMA), total metanephrine and normetanephrine and catecholamines can be studied. The metanephrine study is better than study of VMA (VMA and HVA estimations are more useful for cases of neuroblastoma). Instead of metanephrine and normetanephrine (total), free catecholamines may be studied if laboratory has good experience with these investigations. Stress, illness and strenuous activity, increase excretion of catecholamines and their metabolites in urine. Patients should be kept free from drugs for a few days before the test. Drugs and other factors show maximal interference in plasma catecholamine estimations. Foods containing vanillin, banana, tea and coffee should also be avoided before the test (especially VMA estimation). Also see Table 15.11 for selection of investigations.

Estimation of catecholamines in plasma

In borderline cases, the clonidine suppressor test is done, in which plasma levels of catecholamines before and three hours after administration of a sympatholytic agent (clonidine or pentolinium) are studied. Normally, a decrease of at least 50% is produced while no suppression results in a case of pheochromocytoma.

Levels of chromogranin A (protein co-secreted with catecholamines) has also been used in diagnosis of border line cases. High levels of this protein, however, may occur in renal insufficiency.

Pharmacologic tests

Most of the adrenolytic as well as stimulatory tests have become obsolete because of their non-specificity and the risk involved in their use. However, therapeutic trial with phentolamine is still recommended for screening of pheochromocytoma if the patient presents with a likely paroxysm. Examine the patient after a bolus of 5 mg, following a test dose of 0.5 mg. In case of pheochromocytoma blood pressure should fall by about 35/25 in two minutes and remains so for about 15 minutes. The only stimulatory test which is sometimes used is the glucagon provocative test. Glucagon does not affect plasma catecholamines and blood pressure in normals or hypertensives; but both increase in patients of pheochromocytoma.

Tumor localization

CT and MRI are used to localize the tumor. Scintiscanning using ^{131}I meta-iodobenzyl guanidine (which is taken up by amine uptake process) may also be useful. In case of extra-adrenal tumors if the above tests fail, selective venous sampling with measurement of plasma norepinephrine may help.

Tumor should be excised. Prior to surgery patient is treated with an α and a β-blocker (β-blocker should follow an α blocker; given in the reverse order, blood pressure may further increase) to control his blood pressure and plasma volume. If

Table 15.11. Biochemical tests used for diagnosis of pheochromocytoma.

Patients:

- Young hypertensives (<30 years of age)
- Hypertensives with unusual features
- About 20% patients of pheochromocytoma have intermittent hypertension.
- 4% patients of pheochromocytoma have MEN 2 syndrome. (look for other features of the syndrome)

Studies with urine:

- Normal levels of metanephrines in urine, almost, rule out pheochromocytoma if MEN 2 is not suspected. The test is highly sensitive.
- If metanephrines are increased in urine, increased level of VMA virtually, clinches the diagnosis.
- Urinary catecholamine estimation, commonly, shows false negatives and positives. It, however, is of particular importance in cases of MEN 2 syndrome.
- Urinary excretions in the above mentioned tests are generally increased even if the patient is asymptomatic and normotensive. In rare cases of pheochromocytoma the increased levels are found, only, after a paroxysm. However, diagnosis is never ruled out after a single negative test; repeated testing is important.
- Either a 24h urine sample or a sample collected immediately after a paroxysm should be used. During collection, urine is acidified and refrigerated.

Catecholamines in plasma:

- This investigation is particularly required in MEN 2 cases or when clinical features are quite suggestive of pheochromocytoma but other tests give inconclusive results. This test is also useful in selective venous samples obtained for tumor localization.
- In catecholamine estimation, it is difficult to obtain true basal levels as endogenous catecholamines are easily added to plasma by stimulated sympatho-adrenal system, in stress, exercise, emotions, hypoglycemia, smoking, volume depletion, upright posture and even venous puncture.
- Estimation of catecholamines in plasma may be combined with clonidine suppression test. In a patient of hypertension without the tumor, high basal level is reduced to normal. It remains unchanged in pheochromocytoma.

Interference by drugs/disorders:

- Drugs show maximum interference in plasma catecholamine estimations. These include exogenous catecholamines, catecholamine related drugs (methyl dopa, levodopa etc) and sympathomimetic amines. Monoamine oxidase inhibitors reduce formation of VMA from metanephrines. Certain drugs or their metabolites interfere with chemical estimations. Interference is less with metanephrines and VMA estimations. In case of VMA false increase may occur from food items like vanilla, fruits (especially banana), coffee and tea.

surgery cannot be performed, patient is put on life long treatment with an α blocker (β-blocker is also given along with if tachycardia develops). For chronic treatment metyrosine is used with the above drugs. Metyrosine inhibits tyrosin hydroxylase to reduce secretion of catecholamines.

CASE HISTORY: 15.1

A 20 year old female presented with abdominal pain and vomiting. Her blood pressure was 90/55 mm Hg. History revealed that she had been unwell for the last few months with mild anorexia, excessive tiredness and temporary blackouts, on suddenly getting up from supine position. On examination pigmentation was noted on her buccal mucosa. She was suspected a case of subacute intestinal obstruction but raised serum K^+ (5.8 mmol/L), low blood glucose (65 mg/dL) and HCO_3^- (16 mmol/L)

raised suspicion of adrenal insufficiency. Plasma cortisol level was in the lower part of the normal range.

➢ How to diagnose adrenal insufficiency in this case?

➢ What are important differences between primary and secondary adrenal insufficiencies?

➢ How would you explain a patient of adrenal insufficiency presenting with raised blood glucose (170 mg/dL) and quite low serum Na (110 mmol/L), but with other features quite characteristic of the disease?

• The present case is an early case of adrenal insufficiency. In such cases where plasma levels and urinary excretions of cortisol remain in the normal range, the rapid ACTH stimulation test is helpful. Reduced response to rapid ACTH stimulation test indicates primary or secondary adrenal insufficiency. Study of plasma ACTH level will decide whether the disorder is primary or secondary. In some cases of secondary adrenal insufficiency the rapid ACTH stimulation test does not give reduced response but there is strong suspicion of the disorder. In such cases stimulation tests using insulin induced hypoglycemia, the metyrapone test or the CRH test become useful.

Primary adrenal insufficiency may be due to autoimmune damage, in which total adrenal cortex is destroyed or other causes (infection, metastatic carcinoma, and amyloidosis) which often destroy both cortex and medulla. Thus, generally both glucocorticoid and aldosterone deficiencies are present. Also because of lack of feed back effect of cortisol, ACTH level is increased. In secondary adrenal insufficiency there is atrophy of only cortex excluding zona glomerulosa. Because of this reason the electrolyte abnormalities are seen more commonly in primary adrenal insufficiency cases. Also increased pigmentation is only seen in primary adrenal insufficiency. In secondary adrenal insufficiency, however, one may find evidence of deficiencies of other pituitary hormones. Also see Table 15.1.

- Autoimmune damage of the adrenal gland may be part of PGA II syndrome in which there may be associated damage of islet tissue, the thyroid gland and gonands. In this condition, besides multiple endocrinal changes there can be other associated abnormalities like pernicious anemia and vitiligo. In a patient of adrenal insufficiency, a fasting blood glucose level of 170 mg/dL would mean associated diabetes mellitus. Associated hypothyroidism would explain retention of water much reduced serum sodium level.

CASE HISTORY: 15.2

A 30 year old female presented with irregular menses, central obesity, low back pain, broad striae, mild hypertension and mild hirsutism; features developed gradually, over a period of about one year. Investigations revealed: Blood glucose levels, fasting 105 mg/dL, post prandial (2h) 160 mg/dL; serum Na^+ 140 mmol/L; serum K^+ 3.1 mmol/L; HCO_3^- 32 mmol/L.

➤ How to investigate this patient?
➤ How should this patient be managed?
- In this patient, with the raised level of post prandial blood glucose, sodium in upper part of the normal range, potassium in lower part of normal range and mild alkalosis, along with clinical findings (especially broad striae, irregular menses and mild hirsutism), there is overwhelming suspicion of Cushing's syndrome. For confirmation plasma cortisol level should be studied in the morning sample (9A.M. sample) or free cortisol excretion in 24h urine (some investigators study cortisol (free), creatinine ratio in an overnight urine sample). If the results still leave some doubt, the over night dexamethasone test or the low dose dexamethasone test should be done.

- Cushing's syndrome is most commonly caused by a microadenoma of pituitary and may be located by MRI. A macroadenoma may cause enlargement of pituitary fossa, and is revealed by radiological examination. Properly located adenomas can be resected by trans-sphenoidal surgery. Following successful resection, plasma ACTH should be undetectable (suppression of normal ACTH producing cells around adenoma by excess cortisol). Patient has to be given, daily, dexamethasone till ACTH producing cells resume adequate function (this can be judged by morning plasma cortisol level). The cortisol response to insulin hypoglycemia should also become normal. This will ensure capacity of the patient to deal with stress.

If no adenoma is found but there is no doubt about diagnosis of pituitary dependant Cushing's, radical adrenalectomy is carried out, along with pituitary irradiation to prevent development of Nelson's syndrome. The post operative patients of either of the above two surgical procedures need life long appropriate steroid therapy. If surgery is not advisable, medical adrenalectomy may be indicated by use of steroidogenesis inhibitory drug ketoconazole or some other similar drug. Patient may develop adrenal insufficiency and need replacement steroids. In a primary adrenal cause, adrenal adenoma (and carcinoma if possible), should be removed and patient be kept on sub-optimal steroid replacement therapy, till hypothalamus/pituitary recover from suppression. In case of inoperable carcinoma, tumor is irradiated and patient given mitotane (cortisol suppressor). Patient also receives long term maintenance steroid therapy.

CASE HISTORY: 15.3

A 10 year old boy presented with early sexual development, with the size of penis and presence of pubic hair, quite unusual for his age. His testes were small and of the same size and seminal fluid was scanty.

➤ How to investigate this patient?
➤ How may congenital adrenal hyperplasia (CAH) present in females?
- True precocious puberty (complete isosexual precocity) results from early activation of hypothalamic-pituitary system by some hypothalamic disorder (infection, tumor, trauma). In this case along with early development of penis and pubic hair (virilization), there is also development of testes and spermatogenesis. The present case is that of

precocious pseudopuberty (incomplete isosexual precocity). It may be caused by Leydig cell tumor (rare in children). In the presence of a testicular tumor, the two testes are not of the same size and plasma testosterone levels is high. A hypothalamic germ cell tumor (hCG secreting) could also cause precocious pseudopuberty (only in males). One should look for hypothalamic lesion and increased plasma levels of β-hCG and testosterone (produced by Leydig cell stimulation by hCG which acts like LH). Incomplete isosexual precocity can also occur because of autonomous Leydig cell hyperplasia (without tumor). This inherited disorder comes from an affected father or the carrier mother (male limited autosomal disorder). Plasma testosterone level is increased but LH level and the LH response to LHRH remain pre-pubertal. The most common cause, however, is CAH and the most important investigation would be the study of urinary 17-ketosteroids and suppression with dexamethasone. 17-Ketosteroid excretion is increased in CAH, adrenal and testicular tumors but the increased excretion is suppressed by dexamethasone, only in case of CAH. If the patient is found to be suffering from CAH, the exact enzymatic deficiency may be investigated as per information in Table no. 15.6.

• In presence of CAH in a female fetus, virilization starts at about 5th month of intrauterine life and the new born at birth has ambiguous genitalia (enlargement of clitoris and partial or complete fusion of labia) and condition is called female pseudohermaphroditism. In the postnatal period, the female child may present with virilism. In case of partial deficiency, an adult female may present with hirsutism, amenorrhea, male type built and voice and enlarged clitoris. Virilization of an adult female may however, also occur due to other reasons (polycystic ovary, some ovarian tumors, choriocarcinoma and others). Treatment of CAH essentially, consists of glucocorticoids administration to suppress ACTH secretion and reverse the metabolic abnormalities. A mineralocorticoid may be required in salt losing type of CAH. In the female plastic surgery may be required to correct ambiguous genitalia.

OBJECTIVE TYPE QUESTION

Pick out the wrong statement.

1. The different stimulation tests

i) The rapid ACTH stimulation is useful to diagnose primary adrenal insufficiency.

ii) The rapid ACTH test is also useful to diagnose any case of secondary adrenal insufficiency provided it is more than 3 months old.

iii) The rapid ACTH test is attractive because of convenience and safety for detecting adrenal or pituitary insufficiency.

iv) Pituitary insufficiency in pituitary adrenal axis may be revealed by CRH test or the metyrapone test.

v) In case of primary adrenal insufficiency, the metyrapone test can be dangerous.

2. Steroids, renin-angiotensin system

i) Plasma renin activity (PRA) (involving incubation of plasma and radioimmunoassay of angiotensin-I), is commonly used to evaluate renin angiotensin system.

ii) PRA should be reported in relation to daily urinary Na^+ excretion.

iii) PRA and levels of cortisol and aldosterone, depend upon dietary sodium intake.

iv) DHEA - sulfate level is a good index of adrenal androgen secretion as little DHEA is formed by gonads.

v) These days urinary free cortisol is measured instead of urine 17-hydroxycorticosteroids for assessment of glucocorticoid secretion.

3. Function tests for adrenal cortex

i) To assess cortisol status, use of estimation of 17-hydroxycorticosteroids in urine has been replaced by study of urinary free cortisol.

ii) Urinary excretion of cortisol reflects levels of unbound cortisol in plasma.

iii) Estimation of urinary DHEA-sulfate is a useful index of adrenal androgen excretion.

iv) The rapid ACTH stimulation test is an index of functional reserve of adrenal cortex.

v) In secondary adrenal insufficiency, the response to rapid ACTH stimulation test remains normal.

4. Bilateral adrenal hyperplasia

i) If due to pituitary-hypothalamic dysfunction or pituitary microadenoma, increased ACTH secretion will be suppressed in high dose dexamethasone test.

ii) If due to pituitary macroadenoma or ectopic ACTH or CRH, no suppression will be found.

iii) In idiopathic hyperaldosteronism (or pseudo-primary aldosteronism) there is bilateral cortical nodular hyperplasia.

iv) High dose dexamethasone suppression also occurs in all such cases of idiopathic hyperaldosteronism.

v) In some cases of bilateral adrenal hyperplasia, source of excessive ACTH formation is not apparent.

5. Pseudo-Cushing's syndrome

i) In ordinary obesity fat distribution is different from that of obesity of Cushing's syndrome.

ii) In ordinary obesity, circadian rhythm of cortisol levels remains normal.

iii) In chronic alcoholism and in depression, there is resistance to suppression in the overnight and the low dose dexamethasone tests, along with modest increase in urinary cortisol.

iv) In iatrogenic cases basal state blood or urine cortisol levels are non-informative.

v) In cases of pseudo-Cushing's the response to insulin induced hypoglycemia remains normal.

vi) In acutely ill patients the laboratory tests used in diagnosis of Cushing's syndrome cannot be relied upon.

6. Adrenal cortical tumor

i) In a cortisol producing adenoma a modest decrease in levels of 17-ketosteroids (urinary) and DHEA sulfate (plasma) occurs.

ii) In adrenal carcinoma an abdominal mass may be palpated.

iii) In adrenal carcinoma there is marked elevation of levels of 17-ketosteroids (urine) and DHEA sulfate (plasma).

iv) There is also marked elevation of both urinary and plasma cortisol levels in carcinoma.

v) Adrenal carcinoma is usually resistant to both stimulation and suppression tests.

vi) About 20% adrenal carcinomas are non-functional.

7. Addison's disease

i) In the beginning there may only be anorexia and weight loss.

ii) There may be severe anorexia, vomiting, diarrhea and ill-defined abdominal pain.

iii) Diagnosis may be confused with acute abdomen.

iv) In well developed disease asthenia may be so profound as to require bed rest.

v) In mild cases plasma cortisol may be normal but urinary excretion of cortisol is reduced.

vi) Recent and progressive pigmentation in certain specific areas is important in diagnosis of primary adrenal insufficiency.

8. Addison's disease

i) In women pubic and axillary hair may be reduced.

ii) Hyponatremia occurs only in primary cases of Addison's disease.

iii) Hyperkalemia occurs because of deficiency of aldosterone, low GFR and acidosis.

iv) There may be normocytic anemia, a relative lymphocytosis and a moderate eosinophilia.

v) Mild to moderate hypercalcemia may occur in 10 to 20% patients.

9. Asymptomatic adrenal mass (incidentaloma)

i) Investigate for pheochromocytoma, and for adrenocortical adenoma.

ii) 90% of incidentalomas are non-functional.

iii) In the presence of an extra-adrenal malignancy, there is 30 to 50% chance of adrenal mass being a metastasis.

iv) Chances of an adrenal mass being an adenoma or carcinoma are almost equal.

v) Large size, irregular margins, inhomogeneity, soft tissue calcification (seen on CT), are features of malignancy.

vi) Management alternatives are, to wait and repeat imaging study, fine needle biopsy and surgery.

10. Pheochromocytoma

i) There may be hypertension with adrenergic features.

ii) The single, most useful investigation is estimation of metanephrines in urine.

iii) Diagnosis from study of urinary metanephrines is possible, only, if urine is collected during a paroxysm.

iv) Percutaneous fine needle biopsy of the tumor is contraindicated.

v) Any surgery or even normal vaginal delivery is disastrous unless the patient is properly prepared by stabilizing his blood pressure and plasma volume.

11. Adrenal androgen hypersecretion

i) The most common cause is congenital adrenal hyperplasia (CAH)

ii) Adrenal carcinoma and rarely, adenoma may also produce inappropriate amounts of adrenal androgens.

iii) CAH is the most common adrenal disorder of infancy.

iv) CAH results from autosomal recessive mutations of several enzymes of cortisol biosynthesis.

v) The partial enzyme deficiencies do not express.

12. Hypoaldosteronism

i) Hyporeninemic hypoaldosteronism may occur in

diabetic neuropathy and chronic tubulointerstitial disease.

ii) In hyporeninemic hypoaldosteronism plasma renin level fails to rise following salt restriction.

iii) Hypoaldosteronism is always associated with wastage of salt in urine.

iv) In pseudohypoaldosteronism, hyperkalemia and acidosis, as seen in hypoaldosteronism, are produced in the presence of high renin and aldosterone levels.

v) Hypertension is a usual feature of hyporeninemic hypoaldosteronism while pseudohypoaldosteronism (with salt wasting) is associated with hypotension.

13. The CRH test

i) In Cushing's syndrome caused by hypothalamic/pituitary dysfunction or pituitary microadenoma, there is increase of ACTH level (positive test) in response to CRH.

ii) In most cases of ectopic ACTH production, the CRH test is negative (no increase in ACTH level).

iii) CRH test is also negative in cases of adrenal tumors as tumors are autonomous in secretion.

iv) The CRH test is a well established test.

v) Pituitary macroadenomas (causing Cushing's), also respond to CRH administration by enhanced secretion of ACTH; while response to metyrapone test is variable.

14. Diagnosis of primary aldosteronism

i) Patient has diastolic hypertension and hypokalemia and no edema.

ii) Plasma renin activity is low and fails to rise, adequately, during volume depletion produced by upright posture or sodium depletion.

iii) High plasma aldosterone which fails to decrease, adequately, with volume expansion (salt loading).

iv) Essential hypertension can be easily differentiated from aldosterone hypertension since in the former condition plasma renin activity is not reduced.

v) In primary aldosteronism, although, aldosterone fails to decrease with salt loading, it does increase, in response to potassium loading.

vi) There is poor renal ability to concentrate urine secondary to low K^+.

15. Hyporeninemic hypoaldosteronism

i) Renal insufficiency, as such, may be associated with hyperchloremic acidosis and hyperkalemia.

ii) Acidosis and hyperkalemia are more severe if renal insufficiency is associated with hyporeninemic hypoaldosteronism.

iii) ACE inhibitors, NSAIDs and heparin promote hypoaldosteronism by reducing synthesis of aldosterone.

iv) In hyporeninemic hypoaldosteronism the most significant effect is that of sodium and ECF depletion.

v) In sickle cell disease and obstructive uropathy there may be hyporeninemic hypoaldosteronism as well as tubular resistance to aldosterone.

ANSWERS

1. No.(ii). Not in all cases of secondary adrenal insufficiency. Response may be normal in cases of partial ACTH deficiency. In these patients, there is inadequate pituitary ACTH reserve and there is failure to increase ACTH secretion in stresses of hypoglycemia or surgery.

2. No.(iii). Posture and sodium intake have influence on PRA and the aldosterone levels (the latter is also influenced by dietary potassium). These factors do not influence cortisol levels.

3. No.(v). Response is abnormal provided the central disorder producing adrenal cortical insufficiency is not very recent (it is more than 3 months old). This is due to atrophy of adrenal cortex because of sustained lack of ACTH.

4. No.(iv). Only an occasional patient of nodular hyperplasia may show suppression with high dose dexamethasone. Such a patient may be treated with glucocorticoids.

5. No.(iv). Cortisol levels in blood and urine, in basal state, are low.

6. No.(iv). There is only variable elevation.

7. No.(v). In mild and early cases both basal level (in plasma and urine) remain within normal limits; only adrenal reserve is reduced. Thus the diagnosis should be made by using rapid ACTH stimulation test.

8. No.(ii). It may occur in both, although, severe dehydration, hyponatremia and hyperkalemia are usually indicators of severe primary adrenal insufficiency. In the primary cases hyponatremia is because of aldosterone deficiency (causing loss of sodium in urine) and due to movement of sodium into cells. Elevated angiotensin II and AVP also contribute by reducing free water clearance. In the secondary cases hyponatremia may be dilutional (sodium entering cells) or secondary to subnormal increase in aldosterone secretion in response to severe sodium deficiency.

9. No.(iv). Most of adrenal masses are adenomas (chance of being carcinoma is less than 0.01%).

10. No.(iii). In most patients, increased levels will be

encountered even outside the paroxysms, although, much higher levels occur if urine is collected during a paroxysm.

11. No.(v). Partial enzyme deficiencies (21-hydroxylase, 11β-hydroxylase and 3-hydroxysteroid dehydrogenase) express as late onset adrenal hyperplasia after adolescence. Patients are most commonly women with hirsutism and oligomenorrhea and minimal virilism. Complete enzyme deficiencies express either at birth (female pseudohermaphroditism or male virilism) or in childhood as virilization in female and pseudoprecocity in the male.

12. No.(iii). In cases of chloride shunt (Gordon's syndrome) hypoaldosteronism is associated with increased reabsorption of sodium with chloride. In this case increased plasma volume results in hyporeninemic hypoaldosteronism.

13. No.(iv). The CRH test is not well established at present. Not many studies are available at present (CRH is not readily available). Also position of false positives and false negatives is not properly established as yet (metyrapone test is better, at present).

14. No.(iv). Suppressed renin is seen in about 25% of patients of essential hypertension.

15. No.(iv). The significant effects are hyperkalemia and hyperchloremic acidosis.

CHAPTER 16

Paraneoplastic, MEN & PGA Syndromes and Geriatric Endocrinology

PARANEOPLASTIC MANIFESTATIONS OF TUMORS

Many clinical signs and symptoms of tumors relate to local effects like damage to surrounding cells and pressure on close by structures like nerves, some gland duct or blood vessels. Besides signs and symptoms arising from these effects, tumors may produce clinical features unrelated to their presence in particular tissues. These include, certain systemic features like cachexia, pyrexia, arthropathy, certain central nervous system related syndromes and certain syndromes related to ectopic hormone production, by the tumor cells.

Cancer cachexia

It means malnutrition resulting in wasting, weakness, anemia and general ill health. It often occurs in advanced stage of malignancy, especially in malignancies of gastrointestinal tract, lungs and gonads. Altered tissue metabolism, impaired oxidative phosphorylation, reduced food intake (altered sensations of smell and taste), impaired functioning of gastrointestinal tract produce anorexia, fever, wasting and other features. TNF-α or cachectin produced by tumor cells may partly be responsible for features of cachexia and fever. Tumor tissue may consume important nutrients from the body. This may explain anemia and vitamin deficiencies. Good nutrition may help cachexia partly, but only removal of the tumor reverses cachexia completely.

All malignancies do not produce same degree of cachexia. Not much cachexia may be seen in malignancies of breast, central nervous system, leukemias and lymphomas.

Endocrine syndromes (paraneoplastic)

Most of these endocrine syndromes occur with tumors of non-endocrine tissues which had embryonic origin from neural crest cells. However, paraneoplastic endocrine syndrome also occur in association with tumors that do not appear to be derived from APUD cells (Table 16.1). It may be that oncogenes activate the silent cellular genes encoding these hormones. Alternatively, demethylation of normally methylated inactive genes, in rapidly dividing cancer cells may lead to expression of these genes. Ectopic production of steroid hormones by tumor cells is very rare. Lymphomas, however, may produce calcitriol. Important paraneoplastic endocrine syndromes are given in Table 16.1.

Other paraneoplastic changes

A number of neuromuscular disorders are produced in advanced stage of many malignancies. These include, peripheral neuropathy (both sensory and motor), myopathy/myositis, cerebellar degeneration (with ataxia and nystagmus), myasthenia syndrome, encephalopathy (progressive dementia, brain stem signs) and myelitis (motor neuropathy, spinal cord

Table 16.1. Paraneoplastic endocrine syndromes

Hypercalcemia of malignancy: (most common paraneoplastic syndrome)	Non small cell lung cancer
• Humoral hypocalcemia of malignancy (HMM) ($\uparrow$PTHrP, N PTH, no bone metastases, N phosphate)	Cancer kidney/bladder Cancer head/neck Cancer breast
• Local osteolytic hypercalcemia (LOH) (osteolysis by TGF-α and β, IL-1, IL-6, TNF, PGs)	Cancer breast; Leukemia; Lymphoma; Myeloma
Hyponatremia of malignancy:	Small cell lung cancer
• SIADH	Cancer head/neck
• Some tumors produce ANP	Non-small cell lung cancer
Ectopic ACTH syndrome:	
• Presentation with hypokalemic alkalosis • No suppression in high dose dexamethasone test	Small cell lung cancer: Bronchial carcinoid tumors, Thymic carcinoid: Thymoma
	Pancreatic islet tumors: Neural crest tumors including pheochromocytoma.
Ectopic acromegaly (rare):	
• GHRH	Carcinoids
• GH	Small cell lung cancer
• IGF-1 (no suppression with glucose)	Pancreatic islet tumors
Gynecomastia:	
• hCG (stimulate Leydig cells to produce more estrogens)	Testicular cancer: Lung cancer: Carcinoid tumors of lung/gastrointestinal tract

dysfunction). Other systems may also be affected. Immunologic and metabolic disorders may result. Red cell dynamics, clotting-fibrinolytic system and factors determining ESR may be affected.

NEOPLASTIC DISORDERS AFFECTING MULTIPLE ENDOCRINE ORGANS

Multiple endocrine neoplasia (MEN) are familial disorders with autosomal dominant inheritance. In these disorders, tumors (benign or malignant) develop in two or more endocrine organs. These syndromes are not common. There are two major syndromes, MEN 1 and MEN 2 (Table 16.2). Genetic loci for these two (and also for other less common) are known.

MEN 1

It includes neoplasia of parathyroid, pituitary and pancreatic islet cells. In the particular endocrine organ, the initial lesion is hyperplasia which is followed by adenomatous or carcinomatous change. The neoplasm in one organ may promote develop-

Table 16.2. Tumors present in MEN-syndromes

MEN 1
• Parathyroid/pituitary hyperplasia or adenoma
• Islet cell hyperplasia, adenoma or carcinoma
• Less commonly
  - Fore gut carcinoid
  - Pheochromocytoma
  - Subcutaneous or visceral lipomas

MEN 2A
• Medullary thyroid carcinoma
• Pheochromocytoma
• Parathyroid hyperplasia or adenoma

MEN 2B
• Medullary thyroid carcinoma and pheochromo-cytoma
• Mucosal and gastrointestinal neuromas
  - MEN 2A may be associated with Hirschsprung disease and MEN 2B with marfanoid features.

Mixed syndromes also occur

ment of neoplasm in the other endocrine organs. The syndrome may have total developing period of 30 to 40 years and the presenting features will go on changing during this period.

In MEN 1, the most common manifestation is hyperparathyroidism. Important features to differentiate it from other familial primary disorders of hyperparathyroidism are as under: i) serum calcium is rarely high at birth; ii) histologic features after gland resection and; iii) development of other manifestations of MEN 1 during follow up.

Next to hyperparathyroidism (in frequency), the MEN 1 patients present with neoplasia of pancreatic islet tissue. In these neoplasia, increased level of pancreatic polypeptide occurs in 75 to 85% cases, gastrin in about 60% cases (Zollinger-Ellison syndrome) and insulin in 25 to 35% cases. Less commonly, VIP, glucagon and somatostatin may be produced (Table 16.3).

Pituitary tumors occur in one half of MEN 1 patients. Most commonly the tumors are prolactin secreting. Acromegaly is the second most common syndrome produced, followed by ACTH related syndrome. The tumors tend to be multicentric and difficult to resect. Prolactinomas can be treated with bromocriptine which corrects prolactin level as well as reduces the tumor mass. Octreotide (a somatostatin analogue) is useful for treatment of GH producing tumors.

Less commonly (Table 16.2) fore gut carcinoid may be found. It produces 5HT, other amines and peptide hormones. Features of carcinoid syndrome are flushing, wheezing, diarrhea, alcohol intolerance and hepatomegaly. Some features of carcinoid tumors and syndrome are given in Table 16.4.

The MEN 1 syndrome is believed to be produced by mutations in a tumor suppressor gene (encoding menin) that plays an important role in regulation of cell growth.

MEN 2

It is divided into MEN 2A and MEN 2B. In MEN 2A, medullary thyroid carcinoma is most common, followed by pheochromocytoma (occurs in about 50% cases). Least common is hyperparathyroidism. In MEN 2B, hyperparathyroidism does not occur. Medullary thyroid carcinoma is associated with pheochromocytoma, mucosal neuromas and marfa-

Table 16.3. Manifestations of pancreatic islet tumors

Zollinger-Ellison syndrome (ZES):
- Increased gastric acid production, recurrent peptic ulcers, diarrhea, esophagitis.
- Increased gastric acid secretion, gastrin levels and response of increased gastrin secretion to secretin or calcium are used for diagnosis.
- Treated with H_2-receptor antagonists and H^+, K^+ - ATPase inhibitors.

Insulinoma:
- Hypoglycemia
- Diagnosis is done by demonstrating hypoglycemia along with inappropriate levels of plasma insulin/C-peptide.
- A large tumor may be localized by CT scanning.

Glucagonoma:
- Hyperglycemia, migratory erythema, anemia, diarrhea, venous thrombosis.
- Plasma glucagon level increased in about 50% of patients; although glucagon levels may also be elevated in patients of MEN 1 without above symptoms.

VIP-oma (Verner-Morrison syndrome):
- Watery diarrhea, hypokalemia, metabolic acidosis and hypercalcemia. Watery diarrhea is caused by increased secretion of water and salt by the gut. Hypercalcemia is caused by direct action of VIP on bone.
- VIP levels may be elevated and can be measured to confirm diagnosis.
- Non surgical treatment of VIP-oma includes cytotoxic chemotherapy and use of a somatostatin analogue.

- Islet tumors producing insulin, glucagon, VIP, GHRH, CRH are best resected as medical treatment is ineffective. In families with high incidence of malignant tumors, pancreatectomy should be done.
- ZES and watery diarrhea may also be caused by carcinoids.
- Clinical features, basal and meal stimulated pancreatic polypeptide levels and gastrin levels along with non-invasive methods like high resolution computed tomography and intraoperative ultrasonography are used for diagnosis of pancreatic Islet neoplasms.

Table 16.4. Some features of carcinoid tumors/syndromes

---

* Carcinoid tumors arise from neuroendocrine[1] cells of gut and pancreas. The common feature of these cells is amine precursor uptake and decarboxylation (APUD), a process necessary for secretion of monoamine neurotransmitters like 5HT, dopamine and histamine; cells have also capability of producing and secreting peptide hormones. Tumors of these neurosecretory cells are called APUDomas. Cells of different heritage can acquire the above characters and thus APUDomas can also arise from CNS, thyroid, skin, adrenal medulla and lung, besides gut and pancreas.

• Most common carcinoid tumors arise from structures derived from embryonic foregut (bronchus, stomach, duodenum, jejunum, pancreas and ileum) and rarely from structures derived from mid and hind gut.

• Carcinoid syndrome produces flush, diarrhea, wheezing, hypotension and other features (by tumors of neuroendocrine or enterochromaffin cells, secreting 5HT, histamine, substance P, substance K, VIP and neurokinin).

• Carcinoid tumors produce clinical features because of their secretory products and not by local tissue damage by the growing tumor. Also, generally, frank clinical features occur when hepatic metastases have been produced.

• Diagnosis is based on clinical features and biochemical demonstration of increased urinary excretion of 5-hydroxy indole acetic acid (5-HIAA). In some cases elevated plasma levels of 5-HTP, histamine, or peptide hormones may be helpful (when urinary excretion of 5-HIAA is not high). Barium studies, endoscopy, or CT may help to localize the tumor in the gut. Note that the typical carcinoid syndrome may not be produced by all carcinoid tumors.

• The main aim of the treatment is to relieve symptoms of hormone excess as tumors are generally malignant and difficult to remove. Octreotide (an analogue of somatostatin) is helpful in many syndromes including carcinoid syndrome.

---

[1] The neuroendocrine cells (arising from neural crest) from which APUDomas arise are normally present in intestinal mucosa and secrete regulatory amines and peptide hormones to regulate physiological activities like secretion, absorption and gut motility; also stimulate or inhibit growth of their target cells.

noid features. Medullary thyroid carcinoma occurs in childhood both in MEN 2A and 2B but it is more aggressive in the latter. In early stages, diagnosis can be made by measuring calcitonin level after injection of calcium or pentagastrin. Pheochromocytomas of these syndromes secrete more epinephrine than nor-epinephrine. If adrenalectomy is done on one side, the tumor recurs in the other gland. Peak incidence of hyperparathyroidism occurs in third and fourth decade.

Mutations of the c-ret protooncogene have been identified in about 95% of patients with MEN 2. DNA based technology has been used to identify these mutations. In carriers of MEN 2 related mutations, it is most important to prevent death from medullary thyroid carcinoma by early thyroidectomy (before metastases have occurred); either surgery is undertaken at about 6 years without bothering about the tumor or metastases, or yearly screening is done for medullary thyroid carcinoma by studying serum calcitonin levels before and after pentagastrin injection. Thyroidectomy is performed depending upon the results of the test.

Depending upon the results of the mutation studies and the MEN 2 manifestations in the patient, screening of family may be required for pheochromocytoma and hyperparathyroidism. For

pheochromocytoma both adrenal glands may have to be removed (especially if malignancy is suspected). In case of hyperparathyroidism three glands may be removed fully and also half of the fourth one. The remaining half may be transplanted at some easily approachable site for future surgery (if need arises).

POLYGLANDULAR AUTOIMMUNE (PGA) SYNDROMES (TABLE 16.5)

Autoimmune diseases may be organ specific or organ non-specific. In the latter group the autoantibodies are directed against some component of the cell, in general (cell surface component, cytoplasmic/nuclear component) and in this group there are diseases like rheumatoid arthritis and systemic lupus erythematosus (SLE). In organ specific/tissue specific group, there are diseases like Hashimoto's thyroiditis, pernicious anemia, primary biliary cirrhosis, Sjorgen's syndrome, myasthenia gravis, autoimmune hemolytic anemia and many others. The term polyglandular autoimmune syndrome is used when a disease (in the organ specific group) affects two or more endocrine glands and occurs with some other non-endocrine autoimmune (organ specific) disorder. There are three groups and their disease associations are shown in Table 16.5.

Table 16.5. Polyglandular autoimmune (PGA) syndromes

PGA I
• Hypoparathyroidism
• Adrenal insufficiency
• Hypogonadism
• Hypothyroidism
(associated abnormalities include mucocutaneous candidiasis, alopecia, malabsorption, vitiligo, malabsorption and pernicious anemia)

PCA II
• Adrenal insufficiency
• Hypothyroidism
• Graves' disease
• Type 1, diabetes
• Hypogonadism
(associated abnormalities include myasthenia gravis, vitiligo, alopecia, celiac disease and pernicious anemia)

PGA III
• Autoimmune thyroid disease with another endocrine failure but without Addison's disease.

PGA I

This disorder starts in childhood and requires any two of the following components, for diagnosis: i) mucocutaneous candidiasis; ii) hypoparathyroidism; iii) adrenal insufficiency. Other endocrinal defects may be there, including gonadal failure, hypothyroidism and diabetes mellitus type 1.

PGA II

Important components of this syndrome include adrenal damage, thyroid damage, diabetes mellitus type 1 and hypogonadism. This is also called Schmidt syndrome.

This syndrome presents more commonly in adults with adrenal insufficiency, diabetes mellitus type 1 and thyroiditis. The autoimmune thyroiditis causes either Hashimoto's thyroiditis or hyperthyroidism.

PGA III

Autoimmune thyroid disease with another endocrine failure but without Addison's disease (Table 16.5).

Genetics

PGA I syndrome shows no HLA association. PGA II and III are usually associated with DR3 or DR4 haplotypes (or both) and are inherited as autosomal dominant traits with variable expressivity.

Diagnosis and management

It is crucial to detect adrenal insufficiency as early as possible as it can be fatal if not recognized and treated properly. Screening may be done using rapid ACTH stimulation test (every 1 or 2 years). Patients may be screened for other hormone deficiencies also. Screening by measurement of autoantibodies has not proved very useful.

Besides the above PGA syndrome, involvement of different endocrine secretions can occur in a number of disorders including, acanthosis nigricans, ataxia telangiectasia, pseudohypoparathyroidism, myotonic dystrophy, Noonan syndrome, Fanconi syndrome, Werner syndrome and others.

Biochemical changes in cancer

Malnutrition and blood loss may cause decrease of serum proteins and serum albumin. Fasting blood glucose level may also be reduced. Anemia occurs, commonly, and it may be resulting from hemorrhage, hemolysis, anemia of chronic disease, malnutrition or bone marrow infiltration by the tumor cells.

Serum calcium levels is increased in about 20% of cancer patients (already discussed in this chapter and chapter 10). Elevated serum uric acid may result from rapid lysis of tumor cells and elevated serum lactate because of anaerobic metabolism of tumor cells. Many hematologic malignancies cause low albumin and increase in serum globulin.

Certain malignancies produce immune hemolysis and other immune disorders (glomerular disease). ESR is often normal in cancer patients and significantly high levels are usually associated with metastases. Malignancy may produce a hypercoagulable state resulting in thromboembolism. The paraneoplastic syndromes produced by malignancies have already been discussed.

Tumor lysis syndrome

When a rapidly growing neoplasm (acute leukemia, malignant lymphoma, Burkitt's lymphoma) is effectively treated by chemotherapy, there is rapid cell lysis resulting in hyperuricemia, hyperkalemia, lactic acidosis and hyperphosphatemia. This is called tumor lysis syndrome. Rarely, it may occur without any apparent reason due to sudden necrosis in a malignancy. Dehydration and azotemia promote development of tumor necrosis syndrome.

Lactic acidosis and dehydration promote precipitation of uric acid in renal tubules and produces acute renal failure (uric acid nephropathy). In this acute renal failure, urinary uric acid to urinary creatinine ratio is >1. Hyperphosphatemia may lead to precipitation of calcium phosphate in the kidney to promote renal failure. It also causes lowering of serum calcium and tetany may occur. Hyperkalemia can be dangerous since it may cause ventricular arrhythmias and sudden death.

In leukemias and other disorders with high leukocyte/platelet counts, one should be aware of occurence of pseudohyperkalemia due to lysis of excessive cells in blood after sample has been drawn. It is better to determine plasma potassium in such cases. Also there will be no ECG changes in pseudohyperkalemia.

Before starting chemotherapy risk for tumor lysis syndrome should always be considered. It depends upon tumor burden (high tumor burden will raise serum uric acid >8.0 mg/dL and serum LDH >1500 U/L) and renal functions. For starting chemotherapy, serum uric acid should be <8.0 mg/dL, serum creatinine <1.6 mg/dL and pH of urine should be >7.0. One may be required to correct treatable renal failure (I/V fluids to maintain hydration), lower serum uric acid (use of allopurinol) and maintain proper pH of urine (sodium carbonate administration) before chemotherapy is started. If, however, oliguria and acute renal failure develop, dialysis should be done.

Some considerations of geriatric endocrinology

In the elderly there is age related loss of physiological reserve of each organ system, there is likelihood of presence of one or more diseases and such individuals are likely to be taking a number of drugs. It is because of these factors that an endocrine disorder (as a matter of fact even any other disease)

may present differently, in the elderly people and its diagnosis and management may pose special problems.

Thyroid disorders

Hypothyroidism and hyperthyroidism, each affects 3 to 4% of elderly individuals; prevalence of about twice that in the younger age group. Incidence of sub clinical hypothyroidism is still higher.

In elderly individuals TSH and T_3 are less reliable in diagnosis of thyroid disorders. T_3 levels are often reduced due to some non-thyroid illness.

Thyrotoxicosis is more commonly caused by multinodular goitre or toxic adenoma and less commonly by Graves' disease, in this age group. Clinical features often pertain to cardiovascular system (atrial fibrillation, congestive heart failure, angina, myocardial infarction) and central nervous system (apathy, depression, confusion). Features like frequent bowel movements, weight loss inspite of increased appetite, fine tremor and increased sweating, although less common, are highly suggestive of the disorder, as in the younger age group.

Many patients of multinodular goitre or toxic adenoma will be found to be suffering from subclinical hyperthyroidism (nT_4, nT_3, nFT_4, $\downarrow$TSH).

TSH is suppressed in most of the elderly persons above 60 years of age, and as such diagnosing hyperthyroidism only from TSH levels in this age group may be misleading. Further, differentiation may also be required from euthyroid hyperthyroxinemia caused by some non-thyroid illness or drug/iodide induced hyperthyroidism.

β-Blockers are often required to control symptoms of hyperthyroidism and the actual disease is best treated by radioactive iodine. Patient needs subsequent monitoring for hypothyroidism. Other points which need to be kept in mind are that dose requirements of many drugs depend upon thyroid status of the patient and that a patient with subclinical hyperthyroidism may develop overt disease if he is taking some iodine containing drug for a long time.

Hypothyroidism is often missed in the elderly individuals because the common symptoms of the disorder are often found in euthyroid persons at this age. Further, elderly hypothyroid individuals often present with cardiovascular features (congestive heart failure, angina) or neurological features (cognitive impairment, depression, confusion, deafness and others) which are less common in younger patients. Diagnosis is established by estimating T_4, FT_4I and TSH. Because of reduced reliability of TSH, it may become difficult to differentiate between subclinical (nT_4, nFT_4I, $\uparrow$TSH) and overt ($\downarrow T_4$, $\downarrow FT_4I$, $\uparrow$TSH) hypothyroidism.

Thyroid replacement therapy should be given carefully as excessive drug intake may adversely affect cardiovascular system and worsen the bone loss. Aim should be to keep TSH in the normal range. The same considerations also become important while deciding to treat a patient with subclinical hypothyroidism.

Glucose intolerance and diabetes mellitus

Normal fasting glucose level goes on increasing with age (increase of 1 mg/dL in fasting level and 5 mg/dL in glucose tolerance test, per decade of life).

Diabetes mellitus type 2 is more common in the elderly and the best way to establish diagnosis is to demonstrate the fasting blood glucose level of >140 mg/dL, glycosuria may not always be present because of elevation of renal threshold for glucose. Aim of the management is to keep fasting blood glucose level <150 mg/dL and postprandial level <220 mg/dL.

Chronic complications of the disorder are accelerated by the age related changes. Of the acute complications, non-ketotic hyperosmolar coma occurs, almost, exclusively in the elderly and diabetic ketoacidosis is rare.

Calcium metabolism and bone minerals

Besides the bone loss in perimenopausal women due to loss of sex hormones, there is additional, age related bone loss which continues beyond the perimenopausal period, although rate of bone loss declines after the perimenopausal period. Factors involved in this age related bone loss are: i) reduced vitamin D activation; ii) resistance to intestinal action of 1, 25 $(OH)_2D_3$, reducing calcium absorption;

iii) increased PTH activity (evident from increased urinary excretion of nephrogenic cAMP and osteocalcin). This age related bone loss, leads to an additional effect on the bone i.e., it disturbs its architecture, with the effect that the ability to regain structural integrity with treatment is compromised. Treatment consists of administration of vitamin D, calcium and some regular exercise programme. Vitamin D therapy may cause hypercalcemia if the patient is taking a thiazide diuretic at the same time. In selected cases estrogen therapy (monitor for breast cancer) or estrogen-progesterone therapy (monitor for endometrial cancer) may be used.

Hyperparathyroidism

About 5% of all cases of hyperparathyroidism occur in individuals above the age of 65. Generally, the disease is mild and there may be no symptoms or presenting complaints are vague (weakness, fatigue, depression, confusion). For diagnosis one must rule out other causes of hypercalcemia (vitamin D intoxication, multiple myeloma, metastatic cancer and thiazide diuretics). Besides parathyroidectomy, estrogen therapy may be useful in women. It antagonizes skeletal effect of PTH. Norethindrone has a similar effect. Other alternative in both sexes are oral phosphate or furosemide therapy.

Changes in water and electrolyte balance

There is decline in GFR with advancing age. It is reflected as decrease of creatinine clearance but there is no proportionate increase in serum creatinine because of decrease in muscle mass associated with ageing.

The elderly are more prone to suffer from hyponatremia (with non-specific features like lethargy, weakness and confusion). There are two reasons. Firstly, in the elderly, there is exaggerated response of AVP to hyperosmolar stimuli and secondly, there is salt wasting tendency of the kidney in old age.

Response to stress in the elderly

In the elderly, morning peak of cortisol secretion occurs early and cortisol response to stress is exaggerated and prolonged (cortisol response to CRH is also exaggerated). The exaggerated response to stress in old age may be a factor in glucose intolerance, hypertension, muscle atrophy, osteoporosis and impaired immune response found in such individuals. Inspite of increased incidence of hypertension, glucose intolerance, weight gain and osteoporosis, Cushing's syndrome is uncommon in the elderly.

Reproductive endocrinology in old males

In old age serum FSH and LH levels increase, implying, reduced formation of gonadal hormones (LH response to LHRH is also reduced). However these and other endocrinological changes in the elderly males are less likely to be the cause of increased incidence of impotence with advancing age. Prostatectomy in men over 75 years of age also results in much higher incidence of impotence than in the younger age groups. Drugs used by the elderly might be an important cause of impotence in these individuals.

OBJECTIVE TYPE QUESTIONS

Pick out the wrong statement.

1. Ectopic hormones

i) Production of steroid hormones by non-endocrine tumor cells is rare.
ii) High levels of ectopic hormones (studied by immunoreactive methods) may occur, in the absence of clinical syndromes of the hormones.
iii) In some benign/slowly growing tumors, the ectopic hormone production may be the major cause of morbidity.
iv) Hormones are very good tumor markers for most hormone producing tumors.
v) Most commonly produced clinical syndromes by ectopic hormones are dilutional hyponatremia, hypercalcemia and Cushing's syndrome.
vi) Ectopic calcitonin production is often clinically silent.

2. Hypercalcemia of malignancy

i) It is the commonest paraneoplastic endocrine syndrome.
ii) About 40% patients of hypercalcemia have hypercalcemia of malignancy and out of these

about 80% owe hypercalcemia due to ectopic production of PTHrP by the tumor cells.
iii) Local osteolytic hypercalcemia is produced only by metastases in bone and not in the marrow city.
iv) Lymphoma may cause hypercalcemia by producing $1, 25(OH)_2D_3$ by the tumor.
v) Local bone resorption by tumor metastases is produced by factors like TGF-α and β, IL-1, IL-6, PGs and tumor necrosis factor (TNF).

3. Hypercalcemia of malignancy

i) Non-small cell lung cancer, cancer kidney and bladder and cancer head and neck cause hypercalcemia by producing PTHrP.
ii) Cancer breast may produce hypercalcemia by producing PTHrP or by osteolytic factors produced by bony metastases.
iii) In hypercalcemia of malignancy serum calcium is high but serum phosphate remains normal.
iv) Hyperparathyroidism may account for about 10% cases of hypercalcemia.
v) Other causes of hypercalcemia are, thiazide diuretics, lithium, vitamin D and sarcoidosis.

4. SIADH

i) SIADH is suspected in any patient with serum sodium <130 mmol/L and urine osmolality >300 mosmol/kg.
ii) The most important cause of paraneoplastic SIADH is small cell lung carcinoma, producing AVP.
iii) About 15% of cancer patients producing SIADH, produce atrial natriuretic peptide instead of AVP.
iv) ANP inhibits proximal tubular sodium reabsorption and also inhibits renin (and aldosterone) release.
v) Severe symptomatic cases may be treated with 0.9% saline hydration and furosemide diuresis.

5. Cushing's syndrome of ectopic ACTH

i) The most important cause is small cell lung carcinoma; others are bronchial carcinoid, thymic carcinoid (or thymoma), pancreatic islet cell tumors, medullary carcinoma of thyroid and the neural crest tumors including pheochromocytoma.
ii) Ectopic ACTH produces more mineralocorticoids (compared to pituitary ACTH cases) and therefore presents with hypokalemic alkalosis.
iii) Slow growing tumors producing ACTH are more likely to present with conventional features of Cushing's.
iv) Males suffering from Cushing's are more likely to have ectopic ACTH syndrome compared to females.

v) All patients of ectopic ACTH syndrome show high ACTH levels and lack of suppression with high dose dexamethasone test.

6. Ectopic acromegaly

i) It is produced, more commonly, by increased ectopic secretion of GHRH than GH.
ii) High levels of GHRH, producing acromegaly, may arise from non-neoplastic hypothalamic disorder or ectopic source.
iii) Patients with low GHRH levels and high GH and elevated IGF-1 levels should undergo MRI of pituitary and hypothalamus, for some tumor leading to increased secretion of GH.
iv) Not all GH producing adenomas are detected by MRI.
v) Rarely, a known tumor (of cells other than somatotrops) may be source of ectopic GH.

7. Familial hypercalcemia

i) It may occur in familial parathyroid hyperplasia, familial adenomatous hyperparathyroidism and familial hypocalciuric hypercalcemia (FHH) and in a patient with MEN 1.
ii) Of the causes given at no. i) only FHH is associated with low urinary excretion of calcium.
iii) In all familial conditions serum calcium level is elevated at birth.
iv) Differentiation of hyperparathyroidism of MEN 1 from other familial hyperparathyroidism is based on family history, histologic features of the resected gland and by observing the patient for other manifestations of MEN 1.
v) Other common associations of MEN 1 are adenoma/hyperplasia of islet cells and pituitary.

8. MEN 1

i) Tumors are multicentric; if one tumor is removed another may form.
ii) The most common clinical manifestation is hyperparathyroidism.
iii) Next to hyperparathyroidism, Zollinger-Ellison syndrome (ZES) is the most common feature of MEN 1.
iv) Managements of hyperparathyroidism and ZE-syndrome are totally independent of each other, when present together.
v) In MEN 1, there is greater likelihood of pancreatic islet tumors to be malignant than tumors of other endocrine glands.

9. MEN 1 (pancreatic islet neoplasia)

i) After hyperparathyroidism, this is second most common feature of MEN 1.
ii) Basal level of pancreatic polypeptide (PP), helps diagnosis.
iii) Basal and meal stimulated PP levels make possible early diagnosis.
iv) There is no scope of medical management of pancreatic islet tumors.
v) High resolution CT is the best non-invasive technique for identification of these tumors.
vi) Intraoperative ultrasound is the best method for detection of small tumors.

10. Acanthosis nigricans

i) Patients show hyperpigmented thickened skin.
ii) The condition often occurs in middle aged women and may present with other autoimmune disorders like systemic lupus erythematosus or Sjogren's syndrome.
iii) All patients have antibodies against insulin receptors and present with insulin resistance.
iv) Acanthosis nigricans also occurs in patients with obesity or polycystic ovarian syndrome.
v) Anti insulin antibodies may interfere in insulin assay but not in assay of C-peptide.

ANSWERS

1. No.(iv). hCG is a good tumor marker for choriocarcinoma or testicular teratomas. No other hormone tumor marker is used to quantitate tumor mass.
2. No.(iii). It is caused by cancers spread to bone or bone marrow or tumor present in bone marrow eg; multiple myeloma.
3. No.(iii). This is true if hypercalcemia is produced by local factors produced by tumor/tumor metastases; if PTHrP is the cause, phosphate remains low.
4. No.(i). Only if patient is not edematous, not using diuretics, and has normal thyroid and adrenal functions.
5. No.(v). About 30% patients with carcinoids do show adequate suppression.
6. No.(ii). A patient with elevated GHRH level and acromegaly, must be having ectopic acromegaly (look for cancer in CNS, chest and abdomen).
7. No.(iii). Frequently elevated at birth in FHH but rarely in patients with MEN 1.
8. No.(iv). Hypercalcemia of hyperparathyroidism stimulates gastrin production in ZE-syndrome. In hyperparathyroidism of MEN 1, a special

indication for parathyroid surgery is hypercalcemia with elevated gastrin level.

9. No.(iv). If pancreatic islet tumors can be diagnosed early with the help of basal and stimulated levels of pancreatic polypeptide, surgery may be curative. If they are recognized later (screening, using basal pancreatic polypeptide and gastrin levels), often medical management is done. ZES is managed with H_2 receptor antagonists or omeprazole (H^+, K^+ - ATPase inhibitor); octreotide (a somatostatin analogue) is used to manage watery diarrhea syndrome.

10. No.(iii). Acanthosis nigricans occurring in patients with obesity or polycystic ovarian syndrome has insulin resistance due to post receptor defect. Patients of acanthosis nigricans commonly present with varying degree of insulin resistance but some cases, because of presence of insulinomimetic antibodies, may suffer from hypoglycemic episodes.

CHAPTER 17

Gonadal Hormones and their Disorders

THE TESTICULAR HORMONES

Testes perform two important functions. First, the formation of male germ cells (spermatozoa) and second, formation and development of reproductive organs and development of secondary sex characters. Differentiation of internal and external genital structures is discussed separately (see below).

Before puberty, gonadotropin releasing hormone (GnRH) secreting cells in hypothalamus are inhibited by small amounts of steroid hormones from testes and elsewhere. Puberty starts with pulsatile release of GnRH (also called LH releasing hormone or LHRH), leading to pulsatile release of pituitary gonadotropins, FSH and LH. Under the actions of gonadotropins, testes secrete testosterone (for development of secondary sex characters) and produce spermatozoa. There is feedback effect of testicular hormones at pituitary and hypothalamus (Fig. 17.1).

Biosynthesis of gonadal steroids is shown in Fig. 17.2. Most of testosterone in plasma is bound to serum hormone binding globulin (SHBG) and other serum proteins and only a small fraction is free (Table 17.1). Free hormone is active in tissues. Most of actions of testosterone are due to dihydrotestosterone, to which it is converted in tissues by the action of enzyme of 5-α reductase. There are two enzymes, reductase 1 (present in liver and nongenital skin) and reductase 2 (present in liver and structures of urogenital sinus). There is circadian rhythm of testosterone; higher levels occur during sleep than waking hours. This rhythm disappears with advancing age. After about 40 years of age bio-available testosterone shows gradual decline due to increase of SHBG but total level shows little change until about 70 years of age. In females, most of testosterone, in serum, comes from metabolism of androstenedione, although, small amounts are, directly, secreted by ovary and adrenals.

Aromatization of androgens

Androstenedione from adrenals and testosterone from testes are aromatized to estrone and estradiol, respectively (See under gynecomastia).

SEX DIFFERENTIATION

Sex chromosomes determine whether primitive gonads, during embryonic development, will form ovaries (sex chromosomes XX) or testes (sex chromosomes XY). This is actually determined by SYR gene on Y chromosome that encodes testis determining factor (TDF). Fetal testes produce testosterone, dihydrotestosterone and mullerian inhibitory factor (MIF) while fetal ovaries produce none of these hormones. This difference during embryonic development determines formation of specific internal and external genitalia from common primitive structures in two sexes (Fig. 17.3).

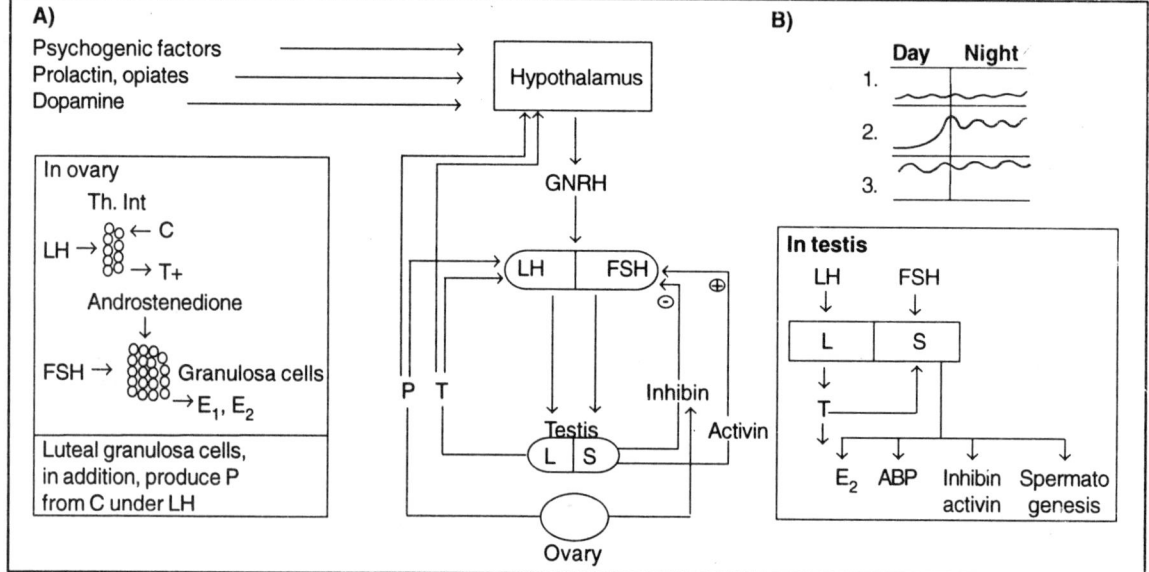

Fig. 17.1. Interactions between hypothalamus, pituitary and gonads.

A) Regulation of gonadal hormones in adults

In the male: LH acts on Leydig cells to stimulate secretion of T while FSH acts on Sertoli cells to stimulate spermatogenesis. T also acts on sertoli cells to influence later stages of spermatogenesis. Note specificity in actions of gonadotropins for gonadal hormones and vice versa.

In the female: E_2 and P have both negative and positive feedback effects. Details are mentioned under hormonal control of menstrual cycle.

B) Gonadotropin levels before puberty, at puberty and later on (in the male)

Note that levels are very low before puberty (1). At puberty, first, increase occurs during night (also note the pulsatile nature of levels) (2). Later on, increased pulsatile levels occur through out 24h (3). In the female the initial changes are somewhat similar as above but with onset of menstrual cycles the pattern of hormone secretion becomes complex (described under menstrual cycle).

L=Leydig cells; T=Testosterone; Th Int.=Theca interna; E_1=Estrone; E_2=Estradiol; S=Sertoli cells; C=Cholesterol, ABP=Androgen binding protein

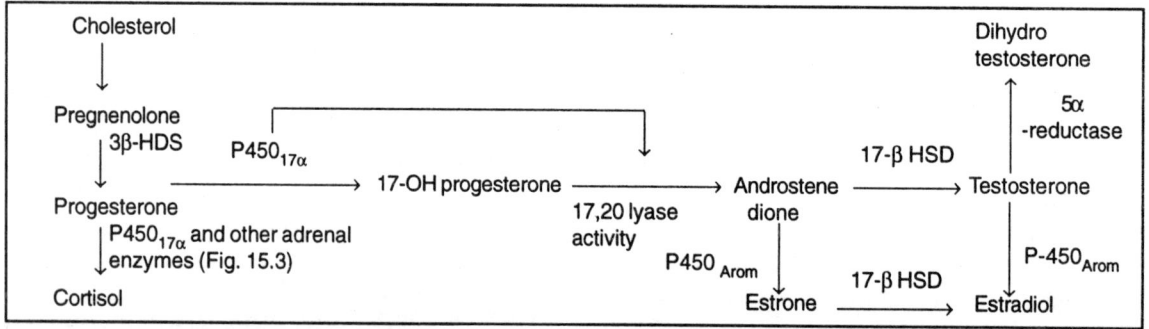

Fig. 17.2. Steroid biosynthesis in testes.

- Figs. 15.3, 17.2 and 17.5 should be studied together, noting the difference in enzymes present on adrenals, testes and ovaries.
- As shown in Fig. 17.2 androstenedione and testosterone are formed in testes which can be converted into estradiol and estrone by aromatase in certain tissues (adipose tissue, skin, liver). In many tissues dihydrotestosterone is the active form of testosterone and is formed from the latter compound in the tissue of action, itself. Also see Fig. 17.7. In ovarian follicles androgens are formed in theca interna (under LH) which are aromatized to estrogens in the granulosa cells (see Fig. 17.1).

Table 17.1. Free & bound fractions of different steroid hormones in plasma

	Plasma	Percentage of total			
	(nmol/L)	Free	SHBG	Albumin	CBG
Estradiol	0.07-0.22	2	37	61	-
Estrone	0.23	<4	16	80	-
Progesterone	1-3(13-64)	>2	<1	79	18
Testosterone	10-35	>1	66	>30	>2
Dihydrotestosterone	0.65	0.5	>78	21	-
Androstenedione	2.8-8	7.5	<7	84.5	>1
Cortisol	140-552	4	<1	>6	90

- In males increased SHBG level, increases free E_2/T ratio (as SHBG binds T more firmly than E_2) to promote gynecomastia.
- Also see Fig. 17.10
- Estradiol, estrone levels are in follicular phase; progesterone levels are in follicular and luteal phases, latter in bracket.

Table 17.2. Some chromosomal disorders

Disorder/Karyotype	Gonad/ Ext. genitalia/ Int. genitalia	Some comments
Klinefelter syndrome (47, XXY or 46, XY/47, XXY) (Defective X-chromosome)	Small firm testes and azospermia/ ext., int. genitalia normal male	• Incidence is 1 in 500 men (most common disorder of sexual differentiation) • One of the two common causes of underandrogenization and infertility in adults (other one is viral orchitis) • Patient is tall (long legs) with gynecomastia. • High LH and FSH (latter is more useful) • Estrogen level increased (from testes under LH); testosterone level low.
XX male (46, XX)	Same as above	• Differences from klinefelter syndrome are; height less than average normal height, mental impairment less common, incidence of hypo-spadias increased. • May be familial
Gonadal dysgenesis or Turner's syndrome. (45, X or 46, XX/45, X)	Gonads as fibrous streaks/ both ext. and int. genitalia normal female but immature	• Incidence is 1 in 3000 newborn females (most common cause of primary amenorrhea; comprises 1/3 of total cases). • Diagnosis is suggested in infancy, by congenital anomalies like webbing of neck, lymphedema of hands and feet, wide apart nipples and mental retardation. • During investigations of amenorrhea, LH is high and estradiol low.
Mixed gonadal dysgenesis (46, XY/45, X or 46, XY)	Testis on one side and streak gonad on the other side/ ext. genitalia variable but always ambiguous (60% grow as females)/ uterus, vagina and one fallopian tube, often present	• Second most common cause of ambiguous genitalia in the new born (after CAH) • High incidence of tumor formation (due to Y-chromosome), especially in streak testis or intraabdominal testis. • Maintenance is eay when diagnosed as females (when patient present in infancy).

- Features of gonadal dysgenesis are primary amenorrhea, sexual infantilism, short stature and multiple congenital anomalies. Allied conditions are pure gonadal dysgenesis (bilateral streak gonads with normal 46, XY or 46, XX karyotype, normal stature and few somatic anomalies, primary amenorrhea), and the Noonan syndrome, an autosomal dominant disorder in both sexes (normal karyotype and gonads, webbed neck, short stature, congenital heart disease and other congenital defects). In Noonan syndrome person is commonly sexually normal but with somatic stigmata of Turner's syndrome; therefore previously called as male turner's or turner's with normal chromosomes. In some cases, it may have associated primary gonadal failure or some other endocrine abnormalities.

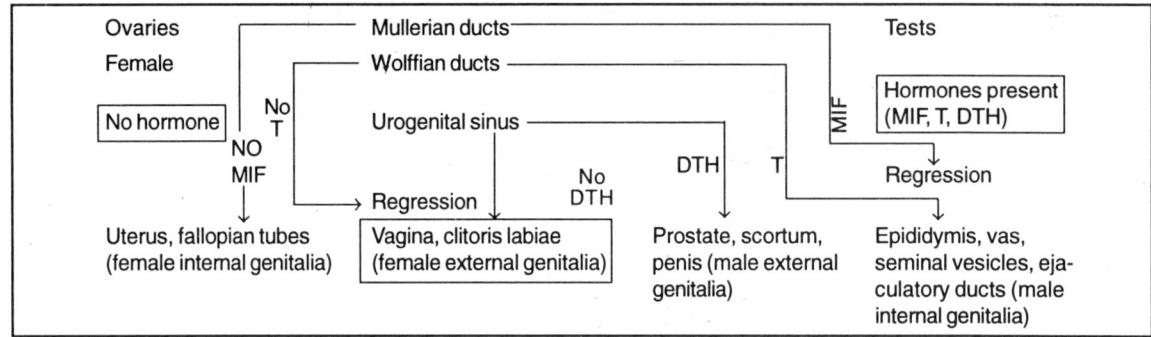

Fig. 17.3. Development of male and female internal and external genitalia.

- In isosexual precocity there is precocious development of gonads as well as genital organs (premature activation of hypothalamic-pituitary system for secretion of gonadotropins).
- In pseudo isosexual precocity there is premature development of genital organs (by some unnatural source of androgens in the male and of estrogens in the female). Gonads are not developed.
- Heterosexual precocity is produced in the female by presence of an unnatural source of androgens (female pseudo hermaphroditism) and in a male by presence of an unnatural source of estrogens.

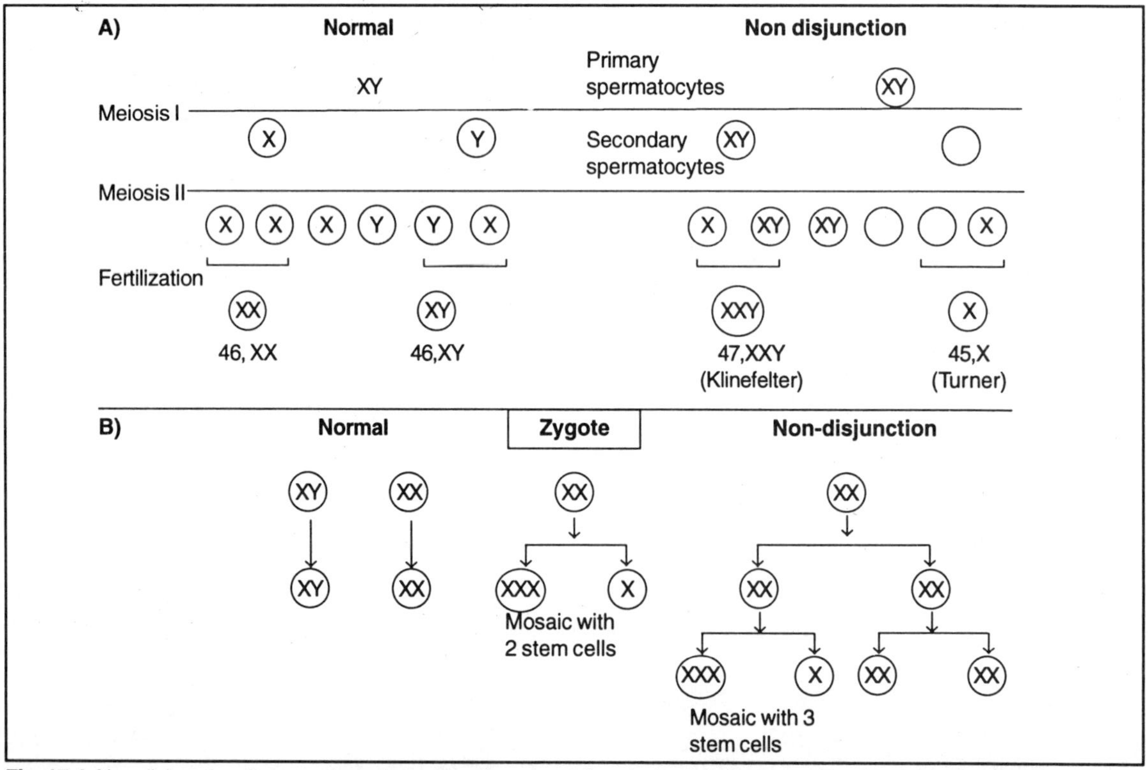

Fig. 17.4. Non disjunction during meiosis (formation of germ cells) and mitosis (after formation of zygote or in a diploid cell).

A) Note formation of haploid gametes with the two sex chromosomes (XY) and without any sex chromosomes (◯) from (XY) diploid cell during spermatogenesis. Also note possibility of formation of diploid zygote with karyotype 47, XXY ((XY)+(X)) or karyotype 45, X (◯+(X)).

B) Note formation of two stem cells due to nondisjunction during the first mitotic division after zygote formation and formation of 3 stem cells due to non dysjunction during second mitotic division.

- It should be remembered that non disjunction is not confined to the sex chromosome pair as shown in figures A and B, it may occur in any other pair.

MOSAICISM AND CHROMOSOMAL DISORDERS (Table 17.2)

Non-disjunction (failure of chromosomes of a pair to separate), during meiosis, in gamete formation can give rise to a chromosomal disorder (Fig. 17.4) and non-disjunction during an early mitotic division after fertilization can produce mosaicism (presence of multiple cell lines with different chromosomal composition). Fetus possessing both XX and XY types of cells will have both ovarian and testicular tissues and will be a true hermaphrodite. Besides non-disjunction other chromosomal alterations can also occur. For example SYR gene (leading to for-

mation of testis determining factor) may be transferred from Y-chromosome to X-chromosome and thus a true hermaphrodite may also have a karyotype 46, XX or a karyotype 46, XY. A true hermaphrodite may have a bilobed gonad (called ovotestis) in inguinal region or in labioscrotal fold. Genitalia are ambiguous. Numerous phenotypes are possible, depending upon Leydig cell function. Secretion of testosterone is inadequate for a male or too much for a female. True hermaphroditism (karyotypes, 46, XX or 46, XY or 46, XX/46, XY) is a rare condition and often, its diagnosis is considered after ruling out all causes of pseudohermaphro-

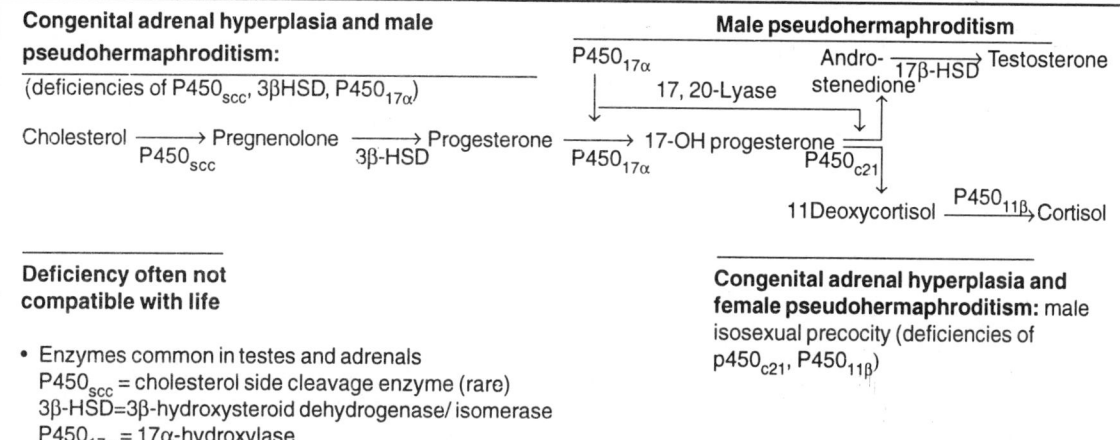

Congenital adrenal hyperplasia and male pseudohermaphroditism:
(deficiencies of $P450_{scc}$, $3\beta HSD$, $P450_{17\alpha}$)

$$Cholesterol \xrightarrow[P450_{scc}]{} Pregnenolone \xrightarrow[3\beta\text{-HSD}]{} Progesterone \xrightarrow[P450_{17\alpha}]{} 17\text{-OH progesterone}$$

Male pseudohermaphroditism

$$P450_{17\alpha} \Big\downarrow \quad 17,20\text{-Lyase} \quad \text{Andro-} \xrightarrow[17\beta\text{-HSD}]{} \text{Testosterone} \atop \text{stenedione}$$

$$17\text{-OH progesterone} \rightleftharpoons \Big\downarrow P450_{c21}$$

$$11\text{Deoxycortisol} \xrightarrow[]{P450_{11\beta}} Cortisol$$

Deficiency often not compatible with life

- Enzymes common in testes and adrenals
  $P450_{scc}$ = cholesterol side cleavage enzyme (rare)
  3β-HSD=3β-hydroxysteroid dehydrogenase/ isomerase
  $P450_{17\alpha}$ = 17α-hydroxylase

- $P450_{17\alpha}$ deficiency reduces androgen/estrogen formation in gonads; cortisol and androgen formation in adrenals, where there is increased formation of DOC and corticosterone. There is male pseudohermaphroditism or female sexual infantilism along with hypertension (latter due to DOC). In 17,20lyase deficiency there is only reduced androgen/ estrogen formation in gonads and androgen formation is adrenals. There is female sexual infantilism or male pseudohermaphrodism but no hypertension.

- In inborn errors of $P450_{scc}$, 3β-HSD and $P450_{17\alpha}$ there is reduced formation of cortisol as well as androgens in gonads (if deficiency occurs both in adrenals and gonads). The result is pseudohermaphroditism in the male and sexual infantilism in the female besides cortisol deficiency.

Congenital adrenal hyperplasia and female pseudohermaphroditism: male isosexual precocity (deficiencies of $p450_{c21}$, $P450_{11\beta}$)

- **Enzymes only in adrenal**
  $P450_{c21}$=21-Hydroxylase
  $P450_{11\beta}$=11β-Hydroxylase
  (deficiency produces female pseudohermaphroditism or male isosexual precocity and congenital adrenal hyperplasia).

  Enzymes only in testes
  17β-HSD=17β-Hydroxysteroid dehydrogenase (deficiency produces male pseudohermaphroditism) 21-Hydroxylase and 11-β-hydroxylase are absent from gonads.

- Other causes of male pseudohermaphroditism include steroid 5α-reductase 2 deficiency and androgen receptor defect.

- Other causes of female pseudohermaphroditism include placental aromatase deficiency, (defective conversion of androgens to estrogens in placeta increases fetal testosterone level), babies born to mothers with virilizing tumors of ovary (arrhenoblastomas) or luteomas of pregnancy or rarely virilizing adrenal tumors. Postnatal armoatase deficiency in women can cause hirsutism and development of polycystic ovaries.

Fig. 17.5.

Table 17.3. Important disorders causing male pseudohermaphroditism (heterosexual precocity in genetic males)

Defective enzymes in testes/Autosomal/ X-linked recessive	Spermatogenesis normal to reduced (testes may be inguinal or abdominal)	• Female internal genitalia (uterus, fallopian tubes) are absent. Variable development of male internal genitalia (epididymis, vas, seminal vesicle). • At puberty virilization and external genitalia variable (male type with hypospadias to female type which is more common). • 17-β-HSD deficiency is more common. There is female phenotype with blind vaginal pouch. Breast usually male type. • LH level is high; testosterone level is low to normal. If testosterone level is normal, increased level of the metabolite behind the block helps specific diagnosis.
Steroid 5-α reductase deficiency/Autosomal recessive	Spermatogenesis normal or decreased	• Internal genitalia male. • External genitalia female type; habitus female but breast male type. • As testosterone levels are normal, masculinization occurs at puberty. No gynecomastia. • As feed back is by testosterone, LH and estrogen levels normal. • High T/DHT ratio, as such or after hCG.
Androgen receptor disorders/X-linked recessive	Spermatogenesis, often absent or reduced (testes small and lie in inguinal canal or else where): may be normal in the mildest form called under-virilized fertile male	• Because of androgen resistance (also at hypothalamus), LH is high (normal in less severe cases); same is true about estrogen and testosterone levels. • Because of androgen resistance and high estrogen level varying degrees of defective virilization and enhanced feminization. • Complete testicular feminization (most severe form) is third most common cause of primary amenorrhea after gonadal dysgenesis and congenital absence of vagina (patient is female in all respets except that there is blind vagina and no uterus and fallopian tubes). • The less severe forms are, incomplete testicular feminization, Reifenstein syndrome (presents as incomplete male pseudo-hermaphroditism, perineoscrotal hypospadias with gyneco-mastia), infertile male syndrome (azospermia with minimum undervirilization and undervirilized fertile man (under virilization with gynecomastia).

- In management whether to rear a newborn as a male or female will depend upon the anatomic defect. In general, the more severely affected should grow as females and less severly affected ones as males. In the former case external genitalia may need corrective surgery. Testes should be removed as early as possible (as there is risk of malignancy) and surgery will be needed for hypospadias. Testosterone therapy may be needed depending upon the plasma androgen level.

ditism (male and female). Confirmation is obtained by demonstrating presence of both ovarian and testicular tissues on laparotomy. Table 17.2 shows some disorders with abnormal sex chromosomes.

PSEUDO FEMALE AND MALE HERMAPHRODITISM

These patients are genetically males or females but have ambiguous genitalia. A genetic female may have ambiguous genitalia because of non-testicular source of androgen during 8th to 13th week of gestation. This is female pseudohermaphroditism (heterosexual precocity). It may happen in congenital adrenal hyperplasia, or in the presence of an androgen secreting tumor, in a female fetus or because of androgen administration to mother (with a female fetus), during pregnancy. In a male fetus,

reduced availability of androgens or their ineffectivity can result in male pseudohermaphroditism. Table 15.6 presents diagnostic features of different disorders of female pseudohermaphroditism, arising from deficiencies of different enzymes of cortisol biosynthesis. Fig. 17.5 shows a unified concept of pathways involved in biosynthesis of cortisol and testosterone and also the relation of different enzymatic defects with congenital adrenal hyperplasia, female pseudohermaphroditism and male pseudohermaphroditism. Besides the enzymatic defects, male pseudohermaphroditism can also be caused by androgen receptor disorders as well as by defective formation of dihydrotestosterone from testosterone (steroid 5α-reductase deficiency). Table 17.3 shows causes of male pseudohermaphroditism (defective virilization of male embryo).

PUBERTY

Puberty starts with pulsatile release of GnRH leading to pulsatile release of gonadotropins. Before puberty, GnRH pulse generator is inhibited by steroid hormones from gonads. At puberty, hypothalamic sensitivity to the hormones is reduced and pulsatile release of GnRH begins. In early puberty, there is pulsatile and mostly nocturnal release of gonadotropins, under the action of GnRH. Subsequently, pulses of similar magnitude occur in sleep and waking hours (Fig. 17.1). The gonadal hormones, released under the actions of gonadotropins, bring about pubertal changes in the two sexes. In the male, FSH and LH releases are fairly concordant (although LH pulses are larger than FSH pulses). In the female the secretory pattern of FSH and LH is more complex as per stages of the menstrual cycle. Pubertal changes start at 9 to 14 years in boys and a little earlier in girls.

Precocious puberty

Precocious puberty is pubertal changes occuring before 10 years in boys and 8 years in girls. Constitutional precocious puberty is more common and occurs close to the above noted ages in the two sexes. Non-constitutional cases may be idiopathic (74% in girls, 41% in boys) or due to known causes. In these cases pubertal changes occur earlier (than constitutional cases) and in girls the normal sequence (breast development → pubic hair growth → general growth → menses) of changes may be disturbed. Known causes include perinatal head injury, abnormal skull development (rickets), lesions of hypothalamus or close to hypothalamus like tumors (craniopharyngioma, optic glioma, astrocytoma, germ cell tumors which cause only male precocity, and hamartomas which are benign growths of fetal rests). Non-tumorous causes include encephalitis, meningitis and granulomata.

Precocious puberty does not prepone menopause in females but short stature occurs in both sexes due to acceleration of skeletal maturation under the actions of sex hormones. Lack of coordination between intellectual and psychosocial development (related to chronological age) and puberty may cause serious problems. Long acting analogues of GnRH are used for treatment. These drugs suppress secretion of GnRH. Pseudoprecocious puberty on the other hand results from inappropriate secretions of androgens in the male (congenital adrenal hyperplasia and androgen secreting adrenal or gonadal tumors) and of estrogens (granulosa cell tumor of ovary) in the female. In pseudoprecocious puberty gonads remain small and undeveloped (as increased gonadal hormones are present without increased gonadotropins) and can be examined to distinguish the condition from precocious puberty in which gonads are also over developed for the age. Read case history 15.3 regarding male isosexual precocity and objective type questions 16 and 17 regarding female isosexual precocity.

Delayed puberty

The hormonal causes are discussed under prepubertal hypogonadism (see below). Some other and more common causes are given in Table 17.4.

Table 17.4. Some causes of delayed puberty without primary disease of gonads or pituitary/hypothalamus

- Constitutional[1]
- Conditions affecting general body growth:
  - Malnutrition
  - Chronic diseases (renal, liver, respiratory, cardiac)
  - GH and thyroid hormone deficiencies and glucocorticoid excess
- Severe emotional deprivation.
- Anorexia nervosa/severe weight loss.
- Excessive physical activity (as in athletes).

[1] Height is less for age but age is appropriate for bone age. Family history is important. Alo see Table 13.4.

ASSESSMENT OF GONADAL FUNCTIONS

Testicular functions

Unlike other hormones, the status of gonadal hormones/functions are better assessed from their biological functions rather than their plasma levels. Thus development of genital structures during embryogenesis and sexual maturity at puberty are best indicators of Leydig cell functions (androgen status) during these periods.

Previously, the biological assays of FSH/LH were considered superior to the immunologic measurements because of multiple isoforms of these hormones (due to varied contents of carbohydrates). However, present days sandwitch techniques for measurements of these hormones, compare well, in results, with old biological measurements. Difficulty however, arises in differentiating levels of these hormones in disease, from the normal levels, because of pulsatile secretion of these hormones. The problem is overcome by pooling a number of blood samples (atleast three samples collected at 20 minute or longer intervals), for studying the levels. Testosterone is also secreted in pulsatile fashion but because of longer half life, the time related variations in its plasma levels are less marked compared to those of LH and FSH. Still, it is advisable to pool three samples collected at 20 minute intervals for this estimation, also.

In gonadal disorders, proper interpretation of low levels is more difficult than high levels. Thus Leydig cell function, prior to puberty is difficult to assess, as levels of both testosterone and LH are low. In this case testosterone response to hCG (which has actions similar to LH) is more useful. If however, basal levels alone are being studied, it is better to measure plasma testosterone (not LH) in a sample collected at early waking hours.

It is always advisable to consider both testosterone and gonadotropin levels together in diagnosis of a disease. For example a low testosterone will give support to a high LH in diagnosis of primary testicular failure. It is also useful to know about prolactin levels, at the same time. Increased prolactin levels reduces gonadotropin levels. Prolactin concentration is stable throughout the day and therefore a single sample is enough. Indications of prolactin estimation are given in Table 17.5.

GnRH stimulation test

LH/FSH response to GnRH (or LHRH) adminis-

Table 17.5. Indications of prolactin estimation

- Galactorrhea
- Unexplained male hypogonadism or infertility.
- Unexplained amenorrhea
- Hyperprolactinemia persisting for >6-12 months after delivery.
- Enlarged sella turcica (or suspected pituitary tumor)

- 10-40% of amenorrheic women have hyperprolactinemia.

tration is some times used. In a normal adult man the response is variable. Usually LH level increases four/five fold after GnRH infusion. Some times, however, the increase may be even less than two fold. In primary testicular failure, measurement of basal LH is sufficient and the stimulation test does not add much to information obtained from the basal value. In cases of failure due to hypothalamic/pituitary disease, a subnormal response establishes the diagnosis while a normal response is without much value. Theoretically, this test should also be useful in differentiating between pituitary and hypothalamic etiologies of gonadal failure. The response is expected to be normal in hypothalamic etiology, while it is reduced if disease is at pituitary level. However, response is commonly, delayed or reduced even in hypothalamic disease (in the absence of GnRH the gonadotrophs are not tuned to respond to GnRH in the test), and cannot differentiate hypothalamic etiology from the pituitary one. However, if daily infusion of GnRH is used for a week and then the test repeated, it will give a normal response, if damage is at hypothalamus. For the provocative test, clomiphene can also be used. It blocks estrogen receptors in hypothalamus to stimulate secretion of GnRH by removing feed back inhibition of estrogen.

Evaluation of functions of seminiferous tubules

A decrease in size of testes in prepubertal period indicates developmental failure or damage to seminiferous tubules. However, in the post pubertal period damage to seminiferous tubules does not result in decrease in size of testes. The functional status of seminiferous tubules is best indicated by semen examination. In the post pubertal period a moderate damage to germinal epithelium of seminiferous tubules is indicated by semen examination. Severe damage, besides being indicated by semen examination, is also indicated by increase in FSH level and decrease in level of inhibin. Size of testes is also useful in differentiating true isosexual from pseudoprecocity (no increase in size in pseudoprecocity).

Female gonadal functions

These are commonly judged from the bodily

Table 17.6. Clinical evaluation of estrogen and progesterone status of the body

Estrogen status:

• Moist rugated vagina; copious, thin cervical mucus that can be stretched/ shows ferning on slide. • Cytological examination of vaginal epithelial cells (cornification with pyknotic nuclei).	Progesterone withdrawl test (menses occur in about 10 days after course of 10mg oral medroxyprogesterone acetate/d for 5 days). Positive test means, normal estrogen status.	In amenorrhea positive test means chronic anovulation with normal estrogen status.

Progesterone status:

• Presence of viscous cervical mucus that does not stretch or fern. • Presence of secretory epithelium or endometrial biopsy during luteal phase	Basal temperature elevation lasting for about two weeks after ovulation (Fig. 17.8).

Status of endometrium/outflow tract:

• Examination of external genitalia and presence or absence of uterus.	Give 1.25 mg oral conjugated estrogen/d for 3 weeks; with 10 mg medroxyprogesterone added for last 10 days: Bleeding should occur in next 10 days Positive test means normal outflow tract.	• Positive test means chronic anovulation with absent estrogen. • Negative test means absent or non-responsive endometrium.

changes produced by the pituitary gonadotropins and the ovarian sex hormones rather than from the actual levels of these hormones (see below). Normal genital structures and secondary sexual characters are a good indication of adequate estrogen status at puberty and earlier on. Regular predictable events in menstrual cycle imply normal pituitary gonadotropins as well as ovarian hormones. In finding a cause for amenorrhea/infertility, it is important to know about the estrogen status of the patient as well as presence or absence of ovulation. All these evaluations are done clinically (Table 17.6). Plasma progesterone levels are evaluated in certain cases of infertility in which a limited defect in the intensity of the luteal phase is suspected (read under infertility).

Inspite of a good specific non-isotopic assay (using antibodies prepared by protein conjugation to estradiol at C-6; which show less cross reactivity with other estrogens), there are many problems with use of estrogen levels in assessment of estrogen status. Plasma levels vary in menstrual cycle and further, there is difficulty in knowing correct day of cycle, when the cycles are abnormal. However, rising levels of estrogens are useful in assessment of estrogen status. Other specific indications

where plasma estrogen levels are useful, include diagnosis of estrogen secreting tumors and to monitor follicular growth (ultrasound is also used) for in vitro fertilization procedure.

DISORDERS OF GONADAL FUNCTIONS IN THE MALE

If hypofunction occurs before puberty, the condition is named as prepubertal hypogonadism and post pubertal hypogonadism, if it occurs after completion of pubertal changes.

Prepubertal hypogonadism and delayed puberty

Causes are given in Table 17.7. Chronic systemic diseases and other disorders (Table 17.4) tend to delay puberty, besides affecting physical growth of the child. Hypothyroidism and growth hormone deficiency are also causes of retarded physical and sexual growth.

Acquired testicular damage caused by infections (mumps, tuberculosis), irridiation and cytotoxic drugs can occur before or after puberty. In prepubertal patients there may be, only, involvement of seminiferous tubules (causing infertility) and secondary sex characters may be normal. If Leydig

Table 17.7. Some causes of male hypogonadism

Testicular disorders:
- Under androgenization and infertility
  - Bilateral anorchia, Leydig cell aplasia
  - Klinefelter syndrome and other chromosomal disorders
  - Acquired damage (viral tuberculosis, leprosy, trauma, irradiation, cytotoxic drugs)
  - Autoimmunity
  - Associated with systemic diseases (sickle cell disease, renal disease and others)
  - Androgen resistance
- Infertility only
  - Cryptorchidism
  - Adult seminiferous tubule failure
  - Varicocele
  - Immobile cilia syndrome
  - Drugs, autoimmunity, febrile illness, celiac disease.
  - Obstruction in epididymus or vas deferens, congenital or acquired.

Hypothalamic pituitary disorders:
- LH and FSH deficiency (underandrogenization and infertility)
  - Panhypopituitarism.
  - Isolated gonadotropin deficiency with anosmia (Kallmann's syndrome) or without anosmia.
  - Cushing's syndrome, hyperprolactinemia.
  - Hemochromatosis
- FSH deficiency (only infertility)
  - Congenital adrenal hyperplasia
  - Isolated FSH deficiency
  - Use of androgen for purpose other than hypogonadism.

cell loss occurs, both functions are lost. However, secondary sex characters are not much altered, if deficiency develops after puberty. Confirmation of partial defects may require testicular biopsy study.

Many of the above causes of hypogonadism can be ruled out from careful history and physical examination and differential diagnosis, generally, remains between constitutional delayed puberty, isolated gonadotropin deficiency commonly occuring as a familial disorder called Kallmann syndrome (other hypothalamic - pituitary causes are discussed, later, under pre-pubertal amenorrhea) and certain testicular causes. Klinefelter syndrome (a testicular disorder) is common and caused by chromosomal abnormalities. This disorder presents as delayed puberty, small testes with lack of spermatogenesis and less commonly underandrogenization. Gynecomastia is, however, common.

Bilateral, untreated cryptorchidism also causes loss of spermatogenesis but other pubertal changes occur as usual (as Leydig cell function is not impaired).

Many cases of male pseudohermaphroditism will also present with puberty defects but these form a distinct category. Only mild cases of androgen resistance may present with incomplete or absent puberty without any evidence of pseudohermaphroditism.

The testicular disorders which, really, need to be differentiated from constitutional delayed puberty and isolated gonadotropin deficiency include Klinefelter syndrome, testicular agenesis or malformation and mild hereditary androgen resistance cases. The autoimmune testicular damage, generally, occurs in adults.

Differentiating constitutional delay in puberty from isolated gonadotropic deficiency

Differentiation between constitutional delayed

puberty and absent or incomplete puberty due to isolated gonadotropin deficiency is, often, a tough job. In both conditions plasma levels of both testosterone and gonadotropins are low. Presence of, respective, family histories and associated anosmia (or hyposmia) and cryptorchidism in isolated gonadotropin deficiency (Kallmann syndrome), may help diagnosis. In constitutional delayed puberty, patient has short stature for chronologic age but bone age is appropriate. In Kallmann syndrome height and growth rate are normal. The major problem is that with suspicion of constitutional delayed puberty, one has to wait for treatment upto about 18 years of age. At this age, if the patient turns out to be gonadotropin deficient, the delay in treatment may leave the patient with permanent reduced bone mass. Also see Table 13.4.

Some times the cause of delayed onset of puberty is quite apparent (Table 17.4). To detect onset of process of puberty before actual physical changes, a useful test is to observe increase in plasma LH level after infusion of 100 µg of GnRH; increase by more than 15.6 IU/L, both in boys and girls indicates that puberty has already set in.

Differentiating hypothalamic, pituitary causes from testicular causes

This mostly depends upon study of levels of gonadotropins, testosterone and prolactin. Increased plasma prolactin levels can cause decrease in levels of gonadotropins. In hypothalamic/pituitary deficiency, gonadotropin and testosterone levels are decreased. In Klinefelter syndrome, plasma testosterone level is low or low normal and levels of LH and FSH are increased. Elevated level of FSH is more consistent, as damage to seminiferous tubules occurs more consistently. One should look for stigmata of the disorder and karyotyping will confirm diagnosis (Table 17.2). This condition is discussed separately and also in case history 17.2. In androgen resistance causes, there is increase of both LH and testosterone levels. In hypothalamic-pituitary deficiency cases, GnRH stimulation test may help to locate the site of disorder. In some cases of testicular failure, testicular biopsy may be required to establish testicular pathology.

Post pubertal hypogonadism

Important clinical features are loss of libido and potency, reduced hair growth (of male distribution) and loss of fertility. Hypoplasia of external genitalia and prostate are rare. Semen examination will show reduced sperm count.

Causes of hypogonadism have already been discussed (see under prepubertal hypogonadism). Hyperprolactinemia in the male causes decrease of libido and impotence. Less commonly other features of hypogonadism may also occur (see Table 17.8).

In differential diagnosis one must first consider commoner causes of loss of libido and potency (Table 17.9). Once these have been ruled out investigations are carried out as outlined in Fig. 17.6. A case of post pubertal hypogonadism may present as a case of infertility alone. This topic is discussed separately.

Androgen deficiency can also cause gynecomastia alone, which is also discussed separately.

Table 17.8. Clinical features of hyperprolactinemia in the two sexes

In females:
- Frequently, amenorrhea or oligomenorrhea and anovulatory cycles. Less commonly, galactorrhea and rarely hirsutism. It may also cause primary amenorrhea or postpill amenorrhea/galactorrhea.

In males:
- Frequently, decreased libido and impotence. Less commonly, hypogonadism and rarely galactorrhea.

- In hyperprolactinemia the cause should be treated. It may mean discontinuation of a drug or surgical resection of a tumor. In inoperable cases bromocriptine is used which stimulates dopamine receptors in pituitary.

Table 17.9. Some causes of loss of potency and libido in differential diagnosis of hypogonadism

- Diabetes mellitus (because of neuropathy).
- Chronic alcoholism.
- Use of certain drugs (sedatives, hypnotics).
- Hyperprolactinemia of any origin.
- Psychological disorders.
- Thyrotoxicosis (level of free testosterone in serum is reduced because of increased level of SHBG although there is increased level of total testosterone). Also hypothyroidism.

In cases of constitutional delay in puberty, a short term therapy with testosterone (in low dose) may be useful, as it will give psychological support to the patient. In actual hypogonadism treatment depends upon the cause. In primary gonadal failure cases there is no treatment to improve spermatogenesis. Androgen deficiency can be treated with androgen replacement therapy. Hyperprolactinemia is treated with bromocriptine (a dopamine agonist). In other hypothalamic-pituitary disorders, gonadotropin therapy (with hCG or hCG/LH along with FSH) is used to induce spermatogenesis and to promote androgenization. This therapy is costly and inconvenient. In cases, where the only requirement is to treat androgen deficiency (and restoration of fertility is not required), androgen replacement therapy is used.

Klinefelter syndrome

It is the most common cause of partial male prepubertal hypogonadism. It is a chromosomal disorder; cell karyotype most commonly is 47,XXY (there is chromatin positive buccal smear). At times, it may be familial. Most commonly there is seminiferous tubular failure. There may also be varying degree of Leydig cell failure. Testes are usually small and firm. Penis and prostate sizes are variable depending upon testosterone secretory status. There is also presence of certain stigmata (Table 17.2). Patients may come with history of delayed puberty or an adult may come with history of infertility. Serum testosterone is low to normal; FSH and LH levels are always raised. Semen examination, karyotyping (to differentiate from mosaicism) and testicular biopsy may be required for diagnosis. Treatment with testosterone may be required if there is only Leydig cell failure. There is no treatment to induce spermatogenesis. Also read case history 17.2.

Gynecomastia (also see Appendix A)

It is breast development in the male. It is caused

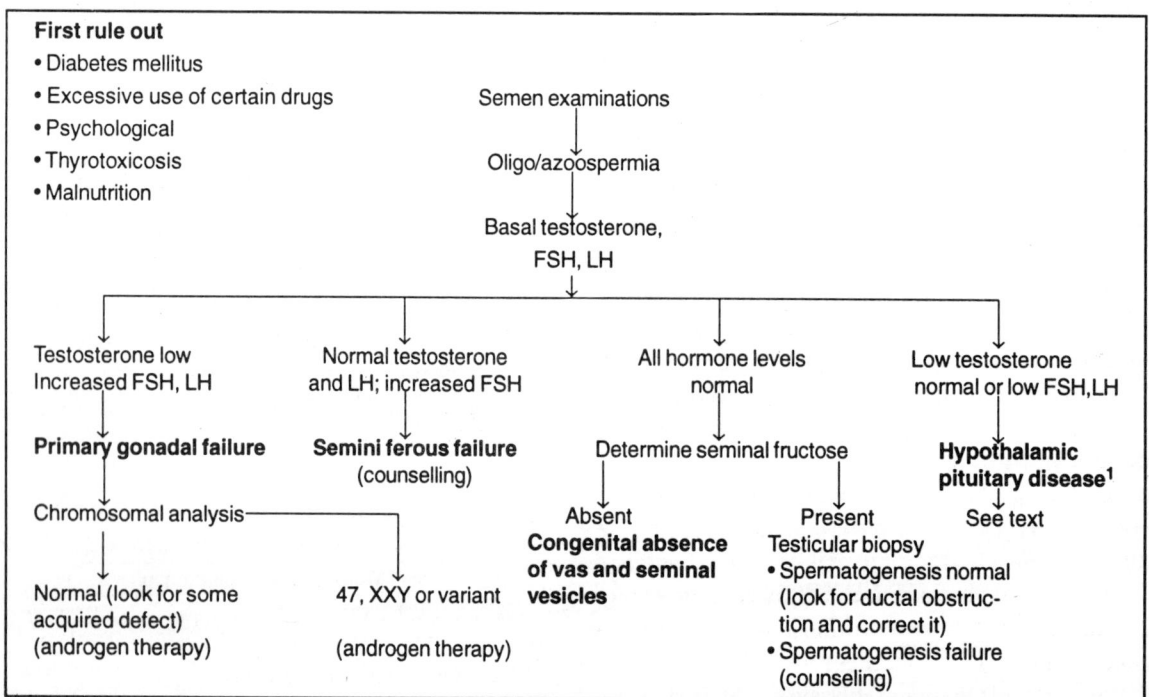

Fig. 17.6. Investigating case of male hypogonadism

---

[1] Besides sellar and other studies, PRL level should be determined.

- In partial androgen resistance cases, LH and testosterone are increased and FSH is normal.

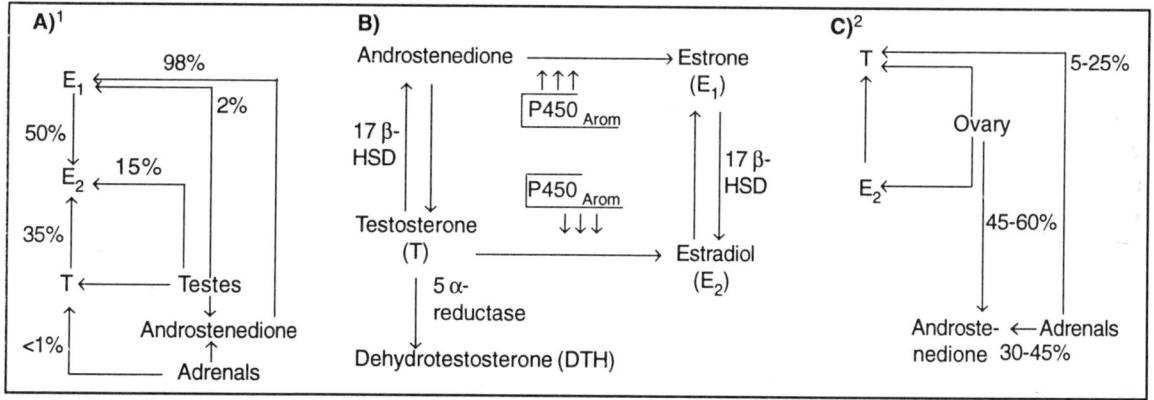

Fig. 17.7. Extragonadal aromatization of androgens (B) and sources of androgens in women (C) and of estrogens in men (A).

---

[1] In males note sources of E_1 (98% from androstenedione, 2% from testes) and E_2 (50% from E_1, 35% from T, 15% from testicular secretion). Elevated LH increases testicular secretion of E_2.

[2] In female note sources of androstenedione (40-60% from ovaries and 30-45% from adrenals) and T (three sources are shown).

- Nongonadal aromatase activity increases in obesity (read under PCOD) and in old age.

- 50% of metabolic products of testosterone and its metabolites (formed in liver) are 17-ketosteroids (androsterone and etiocholonone) and 50% are polar metabolites (diols, triols and their conjugates). Only about 40% of urinary 17-ketosteroids, in men, arise from testosterone and remaining from adrenal androgens.

by increased estrogen production (Fig. 17.7) and decreased testosterone/estradiol ratio in the male. It is regarded as physiological, when seen in a new born, in an adolescent boy and in an old male. In a new born it is due to the effect of maternal estrogens. In adolescence, testosterone/estradiol ratio decreases since aromatase activity (Fig. 17.7) matures earlier than testosterone secretion attains adult level. In old age it is due to increased aromatization of androgens in the adipose tissue. Pathological gynecomastia occurs in Klinefelter syndrome, testicular feminization, liver disease (impaired androgen metabolism) and tumors secreting estrogens or prolactin. Prolactin may have direct action on the breast glandular tissue or it may interfere with peripheral actions of testosterone. In hyperthyroidism increased synthesis of SHBG results in decrease in level of free testosterone. In any systemic illness or in malnutrition gonadotropin secretion declines. During recovery with resumption of normal secretion, there is increased relative production of estradiol (relative to testosterone) by testes. Many drugs also produce gynecomastia by modifying hormonal profile with respect to estradiol, testosterone and prolactin (some drugs interfere

with actions of testosterone or estradiol). Gynecomastia may be idiopathic in some cases.

Investigations are needed where cause is not obvious after careful history and physical examination. Serum levels of testosterone, FSH, LH, prolactin and SHBG may help diagnosis. In some cases, chromosomal analysis (Klinefelter syndrome), thyroid function tests or investigations for pituitary tumor may be needed.

Generally, no treatment is needed except for cosmetic reasons. Antiestrogen drugs (clomiphene citrate) have been used to reduce the swelling. In some cases plastic surgery may be needed.

THE OVARIAN HORMONES

These are estrogens (mainly 17-β-estradiol but also estrone) and progesterone. Besides ovary, estrogens are produced by placenta.

In the female the main androgens are androstenedione (predominently from the ovary in the reproductive period and adrenals in the post menopausal period) and dehydroepiandrosterone (from adrenals). Some testosterone is also produced from the ovary (Fig. 17.7).

Ovarian estrogens bring about puberty in

females including development of secondary sexual characters. Adrenal androgens help development of pubic and axillary hair, at puberty. A very important event at female puberty is start of menstrual cycle. Cyclic secretion of gonadotropins brings about the ovarian cycle (development of ovarian follicles, one of which matures and ovulates followed by formation of corpus luteum which degenerates at the end of ovarian cycle. This results in development of another group of follicles for the next cycle). Cyclic formation of estrogens and progesterone during the ovarian cycle brings about cyclic changes in endometrium (menstrual cycle) and cervical mucus (the cervical cycle). Control of ovarian cycle is shown in Fig. 17.8.

Other areas of female physiology, where estrogens and progesterone play their roles are pregnancy, breast development, lactation and parturition.

As the age of a female, with normal menstrual cycles advances, a time comes when ovaries become unresponsive to pituitary gonadotropins, and the ovarian cycles end. Secretions of estradiol and progesterone from the ovary greatly decline and menstrual cycles also end. The menopause is the last menstrual period. After this stage plasma

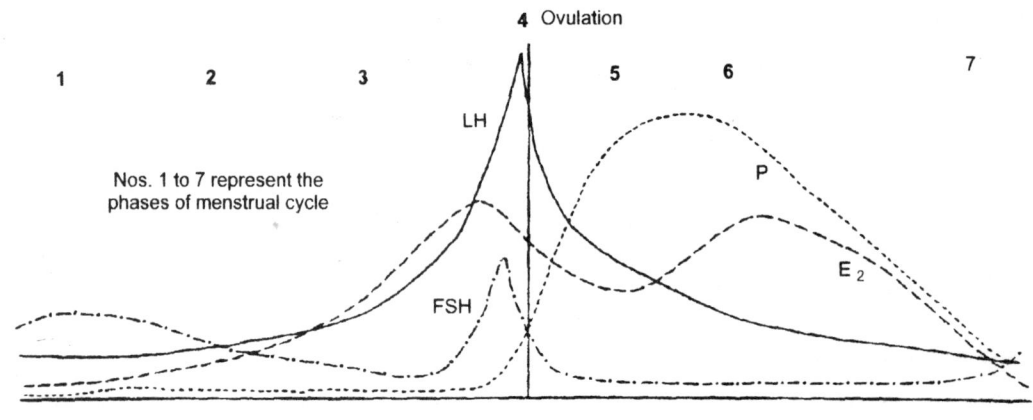

Fig. 17.8. Ovarian, uterine and cervical cycles in the female.

[1] This rise of FSH at the end of previous cycle (low levels of E and P) triggers development of a number of follicles into secondary follicles (with theca and granulosa cells). After this FSH level falls, although follicles keep on growing.

[2] The granulosa cell produced E further suppresses FSH. This causes regression of all developing follicles except one which survives matures and ovulates.

[3] The surviving follicle grows, helped by certain intraovarian factors and starts producing increasing amounts of E. A high level of E maintained for about 36h starts +ive feed back for LH/FSH.

[4] LH surge and a smaller FSH surge are responsible for ovulation.

[5] A reduced level of LH (after the LH surge) maintains corpus luteum.

[6] High E and P levels (from corpus luteum) in the luteal phase further reduces gonadotropin levels especially LH.

[7] (same as 1) Slightly raised level of FSH at the end of cycle.

Note: First day of cycle is the first day of menstrual bleeding. E=Estrogen; P=Progesterone estrogen levels greatly decrease and estrone is the major circulating estrogen derived from peripheral metabolism of androstenedione secreted by adrenals. FSH and LH levels are increased (former more than the latter) because of loss of feed back effects of ovarian hormones.

Biosynthesis (Figs. 17.2 and 17.7)

Estrogens are formed by ovarian follicles, corpus luteum and placenta and by aromatization of androgens in certain tissues (adipose tissue, skin and liver). In ovarian follicles theca interna cells (LH regulated) produce androstenedione and testosterone which are further aromatized in granulosa cells (FSH regulated) to form estrone and estradiol, respectively (Fig. 17.1)

The luteal cells besides producing progesterone (under control of LH), form estrone and estradiol by aromatizing androstenedione and testosterone (under control of FSH) received from theca interna, as mentioned above.

In plasma, only about 2% of estradiol is free and rest is in bound form (about 20% with sex hormone binding globulin (SHBG) and rest with albumin). SHBG also binds testosterone and it has greater affinity for testosterone than estradiol. If SHBG concentration decreases (Table 17.10) ratio of free testosterone to estradiol increases (although free levels of both decreases). Reverse happens on increase of SHBG.

Table 17.10. Factors altering SHBG concentration in plasma

Decrease in concentration:
- In women by androgen administration
- Hypothyroidism
- Corticosteroid therapy
- Obesity
- Acromegaly

Increase in concentration:
- Estrogen therapy/pregnancy
- Hyperthyroidism
- Liver disease (cirrhosis)
- Hypogonadism (in males)

- As binding affinity of SHBG is more for T than for E_2 with decrease of SHBG, there will be increase in ratio of free T and free E_2 (vice versa in case of increase of SHBG).

GONADAL DYSFUNCTIONS IN THE FEMALE

Common problems of gonadal dysfunction in females where laboratory help may be useful are, amenorrhea, hirsutism, virilism and impaired fertility.

Amenorrhea

A patient may present at puberty with the complaint that puberty including menarche has not occurred although the proper age is already over (primary amenorrhea). Second category of cases present with a history that puberty including menarche had previously been established and amenorrhea developed later on. Besides these two categories there are cases of genital tract abnormalities (say poor uterine development). These patients develop pubertal changes normally except that menstruation does not occur. Such cases can be ruled out by physical examination in most cases. In some cases absence of estrogen, progesterone withdrawl bleeding is used to confirm the disorder. Absent estrogen, progesterone withdrawl bleeding is also seen in amenorrhea caused by endometrial damage caused by tuberculosis or excessive curettage.

Diseases causing pseudohermaphroditism and mosaicism form a separate group and in these conditions varying percentage of patients present with amenorrhea. Amenorrhea accompanied by hirsutism/virilism is discussed later.

Prepubertal (primary) amenorrhea

In such patients one must, first rule out constitutional delay in puberty and other causes not involving hypothalamus-pituitary-gonad axis (Table 17.4). In constitutional delayed puberty cases, the hormonal profile resembles that of hypothalamic dysfunction (see later) but there is family history. After ruling out these causes, one must, next, consider, functional hypothalamic causes (Table 17.11).

Isolated hypogonadotropic hypogonadism often occurs as the Kallmann syndrome (as in boys). The affected females are sexually infantile and have a defect in synthesis/release of GnRH. Pituitary tumors cause amenorrhea by decreased secretion of gonadotropins or by increased secretion of prolactin. Tumors occurring early in life, will produce prepubertal amenorrhea. Craniopharyngiomas may

Table 17.11. Important causes of amenorrhea

Anatomic defects:
- Mullerian agenesis (second most common cause of primary amenorhea).
  - Karyotype is 46, XX; normal cyclic ovulation and secondary sex characters; uterus and vagina at different stages of hypoplasia (may present like outlet obstruction).
  - Presence of kidney and bone defects/family history of such defects.
  - In outlet defects (imperforate hymen, vaginal defects), there are cyclic bouts of abdominal pain; blood accumulating behind the obstruction.
- Testicular feminization (Table 17.3)
- Asherman's syndrome
  - Amenorrhea after curettage/endometrial tuberculosis/IUD related infections.

Gonadal failure (increased LH, FSH and low estrogen)**:**
- Gonadal dysgenesis and pure gonadal dysgenesis.
  - Germ cells are absent and ovaries are replaced by fibrous streaks.
  - Characteristics are primary amenorrhea, sexual infantilism short stature and multiple congenital anomalies due to any of the several possible defects in X-chromosome.
  - Some patients may have a few follicles and a short initial period of ovulation.
  - A major group of patients have a 45, X karyotype (Turner's syndrome, Table 17.2). Some patients are mosaics, with no structural abnormality (46, XX/45,X) and the rest have structurally abnormal X chromosome with or wihout moaicism. The patients other than those with classic genotype (45, X), in general , have severity in beween that seen in 45, X variety and the normal. In some of these patients (with clitoric hypertrophy) there is unidentified chromosomal fragment, believed to be an abnormal Y. Gonadoblastoma may develop in these patients. *In pure gonadal dysgenesis the patient has normal XX or XY karyotype (chromosomes are normal) but for some reason gonadal differentiation is abnormal and gonadal sex does not correspond to chromosomal sex. This disorder is much less common than gonadal dysgenesis. Also see note under Table 17.2. All women with elevated gonadotropin levels under 30 years should undergo karyotyping and if a Y-chromosome or its component is present, early prophylactic gonadectomy should be considered except in cases of complete feminization (Table 17.3) where surgery can be deferred until after the time of expected puberty.*
- 17α-hydroxylase deficiency (rare: there is primary amenorrhea with sexual infantilism and hypertension and hypokalemia) and galactosemia (FSH, LH are inactive due to their abnormal carbohydrate components)
- Premature ovarian failure
  - It is also called premature menopause and may be one component of PGA I or PGA II.
- Resistant ovary syndrome
  - Karyotype (XX) and features like pure gonadal dysgenesis. Ovarian biopsy is used to differentiate.

Chronic anovulation without estrogen deficiency:
- Chronic polycystic ovarian disease
  - Most common presentation is infertility, hirsutism, obesity and amenorrhea or oligomenorrhea (polycystic ovarian disease).
  - Some patients present with primary amenorrhea with progesterone withdrawl bleeding present (chronic polycystic ovarian disease).
  - Moderate increase in testosterone, androstenedione, DHEA and LH (LH, FSH ratio is >2): At least 50% decrease in levels of testosterone, androsterone after oral intake of synthetic estrogens and progestins as present in contraceptives for 21 days. No decrease occurs in ovarian tumors or adrenal disorders.

Chronic anovulation with poor estrogen status (Hypogonadotropic hypogonadism; normal or low LH and FSH, low estrogen with or without hyperprolactinemia)**:**
- Isolated gonadotropin deficiency
  - In Kallmann syndrome there is low GnRH release as well as anosmia.
  - There is primary amenorrhea and sexual infantilism.

Contd....

Contd. Table 17.11

- Hypothalamic pituitary lesions (tumors both primary and secondary, trauma, granulomas, irradiation, infarction)
    - Amenorrhea may be accompanied by deficiency of other hormones (GH, ACTH, TSH or AVP) along with deficiency of LH and FSH, with or without hyperprolactinemia.
    - Tumors may act by directly interfering with secretion of gonadotropins or indirectly by increased secretion of prolactin.
    - 50 to 70% of patients of pituitary tumors have associated increased prolactin levels.
    - About 1/10th of amenorrheic women have increased prolactin levels.
- Functional hypothalamic disorders
    - Cause is some sudden stress/ severe physical activity/ weight loss.
    - Functional amenorrhea also occurs in anorexia nervosa.
    - Gonadotropin levels are low or low normal compared to normal women in early follicular phase of the cycle.

- Amenorrhea can also be caused by androgen excess. Examples are PCOD (discussed above; testosterone level usually <200 ng/dL), tumors of adrenal or ovary and use of anabolic steroids (in athletes). These causes are also discussed under 'hirsutism'.
- It is important to rule out pregnancy and thyroid disorders right at the outset.

present with sexual infantilism, delayed puberty and amenorrhea due to gonadotropin deficiency. Secretion of other hormones (TSH, ACTH, GH and AVP) may also be reduced. These tumors constitute about 3% of intracranial neoplasms and frequently extends into suprasellar region. Tumor may calcify and become amenable to diagnosis by conventional X-ray skull.

Ovarian dysgenesis is the commonest cause of ovarian failure resulting in prepubertal amenorrhea. Turner phenotype can be recognized from the associated somatic abnormalities (Tables 17.2, 17.11). The ovarian failure cases are associated with elevated levels of gonadotropins. Other causes of ovarian failure (besides ovarian dysgenesis) are given in Table 17.11. For diagnosis of ovarian dysgenesis, karyotyping, becomes important, besides proper clinical examination.

Patients with anatomical defects, can be diagnosed by proper examination of external genitalia and examining for presence or absence of uterus.

Post pubertal (secondary) amenorrhea

In these cases one has to rule out pregnancy, thyroid disorders and the functional hypothalamic disorders, in the first place. Next, one must consider more common causes given in Table 17.9.

Post pubertal amenorrhea can also be due to pituitary tumors (and other causes) producing deficiency of gonadotropins or increased secretion of prolactin (Fig. 17.11). As already mentioned these

conditions can also produce prepubertal amenorrhea.

Ovarian cause of post pubertal amenorrhea can be premature ovarian failure (uncommon). It may have autoimmune etiology and there may also be associated autoimmune damage to adrenals and thyroid.

Table 17.11 shows different causes which may produce pre-pubertal (primary) amenorrhea and/ or post-pubertal (secondary) amenorrhea. Some causes, mostly result, in primary and others, predominently, in secondary amenorrhea and at places it has been indicated in the Table. For example most women with gonadal dysgenesis, have primary amenorrhea but some may ovulate for short period before becoming amenorrheic. Similarly, polycystic ovarian disease predominently causes secondary amenorrhea but on occasions, it may cause primary amenorrhea. Functional hypothalamic causes should be, especially, looked for and also those given in Table 17.8.

Diagnosis

The first step in diagnosis of the cause of amenorrhea is to exclude pregnancy by some suitable screening test. Next, a proper history and a good physical examination including examination for pubertal changes (development of breasts, pubic and axillary hair), examination of external genitalia and presence or absence of uterus, is undertaken. History of severe stress, weight loss or severe physical stress should be elicited. History of curettage may suggest Asherman's syndrome. Proper physical examination may show some anatomic defect of the outflow tract or sexual infantilism.

In a patient with sexual infantilism and primary amenorrhea, it will be important to differentiate ovarian and hypothalamic/pituitary causes. Even in secondary amenorrhea, many times, this type of differentiation is required.

In case of strong suspicion of a particular cause, it is wise to proceed directly to confirm the cause.

For example in a patient with somatic defects suggestive of Turner's syndrome, chromosomal karyotyping should be done.

In less clear cases, after ruling out pregnancy, initial evaluation requires determination of estrogen status, estimation of prolactin and gonadotropins. Fig. 17.9 summarizes the evaluation procedure.

In constitutional delay of puberty no treatment is required. However, a short term treatment with low dose oral ethinyl estradiol may be used to give psychological support to the individual.

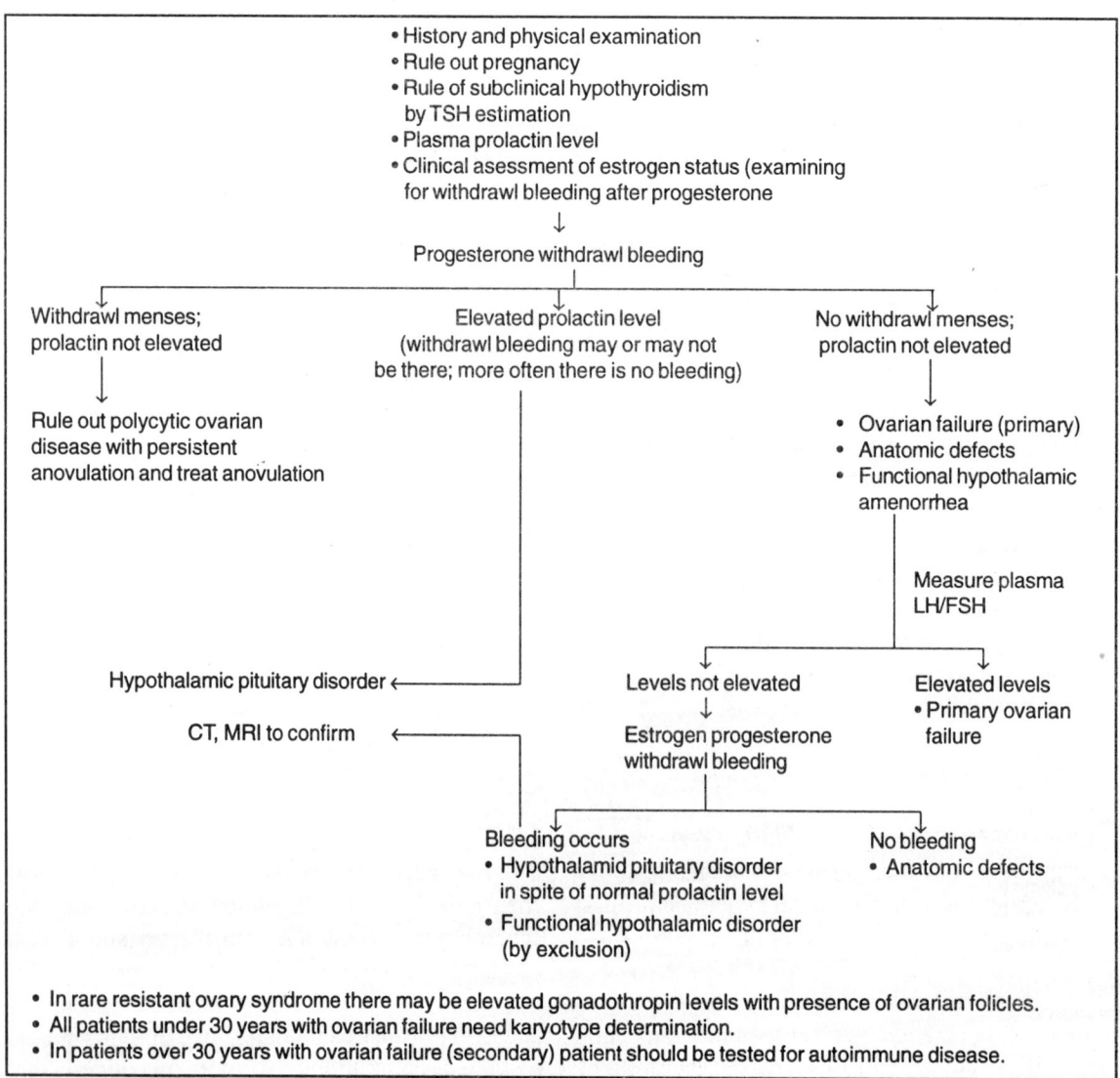

Fig. 17.9. Investigating a case of amenorrhea.

The ovarian causes are treated with estrogen alone or with estrogen and progesterone to initiate menstrual cycles.

In pituitary and hypothalamic diseases when fertility is not required, menstrual cycles can be simulated by the same treatment. This treatment also takes care of osteoporosis. If fertility is desired, cyclic administration of FSH and LH and mid-cycle administration of hCG (to simulate LH peak inducing ovulation) is used. However, administration of excessive amounts of gonadotropins has to be avoided for danger of multiple ovulation and formation of ovarian cysts. Multiple ovulation is less likely to occur with pulsatile therapy of GnRH. In hypothalamic failure clomiphene may also be used to stimulate GnRH secretion (by modulating estrogen receptor activity, in GnRH secreting cells).

Treatment with corticosteroids often restores menstruation in cases of congenital adrenal hyperplasia. In hyperprolactinemia bromocriptine (a dopamine agonist) will reduce secretion of prolactin (see under hyperprolactinemia and polycsytic ovary syndrome).

Polycystic ovarian syndrome

The intraovarian defect, in polycystic ovary syndrome prevents ovulation and this results in formation of large cysts (Fig. 17.10).

Loss of regulatory relationship between gonadotropins and ovarian estrogens which may produce anovulatory cycles, forms basis of many female disorders (Fig. 17.10) including polycystic ovarian syndrome.

There are large cystic ovaries, some times palpable by pelvic examination. Women are often obese. As already mentioned, these women may have menstrual defects and hirsutism without virilization. Some may present with primary amenorrhea, others with infertility because of anovulatory cycles. Mild hirsutism is often present but some may present without hirsutism.

Important laboratory findings are moderately increased serum testosterone, dehydroepiandrosterone, androstenedione and LH and low FSH (LH:FSH ratio ≥ 3 is considered diagnosis) (Table 17.11). Confirmation of large cystic ovaries may be obtained from pelvic ultrasonography or laparoscopy.

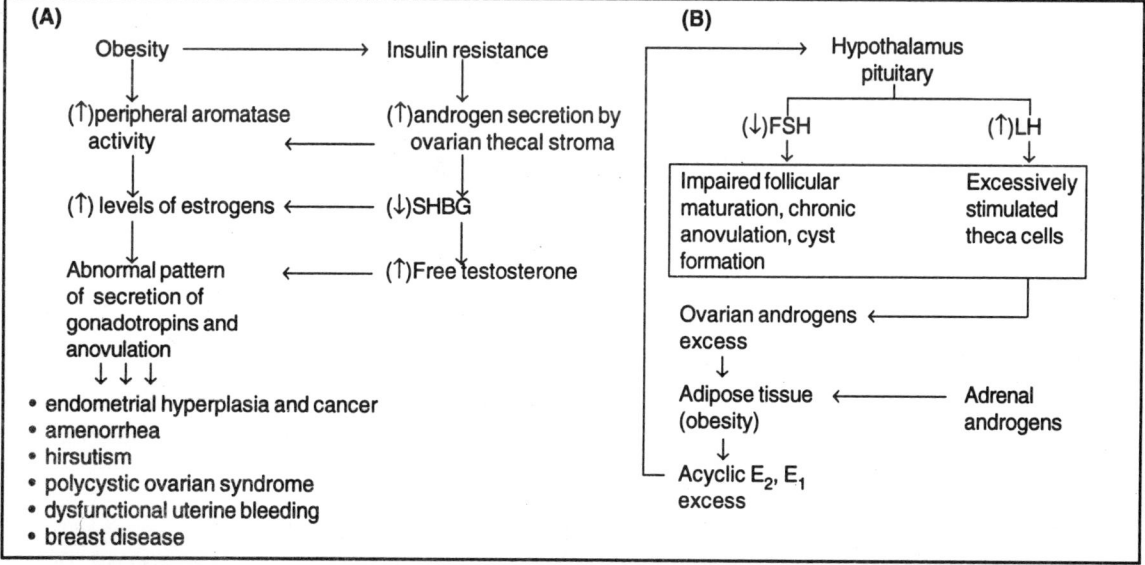

Fig. 17.10. Pathogenesis of chronic anovulation and associated disorders (A) and pathogenesis of polycystic ovarian disease (B)

- The pathological process in (A) maybe initiated by obesity and insulin resistance; increased aromatization (obesity, hyperthyroidism, liver disease); increased androgen levels (androgen secreting tumors, liver disease, stress); increased direct secretion of estrogens (ovarian tumors) and decreased levels of SHBG.

For treatment, ovarian androgen secretion is reduced by use of oral contraceptives, wedge resection of ovary or by increasing FSH secretion by administration of clomiphene or human menopausal gonadotropin (hMG). Use of oral contraceptives can also result in periodic bleeding to simulate menstrual cycles. These drugs also reduce hirsutism and chances of malignant change in endometrium. Clomiphene may be able to establish ovulatory cycles. This may increase chances of pregnancy.

Hirsutism and virilism

Presence of increased number of hair on face, chest, back, lower abdomen and thighs in a female is called hirsutism.

Hirsuitism is a common condition. Most of these women have normal menstrual periods and there is no virilism. In majority of these, it may not be easy to establish any biochemical reason for the abnormality. In some of these idiopathic cases, there may be increased activity of 5 α-reductase or increased concentrations of free androgens because of decreased levels of SHBG (sex hormone binding globulin) (Table 17.10).

1 to 5% of hirsute women may have menstrual abnormalities from adult onset congenital adrenal hyperplasia and polycystic ovary syndrome. A small number from these may also have features of virilism (excessive masculinity including deepening of voice, temporal recession of hair and enlargement of clitoris).

Table 17.12. Causes of hirsutism in women

- Familial
- Idiopathic
- Drugs
- Ovarian causes
  - Polycystic ovarian disease, hilus cell hyperplasia
  - Tumors (arrhenoblastoma, hilus cell tumor, Brenner tumor)
- Adrenal causes
  - Congenital adrenal hyperplasia
  - Cushing's syndrome
  - Tumors (virilizing carcinoma, rarely adenoma).

- In idiopathic cases increased target tissues hypersensitivity/ increased 5 α-reductase activity may have a role to play.
- Relative androgenic potencies of androgens are T(100%), DHT (250%), androstenedione (10-20%), DHEA (5%) and minimal for DHEA-SO$_4$.

Sudden appearance of increased hair growth, amenorrhea and virilization is likely to be due to an ovarian or adrenal androgen producing tumor. Important causes are given in Table 17.12. Some drugs like phenothiazines, minoxidil and phenytoin also produce increase in body hair. Increase in hair, however, is of general type and not specifically, of male type.

Diagnosis

An important objective of investigations in cases of hirsutism is to rule out etiologies with androgen excess (adrenal and ovarian tumors, congenital adrenal hyperplasia, polycystic ovaries). Sudden onset and progressive hirsutism and virilization suggests, an ovarian or adrenal neoplasm. Virilizing adrenal adenomas are rare. Adrenal carcinoma is associated with elevated plasma DHEA-sufate and increased urinary excretion of 17-ketosteroids (cortisol levels in blood and urine are normal or only moderately increased).

Increased DHEA-sufate in plasma and increased 17-ketosteroids in urine may also occur in late onset adrenal hyperplasia. In this case, however, the metabolite levels are suppressed by high dose dexamethasone while no suppression occurs in case of adrenal tumors (see Table 15.5).

The most common virilizing ovarian tumor is arrhenoblastoma (others are adrenal rest tumor, granulosa cell tumor, hilar cell tumor, Brenner tumor). Plasma DHEA-sufate and urinary 17-ketosteroid levels remain, generally, normal. In some cases urinary 17-ketosteroids excretion is increased but remains less than 30 mg/d, except in adrenal rest tumors (in adrenal tumors excretion is more than 30 mg/d). With the exception of adrenal rest tumor, androgen production in ovarian tumors is not influenced by ACTH. No dexamethasone suppression occurs in the adrenal or ovarian Tumors. The virilizing ovarian tumors usually secrete testosterone and androstenedione (which is converted into testosterone in peripheral tissues) (Fig. 17.7). Thus plasma testosterone levels are increased in ovarian tumors. CT-scan and MRI help to locate the tumors.

Polycystic ovarian disease is the commonest cause of androgen excess and is associated with

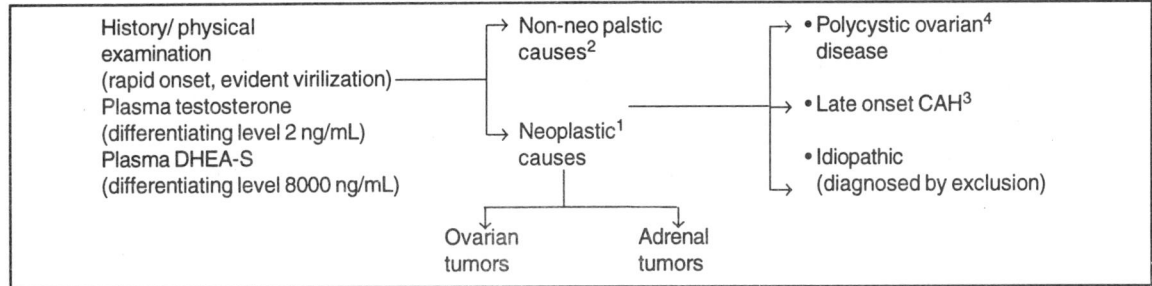

Fig. 17.11. Diagnosis of hirsutism.

---

[1] Urinary 17-ketosteroids and plasma DHEA-SO$_4$ are high in adrenal carcinoma and usually normal in ovarian tumors in which often plasma testosterone level is increased. However, testosterone level may also increase from its peripheral formation from adrenal androgens, in adrenal carcinoma.

[2] Plasma testosterone/DHEA-SO$_4$ levels, differentiating neoplastic from non-neoplastic causes are given in the figure.

[3] Decrease in increased urinary excretion of 17-ketosteroids and plasma level of DHEA-SO$_4$ in response to high dose dexamethasone is a characteristic response in CAH.

[4] There is generally chronic anovulation (presence of progesterone withdrawl bleeding). Also LH/FSH ratio >2.0.

hirsutism but less commonly with virilization. Plasma levels of androstenedione and to lesser extent testosterone, are elevated. Increased urinary 17-ketosteroid excretion is partially reduced by dexamethasone. Low FSH and high LH levels cause increased LH/FSH ratio (see under polycystic ovarian disease). Fig. 17.11 gives a simple scheme to differentiate between common causes of hirsutism.

In majority of cases, all laboratory parameters will be normal. These mild cases of hirsutism without virilization, often, have a family history. In these cases, only, cosmetic treatment is advised.

In late onset congenital adrenal hyperplasia cases with menstrual disturbances, a synthetic glucocorticoid should be tried to suppress androgen secretion. In children, bone growth and maturation need to be properly monitored, since over treatment may cause growth retardation.

In cases of polycystic ovary disease oral contraceptives can be used. This treatment is avoided above 35 years of age, in smokers, hypertensives, those with history of thromboembolic disease or impaired liver functions. In these cases an antiandrogen drug, cyproterone can also be tried. This drug blocks action of androgens at hair follicles. If fertility is required, instead of above drugs, clomiphene or gonadotropins should be tried. Other serious cases need specific treatment.

Infertility

A couple is said to be sub-fertile, if conception does not result after one year of regular and unprotected intercourse. Husband is at fault in about 40% cases and wife in about 60% cases. Infertility may often be caused by multiple factors. Endocrine cause of infertility is very uncommon in the male while in females endocrine defects may be responsible in about one third of the cases. In males the most important cause is defective sperm production and hence the importance of semen examination. Important causes of infertility in the two sexes are given in Table 17.13. Characteristics of normal semen are given in Table 17.14.

Table 17.13. Causes of infertility

In the male (40%):
• Abnormal sperm production -Semen examination

In the female (60%):
• Pelvic factors (tubal disease or endriometriosis) (50%)
  - Hysterosalpingography
  - Laparoscopy
• Failure of ovulation including luteal phase dysfunctions (endocrinal causes) (30%)
  - Testing for presence of ovulation
  - Testing for progesterone levels
• Cervical factors (10%)
  - Post coital test
• Causes not found (10-20%)

- In the male defective sperm formation is the **most important** cause; endocrine causes are rare.

Table 17.14. The criteria of normal semen

Normal ejaculate volume	2 to 6 mL
%age of motile sperms	> 60%
%age of normal morphology sperms	> 60%
Sperm number/ml and number	> 20 million/mL
of total sperms/ejaculate	> 60 million

(in actual experience the relation of above parameters to fertility is often uncertain)

- Semen sample should be obtained by masterbation into a glass container after 24 to 36h of abstinence.
- Motility should be studied in undiluted sample within 30 min. of collection.

A detailed history and clinical examination is extremely important in cases of couples seeking advice on infertility. Information should be sought on previous pregnancies, use of contraceptive devices, use of drugs, sexually transmitted diseases, other serious illnesses (including diabetes mellitus and thyroid disorders), smoking habits, marital relations and other aspects. Detailed menstrual history and complete medical, surgical and gynecological examinations are also of utmost importance. All these aspects and even many investigations (micro-biological, immunological and those concerning patency of tubes) are not in the scope of this book.

Endocrine investigations of the female

Anovulation is responsible for about 15% of infertility problems. If a woman has regular menstruation, especially preceded by certain well defined symptoms, or if she has dysmenorrhea, she must be ovulating normally. Use of rise in basal body temperature is also a useful indicator (Table 17.6). The best way, however, is to measure progesterone levels between days 17 and 23 in three separate cycles. A level more than 30 nmol/L indicates an ovulatory cycle and that less than 10 nmol/L suggests an anovulatory cycle. For levels between 10 and 30 nmol/L, a defect in luteal phase is indicated, although cycles may be ovulatory. This can also lead to sub-fertility.

In case of anovulatory cycles or luteal phase defect, clomiphene administration may bring about conception. If it fails or if there is amenorrhea, one may proceed with further investigations (measure-

ment of prolactin, gonadotropins, etc.) as discussed under amenorrhea.

CASE HISTORY: 17.1

A two week old baby was brought with intermediate genitalia (female pseudohermaphroditism). The baby was buccal smear chromatin positive and chromosomal analysis demonstrated karyotype as 46, XX.

The commonest cause of female pseudohermaphroditism is CAH. Other causes are androgen secreting adrenal and ovarian tumors. It should also be ascertained that no androgen administration was done during pregnancy. True hermaphroditism is a rare condition and its possibility is entertained only after all causes of pseudohermaphroditism, have been ruled out. Final confirmation of this condition requires demonstration of presence of both testicular and ovarian tissues on laparotomy.

Important laboratory features of androgen secreting tumors are discussed under diagnosis of hirsutism. The most common enzymatic defect producing CAH is 21 hydroxylase deficiency. High level of 17-hydroxyprogesterone, in plasma is diagnostic of this condition. Heterozygotes can be detected (in a family) by HLA typing or by studying ACTH induced rise in plasma level of 17-hydroxyprogesterone. Prenatal diagnosis of this condition is also possible. This is done by showing high levels of 17-hydroxyprogesterone in amniotic fluid or by DNA analysis using chorionic villus sample. With proper treatment prognosis of most of the patients is good and fertility is possible. Patients are treated with glucocorticoids (to reduce androgen formation) along with, a mineralocorticoid (in case there is excessive salt loss) and early surgical repair of ambiguous genitalia. In management of CAH babies, cortisol replacement therapy, not only, takes care of cortisol deficiency but also maintains a check on process of virilization. Adequacy of the replacement therapy is monitored by estimating plasma levels of 17 OH-progesterone, androstenedione and ACTH. Renin activity may be monitored if some mineralocorticoid is also being administered.

Gender assignment in difficult cases is best done in early infancy, depending upon chromosomal and gondal sex. The required correction is also applied to external genitalia.

Some other causes of female pseudohermaphroditism are mentioned in Fig. 17.5.

CASE HISTORY: 17.2

A couple after 5 years of their marriage consulted their physician with the complaint that they had no issue. Husband was quite tall (age 32 years) and complained of, lack of libido. He had poor growth of hair on his body. Testes were small and firm. Penis was normal. He also had prominent gynecomastia.

Data of the patient is quite suggestive of Klinefelter syndrome. It is not uncommon (present in one out of 400 to 500 males). Patients are tall (because of long legs) and present with infertility, delayed puberty and occasionally, underandrogenization. Gynecomastia isn common. Other associated abnormalities, in many cases are, obesity, varicose veins, mild mental deficiency, diabetes mellitus, pulmonary disease and abnormalities of thyroid functions. Breast cancer is more common than in normal men.

Plasma testosterone and estrogen levels are lower or in lower part of normal range. Increased estrogen, testosterone ratio promotes development of gynecomastia. Plasma levels of both LH and FSH (increase in FSH is more consistent) are elevated.

Besides hormonal studies, semen examination and karyotyping should be done. Semen is free from sperms and cell karyotype is 47, XXY. Testicular biopsy will show sclerosis of tubules. Condition has to be differentiated from ordinary gynecomastia, mosaicism and XX male syndrome. Karyotyping will detect patients with mosaicism (say 46, XY/47, XXY). These patients have a milder disease. Gynecomastia and azoospermia are less common. XX male has karyotype 46, XX. These patients have height less than normal; mental deficiency is less common but hypospadias is more common, compared to Klinefelter syndrome.

Treatment of Klinefelter syndrome (and XX male syndrome) includes androgen replacement therapy in underandrogenized patients and surgical removal of the breasts. There is no treatment for infertility except invitro fertilization.

CASE HISTORY: 17.3

A 17 year old boy presented with lack of pubertal changes. His penis was infantile, pubic and axillary hair sparse. His physical growth was however, not retarded. He was also not suffering from any chronic systemic disease. Karyotype was normal and there were no somatic abnormalities. Proper family history about age of puberty was not available. Plasma FSH and LH levels were low.

As there is no physical growth retardation, systemic diseases, thyroid hormone and growth hormone deficiencies, are ruled out. Absence of somatic abnormalities and normal karyotype makes primary gonadal failure less likely. Gonadal failure secondary to viral infection or some other reason is also ruled out because of low levels of FSH and LH.

In the present case, constitutional delayed puberty and the Kallmann syndrome are two conditions, one of which is likely to be correct diagnosis. Unfortunately, family history for either of the two disorders is not

available. However, anosmia or hyposmia and cryptorchidism (features associated with Kallmann syndrome) are absent in the present case. Kallmann syndrome is inherited as X-linked recessive trait or as autosomal dominant trait with variable expressivity. Some patients may present with isolated finding of prepubertal microphallus.

It is difficult to differentiate between Kallmann syndrome and constitutional delayed puberty, in the present case. To rule out constitutional delayed puberty the patient should be observed upto 18 years of age. In almost all cases of constitutional delay in puberty signs of puberty appear by this time (in normal girls signs of puberty appear at about 11 years of bone age and in boys at about 12 years of bone age).

With onset of puberty, increased secretions of both gonadotropins and sex hormones occur in episodic fashion. As half life of sex steroids is more than those of gonadotropins, in a random sample, it is better to study the levels of sex steroids than gonadotropins, in evaluation of puberty. If the latter hormones have to be studied, either levels should be studied after GnRH stimulation or their basal levels during sleep. If puberty is in process, 100 µg of intravenous GnRH increases LH concentration by more than 15.0 mIU/mL (both in boys and girls), and this response continues till adulthood. This test may indicate start of puberty when there is no physical sign of puberty.

CASE HISTORY: 17.4

A 30 year old married woman presented with history of irregular periods developing into amenorrhea recently. She had a 6 year old child. She wanted to be investigated for infertility and amenorrhea. Patient did not show progesterone withdrawl bleeding. However, estrogen-progesterone withdrawal bleeding occurred.

As there is no progesterone withdrawl bleeding, the patient is not suffering from anovulatory cycles (chronic anovulation with estrogen present). Further as estrogen, progesterone withdrawl bleeding occurs, damaged endometrium is ruled out. The important conditions that remain for differential diagnosis are, primary ovarian failure, premature menopause, hypothyroidism, hyperprolactinemia and pituitary/hypothalamic disorders. Important investigations required in this case are, serum levels of FSH, LH, prolactin; besides, she should also be investigated for thyroid status. Her pituitary hormonal profile was: FSH 55 IU/L, LH 45 IU/L, and prolactin 50 ng/mL. The investigations revealed a sort of premature menopause due to some ovarian damage. It could be an autoimmune failure of ovaries. In polyglandular autoimmune syndromes, ovarian failure may also be accompanied by thyroid and adrenal failures. Thus patient needs to be further investigated for status of her thyroid and adrenal hormones. Fertility cannot be restored in this case.

CASE HISTORY: 17.5

A 22 year man presented with perineoscrotal hypospadias, cryptorchidism and gynecomastia. His body built was male type and axillary and pubic hair were normal. Testes were small and their position was high scrotal. Karyotype was 46,XY. Plasma levels of both testosterone and estradiol were raised. LH level was also high.

The patient is a pseudohermaphrodite and the hormonal profile suggests diagnosis as incomplete testicular feminization. The condition is caused by the androgen receptor defect.

In androgen resistance cases, because of reduced feed back effect of testosterone, plasma LH level is increased. This in turn, increases production of both testosterone and estrogens by testes. Depending upon the extent of androgen resistance and the plasma estrogen level, different clinical forms are produced. In its severe form, phenotype is female with external genitalia female type and with absence of both Mullerian and Wolffian duct structures. Breast remains female type. Hormonal profile is similar as in this case.

In the present case androgen resistance (due to less severe defect in the receptor) in partial. Treatment of the present case includes surgical correction of hypospadias, and cryptorchidism. Gynecomastia also needs surgical removal.

Other causes of hypospadias and cryptorchidism

Hypospadias is a congenital anomaly in which urethra terminates (along ventral midline of penis), earlier than normal position. It is believed to be produced by some defect in androgen formation or action, during embryogenesis. It is seen in most disorders of male differentiation. Consumption of progestational agents during pregnancy may also cause this condition. In about 75% cases, however, its cause is not known (no relation to any known gene defect, chromosomal abnormality or any hormone intake during pregnancy). Treatment is surgical. In United States it occurs in more than 0.5% of male births.

Testes are formed in abdomen and descend into scrotum subsequently. About 3% of full - term and 30% of premature male infants have, atleast, one cryptorchid testis at birth, but the descent is completed within the first few weeks of life. In cases of permanent cryptorchidism, position of testis may be high scrotal, in the inguinal canal, or intraabdominal. Inadequate intraabdominal pressure or lack of certain hormones (testosterone or MIF) may be responsible for this condition. The exact etiology is not known as only a small fraction of these cases can be associated with known disorders. In the abdominal position of testes, spermatogenesis is affected and in bilateral cases infertility may result. Undescended testis (permanent) is more liable to become malignant and should be removed.

OBJECTIVE TYPE QUESTIONS

Pick out the wrong statement.

1. Sex determination

i) At the first level, sex is determined by sex chromosomes.

ii) Proper sex chromosomes determine proper gonad formation.

iii) Phenotypic sex is determined by proper gonads.

iv) With normal karyotype there is always normal gonad formation and normal sex phenotype.

v) In gonadal dysgenesis, gonads are in the form of fibrous streaks and condition is the most common cause of primary amenorrhea accounting for about one third of total cases.

2. Conditions of absent/rudimentary gonads

i) Gonads are present as fibrous streaks in gonadal dysgenesis.

ii) Gonads are present as fibrous streaks in pure gonadal dysgenesis.

iii) In anorchia or gonadal agenesis testes are absent or rudimentary.

iv) A patient of anorchia presents as a female with primary amenorrhea.

v) Testicular regression could be result of mutant gene, trauma or a teratogen.

3. Leydig cell functions

i) The laboratory help is more important in assessment of Leydig cell functions in the prepubertal period than the postpubertal one.

ii) At the start of male puberty both plasma testosterone and LH levels are higher at night than during the day due to nocturnal LH surge.

iii) Because of pulsatile nature of both LH and testosterone (pulses 60 to 90 min, apart), three samples collected 20 min apart should be pooled for analysis, for either of the two.

iv) Level of plasma LH helps proper interpretation of plasma testosterone level and vice versa.

v) Before puberty testosterone response to hCG stimulation is used to assess Leydig cell function since both LH and testosterone levels are low.

4. Gonadotropin response to GnRH administration

i) Quantitative responses of LH and FSH to GnRH administration, are similar, both before pubertal development and with pubertal development.

ii) LH response to GnRH administration is quite variable in normal men.

iii) Patients of secondary testicular failure can have normal or abnormal response.

iv) In primary testicular failure increased basal LH level is usually sufficient for diagnosis (GnRH stimulation test is not required).

v) In cases of secondary testicular failure, a subnormal response establishes the diagnosis while a normal response does not carry much significance.

5. Seminiferous tubular function

i) A decrease in size of testes, in postpubertal period indicates damage to seminiferous tubules.

ii) Semen examination is the most useful investigation in cases of male infertility.

iii) Moderate damage to germinal epithelium of seminiferous tubules may be indicated by semen examination.

iv) Severe damage to germinal epithelium of seminiferous tubules causes increase in FSH level and decrease in inhibin level.

v) Testicular biopsy is useful in some patients of azoospermia or oligospermia.

6. Assessment of gonadal function in a female

i) Presence of secondary sexual characters, say proper breast development indicates adequate estrogen secretion in the past.

ii) Regular predictable events in menstrual cycle imply normal pituitary gonadotropins as well as ovarian hormones.

iii) In cases of amenorrhea, the progesterone withdrawl test is used to assess functional estrogen status.

iv) No clinical method is available for assessment of functional status of progesterone.

v) In conditions of androgen excess, hirsutism, with or without virilization occurs.

7. Hormone estimations in the female

i) Estimation of plasma estradiol is helpful to establish estrogen status in diagnosis of a number of female reproductive disorders.

ii) Cyclic, predictable menses imply that progesterone levels are adequate in the luteal phase of menstrual cycle.

iii) Estimation of plasma progesterone is helpful to evaluate adequacy of luteal phase in subfertile women.

iv) Serum gonadotropin levels are very useful in supporting diagnosis of hypogonadotropic hypogonadism and polycystic ovarian disease.

v) Serum gonadotropin estimation is also of great help in evaluation of women with suspected primary ovarian failure.

8. Estrogen formation in the male

i) plasma estrone level is higher than estradiol level.

ii) All plasma estrone arises from peripheral aromatization of androstenedione.

iii) Most plasma estradiol arises from peripheral aromatization of testosterone.

iv) Plasma estrogen levels increase in adrenal disease (increased formation of precursor molecules), testicular tumors and the disorder of androgen resistance.

v) Liver disease leads to increased estrogen levels due to reduced metabolic disposal of estrogens.

vi) Relative increase of estrogens to testosterone (higher plasma estrogen, testosterone ratio) may cause gynecomastia.

9. Delayed puberty

i) It may be constitutional.

ii) It may be due to panhypopituitarism.

iii) It may result from hypothyroidism.

iv) In androgen resistance cases, there is always associated male pseudohermaphroditism and increased plasma testosterone and LH levels.

v) Most common testicular cause, the Klinefelter syndrome (a chromosomal disorder) is associated with low testosterone and high LH and FSH levels.

vi) In Kallmann syndrome there is isolated gonadotropin deficiency.

10. Kallmann syndrome

i) There may be severe to partial gonadotropin deficiency leading to low testosterone level.

ii) In partial form there is some pubertal development and some testicular growth.

iii) This is also the most common cause of isolated finding of early pubertal/midpubertal microphallus.

iv) Anosmia/hyposmia and cryptorchidism are common associated findings.

v) Inheritance is X-linked recessive or autosomal dominant with variable expressivity.

11. Constitutional delay in puberty

i) Delayed puberty in boys may commence at 16th year of life or even later.

ii) Constitutional delayed development affects both growth and onset of puberty; bone age is also delayed.

iii) Diagnosis is, often not difficult.

iv) Family history may be suggestive of the diagnosis of delayed puberty.

v) LH response to LHRH may suggest that puberty is imminent.

12. Some causes of hypothalamic/pituitary gonadotropic dysfunction in adults

i) High cortisol levels in Cushing's syndrome can reduce LH secretion.

ii) Infertility of congenital adrenal hyperplasia (adult onset) is explained by suppressed gonadotropin secretion by adrenal androgens.

iii) Hyperprolactinemia may cause combined Leydig cell and seminiferous tubular dysfunction by inhibition of both LH and FSH by prolactin.

iv) Use of androgens for any clinical purpose will increase function of seminiferous tubules.

v) Main effect of hemochromatosis, to impair testicular function, is exerted at pituitary.

13. Klinefelter syndrome

i) The Leydig cell functions and spermatogenesis are equally impaired.

ii) The classical form has karyotype 47,XXY and the mosaic form the karyotype 46,XY/47,XXY.

iii) Mean body height is increased due to long legs.

iv) In some patients obesity/mental retardation may be present.

v) Plasma gonadotropin levels are increased.

14. Male infertility

i) In Klinefelter syndrome, there may be infertility in the presence of normal androgenization.

ii) Varicocele may be responsible for one third of male infertility cases.

iii) Surgical resection of varicose veins restores fertility in 100% cases.

iv) In varicocele the temperature gradient of 2°C between testes and abdominal cavity is lost.

v) Findings of semen analysis in varicocele are non-specific.

15. Male infertility

i) Isolated male infertility may occur in cryptorchidism.

ii) Viral orchitis may produce azoospermia or oligospermia.

iii) Drugs mostly produce isolated male infertility.

iv) Celiac disease and febrile illness also affect spermatogenesis in isolation.

v) Germinal cell aplasia and immotile cilia syndrome are other less common causes.

16. Isosexual precocity in females

i) Breast enlargement before 8 and menarche before 9 means iso-sexual precocity.

ii) In 90% of cases, it is constitutional.

iii) In partial cases, premature pubarche or premature thelarche, in isolation, should be ignored.

iv) About 10% cases of true isosexual precocity occurs due to organic brain disease (encephalitis, tumor, trauma, neurofibromatosis, tuberous sclerosis).

v) Hypothyroidism is another cause of true isosexual precocity.

17. Isosexual pseudoprecocity in the female

i) Most common cause is estrogen secreting ovarian tumors (granulosa and theca cell tumors).

ii) A G-protein defect disorder (McCune-Albright syndrome) produces isosexual pseudoprecocity along with cystic fibrous dysplasia of bones and pigmentary changes in skin.

iii) It may be caused by hypothyroidism.

iv) It may also be caused by CAH and hCG secreting tumors.

v) It may be caused by use of estrogen containing creams for treatment of diaper rash in female infants.

18. Hirsutism

i) History, physical examination, rapid or slow onset of hirsutism, generally differentiate hirsutism due to adrenal/ovarian neoplasms from other causes.

ii) Plasma levels of testosterone (>2 ng/mL) or of DHEA-S (>8000 ng/mL) further add to suspicion of tumor etiology.

iii) In non-tumor cases demonstration of chronic anovulation, along with other features may indicate diagnosis of polycystic ovarian disease.

iv) Of the non-tumor cases elevated plasma level of 17-hydroxyprogesterone occurs in all patients of late onset congenital adrenal hyperplasia.

v) Diagnosis of idiopathic hirsutism is by exclusion.

19. 21-hydroxylase deficiency

i) Most common cause of congenital adrenal hyperplasia.
ii) It causes female pseudohermaphroditism.
iii) It causes virilism in male infant.
iv) All males with the disorder develop early maturation of spermatogenesis.
v) Severe form is associated with excessive salt loss in urine.

20. 3β-HSD, 17 α-hydroxylase, 17, 20-lyase, 17β-hydro-xysteroid dehydrogenase defects

i) Account for about one fifth of cases of male pseudohermaphroditism.
ii) 3β-HSD and 17-α hydroxylase defects produce CAH and male pseudohermaphroditism.
iii) As estrogen synthesis occurs via androgens, 17β-HSD deficiency also produces deficiency of estrogen synthesis.
iv) Many cases of male pseudohermaphroditism occur because of abnormalities in androgen actions.
v) In 17β-HSD deficiency, as estrogen synthesis is reduced proper development of female genital organs in a female fetus will be affected.
vi) 17β-HSD causes sexual infantilism in a female.

21. Steroid 5-α-reductase deficiency/ androgen receptor disorders (male pseudohermaphroditism)

i) In both, there is defective development of external genitalia.
ii) In both, uterus and fallopian tubes are not formed.
iii) Gynecomastia occurs in both.
iv) Male internal genital structures are present in 5α-reductase deficiency but absent in severe form of androgen receptor defect.
v) Patients of 5-α-reductase deficiency have option to live as males or as females.

22. Androgen receptor disorders

i) The receptor disorders, Reifenstein syndrome and the infertile male syndrome cause degree of feminization, in decreasing order of severity.
ii) LH level is increased due to resistance to androgen action at hypothalamic, pituitary level.
iii) Increased LH level, increases levels of both testosterone and estrogens.
iv) Cases with complete feminization should be castrated before puberty, lest they develop male type of pubertal changes at puberty.
v) Those with minimal feminization require surgical correction of hypospadias and gynecomastia.

ANSWERS

1. No.(iv). It is not always true. A normal female and a patient of CAH have no difference in their sex chromosomes as well as gonadal functioning but phenotypes are different. Streak gonads may be associated with different karyotypes, 45,X; 46,XX/45,X (gonadal dysgenesis) and 46,XX or 46,XY (pure gonadal dysgenesis). Further primary gonadal failure/abnormality is present in gonadal dysgenesis (Turner's syndrome), pure gonadal dysgenesis, mixed gonadal dysgenesis (unilateral testis and with other streak gonad) (karyotype 45,X/46,XY).

2. No.(iv). It means karyotype 46, XY with a spectrum of phenotypes. In purest form it is female phenotype, sexual infantilism and there is absence of both mullerian duct derivatives and accessory organs of male reproduction. If testicular failure occurred later in embryogenesis the mullerian duct failure may be more prominent than absence of testosterone influence. In cases with only slight lack of testosterone influence during embryogenesis, phenotype is male with microphallus (failure occurred after formation of male urethra was complete). In 46. XY pure gonadal dysgenesis (compared to patient of anorchia of pure form) there is presence of streak gonads and some evidence of mullerian derivatives.

3. No.(i). Development of external genital structures, during embryogenesis and sexual maturity at puberty are best indicators of Leydig cell functions during the respective periods. The laboratory help is more useful in postpubertal period since many changes, requiring hormones of Leydig cells, during their development, can be maintained without this help.

4. No.(i). The responses are similar before puberty but after this period the LH response increases but the FSH response remains at prepubertal level.

5. No.(i). It is useful indicator of any deviation from normal development or damage in prepubertal period. In post pubertal period damage does not reduce the size of testes.

6. No.(iv). Normal progesterone status is indicated by elevated basal body temperature for about two weeks after the mid cycle. Other tests

showing adequate progesterone status are, presence of viscous cervical mucus (that does not stretch or fern) and secretory epithelium in endomterial biopsy on days 20 to 22, of the cycle.

7. No.(i). In most female reproductive disorders, clinical parameters are used to assess estrogen status of the patient.

8. No.(v). Increased amounts of androgens are aromatized to estrogens in peripheral tissues (adipose tissue), because of reduced metabolic disposal of androgens in liver disease. Obesity alone can also increase this peripheral aromatization and estrogen production.

9. No.(iv). In mild cases there may only be absent or incomplete puberty.

10. No.(iii). Explains only about one fifth of total cases. This condition is caused by fetal testosterone deficiency in the critical period of male differentiation. Testosterone is first secreted under the influence of placental hCG and then (after mid pregnancy) under fetal pituitary LH. Isolated microphallus may also be associated with congenital hypopituitarism, late fetal testicular failure and some cases of GH deficiency.

11. No.(iii). It is one of the most difficult problems in endocrinology.

12. No.(iv). Except when used as replacement therapy, sperm formation is impaired.

13. No.(i). Under androgenization is not common except that gynecomastia is usual.

14. No.(iii). In about 50% of cases.

15. No.(iii). Drugs may block androgen synthesis, androgen action or cause enhancement of estrogen action or cause direct inhibition of spermatogenesis.

16. No.(v). Hypothyroidism leads to increased secretion of TRH, increasing FSH secretion and ovarian production of estrogens to produce pseudo isosexual precocity. In pseudo isosexual precocity, ovulation does not occur.

17. No.(iv). CAH causes heterosexual precocity. hCG (or LH) secreting tumors in the absence of FSH do not induce excessive estrogen secretion, and therefore do not cause pseudoprecocity.

18. No.(iv). It is true for 21-hydroxylase deficiency which, of course is the commonest cause of both CAH and late onset adrenal hyperplasia. In 3β-HSD deficiency, 17-hydroxy progesterone is not formed and there is formation of DHEA via 17-hydroxy pregnenolone. The main secretory metabolite is DHEA. In 11-β hydroxylase deficiency the accumulating precursor is 11-deoxycortisol/11-deoxycorticosterone. 17-hydroxyprogesterone may accumulate to a lesser extent.

19. No.(iv). It may occur if adrenal androgens cause early maturation of hypothalamic-pituitary axis for secretion of gonadotropins. But in some cases adrenal androgens inhibit hypothalamic pituitary gonadotropin secretion and gonads remain infantile inspite of excessive masculinization.

20. No.(v). There is no estrogen requirement for proper development of female genital structures in a female fetus; therefore there is no defect in their embryonic development. However, their further growth at puberty along with other pubertal changes require presence of estrogens. Hence sexual infantilism occurs.

21. No.(iii). In 5-α-reductase deficiency testosterone levels are normal and therefore LH and estrogen levels also do not change. Thus testosterone, estrogen ratio is not changed and therefore there is no gynecomastia.

22. No.(iv). Castration is done after puberty. Because of androgen resistance and because of high levels of estrogens, the pubertal changes are only female type.

CHAPTER 18

Pregnancy and the Newborn

PHYSIOLOGICAL ADJUSTMENTS IN PREGNANCY

A number of physiological and biochemical changes are produced in the maternal body to support growth and development of feto-placental unit. Increased circulatory needs of the body are met with by increasing plasma volume without increasing blood pressure. Formation of angiotensinogen, renin, angiotensin II and aldosterone, are all increased, but there is neither hypertension nor hypokalemia. This may be because of simultaneous increased formation of vasodilatory prostaglandins and also high levels of progesterone in maternal circulation. Progesterone may affect renal action of aldosterone and prostaglandins may decrease sensitivity of maternal vasculature to angiotensin II.

In pregnancy, ventilation also increases, as progesterone stimulates respiratory centre. Pregnancy steroids decrease motility of smooth muscle (intestine, ureter). Decrease in gut motility allows more time for absorption of nutrients from intestine.

Increased cardiac output and increased plasma volume lead to increase in GFR. There is decrease in serum levels of urea and creatinine.

METABOLISM IN PREGNANCY

There is continuous supply of glucose, amino acids and other nutrients to fetus from maternal circulation. Alterations in metabolism of fuel molecules occurs in pregnancy to cater to this need. In the fed state, there is restricted use of glucose by maternal tissues to save it for transport to fetus. Maternal tissues metabolize dietary fat for energy purpose. In the fasting state there is tendency to hypoglycemia since gluconeogenesis is restricted (non-availability of amino acids which are transported to fetus). These metabolic alterations become prominent in second trimester onwards. Basal level of plasma insulin remains almost unchanged in first trimester but increases in second trimester and after that remain high. The above mentioned metabolic alterations are because of insulin resistance produced by placental hormones (human placental lactogen or hPL and progesterone) and cortisol. Inspite of raised insulin levels, lipolysis and ketogenesis are promoted by hPL (also called human chorionic somatomammotropin or hCS). Excessive ketones during prolonged starvation can become harmful to fetus, after entering fetal circulation.

CHANGES IN FUNCTIONING OF DIFFERENT ENDOCRINE GLANDS

Mention has already been made of increased secretion of aldosterone. Production of II-deoxycorticosterone (DOC) also goes on increasing throughout pregnancy but again, this does not cause hypertension. Levels of total T_4 and T_3 increase because of increased synthesis of TBG. Levels of free T_4 and free T_3 do not change.

Of pituitary hormones, levels of TSH and

ACTH remain unchanged, levels of FSH and LH decrease and do not increase in response to GnRH administration. Prolactin level increases in response to raised levels of plasma estrogens. Growth hormone level is not much different but responses to stimulation tests are altered. Increased cortisol binding globulin (estrogen induced) increases cortisol level, free cortisol level also increases.

REFERENCE RANGES OF SOME CHEMISTRIES DURING PREGNANCY

Because of the physiological/biochemical changes mentioned above, reference ranges for a number of blood/serum chemistries change in pregnancy (especially in third trimester) compared to the non-pregnant state (see Appendix B).

PLACENTAL HORMONES AND ROLE OF HUMAN CHORIONIC GONADOTROPIN IN DIAGNOSIS OF PREGNANCY AND PREGNANCY RELATED DISORDERS

Placenta produces a number of hormones, important during pregnancy. Studies of some of these hormones have diagnostic applications. Human chorionic gonadotropin (hCG) helps to maintain corpus luteum of pregnancy and also regulates placental progesterone secretion. Study of levels of this hormone in maternal plasma or urine is used in early diagnosis of pregnancy and also for diagnosis of a number of pregnancy related disorders. hPL has actions like growth hormone and has a major role in producing insulin antagonism in second half of pregnancy. Its exact role in pregnancy is not known. Blood levels of hPL have been related to placental function in late pregnancy. Placental progesterone and estrogens are important for different adjustments and changes required for proper progress of pregnancy. Estriol is the major estrogen present in urine of a pregnant woman. It is synthesized in placenta from dehydroepiandrosterone sulfate (DHEA sulfate) arising from fetal adrenals. Urinary excretion of estriol has been used to monitor well-being of feto-placental unit. However, monitoring of feto-placental unit with biochemical parameters has become obsolete and ultrasonography is currently used to know fetal health and placental blood flow.

Human chorionic gonadotropin (hCG)

It is produced by syncytiotrophoblast cells of placenta. It is a glycoprotein made of α and β subunits. α-Subunits of hCG, FSH, LH and TSH are nearly identical but their β-subunits are different. However, there is still, significant homology among these β-subunits.

A large number of methods are available for estimation of hCG. In the latex particle agglutination and hemagglutination tests, latex particles and red cells, respectively, are coated with hCG. These tests are carried out on slides. The immunoassay methods, using antibodies against β-subunit, are more specific (less cross reaction with LH) than others. Some rapid, sensitive and easy to perform versions of solid phase immunometric assay, are also available.

In early weeks of pregnancy hCG levels rise rapidly (rate of rise of more than 66% in 48h), reaching a level of about 100 mIU/mL at the time of expected but missed menses and a maximal level of 50,000 to 100,000 mIU/mL at 10 weeks of gestation. Level, then declines to 10,000 to 20,000 mIU/mL by 20 weeks and remains at that level till term.

In ectopic pregnancy there are symptoms suggestive of pregnancy. There is abnormal vaginal bleeding and cramping pain in lower abdomen. There may also be a tender mass palpable outside the uterus. The condition may present in acute or chronic form. A negative test for hCG blood assay will rule out ectopic pregnancy. In a positive test, if hCG level is below 6,000 mIU/mL and abdominal ultrasound fails to identify an intrauterine pregnancy, observe increase of hCG level over next 48h. If hCG level increases but less than as expected in normal pregnancy, there is indication of laparoscopy. Using vaginal ultrasonography search for gestational sac can be made earlier (say when hCG level is even less than 1,000 mIU/mL).

In gestational trophoblastic disease (GTD), there is enlarged uterus, excessive nausea and vomiting, no fetal heart and uterine bleeding at 6 to 8 weeks of pregnancy. hCG level is more than expected in normal pregnancy, at the corresponding gestational age. In serial estimations there is no plateauing.

hCG levels can also be used to monitor whether or not abortion has been complete. After spontaneous abortion hCG levels become undetectable in 9 to 35 days while in induced abortion, it may take 16 to 60 days.

The three disorders discussed above, come into differential diagnosis of a very common problem of women in reproductive period of life (patient presenting with vaginal bleeding, after a positive pregnancy test, upto 20 weeks after the last menses). Proper history, physical examination, vaginal examination (state of internal os, presence or absence of products of conception), the ultrasound examination and serial estimations of hCG, are all important in such a case.

Qualitative hCG testing (to rule out pregnancy) is often required in medical practice. It is needed in a woman in reproductive period of life, being evaluated for a medical illness, for surgery or if she has to undergo some procedure like X-ray examination or take some drug for some disease. Hypertension, diseases of heart, liver, lung, kidney and many others are worsened by pregnancy. Also, drugs, X-ray exposure and surgery may harm the fetus.

Urinary gonadotropic factor (UGF) which is a smaller form of β-subunit, is directly secreted by placenta and other tissues. It can also be estimated by a simple radiometric assay and has also been used for following pregnancy and for diagnosis of gynecological malignancies.

Triple marker screen for down's syndrome consists of measurements of hCG, α-fetoprotein and unconjugated estriol in maternal plasma. Role of hCG as a tumor marker is also discussed in Chapter 5.

MATERNAL MONITORING DURING PREGNANCY

Some maternal diseases call for careful biochemical monitoring during pregnancy, as pregnancy may worsen the disease and disease may increase maternal and fetal mortality. Important diseases needing biochemical monitoring during pregnancy are diabetes mellitus, hypertension, liver diseases and thyroid disorders.

Pregnancy induced hypertension

A woman may develop hypertension or her hypertension may worsen during pregnancy. Pregnancy induced hypertension or preeclampsia is characterized by hypertension, proteinuria and edema (Fig. 18.1). Trophoblastic tissue is important in initiating pathophysiological process which results in widespread vasospasm and increasing tendency to platelet aggregation. High blood pressure invokes placental insufficiency (and fetal growth retardation) and impairment of maternal renal function. Increased serum urate level occurs earlier than rise in level of creatinine or urea, in preeclampsia.

Preeclampsia and eclampsia belong to the group of microangiopathic disorders with presence of pathologic lesions in small vessels. After 20th week of gestation, in repeated measurements, blood pressure of 140/85 or more (which was less earlier), increasing further during sleep may indicate pregnancy induced hypertension. In severe cases, blood pressure (diastolic) rises to 110 mmHg or more, proteinuria increases and convulsions may occur. In presence of convulsions the condition is called eclampsia. Other features of severe cases of eclampsia are oliguria, elevated serum creatinine and liver enzymes and thrombocytopenia. In severe cases hemolysis may also occur. The patient is said to have HELLP syndrome, if he develops a combination of hemolysis, elevated liver enzymes and low platelet count. This syndrome shares features of thrombotic thrombocytopenic purpura (TPP) and hemolytic uremic syndrome (HUS). All the three belong to the group of microangiopathic disorders. Damage to vascular endothelium (with release of Willebrand factor and other changes: Fig. 18.1) may be a common feature in all the three conditions. There is also presence of fragmented red cells because of thrombotic obstruction in vessels. Disseminated intravascular coagulation (DIC) is not present (although thrombin time is prolonged and level of fibrin degradation products is increased). If laboratory evidence of DIC is found, it is secondary to severe hemolysis and release of red cell fragments.

Mild cases need close observation and careful conservative management. The objectives of management are, control of convulsions (with $MgSO_4$), control of severe hypertension, avoiding excessive fluids and looking for earliest occasion for delivery. In severe eclampsia cases, it is better to sacrifice the child.

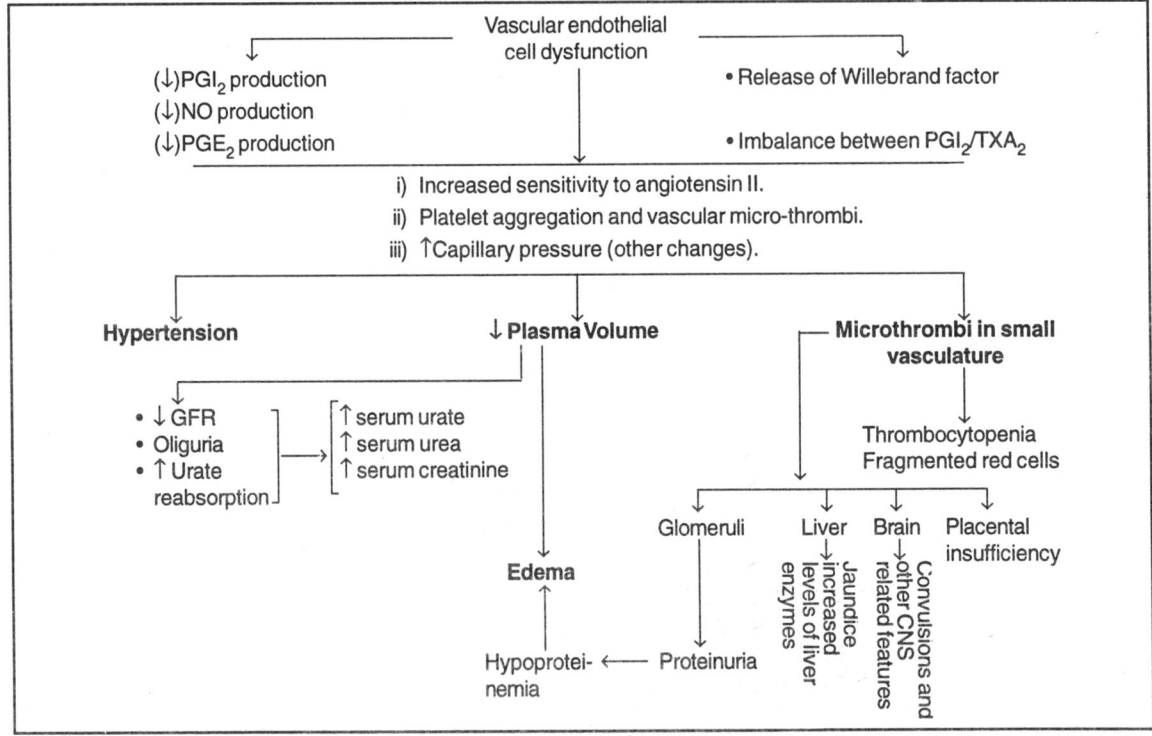

Fig. 18.1. Pathophysiological mechanisms in preeclampsia/eclampsia.

- During conservative treatment biochemical monitoring is done by following proteinuria, and serum levels of liver enzymes, urate and creatinine. Platelet count is also monitored. Rising serum urate is an early sensitive indicator of the disorder.
- Renal biopsy can confirm diagnosis by ruling out primary renal disease or hypertensive vascular disease.

Liver disease and cholelithiasis

In normal pregnancy, there is striking rise of alkaline phosphatase which is placental in origin. There may also be some increase of γ-GT and LDH without rise of ALT or AST. Serum protein level is reduced with reduced hepatic synthesis of albumin, although, there is some increase in other proteins. Increase is also found in plasma levels of TAG and cholesterol.

Intrahepatic cholestasis may occur in third trimester. Bilirubin level remains between 2 to 5 mg/dL and there is pruritis due to accumulated toxic bile acids. Once there is evidence of intrahepatic cholestasis, fetal well-being should be monitored as risk to still birth increases. Formation of biliary stones is promoted because of reduced gall bladder motility and increased concentration of cholesterol in bile.

In acute fatty liver of pregnancy there is increase of hepatocyte microvesicular fat (microvesicular steatosis) in late pregnancy and may be associated with preeclampsia. Serum bilirubin may rise above 10 mg/dL, with moderate increases of ALT and AST. Risk to DIC increases in these cases.

Hepatitis B infection during pregnancy increases risk of fetal death or premature birth; besides there is risk of transmission of infection to the infant, especially if mother is positive for HBe (risk is less if she is only positive for HBs without HBe). Risk of transmission of Hepatitis A is much less and severity of this condition is not increased in pregnancy.

Thyroid disease

In hypothyroidism ovulation may not occur and chances of pregnancy are much reduced. In iodine deficiency areas, a hypothyroid mother, during pregnancy, needs to be given thyroid hormone replacement as well as iodide to reduce incidence of cretinism. In hypothyroid patients dose of thyroid hormone increases during pregnancy.

In Graves' disease the antibodies cross placenta and may produce fetal goitre or transient neonatal hyperthyroidism. Hyperthyroidism in mother, should be treated with propylthiouracil using the minimum possible dose to avoid inhibition of thyroxine synthesis in fetus.

Radio iodine uptake test (or any other radioisotope study) is not undertaken during pregnancy because of risk of malformations in fetus.

Diabetes in pregnancy

About 50% of normal pregnant women show presence of glucose in urine, after the first trimester. This occurs because of increased load on renal tubules due to increased GFR. In the last few weeks of pregnancy, lactose may also appear in urine.

Glucose intolerance in pregnancy affects fetal development. Patient may be a known diabetic with poorly controlled blood glucose during pregnancy. Macrosomia (large fetus) and some other fetal problems can arise even if mother is only a prediabetic (family history of diabetes in a first degree relative), since stress of pregnancy increases her blood glucose to undesirable high levels.

A pregnant woman may develop gestational diabetes. This may occur when insulin secretion is not sufficient to meet increased demands of pregnancy. In gestational diabetes the fasting glucose level is normal. Prevalence of gestational diabetes is between 1 to 3%. It may or may not disappear after delivery. Repeated pregnancies increase likelihood of developing permanent diabetes especially in obese women.

Diagnosis of gestational diabetes

First screening is done at 24 to 26 weeks of pregnancy. 50g of glucose is given orally, and plasma glucose level is measured, 1h later. If glucose level exceeds 130 mg/dL, confirmation is obtained with complete oral glucose tolerance test (see below). If possible, all pregnant women should be screened for gestational diabetes. However, screening must be done in overweight women, those with history of still birth or birth of a macrosomic infant or those who show presence of glucose in urine sample collected after discarding the night urine. In the complete oral glucose tolerance test, 100g of glucose is given by mouth and samples are taken (besides the fasting sample), 1, 2 and 3 hours after glucose ingestion. Normally, fasting, 1h, 2h and 3h values should not exceed (in mg/dL), 105, 190, 165 and 145, respectively. If two or more values are higher, diagnosis of gestational diabetes is confirmed.

In glucose intolerance cases, maternal blood glucose is increased to undesirable high level and as excess glucose passes to the infant, increased insulin secretion will result in macrosomia with increased risk of birth trauma. The same reason can produce neonatal hypoglycemia. During the period of organogenesis in fetus, the abnormal substrate profile, because of maternal glucose intolerance, may result in congenital anomalies. Glucose intolerance during pregnancy may also produce fetal death or respiratory distress syndrome in the neonate.

Pregnancy may not lead to permanent worsening of diabetic nephropathy of the mother (unless pregnancy is complicated by preeclampsia), although temporary increase of proteinuria and serum creatinine level may occur. Hypertension, if present gets worsened.

For glucose intolerance of any type during pregnancy, blood glucose level is controlled by use of appropriate diet or insulin. Strict monitoring is needed to keep fasting glucose at the normal fasting level and post prandial glucose at or less than 140 mg/dL. Glycosylated Hb should also be monitored. Other investigations required may be ultrasound evaluation (in second trimester) and estimation of α-fetoprotein (in 20th week) to rule out neural tube defects.

ASSESSMENT OF FETAL WELL-BEING

Once pregnancy has been confirmed, its progress has to be followed with different objectives in mind. These include assessme   of fetal maturity or gestational age, assessment of fetal size, diagnosis of congenital abnormalities, and monitoring of fetal well-being. Besides, fetus has also to be monitored during labour.

Fetal growth

Clinical assessment is done by monitoring uterine size and maternal gain of weight. However, about half of the growth retarded fetuses may be missed when only clinical assessment is used. Biparietal diameter is widely used to monitor fetal growth but, as head is the last structure to stop growing, measurements of abdominal circumference (and head to abdomen ratio) may be more useful. All these measurements are taken during ultrasound examination.

Fetal gestational age

Prenatal assessment of gestational age is mostly clinical and with the help of ultrasound. Ultrasound measurements of crown-rump length, in the first trimester and biparietal diameter, head circumference and femur length in second trimester correlate well with gestational age of the fetus. Some amniotic fluid studies (concentrations of creatinine, protein, optical density at 450 nm, percentage of fat laden cells, lecithin/sphingomyelin ratio and phospholipid profile) can also be used to assess fetal age (Table 18.1), although with use of ultrasound for the purpose, these studies are seldom required. Estimation of gestational age, in a newborn, is a different matter and more accurate estimates can be made. The Dubowitz method, which uses 11 external criteria and 10 neurological features, to arrive at the gestational age of the newborn, helps proper management of preterm babies.

Diagnosis of congenital and certain other fetal abnormalities

Ultrasound examination has proved very useful in detecting malformations of central nervous system, heart, intestine, limbs and genitourinary system, early enough, to allow safe termination of pregnancy. Amniocentesis, chorion villus sampling (CVS) and fetal blood sampling have been used in diagnosis of fetal inherited disorders and other abnormalities.

Fetal well-being

After confirmation of pregnancy, serum hCG can be used to monitor placental function, as this hormone is secreted proportional to the size of placenta in early pregnancy. Placental isoenzyme of alkaline phosphatase has also been used for the same purpose. Estriol is the dominant estrogen of pregnancy urine. It is produced in placenta from fetal DHEA-sulfate and can be used to monitor well-being of fetoplacental unit. Reduced excretion, more specifically indicates fetal adrenal hypoplasia or placental sulfatase deficiency.

An ultrasound procedure, doppler flow velocity analysis, provides information on blood flow resistance in placenta. This test tells about well-being of fetoplacental unit and is used for evaluation of high risk pregnancies.

The most popular tests to monitor fetal condition in third trimester are, the biophysical profile of the fetus and the non-stress test. Biophysical profile includes, fetal presentation, fetal position, biparietal diameter, fetal heart rate, fetal movements, localization of placenta, amniotic fluid volume and other parameters. In the non-stress test, fetal heart rate, fetal movements and uterine contractions are recorded after stimulating the fetus by palpation.

Besides prenatal diagnosis of inherited disorders, (discussed separately) biochemical help may be required in cases of blood group immunization and fetal lung immaturity, in high risk pregnancies. Such investigations are also important in cases of birth asphyxia (Table 18.1).

Perinatal asphyxia

It is produced by compromised oxygen supply to fetus. Causes may be maternal (toxemia of pregnancy, diabetes, hypotension, dehydration, anemia, malnutrition, some systemic diseases), placental (premature separation, degeneration), uterine (hypertonia) or others (umbilical cord abnormalities, abnormal placentation, prematurity and others). It may be present in fetus before labour but more commonly it develops during labour. When occurring before labour, it may produce fetal distress calling for appropriate management. Tests already

Table 18.1. Diagnostic use of amniocentesis.

FETAL LUNG MATURITY

Lecithin, sphingomyelin(L/S) ratio:

- Levels of the two lipids are similar before 34 weeks of gestation.
- After 34 weeks, L/S ratio of 2.0 means that risk of RDS is slight. However, in a metabolically compromised new born or in the presence of complicated maternal diabetes, the significance of the test is lost.

Presence of phosphatidylglycerol:

- Presence of this lipid (detected by a rapid agglutination test) means that fetal lungs are mature.

Absorbance of light at 650 nm:

- Value of 0.15 or more means normal maturity (correlates well with L/S ratio)

Tests indirectly measuring pulmonary surfactant (In these tests false positives are rare but false negatives occur more often)**:**

- The foam test depends upon surface tension lowering property of the phospholipids.
- The fluorescent polarization (microviscometry) test (Microviscosity of the lipid aggregates in amniotic fluid is assayed by mixing the fluid with a specific dye which incorporates into hydrocarbon regions of the lipids in surfactant; intensity of fluorescence induced by polarized light is measured). Fluorescence falls as L/S ratio rises.

FETAL MATURITY

Amniotic fluid creatinine:

(During later half of pregnancy the amniotic fluid creatinine level goes on increasing as a result of excretion of creatinine in urine by maturing kidneys)

- A level of 2.0 mg/dL means that fetus is mature. The test, however, does not tell about fetal lung maturity.
- High level of creatinine in mother will cause false increase in level of amniotic fluid creatinine.

Lipid staining cells in amniotic fluid:

(Nile blue staining reveals blue particles (shed fetal epithelial cells), and orange particles which appear to reflect maturity of sebacious glands)

- In later stages of gestation, increase occurs in orange bodies (number rises to about 50% near term). False negatives occur commonly.

Amniotic fluid bilirubin:

- Normally, bilirubin levels fall progressively in later half of gestation (level is estimated by study of absorption peak at 450 nm; ordinary chemical method is too insensitive). Normally O.D. becomes almost zero at maturity.
- The test becomes unreliable if maternal plasma starts contributing bilirubin(sickle cell anemia).
- Test is not favoured for judging fetal maturity and is best reserved for monitoring of blood group immunized cases.

FETAL WELL BEING

- A number of parameters including colour, volume, pH, pO_2, electrolyte levels, and hormone levels (estriol, hCG, hPL and others) have been studied in assessment of feto-placental well being. At present these studies have limited value.

FETAL DISORDERS DIAGNOSED BY ESTIMATION OF α-FETOPROTEIN IN AMNIOTIC FLUID

(It is first produced by yolk sac and then by fetal liver. Levels are highest both in fetal serum and amniotic fluid at about 13th week of gestation. Some protein crosses over to mother and in maternal serum the level goes on increasing until late in pregnancy. After 13th week, levels in fetal serum and amniotic fluid decrease sharply).

- Test is of considerable interest in prenatal diagnosis of open neural tube defects (anencephaly, open spina bifida). Mother is first screened for the disorder by estimating serum level of fetoprotein at mid pregnancy. If level is raised amniocentesis is performed.
- Gestational age must be known properly to interpret the levels correctly since there is sharp decrease of levels after 13th week of pregnancy.
- A number of other disorders including congenital nephrosis, bladder neck obstruction, fetal death, abdominal pregnancy,

Contd...

Contd. Table 18.1

fetal blood in amniotic fluid, Turner syndrome, feto-maternal hemorrhage and others can cause increase in fetoprotein levels in maternal serum and amniotic fluid.

DIAGNOSIS OF INHERITED DISORDERS

Chromosomal studies are of value in

i)   Pregnancies in women over 35 years of age

ii) Presence of chromosomal abnormality in either parent or in a close family member

iii) If a previous pregnancy resulted in a chromosomally abnormal infant or an infant with major malformation (without simultaneous chromosomal analysis)

iv) Parent or previous child had a neural tube defect or if maternal serum α-feto protein level is high. The four most frequent chromosomal disorders (in decreasing order of frequency) are the Kleinfelter's syndrome (XXY) (incidence 1:500 male births); Down's syndrome (trisomy 21, non-disjunction, translocation, mosaicism; incidence 1: 600 births); fragile X-syndrome (incidence 1:1000 male births); Turner syndrome (XO; incidence 1:2500 female births).

Fragile X syndrome is the second most common cause of severe mental retardation after Down's syndrome. It is described in male infants but one third of female carriers are mildly affected. It is diagnosed by demonstrating fragile sites on the long arm of a proportion of X-chromosomes.

• Chromosomal studies are also used to identify sex of the fetus in X-linked recessive diseases where prenatal diagnosis is not possible. In carriers of X-linked conditions the detection of the male fetus may be the ground for interruption of pregnancy (although there is 50% chance that the fetus may be normal).

Other methods (discussed in the text later. Also see Table 18.14).

---

mentioned, to monitor fetal condition in the third trimester are used to establish this fetal distress. During labour a continuous record of fetal heart rate can be obtained by applying fetal skin electrode to the presenting part (after rupture of membranes) or non-invasively, with a cardiotocograph. Important indications of fetal distress include alterations in fetal heart rate, fetal movements, and fetal scalp blood pH <7.2. For the last test, fetal blood is actually obtained from the presenting part. The sample should be analyzed immediately, to get fairly reliable pH value. Delay in analysis can lead to loss of CO_2 from the sample and change in pH. The sample is also analyzed for pO_2, pCO_2 and lactate besides pH. Other factors which affect the results include, state of uterus (contracted or relaxed) at the time of sample collection, positioning of the patient, maternal fever, hypertension, maternal plasma pH and lactate level and presence or absence of caput succedaneum. Fetal sample pH of 7.2 to 7.24 means impending fetal distress.

Assessment of birth asphyxia

Asphyxia is defined as hypoxemia, mixed acidosis and hypercapnea. There are different ways of assessing severity of birth asphyxia in a newborn. These include, time taken to establish spontaneous, regular respiration, time taken by the infant to pink up, time before heart rate settles at 100/min, and the Apgar score. However, all these parameters have been found to have limited value, in judging the prognosis of the neonate.

In calculating Apgar score, neonate is given score for each of the following functions: Heart rate (score is zero if absent, one if 100/min and two if >100/min); respiratory effort (zero if absent, one, if cry is weak and two if the cry is strong). Other functions taken into consideration are muscle tone (limp, some flexion, good flexion); reflex irritability (during pharyngeal suction, no response, some motion, cry); colour (pale/overall cyanosis, centrally pink with periphery blue, pink). Generally, an Apgar score of 7 to10 at one min. is normal, 4 to 6 is moderately depressed and 0 to 3 is severely depressed. However many infants can be resuscitated despite an Apgar score of zero at birth and may not suffer from any neurological damage in the long run. Of the clinical criteria, heart rate and respiration are two most important ones, to decide about the degree of resuscitation required.

Cord blood pH, pO_2, pCO_2 and lactate have also been used in assessment of birth asphyxia (Also see Fig 18.2).

Many conditions may affect respiration per se and may reduce reliability of this parameter in assessment of birth asphyxia. Some of the conditions are, drugs (used during labour), fetal immaturity, congenital anomalies, cerebral injury, aspirated meconium and others.

Management requires establishing adequate airway, providing appropriate ventilation and ensuring adequate circulation. Besides, acidosis should be treated and blood glucose level maintained between 60 to 100 mg/dL. Low level will lead to tissue ATP depletion and high level will increase lactate generation.

Surviving baby's fate is the most important consideration in cases of perinatal asphyxia. Survivors of birth asphyxia, often, have a better prognosis than those who suffer hypoxemia before birth. However, only 10% of all cases of cerebral palsy occur because of perinatal asphyxia. Also see Fig. 18.2.

PRETERM AND SMALL FOR GESTATIONAL AGE (SGA) INFANTS

A newborn of gestational age of less than 37 weeks, is termed preterm and the one with gestational age more than 42 weeks is designated as postterm. The preterm newborns are often low birth weight (weight less than 2500g). However, all low birth weight newborns may not be preterm. Many such

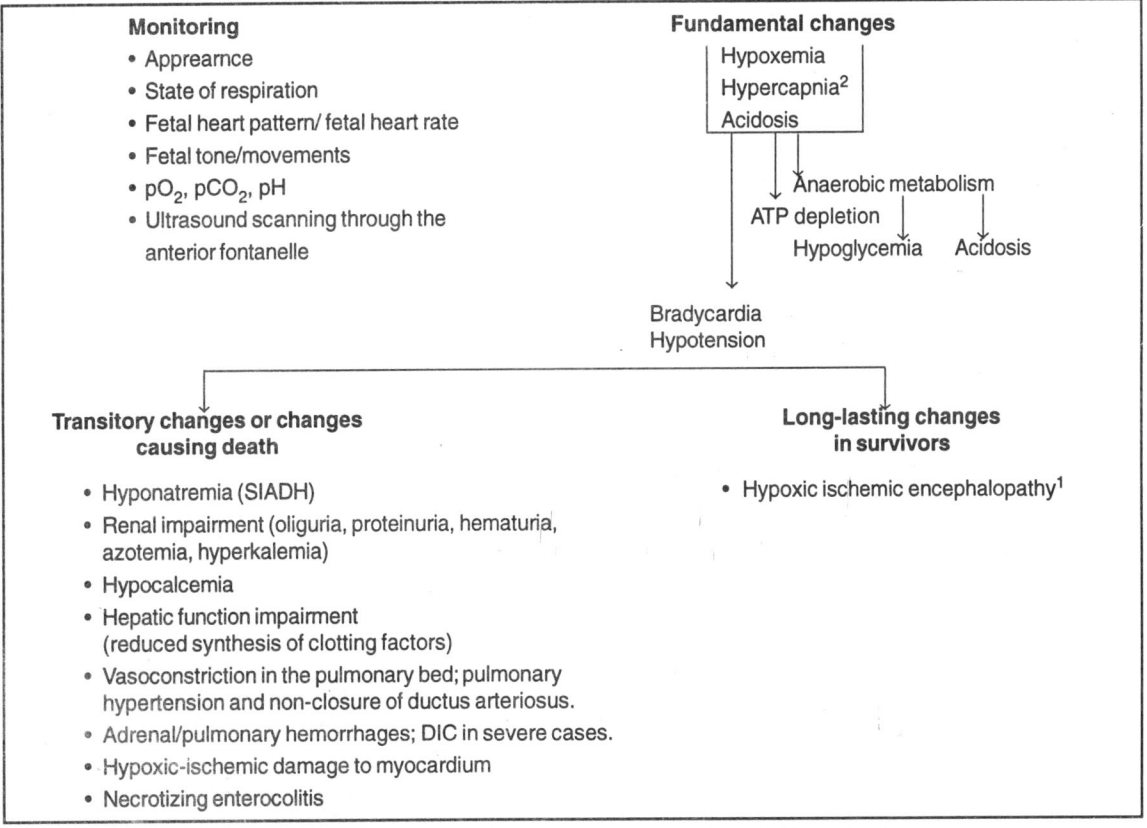

Fig. 18.2. Metabolic and other changes associated with asphyxia.

---

[1] Only less than 10% of all cases of cerebral palsy in term infants are caused by perinatal asphyxia;

[2] Hypercapnia causes cerebral edema; hypocapnia occuring during resuscitation is beneficial by affecting cerebral circulation.

- Survivors of birth asphyxia have a better prognosis than those who suffered hypoxemia before birth.

newborns may have normal gestational age and their low birth weight is because of poor intrauterine growth. Thus low birth weight newborns may be preterm or victims of intrauterine growth retardation (IUGR). These are more appropriately called small for gestational age (SGA).

In case of preterm newborns, different organs are not adequately grown for extrauterine life, leading to higher morbidity rate than those who are appropriate for gestational age (AGA). Preterm neonates have greater predisposition to birth asphyxia and respiratory distress syndrome (RDS). Similarly feeding problems are more because of poor sucking or swallowing reflexes and there is need for feeding through a nasogastric tube.

Because of immaturity of different metabolic pathways metabolic disturbances like, hypoglycemia, hypocalcemia, hypomagnesemia and jaundice are more common. Jaundice of prematurity is diagnosed by eliminating other causes. Chances of bilirubin encephalopathy may be increased in preterm because of hypoglycemia, low albumin levels, acidosis, hypoxia and hypothermia. Certain drugs and starvation also promote bilirubin encephalopathy. Because of renal immaturity, water and electrolyte disturbances, including, hyperkalemia and acidosis occur more frequently. Metabolic acidosis may cause failure to gain weight. Other problems are increased susceptibility to infection, hemorrhagic disease, gastrointestinal intolerance, surgical problems (undescended testis, hernias), and others.

It is important to differentiate SGA due to fetal causes (intrinsic fetal growth retardation) from those due to maternal or placental causes (extrinsic fetal growth retardation). In the latter group (alcohol, smoking, malnutrition, maternal disease, toxemia of pregnancy, multiple pregnancy, small placenta) the causative factors affect fetal growth in the later part of pregnancy while in the former group, (chromosomal abnormalities, dysmorphic syndromes and exposure to viral infection or X-rays) effect is produced, in early part of pregnancy. In SGA due to fetal causes growth retardation is proportionate or symmetrical. In SGA due to maternal or placental causes, growth retardation is disproportionate or asymmetrical. In these babies, weight reduction is more than reduction in height while head circumference is least affected. Catch up growth is more likely in asymmetrically retarded than others.

In SGA newborns, there is greater incidence of congenital malformations and infections compared to preterm ones. Other problems are hypoglycemia and complications during delivery (asphyxia, meconium aspiration and acidosis). Respiratory problem due to meconium aspiration and polycythemia (but not due to RDS), may occur. SGA infants often, are more likely to have long term developmental, behavioural and learning problems than mildly preterm ones.

RESPIRATORY DISTRESS SYNDROME (RDS)

Fetal blood obtains oxygen from maternal blood in placenta. High level of fetal hemoglobin is quite suited to obtain adequate oxygen at low pO_2 of maternal blood, in placenta and also for adequately delivering it to fetal tissues. This system helps fetus to tolerate some degree of hypoxia during labour.

Table 18.2. Fetal respiratory characteristics

- High level of fetal hemoglobin (16 to 17 g%).
- Reduced affinity of fetal hemoglobin for 2,3 -DPG (this property increases uptake of O_2 from maternal sinuses).
- High pCO_2 level (50 mmHg) in maternal blood (high pCO_2 in blood spaces in the decidual tissue of placenta, favours release of O_2 from maternal hemoglobin).
- Shift to left of oxygen dissociation curve of fetal hemoglobin in fetal blood increases O_2 uptake from maternal blood at low O_2 tensions (pO_2 of 60 mmHg).
- Fetal blood arterial pO_2 and fetal tissue pO_2 are such that O_2 releases in tissues operates at the steepest part of the oxygen dissociation curve of fetal hemoglobin.
- After birth blood pO_2 and pCO_2 are normalized and fetal hemoglobin is gradually replaced by adult hemoglobin(fetal hemoglobin is completely absent at 3 to 4 months postnatally).

- Oxygen dissociation curve of fetus is shifted to left (oxygen saturation of Hb is greater at lower pO_2). This helps fetus (living in relatively hypoxic environment) but is of disadvantage to the newborn (as less oxygen is released in tissues at higher pO_2).
- Physiological anemia occurs at 5 to 6 weeks of postnatal life. It is more severe in a preterm infant (Hb about 8 g/dL compared to about 12 g/dL in the full term infant). Lower erythropoietin levels, and poorer stores of iron and vitamin E make anemia more severe in a preterm infant.

After birth, two important changes occur in this oxygen carriage and delivery system of the fetus. Firstly, the pulmonary respiration starts (see below) and secondly, changes occur in type and level of hemoglobin of the neonate (Table 18.2).

Fetal lungs mature quite late. Type II alveolar pneumocytes secrete surfactant (consists of lecithin plus small amounts of other phospholipids and proteins) into alveoli to bring about this maturation. After delivery, surfactant reduces surface tension at the alveolar surface-air interface and the first respiratory movements are able to inflate the lungs, properly. Surfactant reduces resistance to expansion during inspiration and prevents alveolar collapse during expiration.

Deficiency of surfactant produces respiratory distress syndrome, in which there is failure of alveolar expansion at birth and there is alveolar collapse leading to imbalance of ventilation/perfusion. Escape of blood proteins into alveolar air spaces produce hyaline membrane disease.

In an infant having respiratory distress syndrome, breathing is generally fast and each breath is laboured. Peak severity may occur at 48 to 72h (it may occur much earlier in severe cases). As the disease advances, the respiratory distress worsens, cyanosis develops and there is need for oxygen administration. Finally, prolonged apnoea may occur because of muscle fatigue. In a worsening case, breath sounds are decreased and blood pressure falls. There is also oliguria and peripheral edema may occur. If clinical improvement occurs, it is preceded by diuresis. In a worsening case respiratory failure may develop leading to death of the baby.

RDS is related to degree of prematurity and is unusual in fullterm infants. Thus avoiding premature delivery is an important preventive measure in such cases. Other predisposing factors are, hypoxia, acidosis, shock, antepartum hemorrhage and diabetes of the mother.

Lecithin is an important component of pulmonary surfactant and starts appearing in amniotic fluid at about 35 weeks of gestation onwards. Sphingomyelin arises from non-pulmonary sources at a constant rate. Proper assessment of fetal lung maturity requires estimation of lecithin/sphingomyelin (L/S) ratio and also demonstrating presence or absence of phosphatidyl glycerol. L/S ratio of less than 2.0 indicates lung immaturity. Presence of phosphatidyl glycerol indicates completed lung maturation. There are a number of simple tests which give very few false positive results about lung maturity but when the tests are negative, further confirmation may be required (of lung immaturity) by determining L/S ratio. The referred simple tests are the foam stability test and measurement of optical density at 650 nm (value of 0.15 or more indicates that maturity is normal). All these tests are done on amniotic fluid samples. X-ray picture of developed RDS is quite characteristic.

The management modes include, administration of corticosteroids to the mother before delivery (to stimulate surfactant formation) and to maintain adequate levels of pO_2 and pCO_2 in the patient. For the latter purpose, oxygen administration, continuous positive airway pressure (CPAP) and mechanical ventilation may be required. The last method is used if the first two procedures are not able to maintain pO_2 of atleast 60 mmHg, pCO_2 of less than 65 mmHg and pH above 7.2. With mechanical ventilation, there is danger of over inflation and rupture of alveoli, producing interstitial emphysema and other complications. Exogenous surfactant is now available for treating such infants, which has significantly improved their survival.

BLOOD GROUP IMMUNIZATION

Rh-Immunization

An Rh positive fetus produces maternal (mother Rh –ive) sensitization in third stage of labour when Rh positive cells enter maternal circulation due to placental hemorrhage. Accordingly, first child is seldom affected. Following delivery, if Rh positive cells are detected in the mother (these can be stained and their number ascertained), she should be given anti-D Ig within 72h after delivery.

During subsequent pregnancies (some people recommend this routine even, for the first, at risk pregnancy) determination of amniotic fluid amniotic fluid OD_{450} is helpful to predict outcome of Rh immunized pregnancy from 16 to 20 weeks of gestation, onwards. If amniotic fluid (AF) OD_{450} is 0.09 or lower the fetus is unaffected or only mildly affected. If the value is more than 0.15, a serious disease is indicated, needing intrauterine exchange transfusion. Values between the two limits require further evaluation. Ultrasonic evaluation is helpful in such cases. In case OD_{450} is not indicative of fetal hemolysis, at 28 weeks, maternal antibody titre is determined. If no antibodies are present, anti-D Ig is administered. If antibodies are detected and titre is low, the case needs to be followed for fetal hemolysis.

ABO incompatibility

ABO immune disease, commonly (50% cases) occurs in first pregnancy. It is most common if blood group of mother is O, although it may occur even when her blood group is A or B. It is generally a mild disease. Anti-A/Anti-B titres do not help to predict the outcome and amniocentesis is not advised. Moderate hyperbilirubinemia of the baby often needs phototherapy. Early discharge of the patient from the hospital may not allow proper detection of these cases.

NEONATAL HYPERBILIRUBINEMIA

Many full term infants present with jaundice in the first week of life. In premature infants bilirubin levels are higher and take longer time to normalize. Fig. 18.3 shows the mechanisms involved in causation of physiological jaundice and also some factors which affect its intensity and outcome. Fig. 5.2 shows some inherited defects of bilirubin transport through the liver cells.

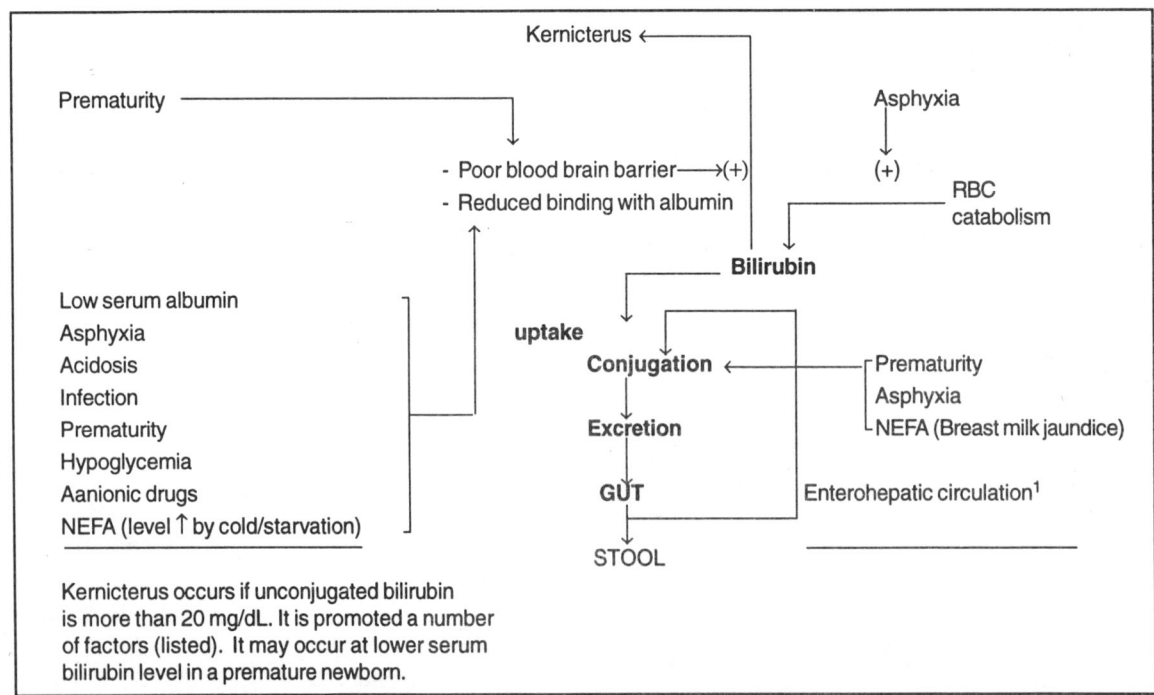

Fig.18.3. Neonatal jaundice and factors which worsen its outcome.

[1] In the new born gut is sterile and there is poor peristalsis, much of conjugated bilirubin is hydrolysed by glucuronidase to enter enterohepatic circulation. This component is enhanced in prematurity and small bowel obstruction (organic/functional) and pyloric stenosis.

- Asphyxia, bacterial infections (sepsis), RDS, prematurity all interfere in bilirubin uptake and the conjugation process to increase unconjugated bilirubin.

- Unconjugated bilirubin also rises in new borns of diabetic mothers.

- Increase of conjugated bilirubin is less common but cause is more serious; jaundice usually presents in 2nd week of life.

Some pathological causes of jaundice should be looked for, under following conditions: (i) if there is clinical jaundice in first 24h; (ii) total bilirubin >12-15 mg/dL in a term infant and >9-12 mg/dL in a preterm infant; (iii) conjugated bilirubin >2.0 mg/dL (or infant has clinical features of obstructive jaundice); (iv) clinical jaundice persists for more than 2 weeks; (v) jaundice is present in an ill infant; (vi) mother has rhesus antibodies.

Inherited defects are indicated in Fig.5.2. Rh and ABO incompatibilities are discussed separately (see above). Bacterial infections (urinary tract infection, septicemia) cause increase of unconjugated bilirubin. In case of intrauterine infections increase of conjugated bilirubin occurs more commonly, since these infections produce neonatal hepatitis. Common intrauterine infections are toxoplasmosis, rubella, cytomegalo virus (CMV) disease and syphilis. Intrauterine infections may cause jaundice immediately after birth. Breast milk jaundice, generally, presents in the second week of life. Stopping of breast feeding may have to be used (for about 48 h) for diagnosis but not for management, as jaundice, generally, regresses within 3 months. Cause of breast milk jaundice is hepatic glucuronyl transferase inhibition by high concentration of non-esterified fatty acids (NEFA) present in breast milk. Short lived jaundice (increase of unconjugated bilirubin) may also be caused by delayed passage of meconium leading to increased enterohepatic absorption of bilirubin. Hyperbilirubinemia of Gilbert's disease should also be kept in mind (Table 18.3). The disorder is harmless.

Increase of conjugated bilirubin is produced by neonatal hepatitis or biliary atresia. Neonatal hepatitis may be produced by intrauterine (and other) infections. If the pregnant woman carries HBs-Ag as well as HBe-Ag (without anti-HBe) then the baby is at risk of developing infection. Risk is only small in the presence of anti-HBe). The baby at risk can be protected by starting immunization at birth. Other causes of neonatal hepatitis are metabolic (galactosemia, tyrosinemia), cystic fibrosis, α-anti-trypsin deficiency and others. A diagnostic approach to neonatal pathological jaundice is shown in Fig.18.4.

SOME METABOLIC AND OTHER PROBLEMS OF THE NEONATAL PERIOD

Fetus lies in a protected environment and in a state of assured nutrition. Many of his systems, which must function efficiently, for independent existence, are still immature. After birth these systems start maturing rapidly but take some time to attain mature levels. It is important to understand functioning of different systems during this transition stage. The subject is briefly discussed below. Some disorders produced during this transit period are also discussed. Many inherited disorders also present in this period and are discussed at the end, as a separate topic.

Many tissue maturity changes are triggered because the adrenal gland starts producing cortisol instead of cortisone. This helps closure of ductus by reducing its sensitivity to prostaglandins. This also helps maturation of many hepatic enzymes and the small intestinal transport processes. Enzymatic changes also result in increased conversion of T_4 to T_3 instead of rT_3 (the latter being inactive), and formation of epinephrine from norepinephrine in adrenal medulla (by inducing PMNT activity). T_3 has important role in activating brown adipose tissue thermogenesis (see below).

In response to exposure to cold, shivering is the main process of thermogenesis in adults. Hormone epinephrine is involved in this process. In neonates, on the other hand, thermogenesis occurs by oxidation of fatty acids in brown adipose tissue. Brown adipose tissue is different from ordinary adipose tissue and is found only in newborns of most species including humans. It is called brown because of rich blood supply. It is present both internally (around

Table 18.3. About Gilbert's disease

- Mild hyperbilirubinemia (<6.0 mg/dL) of uncon-jugated bilirubin with no other evidence of liver disease or increased hemolysis.
- May represent a heterogeneous group (reduced uptake, reduced conjugation or undetected hemolysis) in which there is greater increase in level of unconjugated bilirubin than normals, on fasting or with an infection.
- Quite a common condition , commonly diagnosed in adults (more common in males than females).

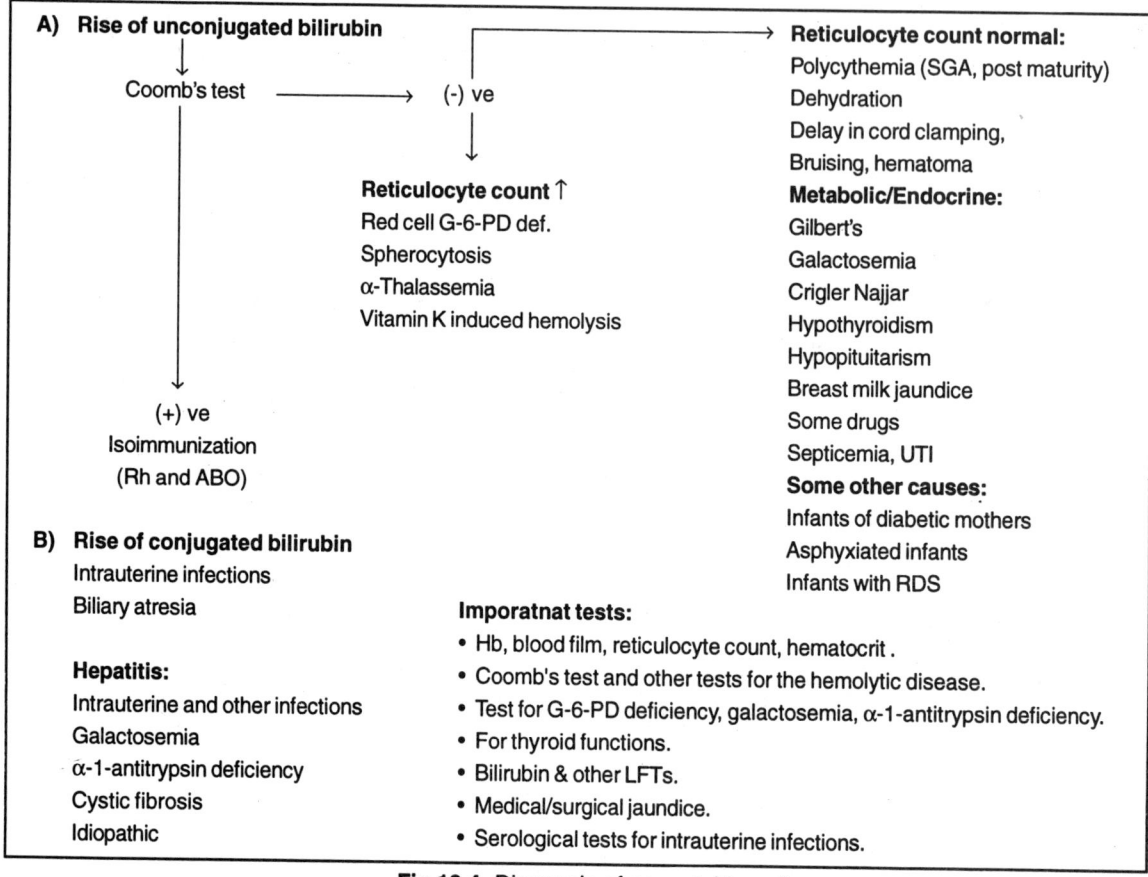

A) Rise of unconjugated bilirubin

Coomb's test ─────────→ (−) ve ─────────→ **Reticulocyte count normal:**
Polycythemia (SGA, post maturity)
Dehydration
Delay in cord clamping,
Bruising, hematoma

Reticulocyte count ↑
Red cell G-6-PD def.
Spherocytosis
α-Thalassemia
Vitamin K induced hemolysis

Metabolic/Endocrine:
Gilbert's
Galactosemia
Crigler Najjar
Hypothyroidism
Hypopituitarism
Breast milk jaundice
Some drugs
Septicemia, UTI

(+) ve
Isoimmunization
(Rh and ABO)

Some other causes:
Infants of diabetic mothers
Asphyxiated infants
Infants with RDS

B) Rise of conjugated bilirubin
Intrauterine infections
Biliary atresia

Hepatitis:
Intrauterine and other infections
Galactosemia
α-1-antitrypsin deficiency
Cystic fibrosis
Idiopathic

Imporatnat tests:
• Hb, blood film, reticulocyte count, hematocrit .
• Coomb's test and other tests for the hemolytic disease.
• Test for G-6-PD deficiency, galactosemia, α-1-antitrypsin deficiency.
• For thyroid functions.
• Bilirubin & other LFTs.
• Medical/surgical jaundice.
• Serological tests for intrauterine infections.

Fig.18.4. Diagnosis of neonatal jaundice.

- Jaundice on day 1 may be due to hemolytic disease of the new born or due to neonatal jaundice because of intrauterine infections (rubella, CMV, syphilis).
- Jaundice on days 2 to 5 may be physiological/prematurity, sepsis, hematomas, G-6-PD deficiency, congenital spherocytosis.
- In jaundice appearing in the second week it is important to differentiate between medical and surgical causes.

aorta) and at body surface (around neck and between scapulae) in human fetus. Oxidation in this tissue is not coupled to ATP formation and dissipates energy as heat. Norepinephrine, in a neonate, causes thermogenesis by activating brown adipose tissue lipase, and sensitivity to norepinephrine is increased by T_3. By the end of the first year of life, thermogenesis becomes adult type. Neonatal cold injury is discussed below.

Changes in sympathetic nervous system lead to increased levels of epinephrine, norepinephrine and dopamine which bring about changes in cardiovascular system (increased cardiac out put and increase in blood pressure).

Tables 18.2 and 18.4, respectively, give characteristics of respiratory and renal systems of the neonate. If the adaptive changes in the transition period, in different systems, are slow or inappropriate (due to immaturity of the newborn or some other reason), neonatal disorders like neonatal cold injury, hypoglycemia, hypocalcemia, hyperbilirubinemia, water and electrolyte disturbances and respiratory distress syndrome may be produced.

Neonatal cold injury

Neonate is prone to suffer from hypothermia because of increased loss of heat and limited ability to shiver. Excessive exposure to cold increases oxygen

Table 18.4. Kidney functions in infancy

1. GFR increases after birth and reaches adult values (corrected for body surface area) in about 6 months.
2. Serum creatinine levels quite fluctuate, in early infancy, and reach adult levels (corrected for body surface area) at about 6 months.
3. Plasma urea is low even with relatively lower GFR because of anabolic state of metabolism.
4. States of nutrition and hydration and the metabolic rate greatly influence plasma urea level.
5. The lower reabsorptive capacity of proximal tubules may cause glycosuria, aminoaciduria and low serum bicarbonate level in a neonate.
6. In a neonate urine cannot be concentrated above 600 mmol/kg.
7. Both sodium conservation and capacity to excrete sodium are low in a neonate.
8. Renal regulation of acidosis is less developed in neonates than older children and adults.

- Because of observtions at serial nos. 6 nd 7, much care is needed during I/V fluid administration, to small infants.
- Because of the observation at serial no. 8, infants readily become acidotic during starvation or fever (increased endogenous protein breakdown produces more acids).

consumption and glucose oxidation leading to hypoxia and hypoglycemia. There is peripheral cyanosis with redness of the face and refusal to feed. It can worsen RDS and severe acidosis produced, predisposes to pulmonary/intracranial hemorrhages. During treatment, as circulation improves, warming occurs and metabolic acidosis worsens.

Hypoglycemia

After birth, till normal feeding process starts, energy is obtained from oxidation of fatty acids and blood glucose is maintained (for providing energy in brain tissue) by glycogenolysis and gluconeogenesis. Neonatal hypoglycemia occurs because of reduced hepatic glycogen stores and immaturity of enzymes of gluconeogenesis. After birth, high glucagon, insulin ratio is required for maturation of these enzymes. In normal infants, proper glucose regulation is achieved in about a week. Prolonged hypoglycemia results from low glycogen stores, presence of more immature enzymes and inappropriate hormonal profile. Neonatal hypoglycemia is encountered in preterm, small for date, infants of diabetic mothers and hypoxic infants.

For other causes of hypoglycemia in early and late infancy, read under the topic of hypoglycemia in chapter 7.

Water and electrolyte balance

In a newborn, body water forms about 75% of body weight (falls to 60% at one year). Thus water requirement (per kg. body weight) is more at this age and fluid depletion is more harmful compared to an adult. In a neonate insensible water loss is high because of higher surface area, less subcutaneous fat and higher water permeation rate. In a dehydrated neonate there is greater depletion of water than sodium because of poor ability to concentrate urine (maximum osmolality attainable in urine is <600 mosmol/L).

As ECF water forms a higher fraction of total body water, any water loss produces more severe hypernatremia than an adult.

In a neonate, history and clinical examination are very important in evaluating water and electrolyte abnormalities. Further, during treatment, monitoring of the baby is very important by repeated clinical examination and recording urine output, fluid balance and urine/plasma osmolality.

Some important characteristics of kidney functions in a neonate are given in Table 18.4.

Hypocalcemia

Active transport of calcium through placenta makes fetus hypercalcemic during pregnancy. Increased calcium level stimulates calcitonin and inhibits parathyroid hormone secretion. Immediately after birth, raised calcitonin level and blunted response to parathyroid hormone (PTH) produces transient hypocalcemia. This is especially marked, if mother had poor vitamin D status during pregnancy. This is called early hypocalcemia. Early hypocalcemia is commonly associated with prematurity, respiratory distress syndrome (RDS), birth asphyxia, sepsis and maternal diabetes. DiGeorge syndrome is a rare X-linked congenital immune deficiency disorder associated with parathyroid hypoplasia resulting in persistent hypocalcemia and hyperphosphatemia, requiring life long vitamin D treatment.

Hypomagnesemia may result from the same

factors which produce hypocalcemia as the homeo-static mechanisms for the two ions are, some what, similar. Maternal magnesium deficiency may also contribute to fetal and neonatal magnesium deficiency. Hypomagnesemia also interferes in secretion of PTH and its actions. At times, newborn infants have convulsions despite correction of calcium level and will need magnesium administration for their control.

Late hypocalcemia or neonatal tetany results from diet induced hyperphosphatemia, which, in turn, produces hypocalcemic tetany. Hyperphosphatemia may be caused by feeding the infant with unmodified cow's milk which is rich in phosphate. Maternal hyperparathyroidism, if present, may also contribute to late hypocalcemia by depressing infant's parathyroids in the second week after birth (because of earlier hypercalcemia induced by maternal hypercalcemia).

Neonatal rickets is a condition of severe bone demineralization, seen in preterm neonates. The main factor is phosphate deficiency due to, prematurity related, impaired placental function. Vitamin D deficiency and end organ resistance to vitamin D play a less important role. Low dietary phosphate adds to severity of this condition. Mother's milk is low in phosphate. Fig. 18.5 compares early and late hypocalcemia.

THE INHERITED DISORDERS

The inherited disorders may be classified into chromosomal disorders, monogenic disorders and multifactorial disorder. Multiple genes are involved in chromosomal disorders. In the monogenic disorders a single gene is involved. These disorders have a predictable pattern of inheritance. The multifactorial disorders are produced by interaction between influence of multiple genes and of environmental factors.

There are thousands of inherited disorders. Some of these are very rare. Some are harmless (alkaptonuria, Gilbert's disease, renal glycosuria etc.). Some are not compatible with life and lead to fetal abortion or failure to thrive. Some are however more important from treatment point of view. Diseases like phenylketonuria, galactosemia, maple

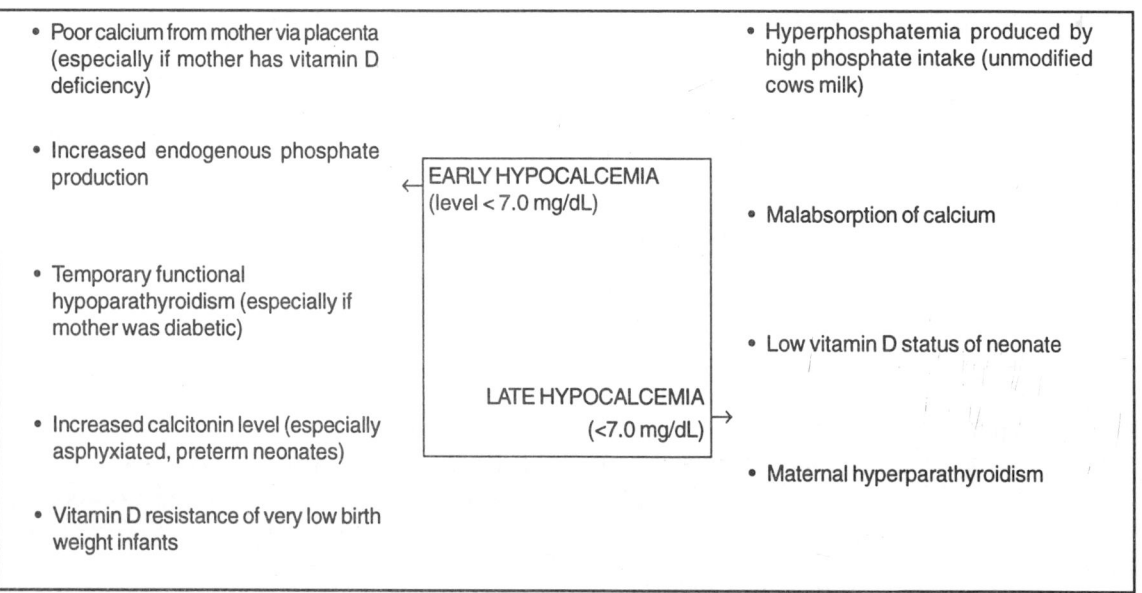

Fig.18.5. Early and late neonatal hypocalcemia.

- Magnesium deficiency also promotes calcium deficiency. Early neonatal deficiency occurs due to maternal magnesium deficiency (maternal diabetes); late neonatal deficiency is caused by malabsorption.
- Base correction of acidosis also promotes hypocalcemia (reduces ionic calcium level).

syrup urine disease and others, if detected early, can be well treated and their harmful consequences avoided. Some can be treated symptomatically (Hartnup's disease, congenital disaccharidase deficiency). In some, almost normal lifespan is possible if the precipitating factors are avoided (acute porphyrias, glucose-6-phosphate dehydrogenase deficiency, certain familial hyperlipidemias, cholinesterase defects, Wilson's disease, hemochromatosis and perhaps cystic fibrosis). In the last category, it is important to look for the disease in close relatives and offer advice on treatment.

Diagnosis depends upon clinical features and certain laboratory tests (Fig. 18.6). Very early in life, clinical features (Table 18.5) are not very specific. Some simple tests (Table 18.6), however, may suggest the presence of an inherited disorder. Once a strong suspicion is obtained, more definitive tests can be done to arrive at the proper diagnosis. In a failure to thrive case (due to a genetic disorder) it is important to establish diagnosis, even after death of the infant, since the information will be useful for genetic counseling.

Besides diagnostic testing of symptomatic individuals, other areas of investigative requirements in medical genetics are: (i) carrier screening (it may be population based in an ethnic group with high frequency of the disease or of individuals with family history of the disorder; (ii) presymptomatic testing in high risk individuals of late onset dominant disorders (Huntingtons chorea, heritable cancer disorders, eg. neurofibromatosis, Marfan's syndrome, adult polycystic kidney disease, tuberous sclerosis); (iii) prenatal diagnosis; and (iv) neonatal screening.

PREVENTION OF GENETIC DISEASE

Genetic screening, counseling and prenatal diagnosis help to prevent genetic disorders.

Genetic screening

For autosomal recessive disorders there are two types of genetic screening programmes. Firstly, there is screening of newborns for certain common genetic disorders (homozygote screening). These disorders are treatable and early detection and institution of treatment prevents development of clinical features. Table 18.7 gives criteria used to select a genetic disease for newborn screening programme. The diseases screened vary from country to country. This programme also identifies couples who would benefit from genetic counseling (see below). Screening for congenital hypothyroidism and phenylketonuria will be described, in some detail, separately (see below).

Besides the newborn screening, there is heterozygote screening (carrier screening). This is recommended for Tay Sach disease, thalassemias and sickle cell anemia in appropriate populations with high frequency of these disorders. Some also favour screening for cystic fibrosis. Carrier screening is

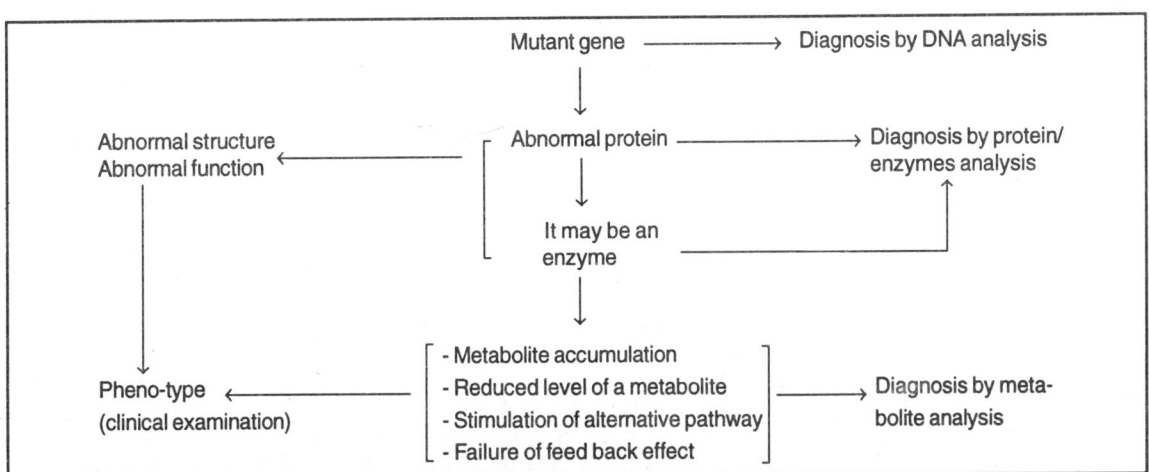

Fig.18.6. Mutant gene producing various changes which help detection of the inborn error produced.

Table 18.5. Important clinical features in a neonate suggestive of an inborn error

- Poor feeding and failure to thrive
- Vomiting with acidosis
- Jaundice or hepatosplenomegaly
  - Galactosemia, α-1 antitrypsin deficiency, tyrosinemia
- Acidosis with increased anion gap
  - Some specific organic acidemia and organic aciduria[1].
- Hypoglycemia
  - Galactosemia, frustosemia, glycogen storage disease, inborn errors of amino acids
- Ketonuria without hypoglycemia
  - Organic acidemia
- Unexpected hyponatremia, neutropenia
- Convulsions, hypotonia, coma
  - Pyridoxine deficiency, non-ketotic hyperglycemia
- In older infants mental retardation, refractory rickets, renal calculi, cataract
- Peculiar smell
  - Maple syrup urine disease
- Characteristic features
  - Pseudohypoparathyroidism
- Ambiguous genitalia
  - Congenital adrenal hyperplasia

[1] Organic acidurias (in born errors of propionate, methyl malonate including biotinidase deficiency; pyruvate, lactate and certain amino acids (branched chain, glycine, aromatic amino acids and others). Collective incidence of these disorders is about 1 in 12,000 births (although individual disorders are very rare). These disorders present in neonatal period with failure to thrive, sudden infant death, vomiting, severe metabolic acidosis, hypotonia, severe hypoglycemia or hepatic damage with encephalopathy.
- There is greater likelihood of presence of an inborn error if there is family history of death in early life and in presence of a consanguineous marriage.

also indicated for some other diseases like Duchenne muscular dystrophy, Huntington disease (may be, also for fragile X-mental retardation), if there is family history. Carrier screening is followed by effective genetic counseling.

Genetic counseling

As described above couples are identified, who are at risk of having a child with a genetic disease. If population is screened, counseling could be useful prior to marriage also. The nature of counseling will depend upon the type or disease (monogenic, multifactorial or chromosomal) and degree of cer-

Table 18.6. Important biochemical features in a neonate suggestive of inherited disorders

- Ferric chloride test positive with urine.
  (reducing organic acids in urine)
- Glucosuria, ketonuria, proteinuria (ketonuria in the absence of hyperglycemia indicates some organic aciduria).
- Abnormal amino acid/organic acid/sugar pattern in urine/plasma.
- Hypoglycemia (some organic acid uria, glycogen storage disease, galactosemia, furctosemia, some inborn error of amino acid metabolism).
- Metabolic acidosis (in metabolic acidosis if anion gap is >25 mmol/L; some specific organic acid could be present).
- Hyperammonemia (urea cycle enzyme defects), lactic acidosis (glucogen storage disease). Lactic acidosis is also caused by perinatal asphyxia.
- Hyponatremia (cystic fibrosis, congenital adrenal hyperplasia). It may cause apnoea and convulsions.
- Hypophosphatemia with increased phosphate excretion in urine.

- Perinatal asphyxia can also cause acidosis and raised serum creatinine and potassium. Similarly sepsis can produce hypoglycemia and hypotension (leading to lactic acidosis, raised serum creatinine and potassium). Hyponatremia may also result from maternal hyponatremia (during labour), inappropriate fluid administration, sepsis, renal failure, congestive heart failure (patent ductus arteriosus), diuretic treatment and SIADH.

Table 18.7. Criteria for selection of cases for newborn screening

- Relatively high incidence of the disease.
- if diagnosed early, effective treatment is available.
- Untreated disease has serious consequences.
- Disease is not clinically evident at birth but laboratory diagnosis is easy.
- Screening programme is cost effective.

- Besides mass screening, it may be done in selective groups, schools of mentally retarded, children in families with an affected members, children of consanguineous marriages and new borns with certain suggestive features as per Table 11.5

tainty in predicting risk to the offspring. Proper counseling requires correct diagnosis (biochemical/molecular testing), knowledge of factors like penetrance and expressivity of the abnormal gene along with the age at which the disease is commonly expressed. Counseling should be used to inform the couple about the behaviour of the disease, management possibilities and aspects like presymptomatic diagnosis, carrier testing and availability of prenatal diagnosis. Counseling is imperfect for common multifactorial disorders like diabetes mellitus, hypertension, atherosclerosis, congenital malformations and psychiatric disorders. In these disorders we are still learning about interaction of various genes and the environmental factors. The genetic loci important in predisposition to such disorders carry polymorphic normal alleles, which respond differently to environmental factors. At the present stage of knowledge the important genetic loci are those which constitute HLA gene complex. In general, risk for inheritance of such disorders depends upon the number of persons already affected in the family and the severity of the disorder. The etiological make up of a multifactorial disorder affecting different families may not be the same in all the affected families. In one family the etiology may involve major contribution from a mutant gene and the risk is predicted as in monogenic disorders. In another family, multiple genes may be involved, in etiology, along with important contribution from environmental factors and the risk is derived from knowledge about behaviour of the disease in the affected families.

Once a couple at risk for having a child with a genetic disease is detected, there are different options, depending upon the disease trait they have. Options are, not to have a child (or to adopt a child), artificial insemination (using donar semen or donar egg) or to proceed with reproduction and utilize prenatal diagnosis with elective abortion of affected fetuses. It may be remembered that risk of having an affected fetus is maximally 50% for heterozygotes with autosomal dominant disorders, less than 10% for nearly all chromosomal and multifactorial disorders and in between for others.

Prenatal diagnosis

It is clear from above that prenatal diagnosis helps when there is risk of having an abnormal fetus because of a genetic disease (Table 18.8). Different situations in which there is risk of having an abnormal fetus are: (i) pregnancy in a woman over 35 years of age (there is increased risk of Down's syndrome in fetus); (ii) when previous pregnancy resulted in birth of an infant with chromosomal abnormality; (iii) pregnancy after three or four abortions;

Table 18.8. Criteria for selection of cases for prenatal diagnosis

- Significant risk of disease to the infant. For example in case of a male fetus when the disorder is X-linked.
- Disease is serious and not amenable to treatment.
- Parents agree for termination of pregnancy if disease is confirmed.
- A reliable method is available for diagnosis.
- If treatment has to be started during pregnancy.
- In pregnancies after carrier screening has identified the couples at risk of getting an affected baby.

(iv) previous child had a neural tube defect. Prenatal diagnosis includes biochemical, cytogenetic and molecular testing and ultrasound examination for anatomic defects including skeletal dysplasias. The doppler ultrasound can assess fetal blood flow and has been used in diagnosis of cardiac anomalies.

Biochemical diagnosis

For prenatal diagnosis of hereditary disorders, tissues used are maternal plasma, amniotic fluid, amniotic fluid cells (AFC) and chorionic villus (CV) biopsy. This amniocentesis is done between 15 to 17 weeks of gestation and is called early amniocentesis. The AFC obtained are used for chromosomal analysis, enzyme studies and DNA analysis. As the number of cells in the amniotic fluid sample is quite small, these have to be cultured for 3 to 4 weeks before study. Unfortunately, with this procedure, when the diagnosis of the hereditary disorder is made, it is already too late for a safe abortion, in case of a serious disorder. More and more experience is becoming available for obtaining amniotic fluid sample at 10 to 14 weeks of gestation, in an ultrasound guided procedure. At present there is increased fetal loss in this procedure, otherwise the diagnosis is established at a time when safe abortion is possible. In an alternative method chorionic villus biopsy can be taken, under ultrasound guidance at 8 to 10 weeks. Cells are cultured, only, for a short period and diagnosis is made quite early in pregnancy. However, a recent study indicates that this procedure is associated with six fold increase in limb anomalies.

Late amniocentesis, is carried out in second half of pregnancy. Indications are, to determine fetal condition in Rh disease or other blood group immunizations (not needed in ABO incompatibility), to determine fetal maturity and to check for infection and maturity in a case of premature rupture of membranes. Lecithin is an important component of pulmonary sufactant and starts appearing in amniotic fluid from 35 weeks of gestation, onwards. Sometimes amniotic fluid sample may be used to study lecithin/sphingomyelin (L/S) ratio to have an idea of fetal lung maturity (Table 18.1).

In fetoscopy, direct inspection of fetus can be done using a fiberoptic endoscope and fetal blood can be obtained for analysis. For obtaining fetal blood, however, cordiocentesis (also called funipuncture) is preferred. In this procedure fetal blood sample can be obtained for analysis from umblical cord by a transabdominal aspiration under ultrasound control (there is very little chance of entering umbilical arteries as their calibre is much smaller compared to that of umbilical vein). Fetal lymphocytes can be used for karyotyping if there is risk of a chromosomal disorder (increased maternal age, low maternal serum α-fetoprotein, previous abnormal fetus or placental translocation). In case of high risk fetus, fetal blood analysis may help management. Blood may be required for estimation of coagulation factors, hemoglobin composition, platelet count, blood gases, and so on). The procedure for obtaining fetal blood can also be used in obtaining fetal liver tissue for knowing liver specific enzyme deficiencies and skin for dermatologic disorders.

Prenatal diagnosis of congenital anomalies

High maternal plasma α-fetoprotein levels during pregnancy may indicate a number of congenital anomalies in fetus especially neural tube and ventral wall defects. As chances of false positive results are high, there is need to follow such positive cases with evaluation of α–fetoprotein level in amniotic fluid and ultrasound examination of fetus. Low maternal plasma α–fetoprotein levels carry increased risk of fetal trisomy (especially trisomy 21). The triple marker screen for trisomy 21 (down's syndrome) is estimation of maternal plasma levels of α–fetoprotein (reduced), hCG (increased) and unconjugated estriol (reduced). To increase predictive value of these parameters for fetal anomalies

Table 18.9. Causes of human births defects

- Single gene disorders (cystic fibrosis, Tay-Sachs, congenital deafness and others) (20%)
- Chromosomal disorders (10%)
- Environmental (5%)
  - Infections (rubella, cytomegalo virus)
  - Maternal factors (diabetes, phenylkelonuria, hyperthermia)
  - Radiations
  - Drugs (thalidomide, alcohol)
  - Multiple gestation
  - Oligohydramnios/polyhydramnios
- Unknown, multifactorial

- Family history of congenital anomalies and abnormal levels of α-fetoprotein in maternal serum also increase likelihood of human birth defects.
- Large dozes of vitamin A (teratogenic in early pregnancy; carotenes are safe) and vitamin D (may cause growth retardation, hypercalcemia) should be avoided in pregnancy.

their levels should be interpreted with respect to gestational age related normal levels (Table 18.1).

It may be mentioned that congenital anomalies are multifactorial disorders (as already pointed out) and some factors (environmental) which increase their likelihood in pregnancy are given in Table 18.9.

Preimplantation prenatal diagnosis

This can be done in cases of invitro fertilization. One of the embryos at 8 cell stage is taken and molecular method of diagnosis is used for a single cell obtained from the embryo. In case the disorder is detected, the embryo is discarded. This method has been used for a number of monogenic disorders including cystic fibrosis and Tay Sachs disease.

Screening newborns for neonatal hypothyroidism and phenylketonuria

Criteria for selecting a disorder for neonatal screening are given in Table 18.7. Phenyl ketonuria, congenital hypothyroidism, galactosemia and cystic fibrosis are the disorders often considered suitable for screening. Incidence of neonatal hypothyroidism is estimated as 1 in 3500 to 4000 live births in developed countries. In iodine deficient regions of the World, incidence is much higher. Further, in these iodine deficient areas, additional milder hypothyroids occur which benefit from early treatment with thyroxine. For screening purpose, blood is collected after about a week after birth, from a heel prick on a filter paper and transported to the laboratory. TSH, is first estimated in the sample and if raised, it is followed by estimation of T_4. Either investigation, in isolation, will be inadequate (see Chapter 14).

Screening for neonatal hypothyroidism is delayed for about a week after birth since TSH and T_4 levels are not suitable for study before that. Also screening should not be done in an ill infant, since the results may be misleading.

For phenyl ketonuria, level of phenylalanine is measured in a sample of capillary blood from heel of the infant. Many centres use microbiological assay of phenylalanine using a mutant strain of B. Subtilis and the growth medium which prevents the growth of the organism unless phenylalanine is added. If the test is positive, more tests are needed to exclude false positive cases (transient tyrosinemia, transient phenylalaninemia) and to establish the type of phenyl ketonuria. In appropriate cases, reduced level of phenylalanine in the diet prevents development of mental retardation. The dietary control must be continued for at least, ten years, although, these days life long dietary control is recommended. Other diseases which could be considered for newborn screening are cystic fibrosis (approximate incidence 1 in 2500), Hartnup disease (1 in 18000), histidinemia (1 in 18000), galactosemia (1 in 62000), homocystinuria (1 in 150000), maple syrup urine disease (1 in 250,000) and hyperglycemia (non-ketotic) (1 in 250,000). The quoted disease incidences are not uniform all over the world.

Baby with ambiguous genitalia

This is not screening in the true sense as it is part of routine examination of the newborn. The baby should be examined in the presence of the parents. In describing abnormal genitalia one should use terms like underdeveloped or overdeveloped and avoid using terms like intersex, and pseudohermaphroditism. The baby should be named as male or female after definitive sex of rearing has been determined.

The child may be a simple undervirilized male, with palpable symmetrical gonads and without any mullerian structures (ultrasound examination). This

condition is called micropenis and further investigations needed will be in relation to pituitary functions, synthesis or actions of testosterone. On the other hand the child may present as a simple virilized female child with no palpable gonads and with normal Mullerian structures. In the presence of abnormal androgens in blood, she might be a case of congenital adrenal hyperplasia. In the absence of abnormal androgens, in blood, there might be a maternal source of androgens during pregnancy or it might be an idiopathic case, provided, in either case her karyotype is 46, XX. Neonates not falling in the above mentioned simple schemes need more detailed investigations for conditions like different forms of gonadal dysgenesis, anorchia, male pseudohermaphroditism and rarely true hermaphroditism (Chapter 17).

DIAGNOSIS OF INHERITED DISORDERS BY DNA ANALYSIS

The most direct method of detecting gene mutations (Fig. 18.6) is by using DNA probes (DNA oligonucleotides complementary to the normal/mutant segment of the gene). The probes are radioactive (^{32}P). Human genomic DNA is extracted from white blood cells and is next, cut into small pieces with the help of restriction endonucleases. Each enzyme recognizes a specific base sequence in duplex DNA and leads to cleavage of both strands. A large number of such enzymes are available (number is also growing with time). The DNA fragments are, next, separated, according to their size on agarose gel, followed by transfer and immobilization on nitrocellulose filter. The labeled specific sequence probes (single stranded) then hybridize with the fragments that contain the complementary sequences and are detected by autoradiography.

In a disease there may be complete deletion of the gene. In this case certain restriction fragments obtained for the normal gene will be missing for the DNA of the patient (Thalassemia A, Fig. 18.7). In another disease a point mutation may occurs at the restriction site of an enzyme. In this case some restriction fragments of normal and mutant genes will differ in size (sickle cell anemia). In ΔF508 mutation of cystic fibrosis there is deletion of

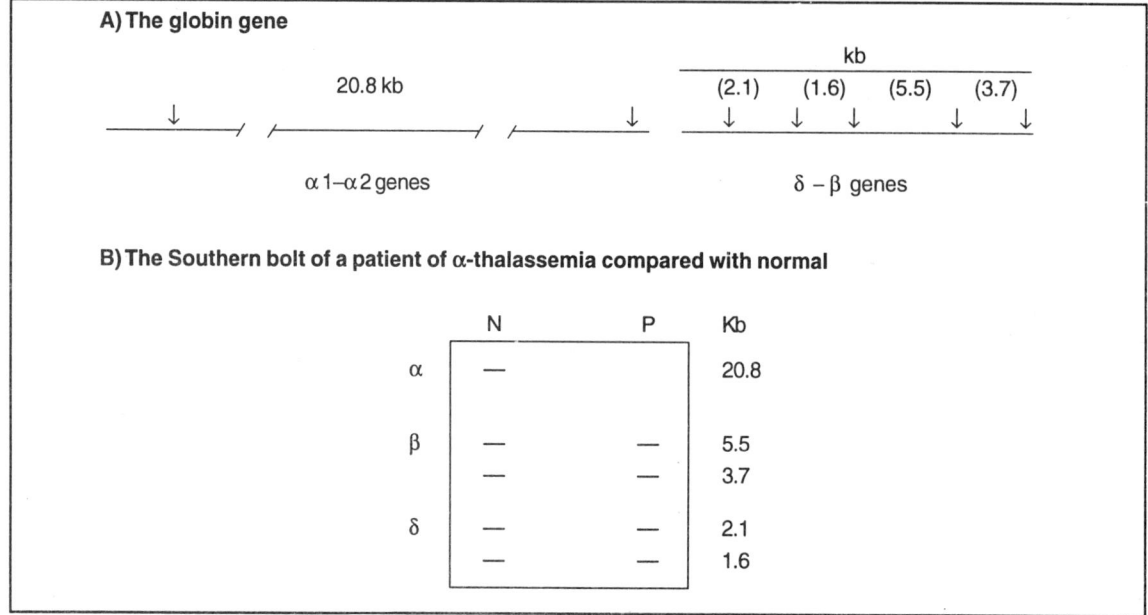

Fig. 18.7. Illustration of Southern bolt analysis of globin gene from a patient of alpha thalassemia.

- DNA obtained from normal reticulocytes and reticulocytes of a patient of α-thalassemia.
- Restriction fragments produced by Eco R1 (fragments of α and δ – β genes shown: sizes in kilobases).
- A mixed DNA probe prepared by reverse transcription of globin chain mRNAs.

phenylalanine codon. The PCR products (see below) of the normal and the mutant genes differ in size and can be separated by acrylamide gel electrophoresis. Restriction enzyme treatment is not required. In some cases the normal and mutant genes are associated with variable tendem repeats. Their PCR products (which include the tandem repeats) also differ in size and can be separated by simple gel electrophoresis.

In many cases there is point mutation and it does not involve any restriction site. In such cases if base sequence at the mutant site is known, small specific probes are constructed, one for the normal gene sequence and the other for the mutant gene sequence. These are called allele specific oligonucleotide probes or ASO probes. Hybridization will occur only under perfect match conditions. Dot blot technique is used in such cases (Fig. 18.8). Also study objective type question no. 28.

Before using ASO probes, portions of DNA containing the normal and mutant sequences are amplified by PCR (PCR produces thousands of

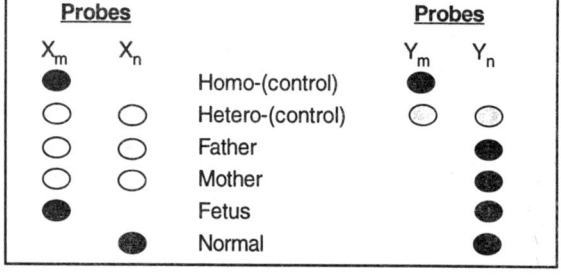

Fig.18.8. Mutation analysis of a patient of β-thalassemia using ASO probes for two mutations.

- Probes X and Y are for two different mutations causing β-thalassemia. The results show that the family has mutation X in the β-globin gene.

X_n = Probe for normal sequence for mutation X
X_m = Probe for mutated sequence for mutation X
Y_n = Probe for normal sequence for mutation Y
Y_m = Probe for sequence for mutaition Y

copies from a very small amount of DNA; say amount extracted from a few cells). In the dot blot technique, the two amplified products are spotted onto nylon membrane and hybridized with oligonucleotide probes to detect the specific mutations. If disease is produced by a number of mutations, the patient's DNA sample is tested with a number of DNA probes (see diagnosis of β-thalassemia).

If the molecular defect of the abnormal gene is not known, it can be detected indirectly. Before explaining principle of this method, a brief note on restriction fragment length polymorphism (RFLP) is important. Polymorphism means normal variations in population. Thus general normal population shows a polymorphism with respect to the lengths of DNA fragment obtained by the actions of certain restriction enzymes. It is interesting in this regard that one base after about every 150 bases (along the total human genome) is polymorphic (but produce no disease). This will give an idea of the large number of polymorphic restriction fragments which could be obtained from the human genome with the action of restriction enzymes (polymorphic base may alter some restriction site). DNA finger printing analysis (useful in establishing identity in the forensic work) is based on RFLP.

Mutation in a gene (causing a disease) may be linked to a specific base sequence at a polymorphic site (see above) (Fig. 18.9), resulting in linkage between the mutant gene and a marker polymorphic fragment. The specific marker fragment should however be close (or even intragenic) to the mutant gene so as to coseggregate consistently with the mutant gene during genetic transmission. Besides the RFLP markers (detected by Southern blot), tandem oligonucleotides (with variable tandem repeats) have also become available as markers for mutant genes. Their detection method is mentioned under trinucleotide repeat expansion disorders.

In this technique (linkage analysis) the family members have to be studied. The marker polymorphic fragment is detected with the mutant allele and not with the normal one. Thus the chromosome carrying the abnormal allele gets marked for the family. Some times the linkage which is true for the parents may not be so, far the children because meiotic recombination between the gene and the marker may disrupt the phase of linkage between the parents and the children. Objective type questions 27 to 30 give some idea of methodological innovations in the field of diagnosis by DNA analysis.

Sickle cell disease

This disease is caused by a single universal mutation in the cleavage site for the restriction enzyme Oxan l. PCR is used to amplify a DNA fragment which traverses the mutant site. Both normal and abnormal amplified fragments are reacted with Oxan l. After acrylamide gel electrophoresis and hybridization with suitable probes two bands are seen for normal DNA and only one band for mutant (homozygous) DNA (Fig. 18.10).

Thalassemia

A number of mutations cause β-thalassemia. Certain mutations are confined to certain ethnic groups. For each mutation a separate intragenic probe is used. Thus if ethnic group of the patient is known, the number of probes required to detect the mutation

---

A) The polymorphic
    fragments/sites ————————————→
    - Do not produce any disease
    - Are inherited according to Mendelian principles
    - Are exactly similar in identical twins

B) Useful marker fragments for linkage analysis.
    - More similar restriction sites/ fragments, more related the individuals
    - Easily detected (say by Southern blot).
    - The marker fragments properly defined for normal and mutant genes after analysis of a number of members (normals and patients) of a family.
    - It should be close to the locus where disease producing allele is located on DNA (it may be intragenic), so that it co-seggregates, consistently, with either normal or disease phenotype.
    - This techniques is helpful when it is not possible to detect the disease producing gene, directly or there are many mutations resulting in the disease phenotype.

Fig.18.9. Characteristics of polymorphic sites/fragemnts and their suitability for diagnosis of a disease by linkage analysis.

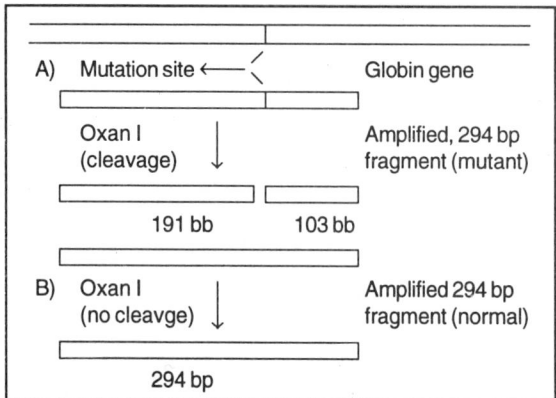

Fig.18.10. Diagnosis of sickle cells disease by DNA analysis.

A) PCR amplified fragment (294 bp) of globin gene from a normal individual is cleaved into 191 bp and 103 bp fragements by the restriction enzyme Oxan 1.

B) The same fragment of the mutant gene remains uncleaved.

- After acrylamide gel electrophoresis and transfer to nitrocellulose filter the fragments are revealed by a suitable probes.

will be reduced. If a family has risk for mutations X and Y (hypothetical), four probes will be required, X_n (normal sequence), X_m (mutant sequence), Y_n (normal sequence) and Y_m (mutant sequence). DNA material is amplified in the region of β-globin gene by PCR and then subjected to dot blot analysis. Results may be as shown in Fig. 18.8.

Trinucleotide repeat expansion disorders

The affected genes in these disorders, normally, contain a repeated sequence of three base pairs say $(CGG)_n$. Where n is variable but limited in range. In the disease state, however, the size of the triplet repeat is expanded outside the normal range (large regions of these sequences are called microsatellites). These sequences can occur in the 5′ untranslated, coding, intronic, or 3′ untranslated regions of the gene. Such mutations are known to cause fragile X-mental retardation [$(CAG)_n$ or $(GCC)_n$], myotonic dystrophy [$(CTG)_n$], Huntington's disease [$(CAG)_n$] and other disorders (spinobulbar muscular dystrophy and other neurodegenerative disorders). Slightly longer than normal repeat sequence may function as premutation in asymptomatic individuals. These premutation (and also mutation) sequences are unstable and may get further enlarged on further genetic transmission. As the repeat sequences enlarge the severity of disease increases and the phenotype onset may also occur earlier.

To demonstrate the expanded sequence regions of the genes. The specific loci are amplified by PCR incorporating ^{32}p-dCTP during the amplication process. The PCR products for normal and mutant genes will differ in size and easily separated by gel electrophoresis.

Future of genetic studied for certain common diseases

Our understanding about genetic aspects of many common diseases like hypertension, diabetes mellitus, atherosclerosis, psychiatric disorders, congenital anomalies, emphysema, various forms of cancer, hemochromatosis and others is rapidly increasing. In some of these major contribution may come from certain genes (Table 18.10 and Fig. 18.11). Molecular methods may become available (hopefully in near future) to screen population for the culprit genes. This will usher a new era of available medical benefit for these common diseases.

Table 18.10. Multifactorial diseases in which a single mutant gene may play predominant effect in disease expressivity in certain families

Diabetes mellitus:
- Glucokinase gene

Early onset coronary disease:
- Gene for familial hypercholesterolmia
- Gene for apo-E
- Gene group including genes for apo-A1, A-IV and CIII.
- Gene for apo-B
- Gene for lipoprotein lipase
- Gene for ACE: There is deletion (D) insertion (I) polymorphism; risk in DD> DI> II.
- Gene affecting homocysteine levels

Hypertension:
- Genes for β and γ subunits of the renal amiloride - sensitive sodium channel
- Gene for 11β-hydroxysteroid dehydrogenase
- Aldosterone synthase, 11β-hydroxylase fusion gene
- Renal thiazide-sensitive Na-C1 cotransporter gene

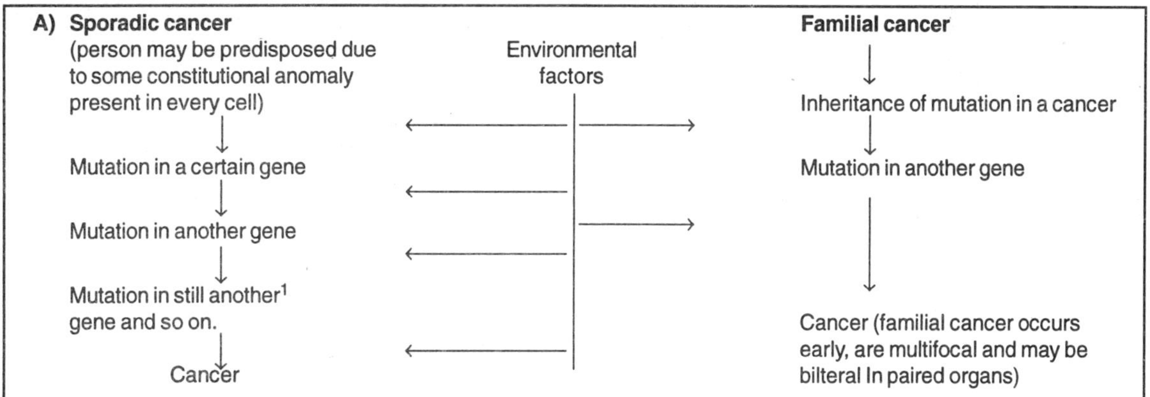

A) Sporadic cancer
(person may be predisposed due to some constitutional anomaly present in every cell)

Environmental factors

Familial cancer
↓
Inheritance of mutation in a cancer
↓
Mutation in another gene

↓
Mutation in a certain gene
↓
Mutation in another gene
↓
Mutation in still another[1] gene and so on.
↓
Cancer

Cancer (familial cancer occurs early, are multifocal and may be bilteral In paired organs)

B) Gene involved in carcinogenesis
- Mutated suppressor genes leading to loss of suppressor control over cell proliferation.
- Genes encoding transcription factors (RBI for retinoblastoma; $BRCA_1$ for early onset cancer breast; P53 for li-Frauemni syndrome and WT_1 for Wilms tumor).
- NF_1, NF_2 involved in causation of neurofibromatosis encodes CTPase activating protein.
- APC involved in causation of Familial polyposis coli encodes a protein which binds to catenin.
- Mutated proto-oncogene[2] lead to increased cell proliferation directly.
- RFT involved in causation of MEN type 2 encodes receptor tyrosine kinase.
- Mutated genes which control DNA repair process.
- MSH2, MHL1, PMS1 and PMS2 (involved in familial polyposis colon cancer

Fig.18.11. Genetic involvement in sporadic and familial cancers.

[1] Presence of one mutated allele (of the pair) in a somatic cell does not lead to its uncontrolled growth. Only, if a rare mutated cell develops mutation in the other allele (generating the homogous), the uncontrolled growth of the cell will occur.

[2] Genes that promote normal cell growth are called the proto-oncogenes. By activation (point mutation, amplification or dysregulation) these may be converted into an oncogenes.

Sickle cell anemia (Hb S replaces Hb A)

Besides American Blacks, there is high incidence in states of Central India especially in tribals. It is caused by a single nucleotide change (GAG to GTG) in sixth condon of the β-globin gene, resulting in incorporation of valine instead of glutamic acid, in β-globin chain of Hb. The genetic defect is transmitted as autosomal dominant trait. Red cells become sickle shaped when O_2 tension is low, resulting in increased viscosity of blood. There is capillary stasis, vascular occlusion and infarction of tissues like bone, lung and spleen. Splenic infarcts followed by fibrosis, explain, why spleen is not enlarged. Pulmonary changes produce pulmonary hypertension and heart failure. There is severe chronic hemolytic anemia.

Episodes of sickling and occlusion are precipitated by hypoxia, infection, fever, exposure to cold and dehydration. If gut is involved patient may present with acute abdomen. Hematuria results from renal involvement. Patient may present with joint pains (Table 18.11). The above type episodes may be accompanied with fever.

Some factors which influence pathological manifestations of sickle cell disease were mentioned above. But these fail to explain the great variability in severity of presentation and also in the dominant organ specific morbidity in different patients. In mixed disorders, concurrent thalassemia seems to protect against clinical manifestation of sickle disease. High level of fetal Hb is also protective. However, there is need to have a sensitive predictors of the course of the disease, in children.

In sickle cell trait (heterozygous state), there is no anemia, red cell morphology is normal and there is no evidence of hemolysis. In some cases

Table 18.11. Different presentations of patients of sickle cell anemia

- Hematuria (D/D gentourinary tumor, tuberculosis/vascular disease).
- Bone/joint pains with fever (D/D rheumatic fever). Patient may present with osteomyelitis.
- Abdominal pain (D/D surgical abdominal conditions). Bowel sound sremain normal in cases of gut infarction, in sickle cell crisis.

  (All above features result from tissue infarction due to vascular occlusion).
- Leg ulcers, cardiac failure produced by chronic anemia.
- Extensive erythropoiesis may produce folic acid deficiency and affect growth. A child may present with stunted growth.
- Chronic hemolytic jaundice may cause cholelithiasis.

hematuria may occur. In pregnancy, chances of pyelonephritis are increased. During high altitude flying, there are chances of getting splenic infarcts.

Treatment of sickle cell disease is prophylactic (adequate hydration, use of vaccines and antibiotics, avoiding high altitudes, chronic transfusion therapy), symptomatic in crisis (use of oxygen, morphine for pain), and curative. In severely affected patients use of hydroxyurea (increases production of fetal Hb by increasing synthesis of γ chains) along with erythropoietin, decreases incidence of crisis. Allogeneic bone marrow transplantation may be undertaken, if severe course is predicted in childhood (mortality rate of procedure is 5 to 10%). Gene transfer therapy is not possible at present.

Diagnosis

There is chronic hemolytic anemia (Hb around 8g/dL, raised LDH, absence of haptoglobin and slight increase of bilirubin), high reticulocyte count (15 to 20%), presence of sickle cells and target cells with normal red cell indices. Screening tests are positive in sickle cell anemia (homozygous state) as well as sickle cell trait (heterozyous state). In a simple screening test, sodium metabisulfite solution causes sickling of red cells on the slide. The screening test is also positive in other sickle diseases (Hb SC diseases, Hb SD disease, Hb S-thalassemia). Hemoglobin electrophoresis is used to demonstrate the presence of HbS, and other hemoglobins.

Sickel cell anemia (SS disease) should be differentiated from sickle diseases (see above). All these disorders have similar manifestations. On the average, sickle cell anemia has the most severe clinical course while splenomegaly is more likely to be found in sickle diseases. Also see Table 18.12. Hb electrophoresis plays an important role in differentiating between these conditions. If there is more of Hb A than Hb S, the patient has sickle cell trait. If both hemoglobins S and A are present but Hb S predominates, the patient has S/B$^+$ thalassemia. If Hb C is present with Hb S, the patient has SC disease. Hemoglobin electrophoresis should also be carried out for the family members. In case of sickle cell anemia both parents will show presence of Hb S while in other conditions, other hemoglobins will also be found. Hb electrophoresis in alkaline

Table 18.12. Hemolytic anemias with positive sickle cell test

Sickle cell anemia:

See the text.Hb S 80 to 100%, Hb A$_2$ 3 to 4%

Sickle cell trait:

See the text.Hb S 22 -48%, Hb A$_2$ 3-4%, rest is Hb A

S/C Hemoglobin disease:

- Racial prevalence. Mode of inheritance of the abnormal HbS is same as in sickle cell anemia. Severity is intermediate between sickle cell anemia and trait. Target cells are present. In contrast to sickle cell anemia splenomegaly is present. Almost equal amounts of Hb S and Hb C are present.

S/D Hemoglobin disease:

- Almost like S/C hemoglobin disease. In oridnary electrophoresis mobility of Hb S and Hb D is the same (Agar gel electrophoresis at pH 6.2 separates the two). HbS and Hb D are present in almost equal amounts.

Sickle cell thalassemia:

- Clinical picture and anemia are variable (often more severe than S/C hemoglobin disease. In HbS/B$^+$ thalassemia Hb S is over 50% and Hb A 15 to 30%; HbF and Hb A$_2$ are also increased. Clinically patients resemble sickle cell trait. HbS/B̊ thalassemia clinically and hematologically resembles sickle cell disease. However, MCH and MCV are lower and HbA$_2$ is increased.

- In proper diagnosis of these conditions (necessary for genetic counseling) race of the patient, clinical hisotry and examination are all important along with the relevant investigations: chains in different Hb S are: Hb A (normal) 2α, 2β; Hb A$_2$ 2α, 2δ; Hb F 2α, 2γ; Hb S 2α, 2β (mutant).

buffer does not sepatate Hb S from Hb D. These two can, however, be separated by agar gel electrophoresis at pH 6.2. Also the screening test for red cell sickling is only present in the presence of Hb S.

Carrier screening and prenatal diagnosis

Carrier screening is done by Hb electrophoresis. About 50% of total Hb is present as Hb S in carriers. Prenatal diagnosis by direct DNA analysis, is done using amniotic fluid cells or chorionic villus samples.

Thalassemias

In these disorders there is impaired synthesis of one of the two globin chains of Hb A. Impaired synthesis of α chain, results in α thalassemia.

α-Thalassemia

When α chains are not produced, the other chains accumulate and form tetramers, hemoglobin Bart's (γ_4) in infants and hemoglobin H (β_4) in adults. These abnormal hemoglobins show marked instability and an abnormal oxygen dissociation curve. Due to lack of cooperativity, in oxygen uptake by these hemoglobins, their oxygen dissociation curves are not sigmoid in shape and are shifted to left. The hematologic manifestations greatly depend upon the extent of accumulation of tetramers which, in turn, is determined by the number of α-chain gene loci deleted.

There are four genes for α-chains, two on either of the chromosomes of the pair 16 ($\alpha,\alpha/\alpha,\alpha$). In homozygous state of thalassemia all the four gene loci are deleted. Because of very poor tissue oxygenation, there develops, high cardiac out put failure, hydrops fetalis and fetal or neonatal death. Deletion of three genes ($--/-\alpha$) results in Hb H disease with increased amounts of Hb H (β_4) and Hb Bart's (γ_4). The patient has moderately severe hemolytic anemia. Unlike most other hemolytic anemias, anemia is microcytic and hypochromic and reticulocyte count is less for the degree of anemia. Deletion of two genes ($-,-/\alpha,\alpha$) or $-,\alpha/-,\alpha$), results in thalassemia trait. There is hypochromic, microcytic anemia with lowered cell volume (MCV).

Deletion of one gene does not produce any clinical features.

Diagnosis of severe forms is easy by demonstration of presence of the abnormal hemoglobins. Hemoglobin H disease presents in adults with hemolytic anemia and splenomegaly. In selected cases splenectomy may be helpful in management. In the milder forms the amounts of these abnormal hemoglobins is too small to be reliably demonstrated.

β-Thalassemias

Impaired synthesis of β-chain results in β-thalassemia. In this case the accumulated chains do not form tetramers but get bound to red cell membrane producing membrane damage. In some mutations there is no formation of β-chains at all (β°) while in others (β^+), there is some formation of these chains. Depending upon which mutations are inherited, different degrees of β-chain deficiencies are encountered in different patients.

When both β-globin genes (one on either of the chromosome pair 11) bear a thalassemic mutation (homozygous state) there is severe anemia (Cooley's anemia). This condition is called thalassemia major. The heterozygous state is called thalassemia minor. These disorders are common in Mediterranean countries, Middle East, South Asia and parts of India and Pakistan. In the homozygous state there is severe anemia starting from infancy (red cells are hypochromic, microcytic alongwith numerous nucleated red cells). There is also severe hepatosplenomegaly. There is high level of fetal hemoglobin. Parents have thalassemia trait. Patients need repeated transfusion and suffer from problems of iron overload.

In thalassemia trait, there is mild hypochromic microcytic anemia (Hb about 9.0 g/dL) with normal serum iron, total iron binding capacity and bone marrow iron (Fig. 11.3). In about one third patients of β-thalassemia trait there is increased level of hemoglobin F (1 to 3%) and most patients also have hemoglobin A_2; about 5% of total. The latter finding is absent if there is associated deficiency of iron and in less common $\delta-\beta$-thalassemia. In the latter condition, hemoglobin F may be 5 to 10% of total Hb. Also see Fig. 11.3. DNA analysis is used

Table 18.13. Molecular variants of G-6-PD, and clinical forms of G-6-PD deficiency

In Africans	In Mediteranean and other regions (Iranians, Arabs, Asians and others)
• Normals have normal B type enzyme and about 20% have variant A+ which is also functionally normal. • About 11% have variant resembling A+ (called A−) and produces moderate hemolytic anemia on exposure to certain agents (oxidant drugs, some bacterial/viral infections, diabetic acidosis).	• Normals have normal B type enzyme • Patients have a variant more unstable than A− and producing more severe hemolytic disease caused by exposure to oxidant drugs, infections, favabeans. Some patients also present with chronic hemolytic anemia (hereditary non-spherocytic hemolytic anemia).

- Other rare forms of G-6-PD variants may also produce congenital non-spherocytic hemolytic disease.
- Deficiencies of glutathione related enzymes (reductase, peroxidase, and synthetase), may also uncomonly, produce drug induced hemolytic anemia.

for prenatal diagnosis and detection of heterozygotes (Fig. 18.8). In selected cases splenectomy may be helpful in management. The homozygous state of β-thalassemia is a serious disorder and untreated, it is usually fatal in childhood. Treatment is in the form of repeated blood transfusions and there is always a danger of iron overload (treated with regular infusions of desferrioxamine). Bone marrow transplantation can also be done. Screening for β-thalassemia combined with counseling has been able to reduce the incidence of disease in certain parts of the World. Heterozygotes of β-thalassemia need no treatment.

Cystic fibrosis

It is a severe autosomal recessive disorder which may present with repeated lung infections and bronchiectasis, pancreatic insufficiency and steatorrhea or as meconium ileus in a newborn. Topic is discussed in chapter 11. Also see Fig. 11.4. Neonatal screening can be done by detecting increased concentration of immunoreactive trypsin in neonatal blood. Prenatal diagnosis, is also possible, although frought with problems at times. Total mutations reported so far are more than 450 but one of these designated ΔF508 accounts for about 70% of mutations occurring in Caucasians (but significantly less in other ethnic groups). ΔF508 can be detected by differential migration in polyacrylamide gel. The detection of 30 mutations in a single sample relies on pooled ASO strategy. The relation between

mutations and their clinical consequences are not properly defined as yet. Not all the mutations cause all the clinical features. Also severity of the disorder caused, cannot be predicted.

Glucose-6-phosphate dehydrogenase deficiency (G-6-PD deficiency)

Activity of this enzyme generates NADPH in red cells which is required to protect red cells against oxidative damage. In a person with G-6-PD deficiency hemolytic anemia occurs, when there is formation of activated oxygen species in excessive amounts (after intake of drugs like primaquin, sulfonamides and vitamin K). 2% of such individuals, however, show chronic hemolytic anemia. There is high incidence of G-6-PD deficiency in Middle and Far East and in North India (also in Central Africa). The gene for the enzyme (with a large number of alleles) lies on the X-chromosome and therefore, it commonly affects males. Several tests are available for detection of susceptible individuals. These include, glutathione stability test, methemoglobin reduction test, cresyl blue reduction test and a dye reduction spot test. In the dye reduction test hemolysate is mixed with a solution of the dye (bromocresyl blue) and time is noted for discharge of the colour. More time is taken in cases of enzyme deficiency.

The African patients generally, have moderate and self limited type of disorder while in other parts of the World, the disease occurs, in more severe form. In these regions, it may appear as hemolytic disease of the newborn or as hereditary non-spherocytic hemolytic anemia (Table 18.13). Pyruvic kinase and phospho hexoisomerase deficiencies may also produce hereditary non-spherocytic hemolytic anemia. Other causes are, acquired autoimmune hemolytic anemia (Coombs test positive), hemoglobinopathies (diagnosed by Hb electrophoresis). A similar picture may occur in hemolytic anemia due to ABO incompatibility. In all these conditions, generally, there is moderate anemia, normal osmotic fragility, high reticulocyte count and slightly enlarged spleen. Some other inborn errors are presented in Table 18.14.

Table 18.14. Selected inherited disorders

INHERITANCE AUTOSOMAL DOMINANT

Achondroplasia:

Skeletal disorders, dwarfism and abnormal body proportions.

Adult polycystic kidney:

- Diseases may present at any age (most commonly in 3rd/ 4th decade with dull flank pain (mass effect of enlarged kidneys), acute pain (due to obstruction/hemorrhage into some cyst) or with some complication (stone, pyelonephritis, end stage renal disease)
- Hypertension, hematuria and impaired urine concentration.
- Extrarenal abnormalities (hepatic/ intracranial cysts, colonic diverticuli).
  - Ultrasound for diagnosis and screening of family members.
  - Genetic linkage analysis, if in a family member, diagnosis is essential (to donate kidney) but ultrasound is negative.

Breast cancer:

- About 10% of breast cancers are directly linked to germ line mutations. Identification of the BRCA-I gene (not used in clinical set up) makes it possible to identify women with 85% to 90% , lifetime likelihood of developing breast cancer.
- Ultrasound, mammography, fine needle biopsy and excision biopsy are used for diagnosis
- Early menarche, late menopaused and nulliparity increase risk of breast cancer.
- Strong family history and increased radiation exposure before the age of 30 years also increases the risk.

Familial polyposis coli and hereditary nonpolyposis colon cancer:

- Heritable gastrointestinal polyposis syndromes (uncommon) and hereditary non-polyposis cancer colon (common), cases occur.
- About 25% of patients of colorectal cancer have family history of disease; in many cases other associated tumors may also be present.
- Screening methods include annual digital examination starting at age 40, screening for fecal occult blood at 50 and sigmoidoscopy every 3 to 5 years at the age of 50 years onwards. Analysis for certain DNA mutations in DNA recovered from stool of patients may also become available in due course.

Hereditary spherocytosis (HS) (incidence 1 in 1000 to 1 in 4500)**:**

- Red cells are spherical due to cytoskeletal defect of red cell membrane (spectrin)
- Major features are anemia (mild to moderate), splenomegaly and jaundice, starting early in life.
- Important to differentiate from spherocytic hemolytic anemia associated with RBC antibodies.
  - Family history of anemia/ splenectomy as splenectomy corrects anemia. Coomb's test negative.
  - Increase in osmotic fragility in HS following sterile incubation for 24 hours at 30°C.
  - Osmotic fragility increased in severe cases.

Huntington disease (incidence 1 in 10,000)**:**

- Degenerative disease of basal ganglia and cortex; presents with choreiform movements and mental retardation in adult life.
- Disease is caused by triplet repeat mutations.
- Diagnosed by family history and detection of caudate nucleus atrophy on CT (or MRI).
- Presymptomatic diagnosis is possible by DNA analysis.

Contd....

Contd. Table 18.14

Marphan's syndrome:

• Long thin extremities associated with other skeletal changes, ectopia lentis, aortic aneurysm (Collagen disorder).

Myotonic dystrophy:

• Incidence is 13.5 per 100,000 live births; the most common adult muscular dystrophy.
• The neck, facial and distal limb muscles are involved (the proximal ones are usually spared except quadriceps)
• Patients may also have occulopharygeal dystrophy (ptosis, limited eye movements and difficulty in swallowing)
    - Serum CK level is normal or shows mild elevation.
    - EMG evidence of myotonia
    - Muscle biopsy shows atrophic changes.
    - Unstable triplet repeat mutation detection can be used for prenatal diagnosis.

Neuro fibromatosis:

• Type-I neurofibromatosis is a common dominant disorder and commonly presents with cafe-au-lait spots, neurofibromas, Hisch nodules of the iris and predisposition to neurofibrosarcoma and glioma. It is caused by mutation of suppressor gene NF-1. Mutation in NF-2 causes neurofibromatisis-type 2 (acoustic neuroma, meningioma).

Osteogenisis imperfecta:

• Fragility of bone causing pathological fractures, blue sclerae, deafness, family history (Collagen disorder).

Tuberous sclerosis:

• It is a multisystem disease, which most commonly present with skin lesions and benign tumors of CNS. Renal involvement is common with cyst formation in the kidney.

Von Willebrand disease (VWD):

• The most common inherited coagulation disorder arising from deficiency of von Wille brand factor (VWF) (it helps platelet adhesion and acts as carrier of factor VIII). Bleeding occurs after trauma (mild cases) or as spontaneous from nose or other mucosal linings (severe cases).
    - Like hemophilia APTT is prolonged, but there is no joint bleeding and bleeding time is prolonged.
    - Reduced plasma factor VIII activity (both coagulative and immunologic activities are low; in hemophilia - A only coagulative is low).

Acute intermittent porphyria(see Chapter 8); **Familial hypercholesterolemia**(see Chapter 9); **Retinoblastoma** (see Table 18.11)

INHERITANCE AUTOSOMAL RECESSIVE

Acatalasia:

• A disorder of catalase deficiency (the enzyme protects against H_2O_2 producing organisms) encountered in Japanese; presents with recurrent ulcers in gums.
    - Blood turns brown on standing.
    - Lack of catalase activity in culture cells.

Galactosemia:

incidence is about 1 in 70,000

• Caused by of galactose-1-phosphate uridyl transferase(GALT) deficiency (more common), galactokinase deficiency and UDP galactose-4-epimerase deficiency(rare).
• Infants develop vomiting and poor nutrition on milk intake within days after birth followed by jaundice, hepatomegaly and cataract(after a month)
    - Screening by demonstrating presence of galactose in blood/urine.
    - Increased level of glycosylated Hb helps diagnosis
    - Diagnosis confirmed by showing GALT deficiency in red cells.

Contd....

Contd. Table 18.14

- Prenatal diagnosis by showing GALT deficiency in cultured amniocentesis cells or increased galactitol in amniotic fluid(if fetus is affected mother should be given lactose free diet in pregnancy).

Glycogenses[1] (also see Chapter 5):

- Type I, type III (debrancher deficiency), type VI (liver phosphorylase deficiency), and type VI a (phosphorylase kinase deficiency) characterized by hepatomegaly and hypoglycemia.
- Type IV (brancher deficiency) and type III (debrancher deficiency) are associated with hepatomegaly and cirrhosis.
- Type V (muscle phosphorylase deficiency), type VII (deficiency of phosphofructo kinase), phosphoglycerate kinase and some other enzyme deficiencies are associated with exercise intolerance, myoglobinuria after severe exercise and increased CK level in plasma.
- Type II (lysosomal α-glucosidase deficiency) and type IIIa and IV are associated with progressive skeletal muscle weakness and atrophy and/or cardiomyopathy.
- The overall incidence is about 1:20,000 live births. The most common is type I which occurs as a childhood disorder; type V is the most common occuring in adults. Type I include type I-a (glucose 6 phosphatase deficiency) and type-1-b (glucose 6 phosphate translocase deficiency).

    - Increased plasma levels of lactate, TAG, cholesterol and uric acid in type I.
    - Administration of glucagon/epinephrine increase level of lactate but not of glucose in type I.
    - In type V, severe exercise causes excessive rise of ammonia but not of lactate.
    - Definitive diagnosis in both type I a and type V involves biopsy studies.
    - DNA diagnosis available for type I a and certain mutations of type V

- Type I requires frequent carbohydrate feeds and type V - use of oral glucose, high protein diet and avoiding severe exercise

Homocystinuria:

Cystathoionine β-synthase deficiency; (incidence 1 in 60,000 in Ireland and 1 in 200,000 elsewhere)

- Dislocation of optical lenses, mental retardation, osteoporosis in childhood and life threatening occlusion of coronary, cerebral and renal arteries in first decade of life.
- Heterozygotes (1 in 70 in population) have only hyperhomocystinemia without any significant homocystinuria (also seen in other variants of forms involving impaired folate/ B_{12} metabolism), have increased risk for thrombotic vascular disease (coronary, cerebral, peripheral).

    - Increased urinary excretion of SH-compounds, demonstrated by cyanide, nitroprusside test: Plasma a methionine elevated.
    - Diagnostic confirmation by measuring cystathionine β-synthase activity in cultured cells (in about 50% patients activity is almost nil and 1 to 5% of the normal, in the rest. In latter cases activity often increases with B_6 administration).
    - Neonatal Diagnosis can be made by showing increase in peak homocysteine levels after methionine loading or by demonstrating low tissue enzyme level. Heterozygotes are also detected in the same way. If the disorder is detected early, effective treatment (as in phenylketonuria) is available.

5,10-Methylene FH_4 reductase deficiency and other errors (5 entities) in methylcobalamine synthesis.

- Varying features including developmental retardation, nervous system defects, megaloblastic anemia and pancytopenia.

    - Elevated levels of homocysteine and methylmalonic acid (in some forms) along with normal or low levels of methionine. In some cases there may be homocystinuria as well. Screening by the cyanide-nitroprusside test.
    - In patients with methylmalonic acidemia serum B_{12} levels are normal (unlike pernicious anemia).

Contd....

---

[1] Most of these disorders are autosomal recessive; phosphoglycerate kinase deficiency and one form of phosphorylase kinase deficiency are X-linked. For most of these diseases the defective genes have also been characterized at molecular level. Classification of glycogenes based on organ involved and clinical manifestations (in preference to old numerical classification) in given in Table 5.5.

Contd. Table 18.14

Hurler syndrome:

- It is one of the mucopolysaccharidoses; a group of diseases due to certain lysosomal enzyme deficiencies, resulting in accumulation of glycosaminoglycans.
- Accumulation of glycosaminoglycans in different tissues (liver, spleen, eyes, central nervous system, cartilage, bone), producing wide variety of clinical features.
- Patients present early in life with coarse facial features; cloudy cornea, hepatosplenomegaly, mental retardation and skeletal changes; death occurs in childhood.
  - Increased urinary excretion of sulfated glycosaminoglycans (dermatan sulfate and heparan sulfate)
  - L-iduronidase deficiency in leucocytes.
  - Enzyme deficiency in cultured amniotic fluid cells establishes prenatal diagnosis.

Maple syrup urine disease:

- There is deficient branched chain ketoacid decarboxylase; accumulation in plasma and increased excretion in urine of branched chain amino acids and their ketoacids (the latter impart a peculiar odour to urine).
- Disease presents in first week of life; if untreated, there develop severe neurological lesions leading to early death.
- Milder forms are helped by a diet low in branched amino acids.
  - Elevated levels of branched amino acids in plasma and urine.
  - Prenatal diagnosis by estimation of branched chain α-ketoacid decarboxylase in cultured cells.

Phenylketonuria:

- Incidence of all disorders taken together is about 1in 10,000 births. Type I (variable deficiency of phenyl alanine hydroxylase depending upon the mutation; more than 200 are known) accounts for 2/3 of total cases (mostly in Whites and Asians rare in Blacks). Type II is deficiency of dihydropteridine reductase and type III is deficiency of synthesis of tetrahydrobiopterin from GTP. Tetrahydrobiopterin is needed as a coenzyme with phenylalanine hydroxylase; the reductase is needed in regeneration of tetrahydrobiopterin from dihydropteridine.
- Feeding problems, vomiting in the first few weeks of life, mental ratardation becoming apparent from delay in early developmental milestones. Final problems are mental retardation, hyperactivity and seizures along with hypopigmentation and eczema of the skin.
- Diet therapy (special diet low in phenylalanine and supplementated with tyrosine)is started within 1st three weeks of life. In patients other than type I disorder, phenylalanine restriction is combined with supplementation of levodopa and 5 HTP. Phenylalanine restriction is also advised during pregnancy in at risk cases.
  - Newborn screening by estimation of plasma phenylalanine level using Guthrie bacterial inhibition assay.
  - Confirmation by quantitative fluorometric assay of plasma phenylalanine.
  - Prenatal diagnosis based on DNA testing is now feasible in families by linkage analysis or by the use of ASO probes.
  - Dihydropteridine reductase can also be estimated in dried blood spots for newborn screening and cultured amniocytes for prenatal diagnosis. These cells can also be used for detection of blocks in synthesis of tetrahydrobiopterin.

Tay-Sachs disease (GM$_2$ gangliosidosis):

incidence 1 in 3,600 in Ashkenazi Jews and French Canadians; 1 in 40,000 in other populations

- Important presenting features are mental retardation, cherry red spot in retina, enlarged liver and spleen and muscular weakness.
  - EMG evidence of myotonia
  - Diagnosis is confirmed by demonstrating low levels of hexosaminidase-A in serum, leucocytes, amniocytes or fibroblasts.
  - Prenatal diagnosis by studying levels of hexosaminidase in cultured cells.

Adrenal hyperplasia (see Chapter 15); Cystic fibrosis(see Chapter 18 Text); Congenital Hypothyroidism (see Chapters

Contd....

Contd. Table 18.14

14, 18 Text); Sickle Cell disease (see Chapter 18 Text); Thalassemia (see Chapter 18 Text); (α_1 antitrypsin deficiency (see Chapter 5); Hemochromatosis (see Chapter 5, 11); Wilson's disease (see Chapter 5, 11)

INHERITED X-LINKED

Chronic granulomatous disease:

- Granulocytes are deficient in the enzyme system producing burst of singlet oxygen needed to kill certain bacteria (Proteus, Staphylococcus). Thus childhood infections caused by these bacteria occur in males.
- A milder form(autosomal recessive) occurs both in boys and girls in which granulocytes fails to mediate H_2O_2 - myeloperoxidase killing of certain bacteria (which lack catalase; Streptococcus).

Duchenne/Becker muscular dystrophy (incidence 1 in 3,300 male births):

- Disease starts in the first 3 years of life.
- Pelvic girdle and lower limbs are involved first.
- Family History
- After ruling out diabetes, hyperparathyroidism, renal failure and electrolyte abnormalities.
- CK levels are useful;
  - i) For clinical diagnosis
  - ii) Preclinical diagnosis of Duchenne and Becker in families with history of   disease.
  - iii) For screening
  - iv) To identify female carriers
- Presence of Abs to dystrophin (means absence of protein dystrophin in Duchenne's dystrophy and decrease in its amount in Becker's dystrophy).
- Muscle biopsy shows degenerative changes but no cellular infiltration. Enzymes CK, AST, aldolase may also be evaluated in the biopsy material.
- Molecular methods are also useful;
  - i) Prenatal diagnosis
  - ii) Diagnosis of carriers.
  - iii) For differential diagnosis.

Fabry's disease:

- It is one of the sphingolipidoses in which there is accumulation of a ceremide in neurons of CNS and peripheral ganglia and media of small blood vessels.
- Presents with skin lesions, episodic fever, paraesthesia and proteinuria. Early death from strokes or renal failure.
- Deficiency of α-galactosidase in leukocytes and fibroblasts of patient and carriers.
- Prenatal diagnosis possible.

Hemophilia A (factor VIII deficiency) and B (factor IX deficiency):

Incidence is about 1: 10, 000 in male population

- Both are X-linked congenital disorders. Hemophilia A is more common(about seven times) and usually more severe compared to hemophilia B.
- In mild cases surgery results in excessive bleeding; in moderately severe ones, trauma produces hematomas and in severe cases there occur spontaneous muscle hematomas and hemarthroses.
  - Clotting time and activated prothrombin time (APTT) are prolonged. APTT depends upon most factors except factor VII. In mild cases clotting time may be normal.
  - Prothrombin time ,(depends upon factors II, V, VII, X), platelet count, bleeding time and fibrinogen levels are all normal.
  - Specific assays of factors VIII and IX are needed to differentiate between hemophilias A and B since the plasma factors needed for management are different.
  - Defective alleles in factor VIII deficiency in different families can be detected by linkage analysis or by using ASO probes after gene amplification.
  - Fetal blood can also be used (plasma factor assay) for prenatal diagnosis.

Fragile-X (Table 18.1); Glucose 6 phosphate dehydrogenase deficiency (see Chapter 18 Text); Hypophosphatemic rickets (Chapter 10); Testicular feminization (Chapter 17); Lesch-Nyhan Syndrome and partial deficiency of HRPT (Chapter 8).

OBJECTIVE TYPE QUESTIONS

Pick out the wrong statement.

1. Toxemia of pregnancy

i) In normal pregnancy plasma flow and GFR increase by 30 to 50%.

ii) A pregnant woman with serum creatinine level above 0.8 mg/dL and BUN over 13 mg/dL needs to be investigated for pre-eclampsia.

iii) In repeated measurements, a blood pressure of 140/85 or more, during early pregnancy, which increases during the night may indicate pregnancy induced hypertension.

iv) In a previously hypertensive patient there is rapid increase of blood pressure, if preeclampsia supervenes.

v) To avoid worsening of renal disease during pregnancy, the aim should be to keep blood pressure under control.

2. Gestational changes

i) Gestational hypertension develops in later half of pregnancy, and disappears within 10 days, following parturition.

ii) Gestational proteinuria is proteinuria during pregnancy without hypertension, edema or renal disease.

iii) Gestational proteinuria is a common finding.

iv) Gestational diabetes should be treated with dietary treatment or insulin.

v) Gestational diabetes disappears after delivery and there is no chance that it will change into permanent diabetes.

3. Fetal functions

i) Fetal liver produces albumin, coagulation factors and red cells.

ii) Fetal kidney produces urine which enters amniotic fluid.

iii) Development of a number of endocrine glands is completed by 12 to 14 weeks of gestation.

iv) Maturation of hypothalamic-pituitary axis is completed by about 20 weeks of gestation.

v) Proper thyroid function starts at about 20 weeks of gestation.

vi) Main fetal thyroid hormone is T_3.

4. Fetal hormones

i) Fetal pattern of low T_3 and high rT_3 is similar to that seen in PEM.

ii) After delivery hypothalamic-pituitary-thyroid axis is stimulated by environmental cold, with peaking of T_3/T_4 in 24 to 48h.

iii) rT_3 level is reduced to adult levels in about 2 weeks.

iv) Endemic cretinism is goitrous while sporadic cretinism is non-goitrous.

v) With neonatal screening, treatment of cretinism can be started when the neonate may look clinically normal.

5. Neonates with maternal hepatitis B infection

i) Acute hepatitis B infection in third trimester passes to neonate in about 70% of the cases.

ii) Neonate getting infection from mother, in third trimester generally, gets a severe infection and dies.

iii) Mothers positive for Australia antigen (HBsAg) and also positive for HBeAg, have risk of infecting their babies.

iv) Mothers positive for HBsAg but negative for HBeAg and having anti-HBe, have very small risk of infecting their babies.

v) Infants of mothers positive for HBsAg, negative for HBeAg and having anti-HBe may become carriers of HBsAg and will be at risk of developing carcinoma of liver.

6. Maternal smoking

i) Maternal smoking has dose dependant effect of decreasing fetal weight.

ii) Passive smoking because of a smoker father has a similar effect but about 60% as strong as produced by maternal smoking.

iii) Maternal smoking also produces a number of congenital anomalies.

iv) Reduced uterine perfusion, increase in carboxyhemoglobin and structural changes in placenta are some factors which produce intrauterine growth retardation in case of smoker parents.

v) In follow up studies, such babies (retarded during intrauterine growth because of maternal smoking) run an increased risk for deficient stature and mental dysfunctions.

7. In a diabetic mother

i) Blood glucose level should be maintained below 140 mg/dL and hypoglycemia avoided.

ii) In poorly controlled diabetes, risk of intrauterine fetal death is increased.

iii) In poorly controlled diabetes, there is increased risk for birth asphyxia, RDS, and polycythemia.

iv) Infants are frequently large for gestational age even if mother has gestational diabetes or she is simply prediabetic.

v) In cases of severe maternal diabetes (diabetes started in childhood, with duration of about 20 years with retinopathy), the newborn suffers from severe RDS and becomes difficult to manage.

8. Neonatal jaundice (indirect bilirubin)

i) It may be physiological jaundice, if it occurs in first 24 hours after birth.

ii) Blood film for red cell morphology may indicate hereditary spherocytosis, as the cause.

iii) It may be due to delayed cord clamping which increases hematocrit.

iv) In preterm and SGA, reduced activity of glucuronyl transferase is the cause.

v) Haemorrhage, bruising and delayed passage of meconium may be the causative factors.

vi) Septicemia and urinary tract infection can also increase level of indirect bilirubin.

vii) Intrauterine infections can increase indirect (due to hemolysis) as well as direct (neonatal hepatitis) bilirubin.

9. Neonatal jaundice (direct bilirubin)

i) Neonatal hepatitis caused by intrauterine infection, galactosemia or α-antitrypsin deficiency may be the cause.

ii) Cystic fibrosis may be the cause.

iii) It may be breast milk jaundice.

iv) Biliary atresia which may·be intrahepatic or extrahepatic, may be the cause.

v) Dubin-Jonson and Rotor syndromes also cause increase of direct bilirubin.

10. Neonatal jaundice

It may not be physiological jaundice if:

i) Jaundice is present at birth.

ii) Total bilirubin >15 mg/dL in a term infant or >12 mg/dL in a preterm infant.

iii) Jaundice persists for one week in a preterm infant.

iv) Jaundice present in an ill infant.

v) Conjugated bilirubin is more than 2 mg/dL.

11. Neonatal hypoglycemia

i) It may be because of reduced substrate availability, in SGA infants and in preterm infants.

ii) It may be due to hyperinsulinemia in an infant of a diabetic mother.

iii) In nesidioblastosis, hypoglycemia is temporary and clears up in about a week.

iv) In many inborn errors (glycogen storage disease, galactosemia, inborn errors of amino acids), hypoglycemia is due to inability to produce glucose.

v) It may be caused by birth asphyxia.

vi) It may be caused by deficiency of GH or cortisol.

12. Hypoglycemia

i) In infants at risk, frequent checks of blood glucose should be carried out to prevent severe hypoglycemia.

ii) At risk infants should be fed within 2h after birth.

iii) If hyperinsulinemia is suspected clinically, the baby should have the sample taken, for estimation of only insulin, immediately and treated promptly.

iv) Asymptomatic hypoglycemia should be first managed by early, frequent feeds and if it persists, be treated with infusion of 10% dextrose.

v) Symptomatic hypoglycemia requires dextrose infusion.

13. Hypoglycemia

i) Because of autonomic nervous system response (sweating, pallor, tachycardia), it is quite easy to diagnose neonatal hypoglycemia.

ii) Plasma glucose level should not be allowed to fall below 46 mg/dL otherwise, the cerebral functions will get compromised.

iii) Severe hypoglycemia can produce apnoea, convulsions and coma.

iv) Prolonged hypoglycemia may some times cause congestive heart failure or persistent pulmonary hypertension.

v) A low blood glucose level detected by a stick test should be checked by a laboratory assay method.

14. Selecting a disease for newborn screening

i) Relatively high incidence of disease.

ii) Disease is serious and not amenable to treatment.

iii) Disease is not clinically evident at birth.

iv) Disease easily diagnosed by an available laboratory method.

v) Screening programme is cost effective.

15. Autosomal recessive disorders

i) Most of inborn errors are inherited as autosomal recessive disorders.

ii) In family history it is important to enquire about consanguinity.

iii) Heterozygotes are often clinically normal.

iv) Heterozygotes of most of the inborn errors can be diagnosed by ordinary biochemical tests.

v) There is vertical transmission of the disease.

16. Autosomal dominant disorders

i) The patient has normal parents.

ii) Half the offspring of the affected patient can have the disorder.

iii) There is marked variation in expressivity of the disorder.

iv) Most malformations are either polygenic or autosomal dominant disorders.

v) New cases commonly arise as spontaneous mutants.

17. X-linked recessive disorders

i) In these inherited disorders, males suffer and females act as carriers.

ii) Commonly the affected male passes on the trait to his offspring.

iii) Half the female offspring of a carrier female will become carriers of the disease.

iv) All the female offspring of the affected male will be carriers.

v) These disorders are often expressed as a new mutation, making genetic counseling difficult.

18. Multifactorial (polygenic) mode of inheritance

i) These disorders do not show the characteristic patterns of Mendelian inheritance.

ii) The occurrence of these diseases within affected families is greater than that predicted for general population.

iii) In these disorders both genetic and environmental factors interact to produce the disease.

iv) Incidence of these disorders, in general population is about 1 in 1000 live births.

v) If the disease has occurred in a family, the risk of recurrence in first degree relatives of the proband is about 1 in 20-40.

19. Molecular diagnosis of genetic diseases

i) Genotype/phenotype correlation for genetic diseases is straight forward.

ii) Genotype/phenotype correlation and confirmation of diagnosis should be based on mutation analysis and not linkage analysis.

iii) Molecular diagnosis can be used for heterozygote detection.

iv) Molecular diagnosis may be used for presymptomatic diagnosis.

v) Molecular techniques have been used for prenatal diagnosis.

20. Family history in genetic disorders

i) First obtain information on the index case (proband).

ii) First degree relatives include, parents, siblings and offspring of the proband.

iii) Enquiring about more distant relatives is more relevant in autosomal recessive disorders.

iv) Consanguinity is also of special interest in autosomal recessive disorders.

v) Ethnic origin of family members may also be relevant in establishing diagnosis.

21. Genetic diseases in certain ethnic groups

i) β-Thalassemia in Mediterranean populations.

ii) Sickle cell disease in populations of African descent.

iii) Cytic fibrosis in Scandinavians.

iv) Porphyria variegata in South African Whites.

v) Familial hypercholesterolemia in Lebanese.

22. Genetic heterogeneity

i) Allelic mutations (at a single locus) can produce dominant and recessive variations.

ii) Genetic heterogeneity in a disease can also result from mutations at different genetic loci.

iii) Most genetic diseases are genetically homogeneous.

iv) Compound heterozygotes have two different mutant alleles at a locus.

v) SC hemoglobinopathy is an example of compound heterozygous state.

23. Dominant/recessive genetic diseases

i) Null mutations in tolerant systems produce recessive phenotypes.

ii) Null mutations in less tolerant systems produce dominant phenotypes.

iii) New mutations is germ cells of a person are quite common but have no relevance to the person himself.

iv) Sibs of a person with a new germ cell mutation may be normal since only a few germ cells may be affected.

v) All lethal recessive disorders are rare.

24. Phenotypes of heterozygotes

i) Heterozygotes for α_1- antitrypsin deficiency (a recessive disorder) are predisposed to pulmonary disease.

ii) Heterozygotes for telangiectasia (a recessive disorder) are at increased risk of malignancy.

iii) Heterozygotes for homocytinuria (a recessive disorder), have risk for vascular disease.

iv) In heterozygotes of dominant traits phenotype is indistinguishable from those of homozygotes.

v) Heterozygotes of sickle cell anemia (a recessive disorder), are resistant to malaria and have subtle abnormality in urine concentration ability.

25. Mitochondrial inheritance

i) Mitochondrial DNA is maternally inherited; an egg containing 200,000 to 300,000 copies, and contribution from sperm is insignificant.

ii) The mutant DNA is present in all copies of mitochondrial DNA, present in the cell.

iii) Woman transmits the trait to all her children.

iv) Man will not transmit the trait to any of his children.

v) Myoclonic epilepsy and several forms of mitochondrial myopathy and Leber's hereditary optic neuropathy are some of the diseases caused by mutations in mitochondrial DNA.

26. Coagulation disorders

i) Hemophilia A and hemophilia B are X-linked recessive disorders.

ii) In hemophilia, prothrombin time (PT) is prolonged while partial thromboplastin time is normal.

iii) PT assesses the intrinsic clotting pathway.

iv) Liver immaturity in a neonate prolongs PT and PTT.

v) Thrombocytopenia, prolonged PT, PTT and thrombin time, low fibrinogen and increased fibrin degradation products (FDPs) occur in disseminated intravenous coagulation (DIC).

vi) In DIC blood film shows hemolysis along with presence of fragmented and distorted red cells.

27. Allele-specific PCR product

i) Method used for PCR of normal gene will also form the PCR product for the mutant gene.

ii) The PCR product may be digested with a restriction enzyme and the fragments analyzed.

iii) The PCR product may be hybridized with allele specific oligonucleotide probe.

iv) PCR product may be allowed to express, invitro, to study presence of truncated protein product.

iv) The protein truncation test can be used to detect any mutation that results in premature termination of the peptide chain during protein synthesis.

28. Mutation analysis

i) Large mutations include expansion of triplet repeats, deletions, insertions and other rearrangements.

ii) Large mutations are easily detected using Southern blotting or PCR.

iii) A large mutation may reduce level of m-RNA.

iv) If two alleles of heterozygous DNA are subjected to RT-PCR (reverse transcriptase-PCR), the ratio of the m-RNA's from the two alleles may help to detect a mutation which tends to reduce the level of m-RNA.

v) The only method available for detection of point mutation is by using hybridization with an ASO probe.

29. PCR

i) It is an, invitro, method used to amplify a selected nucleic acid sequence.

ii) The method can be used for detection of presence of given DNA (virus, bacteria) in a given DNA test sample.

iii) PCR based approaches may help early detection of cancer.

iv) The PCR procedure is highly sensitive and totally problem free.

v) Other less commonly studied amplification techniques include the ligase chain reaction and the isothermal target amplification methods.

30. DNA-chips

i) A large number of oligonucleotides of known sequences are arranged on a solid miniature support.

ii) In total 65,536 combinations are possible for an octamer.

iii) DNA to be analyzed is amplified and fluorescent labeled.

iv) After hybridization, an optical system is used to detect hybridization.

v) The only use of the method can be to detect mutations 3 to 4 nucleotide long.

ANSWERS

1. No.(iii). Elevated blood pressure developing after 20th week of gestation is called pregnancy induced; if it is observed earlier, it is characterized as chronic hypertension.

2. No.(v). 30% or more of women with gestational diabetes develop diabetes mellitus within next 5 years.

3. No.(vi). The main fetal thyroid hormone is T_4 which is largely changed into rT_3.

4. No.(iv). Both can present with or without goitre.

5. No.(ii). The neonatal disease is rarely severe.

6. No.(iii). There is no association with any specific congenital anomaly. There is increased risk for infertility before pregnancy and certain complications during pregnancy (spontaneous abortion, abruptio placentae, premature rupture of

membranes). There is increased risk of SIDS (sudden infant death syndrome) and malignancy, in later life of such children.

7. No.(v). Such children are born SGA and do not develop RDS but have a higher incidence of congenital anomalies.

8. No.(i). Jaundice in first 24 hours after birth is not physiological.

9. No.(iii). In breast milk jaundice there is increase in the level of unconjugated bilirubin.

10. No.(iii). If it persists for more than one week or ten days in a full term or more than two weeks in a preterm infant.

11. No.(iii) This hypoglycemia requires a large infusion of glucose to control. Hypoglycemia is without ketosis. Treatment requires total or sub-total pancreatectomy (with removal of about 95% of pancreas). It is a condition with increased number of islets which have excessive number of B-cells. Severe hypoglycemia of this disorder is temporarily, reversed by glucagon.

12. No.(iii). In cases of hyperinsulinemia, insulin level is informative, only, in the presence of hypoglycemia. Thus both insulin and glucose should be estimated.

13. No.(i). This response is unusual in infants. Early features are irritability, tremors, cynotic spells and temperature instability. It is, often, not possible to diagnose hypoglycemia from clinical features as these are non-specific.

14. No.(ii) The disease should have an effective treatment if diagnosed early. For a disease not amenable to treatment, prenatal diagnosis is required.

15. No.(iv). The usual biochemical tests are available only for some inborn errors. Generally it requires DNA analysis.

16. No.(i) One of the parent has the disease.

17. No.(ii). Many X-linked recessive disorders are lethal and thus vertical transmission occurs via female carriers rather than the affected males.

18. No.(v). In contrast to monogenic disorders, in which 25 to 50% of the first degree relatives of the proband are at risk, it is only 5 to 10%, in case of polygenic disorders.

19. No.(i). Prediction of phenotype, future risks and severity of disease are complicated and not straight forward issues.

20. No.(iii). It is important in case of autosomal dominant, X-linked and chromosomal translocations.

21. No.(iii). In Europeans. In Scandanavians there is increased frequency of α_1-antitrypsin deficiency and LCAT deficiency.

22. No.(iii). Most genetic diseases are genetically heterogeneous.

23. No.(v). Not all lethal recessive disorders are rare. Lethal disorders like cystic fibrosis, thalassemia, and sickle cell anemia are common. Generally, autosomal recessive disorders are rare because of reduced fitness of homozygotes. In the above mentioned disorders although the homozygous states are lethal the heterozygous states have biological benefits.

24. No.(iv). In case of null mutations the disease of homozygous state is more severe than that of heterozygous state. In mutations other than null mutations, the phenotypes (of heterozygotes) are because of special properties of the mutant gene products. A mutation may produce a protein which interferes in function of the normal protein (negative mutation). In amyloidosis the mutant gene product has a novel function of abnormal protein folding (leading to extracellular deposition), producing the disease.

25. No.(ii). Mutant DNA is present as a proportion of total mitochondrial DNA per cell. This heterogeneity of mitochondrial DNA in a cell is called heteroplasmy.

26. No.(iii). PT assesses extrinsic clotting pathway (factors II, V, VII and X). This is not markedly affected by heparin. PTT assesses intrinsic pathway (most factors except VII and XII). This is the most sensitive test of coagulation disturbances and is prolonged by heparin. Thrombin time assesses fibrinogen activity and requires calcium for activation.

27. No.(i). Using particular oligonucleotide primers the mutant gene may not yield PCR product. This may be used for its detection.

28. No.(v). Other methods include, denaturing gel electrophoresis, (the mutant is slower in gel because of increased tendency for the mutant to get denatured), carbodiimide modification (carbodiimide conjugates at the unpaired bases in the mutant and reduces its movement in gel), ribonuclease cleavage (RNase cleaves strand at the mutant site), and others.

29. No.(iv). Due to high sensitivity of the method, either exogenous or previously amplified DNA can cause interference. Extreme precautions are required to avoid these contaminations and that has prevented many laboratories in adapting PCR technique for routine use in diagnosis.

30. No.(v). Through alignment of overlapping sequences large sequences can be analyzed/detected.

Appendix A

Drugs causing positive Benedict's test with urine

- Acetylsalicylic acid, vitamin C, cinchophen, nitrofurantoin, PAS, streptomycin, sulfonamides, chloral hydrate, cephaloridine, cephalothin. Degraded tetracycline may cause renal damage and renal glycosuria.

Drugs modifying urinary calcium

- Sodium phytate and thiazides reduce urine calcium while corticosteroids, androgens, anabolic steroids, dihydrotachysterol, vitamin D, viomycin increase urine calcium.

Drugs causing positive test for hematuria or hemoglobinuria

- Amphotericin B and bacitracin produce nephrotoxicity; phenylbutazone, indomethacin and coumarin may cause actual bleeding and acetylsalicylic acid, acetophenetidin and acetanilid produce hemolysis.

Drugs causing increased blood glucose/ impaired tolerance

- Oral contraceptives, glucocorticoids, progestins, thyroid hormone, GH.
- Diuretics and antihypertensive drugs (thiazides, chlorthalidone, clonidine, furosemide).
- Phenothiazines, phenytoin, tricyclics, lithium and haloperidol).
- Anti-inflammatory drugs like indomethacin; isoniazid, heparin, cimetidine, nicotinic acid; adrenergic agonists.

Drugs producing hypoglycemia

- Alcohol, propranolol, salicylates (Impair glucose formation), quinine, disopyramide, pentamidine, insulin, octreotide, oral hypoglycemics.

Drugs affecting serum calcium level

- Loop diuretics and anticonvulsant drugs (phenobarbital, phenytoin) in long term therapy, lower serum calcium level.
- Vitamin D, vitamin A, thyroid hormone, androgens, progestins, estrogens, and lithium elevate serum calcium level.

Drugs increasing serum uric acid

- Cytotoxic drugs; drugs which reduce renal clearance (diuretics); nephrotoxic drugs (mitomycin C); drugs interfering in the method (vitamin C, L-dopa, methyldopa).

Drugs that may increase serum creatinine

- Acetohexamide, cephalosporins, cimetidine and trimethoprim by acting at renal tubular level.
- Vitamin C and L-dopa by interfering in the method.

Drugs increasing serum triglycerides

- Thiazide diuretics, oral contraceptives, amiodarone, β-blockers, corticosteroids, interferones, cholestyramine.

Drugs that increase serum cholesterol

- Drugs producing cholestasis (androgens, anabolic steroids, thiazides, sulfonamides, promazines, chlorpropamide, cinchophen). Other drugs include corticosteroids, oral contraceptives, amiodarone and long term therapy of L-dopa.

Drugs that lower serum cholesterol

- Drugs include androgens, clomiphene, phenformin, chlorpropamide (inhibit synthesis), oral estrogens, azathioprine and certain drugs acting through their hepatotoxic effect (tetracyclines, erythromycin, isoniazid, MAO inhibitors and allopurinol).

Drugs which increase serum potassium

• ACE inhibitors, amiloride, digitalis overdose, lithium, spironolactone, potassium salts of drugs, nonsteroid anti-inflamatory drugs, succinylcholine, triamterene, trimethoprin antineoplastic agents and drugs causing renal toxicity (amphotericin B, methicillin, tetracycline).

Drugs which decrease serum potassium

• Amphotericin B, carbenoxolone, corticosteroids, diuretics (ethacrynic acid, furosemide, thiazides), gentamicin, chronic laxative abuse, licorice, corticosteroids especially mineralocorticoids, insulin, alkali induced alkalosis, sympathomimetic agents and theophylline.

Drugs producing hyponatremia

• Salt wasting by diuretics and enemas. Other drugs are antipsychotics, carbamazepine, chlorpropamide, desmopressin, vincristine, octreotide, cyclophosphamide.

Drugs causing hypernatremia

• Corticosteroids, guanethidine, phenylbutazone (retain salt and water), mannitol (loses more water than salt), clonidine, methoxyflurane, tetracycline and inappropriate fluid administration.

Drugs producing metabolic acidosis

• Metformin, phenformin, salicylates and spironolactone; acetazolamide, amphotericin B and outdated terracycline may cause RTA.

Drugs interfering in management of porphyrias

• May exacerbate the disorder: barbiturates, sulfonamides, metphentoin, succinimide, carbamazepine, valproic acid, meprobamate, glutethimide, oral contraceptives, alcohol.
• May interfere in diagnosis (tetracycline, ethoxazene, phenazopyridine, sulfamethoxazole).

Drugs increase or decrease plasma serum renin activity (PRA)

• Diazoxide, furosemide, hydralazine, spironolactone, estrogens, minoxidil, thiazides, saralasin, guanethidine increase PRA.
• Clonidine, propranolol, reserpine reduce PRA.

Drugs increasing ADH secretion

• Chlorpropamide, vincristine, vinblastine, carba-

mazepine, general anesthetics, narcotics, tricyclic antidepresants, cyclophosphamide, oxytocin.

Drugs producing euthyroid hyperthyroxemia

(FT$_4$, or FT$_4$I($\uparrow$), T3 ($\downarrow$)/N and TSH is variable).
• Drugs which block T$_4$($\rightarrow$)T$_3$ and produce (FT$_4$ ($\uparrow$), FT$_4$I($\uparrow$), T$_3$($\downarrow$), TSH($\uparrow$).
Propranolol, propyl thiouracil, dexamethasone, amiodarone, radiographic contrast media.
• Drugs which increase T$_4$ binding and produce T$_4$($\uparrow$), FT$_4$N, T$_3$N, TSH N- Oral contraceptives pherphenazine, estrogen therapy.

Drugs which cause abnormal thyroid function

• Acetazolamide, chlorpropamide, clofibrate, colestipol and nicotinic acid, dimercaprol, iodides, lithium, phenindione, phenytoin, phenothiazines (long term use), tolbutamide, sulfonamides, oral contraceptives, amiodarone and phenylbutazone.

Drugs interfering in estimations of catecholamines, metanephrines and VMA.

• Exogenous catecholamines, sympathomimetic amines and certain related drugs like β-blockers (propranolaol), drugs used in treatment of hypertension (methyldopa, clonidine, calcium channel blockers, guanethidine) and drugs used for treatment of Parkinson's disease (levodopa, carbidopa) affect plasma levels of catecholamines and urinary excretions of catecholamines and metanephrines. Excretion of VMA is much less affected.
• Carbidopa (an aromatic aminoacid decarboxylase inhibitor) increases excretion of VMA and excretion is reduced by MAO inhibitors (which increase excretion of metanephrines).
• Certain drugs like propranolol, phenothiazines, imipramine (tricyclic antidepressant), methyl glucamine (in radiographic contrast media), tetracyclines, erythromycin and ampicillin may produce interference in certain methods. Such an interference needs to be notified by the laboratory itself.

Drugs increasing prolactin levels

• Drugs which block dopamine receptors include antipsychotics, phenothiazines (chlorpromazine, thioridazine), haloperidol, sulpiride and antiemetics (metoclopramide, butyrophenone).
• Dopamine depleting agents (alpha-methyldopa, reserpine).
• Estrogens and oral contraceptives. Other drugs are opiates, isoniazid, verapamil, amphetamine.

Drug induced hypothyroidism

• Lithium carbonate, amino salicylic acid, phenylbutazone, iodoantipyrine, iodides.

Drugs causing hyperbilirubinemia

- Novobiocin, rifampin: drugs producing cholestatic hepatitis include, phenothiazines, chlorpropamide, nitrofurantoin, methimazole, erythromycin estolate, cyclosporine, anabolic steroids, acetonexamide.

Drugs causing renal dysfunction

- ACE inhibitors, cyclosporine, NSAIDs, pentamidine, triameterene: drugs producing nephrotic syndrome include, captopril, ketoprofen, pencillamine, probenecid, phenindione.

Drug induced gynecomastia

Drugs increasing estrogen activity
- Oral contraceptives, digitalis, estrogen containing cosmetics, estrogen containing foods
- Clomiphene (increases estrogen secretion).

Drugs inhibiting formation/action of testosterone
- Ketoconazole, metronidazole, cisplatin, alkylating agents, spironolactone, cimetidine, flutamide, etomidate

Produce gynecomastia by some unknown action
- Isoniazid, methyldopa, tricyclic antidepressants, diazepam, omeprazole, calcium channel blockers, angiotensin coverting enzyme inhibitors, busulfan, penicillamine, heroin, marijuana.

Drugs have potential of fetal toxicity

- Antineoplastics, antithyroid durgs, benzodiazepines, coumarin anticoagulants, lithium, immunosuppressants.

Teratogens

- Thalidomide, coumarin derivatives, hydantoin, valproic acid, trimethadione, tetracycline, isotretinoin, lithium, androgenic hormones, synthetic estrogen DES.

Information in Appendix A is meant to produce awareness in the minds of clinicians and laboratory people about an important factor (drug interference in interpretation of test results) which could disturb the expected changes in test results in different disease. It is in no way a complete list and it should not be presumed that a drug not included in the list cannot produce drug induced change in a particular test result.

Appendix B

> - Values in brackets are in SI units (mmol/L = mg/dL × 10/mol.wt.)
> - 1 mg = 10^3 µg (micro) = 10^6 ng (nano) = 10^9 pg (pico)
> - Along with normal values, at places, useful key points are mentioned which are important in different diagnostic issues.

Bilirubin: conventional units (SI units)

Adult 0.1-1.2 mg/dL (2-21 µmol/L) out of which <0.3 mg/dL is direct: Newborn 1.0-12 mg/dL: Jaundice appears at about 2.5 mg/dL of serum bilirubin

- In case of hemolytic jaundice or ineffective erythropoiesis, Gilbert's and Crigler-Najjar, <20% of bilirubin is direct; 20-40% is suggestive of hepatic jaundice and >50% of post hepatic jaundice.
- Three important causes of neonatal hyperbilirubinemia (nonphysiological) are haemolytic disease, hepatitis and exaggerated enterohepatic circulation of bilirubin
- Neonatal hypothyroidism is associated with excessive and prolonged hyperbilirubinemia (unconjugated bilirubin) in about 10% of jaundiced newborns.

Alkaline phosphatase (ALP serum)

ALP (p-nitrophenyl phosphate in AMP buffer) 20-130 U/L at 37°C (20-130 U/L). 40-300 U/L in a neonate.

- Biliary obstruction is best indicated by elevated ALP (often 5 times the normal value). However, it does not differentiate between intrahepatic and extrahepatic obstruction.
- ALP, 5′-nucleotidase and γ-GT are elevated in biliary obstruction, only ALP is elevated in bone disease and pregnancy.
- Increased bilirubin with normal ALP suggests constitutional hyperbilirubinemia (Gilbert's, Crigler-Najjar) or hemolysis.

ALT, AST, γ-GT, LDH

ALT 4-36 U/L at 37°C (4-36 U/L); AST 8-33 U/L at 37°C (8-33 U/L); γ-GT 5-40 IU/L (5-40 U/L at 37°C); LDH (lactate to pyruvate at 37°C) 100-190 U/L (100-190 U/L).

- Normal AST, ALT with elevated ALP and LD suggest obstruction in one hepatic duct, metastatic or infiltrative liver disease.
- γ-GT is also used to establish hepatic origin of elevated ALP.

Creatinine kinase (serum)

Total 55-170 U/L at 37°C (55-170 U/L at 37°C) in male; 30-135 U/L at 37°C in female: 3 × adult level in a new born; adult level reached in 1 year.

Albumin (serum)

By the dye binding method: 3.8-5.0 g/dL (38-50 g/L).

Ammonia (Blood)

Enzymatic method 40-80 µg/dL (23-47 µmol/L).

PT (Prothrombin time)

One stage: ±2 second of control (control should be 11-16 seconds).

Ceruloplasmin

1-9 years 24-40 mg/dL and reduced to adult level at 14-19 years: 14-34 mg/dL (140-340 mg/L). In Wilson' disease level is <20 mg/dL and there is increased hepatic copper.

Alpha-fetoprotein (serum)

Adult <30 ng/mL (<30 µg/L)

- Alpha fetoprotein is used for screening for hepatoma in patients of chronic active hepatitis or cirrhosis positive for HbsAg and certain high risk groups (Chinese,

Eskimos). Can be used to differentiate neonatal hepatitis from neonatal biliary atresia. Can be used for fetal defects (Chapter 18). In case of primary cancer of liver, after surgery, the level should return to normal, if not, resection might be incomplete or metastases might be there.

- Diagnosis of hepatic encephalopathy is clinical, the laboratory findings are supportive; blood ammonia is increased in 90% of patients but does not reflect degree of coma; other laboratory findings due to hepatic failure are progressively increasing bilirubin, elevated AST, ALT (which may abruptly decrease), low blood glucose, low albumin (especially if course of illness had been prolonged, rapidly prolonging PT (the test with great prognostic value), and variable ALP.
- Metabolic complications of fulminant hepatic failure arise from renal failure, pancreatitis, and other changes. Hypokalemia, hypocalcemia, hypomagnesemia, acid base disturbances and other changes need monitoring with creatinine, BUN, sodium, potassium, pCO_2, calcium, magnesium, glucose and PT(also platelet count and other peripheral blood counts).
- In a newborn AST 16-74 U/L, γ-GT 10-103 U/L, LDH upto 2 × adult level.

❑

Amylase (serum) (adult level, 1 year after birth)

16-120 Somogyi units/dL (30-220 U/L): Urine amylase: 35-260 Somogyi units/h: Amylase -creatinine ratio: $(Cl_{am}/Cl_{cr}) \times 100 = 1\text{-}5\%$.

Lipase(serum)

14-280 mIU/mL (14-280 U/L).
- The main use of estimation of these enzymes lies in diagnosis of acute pancreatitis. The enzyme levels may also be helpful in diagnosis of acute exacerbation of chronic pancreatitis.
- Magnitude of high levels of amylase and the rate of fall do not correlate with severity of disease, its prognosis or rate of resolution.
- Increase of amylase for >8-10 days is suggestive of associated cancer, pseudocyst, pancreatic ascites or non-pancreatic etiology.

❑

Malabsorption

- Laboratory evidence of malabsorption is obtained from low plasma levels of carotene; iron and albumin and raised ESR, besides, history of weight loss, diet and drug intake is also important. Stool weight is >300g/24h.
- Clinical or laboratory evidence of vitamin K (pro-

thrombin time) and B_{12}/folate deficiences and hyperthroidism needs to be obtained.
- If laboratory evidence of steatorrhea is absent, lactase deficiency (less commnly other carbohydrate malabsorption defects) should be investigated.
- In the presence of evidence of steatorrhea, cause is commonly chronic pancreatitis or small bowel disease.

Fecal fat test

Collect 3d stool sample after 60-100g fat intake/d. Normally <6-7g fat/d is excreted (<5g/d with intake of 50g fat/d). It is best test to establish presence of steatorrhea. A new born excretes about 20% of ingested fat.

Xylose excretion test

25g D-xylose in water is ingested; urinary excretion in next 5h or blood level after 2h is determined. Normally 16-23% of the ingested dose is excreted in next 5h; blood level at 2h is 30-52 mg/dL. In infants and children only 5g dose is used and 1h blood xylose level (normally) is ≥15 mg/dL in infants and ≥20 mg/dL in children ≤ 9 years of age.
- The test has 90% accuracy in differentiating chronic pancreatitis (test is normal) from intestinal mucosal disease and intestinal bacterial overgrowth (test is abnormal)
- Test also result in low values in renal disease, delayed gastric emptying, myxedema and the elderly (false positive test).

Serum trypsinogen (RIA)

10-75 ng/mL.
- In about 80% of patients of severe chronic pancreatic insufficiency (with steatorrhea) and 15-20% of those with mild to moderate disease serum trypsinogen level is <10 ng/mL; in non-pancreatic causes level remain normal.

The bentiromide test

500g of bentiromide is ingested after an overnight fast; chymotrypsin releases PABA and more than 50% of the dose is excreted in next 6h in urine in normal individuals.
- Along with D-xylose excretion test, this test is used to differentiate pancreatic exocrine insufficiency from intestinal mucosal disease. Renal insufficiency and delayed gastric emptying, however affect the results.

Secretin-cholecystokinin (CCK) test

Secretin is 27 aminoacid peptide and acts mainly on ductal cells while CCK-Pz acts on acinar cells. Addition of CCK-Pz to secretin gives extra secretion of enzymes. In chronic pancreatitis volume, bicarbonate and amylase levels of duodenal juice are reduced, more so after stimulation. In this test three above mentioned parameters are studied after I/V adminstration of CCK. As rates of secretions give better discrimination between normals and patients of chronic pancreatitis, duodenal juice is aspirated continuously (avoiding mixing of gastric juice) and timed samples are obtained. Wide variations are found in results of different laboratories and therefore it is best to compare patient's results with normal values obtained for the laboratory.

- In chronic pancreatitis maximal HCO_3^- concentration is reduced early than that of enzymes. Reverse is true in early carcinoma.
- The test is going out of favour because of difficulties in collection of accurate duodenal juice sample

Lactose intolerance test

After intake (oral) of 50-100g of lactose, blood samples are collected at 15,30,60 and 90 min. In normal individuals peak rise of reducing substances expressed as glucose level, is more than 24 mg/dL. In lactase deficiency cases increase is less than 20 mg/dL over the fasting level. The abnormal test is followed by a similar test in which equivalent amounts of monosaccharides are used (instead of say 50g of lactose, 25g of galactose and 25g of glucose). This will differentiate lactase deficiency from monosaccharide absorption defect and general mucosal absorption defect.

- Alternatively, in hydrogen breath test H_2 exhaled at 2h after ingestion of 50g of lactose in fasting state is found out.
- The lactose tolerance test may become abnormal because of delayed gastic emptying or reduced small bowel transit.
- In this test stool examination can also help in proper interpretation of the test. Typically the stool, in lactase deficiency, is frothy, with low pH (4.5-6.0) high osmolality and positive for presence of reducing substances.

The sweat test

Normal level of Cl⁻ in sweat, collected after pilocarpine stimulation is 8-43 mEq/L in children.

- In children chloride level of 60 mEq/L or higher is considered as a positive test; 40-60 mEq/L as borderline (needing further investigatin) and <40 mEq/L as normal. Upto 80 mEq/L may be normal for adults.
- As test cannot be easily performed, the abnormal results must be obtained in repeated (at least twice) tests, for firm diagnosis.
- Immunreactive trypsin is reduced in about 90% infants of cystic fibrosis.
- Reduced trypsin in stools is also used to screen infants for cystic fibrosis. This test is useful upto age of 4 years.
- The bentiromide test can be used to show reduced chymotrypsin production

- Biochemical evidence of hypochloremic alkalosis, hypokalemia, impaired glucose tolerance, malabsorption and chronic lung disease may be there, as well as evidence of aspermia.

Gastric acid

Normal, basal <2 to 5 mEq/h. After stimulation with histamine 5-20 mEq/h; ratio of basal to post-stimulation; normally 20% increase over basal occurs after stimulation.

Basal secretion may be >5 mEq/h in duodenal ulcer (not in all cases); >20 mEq/h in ZE syndrome and nil in achlorhydria, gastritis and gastric carinoma.

- Ratio of basal to post stimulation may be increased (20 to 40%) in duodenal ulcer and still more in (>40 to 60%) in ZE syndrome and some cases of duodenal ulcer.

Serum gastrin

Normal and duodenal ulcer 0-≤200 pg/mL; no change occurs after infusion of secretin (2 units/kg body weight). In ZE syndrome basal level is elevated and further increases after secretin infusion.

Serum sodium

Normal level 136-145 mEq/L (136-145 mmol/L)
- Levels requiring prompt treatment <120 mEq/L: >160 mEq/L
- Spurious hyponatremia is caused by hyperlipidemia and hyperproteinemia (if flame photometric levels are used: since the aqueous phase is less than the sample volume); also in the presence of increased plasma osmolality (water is drawn from the cells).
- Depletion of body sodium is indicated by urine sodium <10 mEq/L; increased urinary loss of sodium (>20 mEq/L) is caused by reduced excretion of water (SIADH) or reduced sodium reabsorption (increased salt loss) by low aldosterone level or effectivity.

Serum potassium

Normal level 3.5-5.0 mEq/L (3.5-5.0 mmol/L): levels requiring prompt treatment <2.5: >6.5 in adults, >8.0 in infants.

- Serum, potassium levels are important during management of diabetic coma, renal failure, diuretic therapy and severe water and electrolyte abnormalities; also in diagnosis of hypokalemic and hyperkalemic periodic paralysis.
- Hyperkalemia is a medical emergency and two most important causes are renal failure and diabetic ketoacidosis, after ruling out hemolysis, trauma, iatrogenic and pseudohyperkalemia.

Osmolality

Normal serum osmolality, 280-295 mOsmol/kg.
- See urine osmolality in Part III.
- Used in diagnosis of nonketotic hyperlgycemic coma, in water electrolyte disturbances, in evaluation of hyponatremia and state of hydration (urine and plasma osmolality changes are more useful than changes in hematocrit, serum protein and BUN).
- Osmolal gap is the difference between the measured and the calculated values:
- Calculated serum osmolality in mOsmol/L = (1.86 × serum Na) + Serum glucose/18 + BUN/2.8 (all values in the conventional units).
- Osmolal gap may be used in estimation of blood alcohol: Blood alcohol (mg/dL) = osmolal gap × 100/22 (every 100 mg/dL of alcohol in serum increases osmolality by 22 mOsmol/kg).

Acid-base parameters

Normal pH 7.4; range pH 7.38-7.44: levels beyond which urgent treatment is needed pH <7.2 and >7.6; Venous blood pH 7.36-7.41 (For H^+ concentration unit is mEq/L and SI unit is nmol/L).

pCO_2 adults 32-48 mmHg, infants 27-41 mmHg. Urgent management is needed when pCO_2 <20 mmHg, >70 mmHg; Bicarbonate adults 21-29 mEq/L (21-29 mmol/L); at 1-2 year 17-25 mEq/L gradually increase to adult levels at about 8 years in males and at about 10 years in females.

pO_2 while breathing room air in children/adults >85 mmHg, newborns 60-75 mmHg; after 60 years gradually decreases to >50 mmHg at 90 years; Urgent treatment is need at pO_2 <40 mmHg; Normal oxygen saturation is 96-100% of capacity.
- For gas tensions concentional units (mmHg) are multiplied by 0.133 to SI units (Kpa).
- Clinical data of the patient must be available for proper interpretation of blood gases, pH and electrolytes.
- Acid-base disorders in actual practice are more often mixed than simple.
- In severe metabolic acidosis respiratory compensation can not bring pCO_2 <20 mmHg (H^+ oppose hyperventilation); in metabolic alkalosis respiratory compensation cannot raise pCO_2 >60 mmHg (retained CO_2 stimulates breathing).
- Respiratory acidosis is associated with pCO_2 of >45 mmHg and respiratory alkalosis with pCO_2 of <35 mmHg.

❑

Glucose

Fasting blood glucose 60-100 mg/dL (3.3-5.6 mmol/L); plasma/serum glucose 70-110 mg/dL; if estimation is delayed beyond 1h, add sodium fluoride 3 mg/dL. In new borns: (serum, mg/dL) 20-110, preterm 20-66.

Critical levels (serum) <40 mg/dL and >450 mg/dL. In infants (at 72h $\leq$30 mg/dL, at >72h <40 mg/dL and in premature <20 mg/dL. In new born level >300 mg/dL is also critical. However, recently the above mentioned low levels in infants have been challenged as too low. In a preterm, brain function may get compromised below 47 mg/dL.
- Three important uses of serum glucose level measurement are in diagnosis of diabetes mellitus, monitoring of treatment of diabetes and diagnosis of hypoglycemia.
- In infant blood glucose level should be estimated by a specific method, non-glucose reducing agents concentration may be upto 60 mg/dL.
- Plasma glucose values are 14% higher than whole blood.
- At room temperature blood glucose decreases by 7 mg/dL per hour.

Serum cholesterol

Desirable level <200, moderate risk 200-239 and higher risk $\geq$ 240 mg/dL; In children and adolescents with family history of premature cardiovascular disease or at least one parent with high cholesterol, the levels (mg/dL) are: acceptable total cholesterol (C) <170, LDL-C <110; borderline (needing repeat measurement) C 170-199, LDL-C 110-129; high C $\geq$200, LDL-C >130.
- Desirable, with moderate risk and with higher risk for CAD, respectively, ratio of LDL-C, HDL-C is 0.5-3.0, 3.0-6.0 and >6.0:
- These lipid studies are used as markers of risk for CAD for primary and secondary hyperlipidemias and for monitoring treatment of hyperlipidemias.
- Risk for CAD may be defined, in terms of total-C, HDL-C ratio, as follow: 3.3-4.4 low risk 4.4-7.1 average risk, 7.1-11.0 moderate risk and >11.0 high risk. More useful is HDL-C/(total-C minus HDL-C) ratio: <0.2 is atherogenic (>0.25 is desirable): For other values see Chapter 9.
- Positive risk factors for CAD include male gender, $\geq$55 years of age, premature menopause, family history of premature CAD (CAD in a parent or grand parent before 55 years of age), smoking, hypertension, diabetes mellitus and HDL-C <35 mg/dL.

Serum triglycerides (80% in VLDL, 15% in LDL)

Normal <200 mg/dL, desirable <165 mg/dL (<1.9 mmol/L); levels in serum are higher than plasma by 5%.
- Sample should be taken after 12h fast
- Levels vary during the day, lowest in the morning and highest at mid day.
- Analytical variations 5-10% and intra individual variation 12-40%

- Levels >500 mg/dL are associated with risk of pancreatitis and need treatment
- TAG: C ratio in different hyper lipoproteinemias is as under: about 8 in lipoprotein lipase deficiency (rare): about 1 familial hypercholesterolemia (common) <2 in familial dysbetalipoproteinemia (uncommon) 1-5 in familial hypertriglyceridemia (most common); variable in familial combined hyperlipidemia (common)
- Triglycerides level in the range 250-500 are associated with peripheral vascular disease and may be markers for patients with genetic forms of hyperlipoproteinemias and in this range, particularly, TAG levels are inversely related to HDL-C.
- Level <250 mg/dL has no disease association.

Uric Acid (serum)

4.0-8.5 mg/dL (0.24-0.51 mmol/L) in males and 2.7-7.3 in females. In females, levels approach those in males after menopause.
- There are day to day and several other variations
- Level is increased by stress, fasting and increased body weight
- It is used in diagnosis of gout and in monitoring treatment of gout and of neoplasms treated with chemotherapy.
- About 10% of normal adult males have elevated serum uric acid levels
- In toxemia of pregnancy serum uric acid levels are used to monitor therapeutic response to treatment.
- Hyperuricemia occurs in 25-35% of untreated hypertensive patients; incidence increase to 65-75% with use of oral diuretics (benzothiazides) in these hypertensives. Also 80% patients with elevated serum TAG have hperuricemia.

Serum Iron

In case of infant 40-100 µg/dL, increases to 50-150µg/dL (9-27 µmol/L) in an adult

Transferrin

Serum transferrin may be measured as total iron binding capacity (1µmol of transferrin corresponds to 2 µmol of iron). Normal TIBC 250-370 µg/dL (45-66 µmol/L). A TIBC of 60 µmol/L corresponds to 2.43 g/L of transferrin (in terms of protein concentration) assuming a mol. wt. of 81000 for transferrin. Its normal level is 240-480 mg/dL. As for TIBC, transferrin protein concentration can also be used for differential diagnosis of anemias. It is increased in pregnancy and reduced in conditions of protein dificiency (chronic disorders, malnutrition, nephrotic syndrome).

Serum transferrin saturation = (Serum iron/TIBC) × 100. Normal transferrin saturation is 20 to 55% (values below 15% indicate iron deficiency anemia) especially with increased TIBC.

Ferritin

Adult male 15-200 ng/mL (15-200 ug/L). Adult female 12-150 ng/mL (12-150 ug/L). Levels are quite variable in early years of life

Free erythrocyte protoporphyrin (FEP)

Normal level 1-10 µg/dL of packed RBCs (FEP) and 10-38 µg/dL (Zinc protoporphyrin) of packed RBCs. FEP level >100 µg/dL of packed RBCs suggests diagnosis of IDA, ACD, most sideroblastic anemias and lead poisoning.
- Ferritin correlates with total body iron stores and is used in diagnosis of iron deficiency or excess and in monitoring therapy. The transferrin however, is an acute phase protein and therefore, increases in malignancies, infections, inflammatory disorders, alcoholism, liver disorders and hyperthyroidism. In these conditions transferrin levels do not decrease in the coexisting iron deficiency and for iron status bone marrow should be stained for iron.
- Ferritin is also used to differentiate iron deficiency from anemia of chronic disease. In uncomplicated iron deficiency anemia, ferritin is low and normal or high in chronic disorders.
- In IDA with no stainable bone marrow iron, ferritins level is 50-100 µg/L in the presence of inflammation/infection (level will in higher without iron deficiency and lower in pure iron deficiency).
- Ferritin level is also used to detect iron overload conditions.
- Transferrin saturation is used in screening for hemochromatosis and differential diagnosis of anemia.

B$_{12}$ (Serum) and folic acid

B$_{12}$ normal reference range is 200-900 ng/L (150-670 pmol/L); depends on the assay method. Serum folate is 5-21 µg/L (11-48 nmol/L), red cell folate is 150-600 µg/L of red cells.
- Level of 100 pg/mL or less means B$_{12}$ deficiency even without macrocytosis.
- RBC folate is low in many patients of B$_{12}$ deficiency; serum folate serves to differentiate folate plus B$_{12}$ deficiency from B$_{12}$ deficiency alone.
- RBC folate deficiency indicates tissue deficiency as RBC level does not fall till stores are depleted.
- Transcobalamin I (TC I) and II (TC II) are B$_{12}$ binding proteins. Congenital deficiency of TC II causes megaloblastic anemia without affecting serum B$_{12}$ level. Reverse in true about deficiency of TC I.

Haptoglobin

Absent in 90% newborns; gradually increases to 30 mg/dL by 6 months; levels upto adulthood 40-180 mg/dL; adults 40-270 mg/dL
- Genetic absence in 1% individuals
- Helps diagnosis of hemolytic anemia
- It is marker of chronic hemolysis. In hereditary spherocytosis a very low level (<40 mg/dL in the absence of any infection/Inflammation, which increase the level of this acute phase reactant) may be an indication for splenectomy.
- It can also be used to diagnose a transfusion reaction as the level is reduced in the sample collected after transfusion compared to the pretransfusional sample.
- Important tests in hemolytic anemias are increased plasma hemoglobin along with increased urinary excretion of hemoglobin and hemosiderin (intravascular hemolysis), increased reticulocyte count, blood film polychromasia, bone marrow erythroid hyperplasia, and increased plasma unconjugated bilirubin (in both intravascular and extravascular hemolysis)
- If Combs' test is positive, three important conditions to look for are incompatible blood transfusion, acquired autoimmune hemolytic anemia and hemolytic disease of the newborn.

Part II

Calcium (serum)

Total: With the realization that calcium levels are easily increased by sample contamination (dust especially from chalk particles) the new normal range is reported lower than the previous normal range of 9.2-11.0 mg/dL (2.30-2.74 mmol/L); new range is 9.0-10.5 mg/dL in adults. Critical levels <6mg/dL and >14 mg/dL.
- Calcium estimation should be done in a fresh sample as the stored sample may yield artifactual decrease
- Ionized calcium levels are generally not required in clinical setting.
- Hypercalcemia generally becomes symptomatic at or above 11.5-12.0 mg/dL (fatigue, depression, mental confusion anorexia, nausea, reversible renal tubular defects, polyuria, shortened QT interval in ECG); at higher levels soft tissue calcification may occur (depending upon phosphate levels); renal insufficiency may also develop; at 15 mg/dL and higher levels there is medical emergency (coma, cardiac arrest).
- Acute hypocalcemia may be produced with multiple transfusions of citrated blood (reduced ionic calcium) cancer chemotherapy, any serious illness, toxic shock, rhabdomyolysis (rhabdomyolysis producing acute renal failure causes hypercalcemia).

- Neonatal hypocalcemia (early) may be caused by RDS, asphyxia, prematurity, sepsis or if mother had diabetes. Normal levels: neonate 70-120 mg/dL, preterm 60-100 mg/dL.
- Ionized calcium is reduced during hyperventilation, administration of bicarbonate (to control metabolic acidosis), and conditions causing elevated serum fatty acids (diabetic ketoacidosis, sepsis, AMI, acute pancreatitis)and with use of certain drugs (heparin epinephrine, norepinephrine, isoproterenol and alcohol).
- 90% cases of hypercalcemia are due to PHPT, neoplasms and granulomatous disease.

Urinary calcium

On a low calcium diet excretion in 24h urine is <150 mg/d; on diet with average calcium 100-240 mg/d and on diet with high calcium 240-300 mg/d (6.0-7.5 mmol/d).
- Hypercalciuria is calcium excretion of >300 mg/24h in males and >275 mg/24h in females.

Phosphate (serum)

Children 4.0-7.0 mg/dL (1.29-2.26 mmol/L); first week of life 4.6-8.0 mg/dL; Adults 2.3-4.7 mg/dL.
- Sudden intracellular shift of phosphate may produce very low serum levels (about 1 mg/dL), in recovery from diabetic ketoacidosis, alcoholism, rapid refeeding after prolonged starvation and hyperalimentation. Use of phosphate binding antacids also produce quite low serum levels.
- Hyperphosphatemia (>5.5 mg/dL) may be caused by impaired renal function. If renal function is normal, it may be produced by increased phosphate load (urine phosphate >1g/d) because of hemolysis, neoplasms, phosphate enemas and excessive vitamin D intake. *With absent excessive load and normal renal function* the cause may be increased phosphate reabsorption as in PTH deficiency, acromegaly, thyrotoxicosis and sickle cell anemia. In these cases renal excretion will be generally less than 1g/d. High phosphate level in neonates (8 mg/dL) may produce hypocalcemia.

Alkaline phosphate (ALP)

New born (40-300 IU/L at 37°); child 60-270 IU/L; adult 20-130 IU/L (p-nitrophenyl-phosphate in AMP buffer)
- ALP levels are used in diagnosing cause of cholestasis and for its management monitoring; also helpful in bone disorders with increased osteoblastic activity (in osteogenesis imperfecta due to healing fractures; in osteoblastic bone tumors, osteogenic sarcoma and metastatic carcinoma)
- Marked elevation in Paget's disease (rare in our country) or metastatic carcinoma (in bone) from prostate

Serum magnesium (serum)

1.8-3.0 mg/dL (0.74-1.23 mmol/L).
- Disorders of Mg level are common in renal failure, gastrointestinal disorders and alcoholism.
- Mg deficiency may produce hypocalcemia and hypokalemia.
- 90% patients of elevated or low Mg levels are not clinically apparent.
- If hypokalemia and hypocalcemia coexist, correction of hypokalemia may provoke tetany.
- Serum Mg should always be measured in any patient of hypocalcemia since a patient with low Ca as well as Mg does not respond to calcium administration unless magnesium level is corrected.

Parathyroid hormone (intact hormone assay)

11-54 pg/mL (1.2-5.6 pmol/L)
- Level is low in the morning and maximum at about midnight.
- Level is reduced to 1 pmol/L in 95% cases of HHM (humoral hypercalcemia of malignancy).
- In about 4% cases of HHM (cancer breast cases) PTH may not be reduced because of co-existing parathyroid adenoma.
- Differentiation between PHPT (primary hyperparathyroidism) and occult cancer is a common problem in diagnosis of cause of hypercalcemia.
- Daily urinary excretion of <200 mg/24h (in a case of hypercalcemia) makes diagnosis of familial hypocalciuric hypercalcemia likely; in PHPT calcium excretion lies between 250-300 mg/24h and >500 mg/24h supports diagnosis of malignancy.
- In hypercalcemia of familial hypocalciuric hypercalcemia, the inappropriateness of calcium excretion to serum calcium level can be demonstrated by determining calcium-creatinine clearance. In this condition the value is <0.01 (the ratio in PHPT and other hypercalcemic conditions is >0.02). This test is done in a 4h urine sample, collected in a fasting patient.
- Decrease of nephrogenic cAMP excretion within hours after parathyroidectomy is used to judge success of the operation.
- Serum protein electrophoresis may help to rule out sarcoidosis and multiple myeloma as cause of hypercalcemia.
- Consistent, distinct hypercalcemia, even with PTH in the upper part of normal range, is also enough to diagnose PHPT. However, hypercalcemia with normal (not in upper part of normal range), or low PTH level goes against the diagnosis. In essence, both serum PTH and calcium levels should be interpreted together.
- In PHPT serum calcium level may be normal if there is coexisting condition that could reduce serum calcium (malabsorption, nephrotic syndrome) or with intake of high phosphate diet.
- In diagnosis of PHPT serum calcium level should be confirmed repeatedly, in fasting state and after stopping thiazide diuretics, (or any other similar drug which could increase serum calcium).

❑

Prolactin

Adult female, follicular phase < 20 ng/mL (<0.9 nmol/L); Adult male, <15 ng/mL (<0.7 nmol/L); Prolactin level starts increasing from normal (10-25 ng/mL) in second trimester of pregnancy and peaks at term (100-300 ng/mL). In post partum period basal levels are higher than normal which further increase with suckling. In 4-6 months the basal levels normalize and the sukling induced increase also greatly declines
- High doses of estogens cause hyperprolactinemia but it is not seen with oral contraceptives containing low doses of estrogens.
- A number of drugs increase plasma prolactin level but it generally remains below 100 ng/mL. Diseases of hypothalamus or pituitary stalk cause moderate increase in prolactin level (50-100 ng/mL). Other common causes are renal failure, hypothyroidism, cirrhosis and stress. Food and stress cause minimal elevation (<30 ng/mL).
- Large pituitary tumors (not secreting prolactin) cause modest increase in prolactin level (50-100 ng/ml).
- Levels > 150 ng/mL generally indicate a prolactinoma (micro on macro; larger the tumor, higher the level). Some microprolactinomas may produce lower levels (<100 ng/mL) and cause diagnostic problems.
- Antiprolactin antibodies interfere in prolactin estimation in radioimmunoassay methods but not on immunoradiometric assays.

Growth hormone

Fasting level: children <10 ng/mL (<465 pmol/L): adults <5 ng/mL.
- GH estimation helps in finding cause of short stature or retarded growth and to evaluate pituitary function.
- For screening of acromegaly IGF-1 levels are better than GH levels. The latter test is not reliable in women, in uncontrolled diabetes, renal failure or stress, as false elevations may occur.
- In all patients of acromegaly prolactin should be estimated as 40% of adenomas secreting GH also secrete PRL. Similarly in all cases of hyperprolactinemia thyroid functions should be evaluated since about 20% cases of hypothyroidism also show hyperprolactinemia.
- GH deficiency is diagnosed by showing failure of GH

response in atleast two provocative tests. The best provocative test is the one using insulin induced hypoglycemia (blood glucose <40 mg/dL), but carries risk of producing seizures.

- Other provocative tests use oral levodopa, oral clonidine or 1/ V L-arginine. In all those tests GH level of >10 ug/L rules out GH deficiency.
- Obesity, thyroid disorders, other endocrine disorders and drugs may impair the GH response in provocative tests. Response may be normal in partial deficiency cases; normal or increased in GH resistance (Loran's dwarfisin)
- Measurements of levels of IGF-I and IGF BP-3 are used to screen for GH deficiency.
- In GH insensitivity syndrome, GH is not able to generate IGF-1 because of GH receptor deficiency. In such cases GHBP (growth hormone binding protein) which is structurally related to GH receptor is absent from plasma.
- Constitutional delay is often seen in a familial pattern and normal (although late) growth and reproductive function is expected in these cases.
- Generally, endocrine disease is an uncommon cause of impaired growth. Of the endocrine causes hypothyroidism is the commonest and others are hypopituitarism, and increased cortisol secretion.

TSH/T$_4$/T$_3$

TSH
Serum level 0.5-5.0 µU/mL (0.5-5.0 mU/L)

T$_4$
Cord blood 4.6-13 ug/dL (59.2-167 nmol/L); 1-3 days 11.8-23.2 ug/dL, adults 5-12 ug/dL

Free T$_4$
0-4 days 2.2-9.3 ng/dL (28-68 pmol/L) >2 weeks 0.9-2.0 ng/dL

Free T$_4$ index (FT$_4$I)
T$_4$×RT$_3$U = 1.3-4.2 arbitrary units: adjusted FT$_4$I (for TBG binding) = 5-12 arbitrary units). Can be similarly calculated and expressed in SI units. RT$_3$U (resin T$_3$ uptake) is expressed as % (normally 25-35%). RT$_3$U may also be expressed as ratio to normal.

T$_3$
Cord blood 15-75 ng/dL (0.23-1.2 nmol/L); 1-3 days 32-216 ng/dL adults 95-190 ng/dL.

Free T$_3$
0.2-0.52 ng/dL (3-8 pmol/L).

Free T$_3$ index
T$_3$×RT$_3$U = 24-67 arbitrary units (see for free T$_4$ index)

TRH Test

200 µg or 500 µg of TRH is given I/V and TSH is measured at 0, 20 and 60 min. Normal response is an increase to 16-26 mU/L in women and levels dropping to basal level in 2 to 4h. Response is slightly lower in men.

- Response to TRH test suppressed by starvation, renal failure, depression, certain drugs (glucocorticoids) and in old age.
- The TRH stimulation tests is rarely needed with availability of sensitive TSH assay.
- Glucocorticoids reduce TSH secretion. Levels of TSH also reduce in severe illness
- In hyperthyroidism (primary) TSH is suppressed and TSH response to TRH absent; in primary hypothyroidism basal TSH level is elevated and response to TRH is increased.
- In primary hypothyroidism serum TSH, commonly, increases before thyroid hormone level decrease.
- In severe cases of central hypothyroidism, there may be mild elevation of TSH (TSH is biologically inactive but immunologically active). In such cases however, T$_4$ levels are very low and this helps differentiation from subclinical cases of primary hypothyroidism in which elevated TSH is associated with normal or near normal T$_4$ level.

Human chorionic gonadotropin (hCG)

- It is assayed using immunological methods using antibodies against β-subunits and levels are referred as β-hCG. Plasma may also contain free α and β-subunits which can also be measured. Qualitative assay of hCG in urine (with the help of kits) is available for diagnosis of pregnancy. Quantitative determinations by immunoassay methods are used to know about progress of pregnancy and may also aid in diagnosis of threatened abortion and ectopic pregnancy. hCG determinations are also useful in diagnosis of gestational trophoblastic disease (GTD) and Down's syndrome and in evaluation of germ cell tumors. Free β-hCG is present in normal pregnancy (<4% of total hCG) but levels are higher in GTD. Free β-hCG/hCG ratio also correlate with degree of immaturity of trophoblastic cells in GTD (lowest in hydatidiform mole and highest in choriocarcinoma).
- Kits in the past (not estimating β-hCG) gave false positives due to cross reactivity with LH.
- hCG is also a reliable tumor marker in some forms of testicular cancer.

ACTH (Plasma sample: 8 A.M.)

Plasma: 10-50 pg/mL (2.2-11.1 pmol/L). Heparinized sample is collected in plastic syringes and centrifuged in cold in a plastic tube and analyzed without delay.

- Helpful in differentiating pituitary from adrenal causes of adrenal insufficiency. In primary adrenal disease ACTH level is >200 pg/mL with wide variations in morning and evening levels) and <20 pg/mL in pituitary deficiency cases.

- ACTH levels are also markedly elevated in congenital adrenal hyperplasia (common forms)
- Helpful in finding cause of Cushing's syndrome: In adrenal tumor (glucocorticoid secreting) ACTH level is <10 pg/mL, in hypothalamic pituitary dysfunction cases there is modest increase, 20-200 pg/mL (in 50% cases the level lies in the normal range), in cases with ectopic source of ACTH, the levels range from above 200 pg/mL to over 500 pg/mL. In pituitary macroadenomas levels are less than those with ectopic source of ACTH but higher than hypothalamic pituitary dysfunction (however, there is lot of overlap).

Cortisol

Plasma: 5-20 ug/dL (140-552 nmol/L). Collect sample (morning) in cold; separate sample without delay; Free cortisol in urine: 25-95 ug/g creatinine (8-30 umol/mol creatinine) 20-100 µg/d (55-275 nmol/d). At 1-10 years 2-27 µg/d; 17-Hydroxycorticosteroids, 2-10 mg/d (5.5-28 µmol/d); Plasma 11-deoxycortisol <1 µg/dL (<30 nmol/L).

- Collect 24h urine with 8g boric acid
- Single plasma cortisol level has limited utility because of its pulsatile secretion; from this angle level of free cortisol in urine is more useful.
- Stress of acute illness, surgery, trauma increase plasma cortisol level in the range of 40-60 µg/dL. Level may increase to 2-3 times the normal in pregnancy or with use of oral contraceptives because of estrogens. Other conditions in which plasma cortisol increases are severe anxiety, endogenous depression, starvation, alcoholism, chronic renal failure. Urinary free cortisol excretion is not useful in diagnosis of adrenal insufficiency as the method has low sensitivity at low levels. Method is of particular use in differentiating simple obesity from Cushing's

Dexamethasone suppression test

- In the screening overnight test, baseline sample at 6 A.M.; 1 mg dexamethasone orally at 11 PM and serum sample at 8 AM next morning.
- Level <5 µg/dL excludes Cushnig's syndrome; a level of >10 µg/dL is suggestive of Cushnig's in the absence of conditions causing false positive response.
- In the definitive low dose test 0.5 mg dexamethasone is given every 6h for 2 successive days. On second day urinary 17.OHCS or free cortisol, normally should fall to <3 mg/d or <20 µg/d, respectively or plasma cortisol level to less than 5 µg/dL.
- The low dose dexamethasone test may not be useful in diagnosis of Cushing's syndrome in the presence of obesity, chronic alcoholism and severe depression (pseudo Cushing's) or in an acutely ill patient.
- In the high dose dexamethasone test 2 mg dose of dexamethasone is used everey 6h for 2 days. In normals

and hypothalamic-pituitary cases (Cushing's disease) there is fall of 17-OHCS to 50% of baseline (free cortisol to 20%); no suppression in other causes.
- The overnight dexamethasone test is used for initial screening of patients of Cushing's syndrome. In differntiating simple obesity, 24h urine free cortisol may also be helpful (excretion of > 100 µg/d is suggestive of Cushing's syndrome.) The definitive low dose dexamethasone test is used for proper diagnosis. The high dose test further confirms the diagnosis and also helps to arrive at the cause of disorder. Dexamethasone suppression also helps to find cause of androgen excess related disorders of women (see under hirsutism).

The provocative test

- ACTH stimulation test: 0.25 mg cosyntropin ($ACTH_{1-24}$) I/V or I/M; serum cortisol measured at 0, 30 and 60 min; minimum peak level increment of >7 µg/dL in a normal person (peak level >18 µg/dL is clear cut normal response).
- Poor response means lack of adrenal reserve (primary cases) or adrenal atrophy due to poor ACTH levels (secondary cases). However, if in cases of partial deficiency of ACTH (not resulting in adrenal atrophy) response may be normal, such patients are further tests with metyrapone or insulin induced hypoglycemia. Insulin induced hypoglycemia is also used in suspected hypothalamic/pituitary tumors since it can assess both GH and ACTH responsiveness.
- The ACTH stimulation test is not recommended to differentiate between primary and secondary adrenal insufficiency.
- The overnight metyrapone test is used in cases of suspected hypothalamic/pituitary disorders when hypoglycemia carries risk to the patient (Chapter 13). Metyrapone (30 mg/kg body weight) is given orally at midnight and plasma 11-deoxycortisol is measured at 8 AM. Metyrapone stimulation occurs at hypothalamus and normal response is increase of 11 deoxycortisol level to more than 7 µg/dL; cortisol level should be <10 µg/dL to ensure adequate inhibition of 11-β-hydroxylation (reducing cortisol formation). Because of effect on cortisol level, this test is not done in sick patients or where primary adrenal insufficiency cannot be ruled out.
- Metyrapone test discovers partial ACTH deficiency cases but its main use is an a substitute of high dose dexamethasone test to differentiate Cushing's disease from ectopic ACTH cases.

CRH test

- 1 µg/kg CRH is given I/V and blood samples for cortisol/ACTH are collected at 0, 15, 30 and 60 min. Peak increase of cortisol >10 µg/dL occurs normally. ACTH response is exaggerated in primary adrenal failure and absent in hypopituitarism. Delayed response may occur in hypothalamic disorders.

Aldosterone and renin activity

(For all studies, Na intake 100 mmol/d; K intake 60-100 mmol/d; plasma sample, 8 A.M., supine). Plasma aldosterone: <8 ng/dL (<240 pmol/L). Aldosterone (urine/d): 5-19 ug/d (14-53 nmol/d). Plasma renin activity (PRA): 1-2.5 ng/mL/h (1-2.5 ug/L/h). Normal plasma aldosterone/PRA ratio should be <20.

Stimulation and suppression tests for renin-angiotensin system.

After low sodium intake (10 mmol/d) for 3-5 days, aldosterone execretion should increase 2-3 fold over control value. Alternatively, 40-80 mg furosemide followed by 2-3h of upright posture, normally, causes 2-4 fold rise in plasma aldosterone level.

After I/V infusion of 500 mL/h of normal saline for 4h, plasma aldosterone level is suppressed to <5 ng/dL. This test is not done in K depleted individuals..

- A patient of diastolic hypertension (not on diuretic therapy) and on his usual salt intake, takes extra 1g sodium chloride with each meal for four days and investigations show that he is hypokalemic, with sodium concentration more than 142 meq/L (in the presence of reduced hematocrit because of increased ECF volume), needs to be assessed for plasma renin activity. If renin activity is suppressed, primary aldosteronism is likely to be present.

- In diagnosis of primary aldosteronism: serum K^+ <3.6 mmol/L $\longrightarrow$ PRA $\leq$1.0 ng/mL/h $\longrightarrow$ urinary K^+ > 40 mmol/d; aldosterone >15 µg/d $\longrightarrow$ CT scan and adrenal vein sampling. In equivocal cases the postural stimulation test as well as study of serum level of 18-hydroxycorticosterone (>60 µg/dL) (which is increased in adenoma cases) are needed. Plasma aldosterone level >25 ng/dL usually indicates adenoma and <25 ng/dL, hyperplasia.

Catecholamines and metabolites

Total free catecholamines 4-126 µg/d (24-745 nmol/d). In adrenal tumors and those associated with MEN, epinephrine, excretion is usually > 50 µg/d (the sole metabolite in MEN).
Total metanephrines 0.1-1.6 mg/d (0.5-8.7 µmol/d), usually <1.3 mg/d; VMA 1.5-7.5 mg/d (7.6-37.9 µmol/d).Plasma norepinephrine upto about 500 ng/L, epinephrine upto about 100 ng/L (sample taken in supine position).

- In diagnosis of pheochromocytoma, plasma studies of catecholamines are much less used than urinary studies. It is difficult to determine basal plasma cate-

cholamine levels as even a mild stress affects these levels.

- For all (catecholamines or metabolites) urinary assays, (preferably 2-3 repeated assays), 24h urine sample is better than a random sample); sample collection started during a paroxysm is still more useful. Drugs should be stopped (if possible) before sample collection. Drug and dietary restrictions depend upon the method used and should be known from the laboratory. During collection urine should be acidified and refrigerated.

DHEA (plasma)

2-9 µg/L (7-31 nmol/L)

DHEA-SO₄ (Plasma)

500-2500 µg/L (1.3-6.7 umol/L)

Androstenedione (plasma)

Adult male/female 0.8-2.3 ng/mL (2.8-8.0 nmol/L). Postmenopausal female 0.3-0.8 ng./mL. 6-10 years 0.1-0.5 ng/mL

17-Ketosteroids (urine) (pregnanediol, androsterone, etiocholanolone, DHEA, Δ5-pregnanetriol, 11-ketoandrosterone, 11-ketoetiocholanolone, 11-ketopregnanetriol)

Adult male 9-22 mg/24h (31-76 µmol/24 h). Adult female 5-15 mg/24h (17-52 µmol/24h). Birth to 8 years 0-1 mg/24h; 8 years to puberty 1-10 mg/24h. During collection of urine, 10 mL of 6 N HCl is used as preservative.

17-OH Progesterone (plasma)

Adult male 0.06-3.0 µg/L (0.2-9.0 nmol/L). Adult female follicular phase 0.2-1.0 µg/L. Infant upto one year <2.2 µg/L.

- 17-hydroxy progestrone has replaced study of urinary pregnanetriol for diagnosis of adrenal enzyme defects. Similarly radioimmunoassay of DHEA-SO₄ has replaced study of urinary 17-ketosteroids in evaluation of adrenal androgen production.

- In ovarian and adrenal tumors marked elevations of testosterone, androstenedione and DHEA-SO₄ occur (major amount of testosterone arises from peripheral formation). DHEA-SO₄ arises from adrenal tumors or adrenal rest tumors of ovary. Patients of CAH may present with marked elevation of testosterone/androstenedione and minimal elevation of DHEA-SO₄ (↑ 17-OH progesterone will differentiate from ovarian/adrenal tumors) or with marked elevation of DHEA-SO₄ and normal or elevated levels of the other two hormones (dexamethasone suppression test will differentiate from the tumors). Adrenal tumors and virilizing tumors of ovary other than the adrenal rest tumors can be differentiated from each other as the main androgen in the latter tumors is testosterone and DHEA-SO$_4$ level is not much elevated; also 17-keto-steroids excretion is rarely >30 mg/d. In rare Leydig cell tumors DHEA-SO$_4$ (and 17-ketosteroids) is elevated. Serum testosterone level is low or normal.

- Important clinical condition where adrenal androgen studies are likely to be useful include hypertension (see under primary aldosteronism), female hermaphroditism, male isosexual precocity, hirsutism, polycystic ovarian syndrome, gonadal tumors.

Testosterone (T)

Adult male 300-1000 ng/dL (10.4 -34.7 nmol/L) Prepubertal 8-14 ng/dL; pubertal 84- 180 ng/dL. Adult female 30-70 ng/dL (level >160 ng/dL usually reflects virilism); prepubertal, 5-13 ng/dL; pubertal 9-24 ng/dL.

- In the male low T level is suggestive of hypogonadism and high T level of sexual precocity. Further evaluation of gonadotropin levels is required to localize the cause in either condition.
- In hypogonadism due to T resistance, T is ↑/N, LH ↑/N and FSH N/↑. In isolated germinal cell disease T and LH are normal, FSH ↑/N.
- Plasma T level and response to LH stimulation (see chapted 18) is useful in evaluation of a patient of delayed puberty.
- Levels of E$_2$, T and LH are also useful in evaluation of a patient of male pseudohermaphroditism.
- Plasma estrogen levels are increased in the male in the liver or adrenal disease (due to increased accumulation or formation of precursor androgens for aromatization), in obesity (increased extraglandular aromataze activity) and in testicular tumors or androgen resistance (increased E$_2$ formation by testes).
- Leydig cell tumors (interstitial cell tumors) may be associated with increased or low levels of tesostrone (Chapter 17).

Estradiol; E$_2$

Adult female: normal level (follicular phase) 20-60 pg/mL (70-220 pmol/L): in men <50 pg/mL: in prepuertal children upto 20 pg/mL. Mid cycle ovulatory peak is about 3 times the basal level.

Urine (Non pregnant mid cycle: μg/d)

Total estrogens 28-100 μg; E$_2$ <10 μg, E$_1$ (estrone) 2-25 μg; E$_3$ (estriol) 2-30 μg: Post menopausal total estrogens upto 10 μg: in pregnancy total estrognes upto 45000 μg. Total estrogens in male is 5-18 μg/d.

Progesterone

Serum level (follicular phase) 0.3-0.8 ng/mL (1-3 nmol/L); (luteal phase) 4-20 ng/mL. In male 0.12-0.3 ng/mL. Urinary pregnanediol female 1-8 mg/d (3-25 μmol/d): male

<1.5 mg/d: pregnancy <50 mg/d: pregnanetriol female 0.5-2.0 mg/d: male 0.4-2.4 mg/d.

- Plasma level of 12 to 15 ng/mL, a week prior to onset of menstruation is considered a good evidence of adequacy of luteal phase. This investigation may be required in female infertility because of inadequate luteal phase in spite of normal menstruation. Endometrial biopsy however, is a preferable method of correct diagnosis.
- Pregnanediol (in urine) is main metabolite of progesterone and was used in the past to document well-being of early pregnancy. Urinary pregnanetriol arises from 17-hydroxy progesterone and was used in diagnosis of CAH when estimation of the latter was not easily available.
- Plasma estradiol estimation is useful to monitor a patient for risk of development of ovarian hyperstimulation syndrome while trying to induce ovulation with human menopausal gonadotropins. Hyper-stimulation syndrome results from excessive estrogen secretion by ovaries (during treatment) resulting in excessive leakage of fluid and protein from ovaries and peritoneal capillaries producing hypovolemia and renal insufficiency
- Estradiol estimation is also useful along with ultrasound for monitoring follicular growth in women, who are to undergo in vitro fertilization.
- E$_2$ estimation may also be useful in diagnosis of tumors producing this hormone. Important tumor is granulosa cell tumor of ovary which causes precocious puberty or menstrual abnormalities in females.
- Levels of T and adrenal androgens (DHEA-SO$_4$, androstenedione) are useful in evaluation of female pseudo-hermaphroditism, hirsutism and polycystic ovarian syndrome. Plasma T level >2 ng/mL or DHEA-SO$_4$ level >8000 ng/mL suggests neoplastic (ovarian/adrenal) source of androgens.

Gonadotropins

Serum LH: in menstruating women (follicular phase) upto 10 mIU/mL (10 IU/L); post menopausal 30-200 mIU/mL; children upto 12 mIU/mL; men upto 15 mIU/mL. Serum FSH: In menstruating women (follicular phase) upto 10 mIU/mL (10 IU/L); postmenopausal upto 200 mIU/mL; children upto 12 mIU/mL; men upto 15 mIU/mL.

- Plasma testosrone levels in the male and plasma E$_2$ levels in the female (in the female, oligomenorrhea or amenorrhea is generally adequate evidence of low E$_2$ status) will suggest hypogonadism. Gonadotropin levels are required to localize the cause of hypogonadism, if cause is in the ovary (post menopausal, castrate and ovarian failure), high FSH (>40 mIU/mL) and LH levels occur (FSH higher than LH). Contrary to this, higher levels of LH (>35 mIU/mL) and normal to depressed levels of FSH occur in polycystic ovary syndrome. If cause of hypogonadism is hypothalamus/pitutary or in prepubertal stage, LH is <5 mIU/mL, FSH is also low (actual level slightly higher than LH).

- Gonadotropin secreting pituitary tumors are rare. However, some chromophobe cell tumors (chromophobe adenomas are generally large when detected) do produce gonadotropins (generally FSH, less commonly LH which may be inactive). Generally, the clinical syndromes are not produced. These patients may occasionally require differentiation from primary hypogonadism. In these tumors normal testicular response to hCG may help in men and exaggerated FSH response to TRH in both sexes. The latter increased response is not seen in normals individuals and hypogonadal men or postmenupausal women.

Part III

Urinary constituents

- Volume (24h) 600-2500 mL (0.6-2.5 L/d).
- Ratio of night to day urine 1:2 to 1:4.
- Infant 15-60 mL/d (premature 1-3 mL/kg/h): Increase to 500-600 mL/d at 1 year.
- Osmolality (random) 500-800 mOsmol/kg (500-800 mmol/kg) (range) 50-1400 mOsmol/kg.
- Specific gravity (random) 1.016-1.022 (1.016-1.022) (relative density U20°C/water 20°C), range 1.001-1.035.
- pH 4.6-8.0.
- Ammonia nitrogen 20-70 mEq/d (20-70 mmol/d).
- Titrable acidity 20-50 mEq/d (20-50 mmol/d).
- Total solids 55-70 g/d (multiply last two figures of specific gravity by 2.66 to get total urinary solids in g/L).
- Chloride 140-250 mEq/d (140-250 mmol/d).
- Creatinine (in male) 1.0-2.0 g/d (8.8-17.7 mmol/d); 0.8-1.8 g/d (in female).
- Creatine (in male) <40 mg/d (<305 μmol/d); (in female) <100 mg/d.
- Uric acid 250-750 mg/d (1.5-4.5 mmol/d).
- Anuria (urine volume <100 mL/d); occurs in acute cortical necrosis, bilateral complete urinary tract obstruction and some cases of acute tubular necrosis.
- Oliguria (urine volume <400-500 mL/d, less than 15-20 mL/kg/d in children). In glomerular cause of oliguria urine protein excretion is >1.5 g/d (WBCs, RBC casts are also present); in tubulointerstitial disease urine protein is ≤1.5g/d (WBCs and WBC casts are present).
- Potassium 40-80 mEq/d (40-80 mmol/d)
- Phosphorous 0.9-1.3 g/d (29-42 mmol/d) depends on diet
- Pregnanetriol female 0.5-2.0 mg/d(1.5-5.9 umol/d); in males 0.4-2.4 mg/d; children upto 1 mg/d)

- Urobilinogen 0.05-2.5 mg/d (0.1-4.2 μmol/d) or 0.5-4.0 Ehrlich units/d.
- Sodium 75-200 mEq/d (75-200 mmol/d).
- Magnesium 6.0-8.5 mEq/d (3.0-4.3 mmol/d).

Urine sample

For quantitative work 24h urine sample is used because of great variations in its concentration, occurring during the day and because of diurnal variations in excretion of some substances. Difficulty, however, arises in collection of accurate 24h urine sample. Creatinine content of the 24h urine sample can be used to check on reliability of collection. Five mL of a 100g/L solution of isopropanol can be used as a satisfactory preservative for a large number of urinary constituents including inorganic ions, urea, amino acids, creatinine, protein, reducing substances, ketones and amylase. For catecholamines and their metabolites, urine should be preserved at pH of 1 to 2 with 6N HCl. For porphyrins and related compounds pH is maintained at 6 to 7 using acetic acid or sodium bicarbonate. About 0.5g of sodium fluoride may be used for 24h sample for estimation of glucose. Fluoride inhibits bacterial growth and cell glycolysis but does not inhibit activity of yeast. It also inhibits glucose oxidase used in strip test. Boric acid is used for preserving urine for estrogens.

Reagent strips

Outside the laboratory, reagent strips are available to detect (also for semi-quantitative evaluation), a number of clinically relevant substances in urine and in some cases in plasma as well. The strip methods keep on changing, altering colour reactions and sensitivities. The manufacturer's information including interferences and precautions for use should be strictly followed. The constituents tested include pH, glucose, protein, blood, ketones, bilirubin, urobilinogen, nitrite, leukocyte esterase, specific gravity and ascorbate. Strips are available for constituents singally or in combinations.

- Some important precautions for use of these strips are; use the strip test on a fresh sample without delay; after removing the required number of strips for use, recap the container; use un-spun urine brought to room temperature, do not touch the test area of the strip with fingers, dip the reagent strip into urine only briefly (not more than one second), drain off the excess urine by running the edge of the strip on an absorbent paper and compare with the chart provided after exact specified time in suitable light. Information provided by the manufacturer regarding sources of errors, specificity and sensitivity of the test should also be carefully, read.
- Leucocyte esterase in urine is a marker of significant number of neutrophils in urine and nitrite in urine

indicates presence of significant number of nitrate reducing bacteria in bladder urine (many gram negative organisms are nitrate reducing).

- Ehrlich reacting strip test is positive for urobilinogen or porphobilinogen (Chapter 8). The test is not considered reliable for the latter compound. In hemolytic jaundice urine contains increased urobilinogen but no bile pigments. In complete extra-hepatic obstruction urine may be free from urobilinogen. Inappropriate increased excretion of urobilinogen in urine may result during convalescence after infective hepatitis or during cirrhosis. Urinary excretion may also be increased due to bacterial overgrowth in the intestine, leading to increased formation of urobilinogen. In acid urine there is increased tubular reabsorption of urobilinogen and reduced excretion in urine.

Melituria (Benedicts reaction positive)

- 5% persons in normal population show melitura due to renal glycosuria, pentosuria and essential fructosuria.
- In hereditary disorders, galactose (galactosemia), fructose (fructose intolerance and other disorders), xylulose (pentosuria), lactose (lactase deficiency, lactose intolerance) and reducing phenolic compounds (phenyl ketonuria, tryrosinosis) appear in urine.
- In neonatal period urine may show reducing reaction due to physiological lactosuria, sepsis, hepatitis and gastroenteritis.
- Lactosuria may occur during lactation and xylulose appears in urine with excessive intake of fruits.
- Reducing drugs in urine (ascorbate, glucuronates, salicylates) will give Benedicts reaction with urine.
- Renal glycosuria may be seen in Fanconi syndrome, toxic renal disease (due to lead mercury, outdated tetracycline) or may be idiopathic.

Glycosuria

Reducing substances 0.5-1.5 g/d. Total sugars, average 250 mg/d. Glucose, average 130 mg/d (0.72 mmol/d). At glucose <0.3 g/d; protein 40-150 mg/d; qualitative tests are negative (protein and glucose in normal urine).

Ketonuria

- Qualitative examination of urine for ketones is needed in diagnosis of diabetic ketocidosis and insulinoma.
- Besides dibetes mellitus, ketonuria may also occur in renal glycosuria, glycogen storage disease, starvation, high fat diet, and in conditions of increased metabolism (fever, hyperthyroidism, pregnancy and lactation)
- In insulinoma, glycogen storage disease and starvation there is ketonuria without glycosuria.

Hemoglobinura (renal threshold 100-140 mg/dL)

- In hemoglobinuria and myoglobinuria urine gives positive stick test (test for pseudoperoxidase). Next serum is used to differentiate between Hb and myoglobin (Page 94).
- Hemolysed blood may come from genitourinary tract (infraction of kidney) or due to intravascular hemolysis (malaria, Clostridial/E coli bacteremia, DIC, hemolytic disorders, chemical or thermal burns and other causes.

Myoglobinuria (renal threshold 20 mg/dL)

- Indicates recent necrosis of skeletal or cardiac muscle. Serum is clear and haptoglobin is normal (in hemoglobinuria serum is pink and haptoglobin is reduced). Some enzymes of muscle are increased.
- Causes are crush syndrome, ischemia, other physical causes (convulsions, electric shock, march hemoglobinuria), metabolic (alcohol, CO poisoning, diabetic acidosis, barbiturate poisoning) and hereditary disorders,

Porphyrins and their precursors

ALA (γ-amino levulinic acid) 1.5-7.5 mg/d (11.2-57.2 µmol/d).

PBG (porphobilinogen) <1.0 mg/d (<4.4 µmol/d) (qualitative test is negative). Coproporphyrin 50-160 ug/d (0.075-0.24 µmol/d) fecal; 0-500 ug/d; erythrocyte 0.5-2.0 µg/dL. Uropoprhyrin 10-30 ug/24h (0.012-037 µmol/d). Protoporpysin in feces 0-600 µg/d (0-1.08 µmol/d); erythrocytes 4-52 µg/dL.

- The strip test is first done and if reaction of >1 Ehrlich unit is shown, the qualitative test is performed. The Waston-Schwartz test is used to give idea about the amounts of PBG or urobilinogen in presence of each other. A positive result for porphobilinogen in this test is confirmed by Hoesche's test
- For study of porphyrins and their precursors, urine must be fresh.

Secreening of urine for metabolic inherited disorders (Also see Chapter 18)

- These disorders give rise to accumulation of certain metabolites in blood which then spill over in urine (over flow mechanism). In some cases the reabsorption process for the metabolite may be defective (cystinlysinuria is an example). The metabolites involved in the above processes are amino acids, ketoacids, sugars, phenolic and other compounds. The individual inborn errors are rare but collectively they become important. In most cases, the disorder is first suggested by a screening test (reducing test for sugars, dinitrophenyl hydrazine test for keto acids and the ferric chloride test for mild reducing agents) and definitive diagnosis needs some chromatographic or enzymatic study.

• In a neonate presence of anemia, thrombocytopenia, hypoglycemia, metabolic acidosis or hyperammonemia may indicate an acute metabolic illness. *Hyperammonemia* (besides transient i.e.; RDS associated), may be due to organic aciduria (there is associated metabolic acidosis and thrombocytopenia) or due to urea cycle enzyme defects (specific enzyme deficiency can be demonstrated in cultured fibroblasts). Organic acidemias include methylmalonicacidemia, isovalericacidemia, propionicacidemia, multiple carboxylase deficiency (one cause being biotinidase deficiency) and others. Incidence of biotinidase deficiency is about 1:40,000. Important biochemical features of organic acidemias are metabolic acidosis and ketosis, hyperammonemia, hypoglycemia and a peculiar odour of urine and sweat.

Some biochemical parameters used to assess kidney functions

Evaluation of GFR

Clearance of a substance which is completely filtered (not being associated with plasma proteins) and is neither secreted nor reabsorbed by the tubules, is equal to GFR. Renal clearances of urea and creatinine are meant for evaluating GFR. These days, however, urea clearance is, hardly ever, used for the purpose since it, quite varies with rate of urine flow, even in a normal person. Creatinine is partly secreted by the tubules and, therefore, overestimates GFR. There is, however, analytical over estimation of serum creatinine (presence of chromogens in serum) but not of urinary creatinine. The two factors, affect creatinine clearance value in opposite directions, making creatinine clearance value close to GFR when serum level is not much above the normal range. When serum level is high (renal failure) tubular secretion becomes very significant component of urinary creatinine excretion. Under these circumstances creatinine clearance overestimates GFR.

Serum levels of urea and creatinine are inversely, related to their respective clearance values since decrease of clearance, increases the serum level. Serum levels of the two compounds are also used as indicators of GFR. However, difficulties arise when assessment of GFR is made from these levels. The relationship between serum levels of urea and creatinine and their clearances is such, that when clearance (or GFR) is reduced by more than 50%, there is only slight increase in the serum level. On the other hand, If GFR (and clearance) is already, considerably reduced, a small further decrease causes marked increase in serum levels. Further, there are wide variations in serum levels of urea (due to variation in protein intake) and creatinine (due to variations in muscular bulk). Thus in a person with poor muscular bulk, normal serum creatinine level may be 0.4 mg/dL, and with two third loss of GFR, serum creatinine level will rise to about 1.2 mg/dL; a serum level which may be perfectly normal for a person with large muscular bulk. See the box below.

BUN(mg/dL)		GFR(mL/dL)	Serum creatinine (mg/dL)	
High protein intake	Low protein intake		Small muscle bulk	Large muscle bulk
40	8	120	0.5	1.5
60	12	60	0.9	3.5
120	20	30	1.5	6.0

As creatinine clearance varies with age and muscle bulk, normal value for an individual of a particular age and weight should be suitably worked out.

• Theoretically, creatinine clerance gives more precise information about GFR (compared to serum levels of urea or creatinine). However, there is greater, likely, imprecision in the reported clearance values than the reported serum values (reported serum levels have imprecision of only one analysis whereas in the reported clearance values, imprecisions of two analyses are compounded by imprecision of urine collection). In evaluation of GFR serum creatinine is better than serum urea, since in the latter case serum levels depends upon protein intake, endogenous protein break down and state of hydration,besides, the renal clearance.

• Serum creatinine is preferred over serum urea as a single test for assessment of renal function (Fig 4.6). However, it is useful to estimate both serum urea (serum urea nitrogen also called blood urea nitrogen or BUN) and serum creatinine and work out ratio of BUN to serum creatinine. This ratio may provide some additional information about the case.

• With progressive nephron damage in renal disease, there is progressive decrease of GFR which is reflected in progressive increase of serum creatinine levels which may go upto 20 mg/dL. There is also fluctuating increase of serum urea levels. These levels fluctuate because of influence of a large number of factors, besides, GFR on levels of serum urea (Fig.4.6).

Evaluation of integrity of glomerular filtration membrane

Normal urine contains about 150 mg of protein per day in an adult and about 100 mg/d in a child under 10 years of age. More than 300 mg/d is taken as significant proteinuria in an adult. About one third or protein in normal urine is albumin. Other proteins present in normal urine arise from plasma (retinol binding protein, β_2-microglobulin, immunoglobulin light chains and lysozyme) as well as from nephron and urinary tract. Tamm-Horsfall glycoprotein is derived from cells of ascending limb of loop of Henle and cells of distal tubule and constitutes about one third of total protein loss in urine. Other proteins present in small amounts are IgA (secreted from urinary tract) and proteins and enzymes of tubular cells. Protein excretion can increase, in a febrile illness, in dehydration after hemorrhage and after strenuous exercise.

Isolated proteinuria

It is defined as proteinuria (generally <2 g/d) in the absence of any known disease of kidney or urinary tract and without any urinary sediment. Important types are as under:

Benign intermittent proteinuria

Proteinuria is said to be intermittent if, about half the number of urine samples tested, show presence of protein, and transient, if very few samples are positive for protein. A patient of intermittent proteiuria needs check up,once a year, for hypertension or some other renal abnormality. Intermittent proteinuria in pregnancy, however, needs proper work up of the patient for preeclampsia.

Benign functional proteinuria (<0.5 g/d)

It occurs after fever, a bout of sever exercise, following exposure to cold or in congestive heart failure. Some times hyaline/granular casts may also be present along with protein in urine. Rest greatly reduces urinary excretion of protein which disappears with resolution of the causative disorder.

Postural proteinuria (<1 g/d)

Proteiuria is present only in upright posture and is seen in 3 to 5% of adolescents. The condition resolves latest after a period of 10 to 15 years. It is also a benign disorder.

Persistent proteinuria

Protein excretion is 1 to 2 g/d. Prognosis is less favourable than that in cases of benign proteinuria, especially when accompanied with hematuria. Renal biopsy may show some histopathological change (glomerulopathic/interstitial nephritis). Renal insufficiency may develop in 20 to 40% cases after about 20 years.

Proteinuria in renal disease (glomerular, tubular and overflow types of proteinurias)

Barriers to protein filtration is mostly constituted by basement membrane (size restriction) and negatively charged slits of the epithelial cells. Slight damage of filtration membrane leads to leakage of albumin in urine. With increased damage, besides other proteins, there is

leakage of red cells and other type of cells in urine. Presence of excessive protein in the tubular fluid gives rise to hyaline casts. Red cell casts appear if red cells are also present along with protein in the tubular fluid. Other types of casts arise from damaged tubular cells in case of superimposed tubular damage.

- Proteinuria produced by disrupted barrier function of the filtration membrane is called glomerular proteinuria. It is generally moderate to heavy (>1.5 g/d). It may be selective (mostly albumin and transferrin) or non-selective, resembling serum pattern (see Table 4.10). In glomerulopathies presenting as nephritic type syndromes, proteinuria is generally moderate and is associated with nephritic type of urinary sediment (red cells, red cell casts with or without WBCs and other types of casts). In glomerulopathies presenting as nephrotic type syndromes, proteinuria is heavy but occurs in the absence of nephritic type of urinary sediment.

- In case of tubular proteinuria, the urinary proteins do not arise from plasma but are secreted from cells from different parts of nephron and urinary tract (predominantly $\alpha_1, \alpha_2, \beta$ and γ globulins without marked albumin). This type of proteinuria is seen in early diabetic nephropathy, in chronic pyelonephritis, interstitial tubular nephritis, congenital tubular nephropathies and polycystic kidney. Tubular proteinuria is generally mild (≤ 1.5 g/d).

- In over flow type of proteinuria certain plasma proteins appear in urine due to their elevated levels and there is no filtration membrane barrier for these small molecular weight proteins. This occurs in multiple myeloma, primary amyloidosis, heavy chain disease and others. The over flow type of proteinuria is generally moderate to heavy.

Protein and urinary sediments of some other disorders

Minimal proteinuria (see below) along with WBCs, WBC casts (red cells, may or may not be there) in the presence of bacteria in urine indicates chronic pyelonephritis and in the absence of bacteria but with presence of eosinophils indicates interstitial renal disease. Minimal proteinuria (>150 mg/d) with broad casts (due to dilated nephrons) and granular cellular casts, indicates advanced chronic renal disease.

Magnitude of proteinuria

Most renal diseases are associated with proteinuria which may be minimal (≤ 1.5 g/d), moderate (1 to 3 g/d) or heavy (>3 g/d). Magnitude of proteinuria may be expressed in terms of protein, creatinine ratio. The first morning urine sample is tested and protein, creatinine ratio of <0.2 is normal; 0.2-1.0 (or 1.5) indicates low grade proteinuria; 1.0 to 3.0 is taken as moderate and >3.0 as heavy proteinuria.

Heavy proteinuria (>3g/d)

Important disorders in this group are nephrotic syndrome (diabetes and SLE are important secondary causes); amyloidosis including that with multiple myeloma; toxemia of pregnancy, malignant hypertension, renal vein thrombosis (often complicates nephrotic syndrome); severe congestive heart failure and constrictive pericarditis.

Moderate proteinuria (1 to 3 g/d)

It is found in nephritic disorders (in some cases protein excretion may be heavy) and toxic nephropathies.

Minimal proteinuria (≤1.5 g/d)

Important causes are chronic pyelonephritis (proteinuria may be intermittent), inactive phase of glomerular diseases and microalbuminuria of early diabetic nephropathy. Also interstitial nephritis and chronic renals failure.

Renal diseases without proteinuria

Important examples are phases of acute/chronic pyelonephritis, obstructive uropathy, kidney stones/tumors (urine may contain red cells) and congenital malformations.

Evaluation of protein in urine

- The reagent strip test is now readily available for detection of protein in urine. A small area on the strip carries tetrabromophenol blue buffered to a pH of 3.0. (the dye gives yellow colour due to undissociated molecules). When dipped in urine, proteins (if present) change pH in the area. Increase in pH causes dye to dissociate and colour changes to green. Colour is read in 30 to 60 seconds. Alkaline urine due to medication or bacterial contamination will give a false positive reaction. Excessive wetting, by removing buffer from the impregnated area of the strip, will also invalidate the result. The strip test is more sensitive for albumin than globulins or Bence Jones protein. *These strips can not be relied upon for absence of protein in urine or for degree of proteinuria.* A number of acid precipitation tests (sulfosalicylic acid (SSA) and trichlor acetic acid (TCA) are also available for qualitative, semiquantitative or quantitative analysis of urine protein. These are more sensitive than the strip test but give positive results in presence of X-ray contrast media or many drug metabolites. For quantitative work, turbidity is produced with SSA or TCA and read with a photometer or a nephlometer. For more precise measurements TCA precipitate is dissolved in sodium hydroxide solution and measured by the use of biuret reaction. Automated methods based on biuret reaction or turbidimetry are available. Albumin and β-microglobulin can be measured by radio-immuno assay or by immunogenic nephlometric methods.

Hematuria

- Less than 3% normal individual may show ≤3 RBCs per high power field (>3 are taken as abnormal). After strenuous exercise about 18% of normal persons show hematuria. Dipsticks detect (designed to detect pseudoperoxidase) RBCs, Hb and myoglobin in urine.
- If in a dipstick positive urine no RBC are seen, the cause may be hemoglobinuria or myoglobinuria.
- If in a dipstick positive urine, only RBCs are seen microscopically, cause may be calculi, papillary necrosis, polycystic kidneys, sickle cell disease, genitourinary tract trauma, neoplasm or parasites.
- If in a dipstick positive urine, RBCs and WBCs are present, the cause may be lower genitourinary tract disease.
- If in a dipstick positive urine RBCs are seen with WBC's casts, diagnosis may be pyelonephritis, tuberculosis, sarcoidosis or drug reaction.
- In dipstick positive urine, if microscopic examination shows presence of RBCs, RBC casts/Hb casts or dysmorphic red cells, it indicates glomerular disease (immune complex disease or post infection glomerulonephritis), hypertension, diabetes mellitus, drug reaction, endocarditis or embolic disease.
- Microscopic hematuria with dipstick 2+ proteinuria, means glomerular involvement. Daily excretion >1.5g.

Plasma and urine osmolalities

On average water intake, plasma and urine osmolalities vary between 280 to 295 and 500 to 800, respectively (all values expressed as mOsmol/kg). Urine to plasma osmolality ratio (in a random sample) varies between 1.0 and 3.0. Comparing osmolality of a random urine sample with that of a similar plasma sample, gives an idea about ability of kidney to concentrate urine. Indication of poor concentrating ability may need confirmation by the urine concentration test. Second important use of urine and plasma osmolality studies is, for differentiating between prerenal azotemia and acute tubular necrosis (Table 4.5).

In glomerulonephritis and congestive heart failure, tubular functions remain intact and therefore U/P osmol ratio remains above 1.2 and urine Na^+ concentration less than 20 mmo/L (due to retained effectivies of ADH and aldosterone).

The osmolality studies may also help to find caus in a case of polyuria. In osmotic diuresis the ratio c urine/plasma osmolality (U/P ratio) remains higher then 1.0. This ratio is less than 1.0 in water diuresis. In complete diabetes insipidus U/P ratio is <1.0 and does not change on water deprivation. In incomplete diabetes insipidus or psychogenic polydipsia the ratio may be less than 1.0 but increases on water deprivation.

Urine and serum (or plasma) osmolalities can be determined with the help of an osmometer. Serum osmolality can also be calculated as follows:

Osmolality (mOsmol/kg water)=1.86 (Na+)+ Glu/18+BUN/2.8 (concentrations expressed in conventional units). Difference between measured and calculated osmolalities of serum is called delta osmolality (Δ osmolality or osmolar gap). Study of delta osmolality can be used to indicate the presence of some non-conventional substance in serum. In a patient of polyuria it may also help to find the cause of the disorder.

In a normal individual urine osmolality varies depending upon state of hydration. This variation may be expressed as osmolality or as specific gravity, as there is a good correlation between the two in a normal person. In a healthy young adult maximally diluted urine may have osmolality of 50 mOsmol/kg and specific gravity of 1.003, and a maximally concentrated urine may have osmolality of 1400 mOsmol/kg and specific gravity of 1.040. The correlation between osmolality and specific gravity observed in a normal individual is missing in a patient of renal failure because of presence of a number of high mol. wt. substances which contribute to specific gravity but not much to osmolality.

Certain parameters and tests concerning kidney function evaluation

Serum creatinine

1-2 years (0.2-0.6 mg/dL); gradually increase to adult range 0.8-1.2 mg/dL; Blood urea nitrogen (BUN); 1-3 year, 5-17 mg/dL gradually increase to 8-21 mg/dL in adults; BUN/creatinine ratio; normal range is 12-20; Creatinine clearance: adults male 94-140 mL/min/1.73 sq m; value is 72-110 mL/min/1.73 sq m, in females. The creatinine clearance values gradually decline to 30-60 mL/min/sq m in males and 27-55 mL/min/sq m in females at 80-89 years of age; Value at 1-2 years, 50 mL/mt/1.73 sq m; gradually increase to adult levels.

For practical purposes range of creatinine clearance in a young male adult is 90-139 mL/min, It starts decreasing gradually from the age of 20 onwards. Normally clearance is less in women than men.

Urine concentration test

Three urine samples, 1,2 and 4 hours after a fluid restriction of about 14 hours are collected and specific gravity determined. In one of the samples specific gravity should be $\geq$1.025. In the presence of renal disease specific gravity will be less than 1.020. As the disease severity increases, specific gravity declines to approach 1.010.

- The test is useful to detect early loss of renal function. However a normal result does not necessarily rule out active renal disease.
- Fluid restriction is harmful in early renal failure and heart disease.

Urine osmolality test

After high protein diet for three days, paitent takes a dinner with minimum amount of water and no water afterwards; urine is passed and discarded at 6 A.M. and then urine sample is collected at 8 A.M. Normally it should show an osmolality $\geq$800 mOsmol/kg.Osmolality of 400-600 indicates moderately impairment or renal function and <400, a severe impairment. The test is especially useful in cases of pyelonephritis and hypertension. To increase test sensitivity, serum osmolality should also be determined and urine, serum osmolality ratio calculated, which normally should be $\geq$3.0.

- In the presence of edema or ascites no water restriction is undertaken and urine samples are collected 1 and 2h after s/c injection of 10 units of AVP after emptying the bladder. Normally specific gravity should reach $\geq$1.020.
- Usually there is good correlation between GFR (creatinine clearance) and concentrating ability in cases of impaired renal functions; however, impaired concentrating ability may exist with normal GFR in certain disorders (diabetes mellitus, nephrolithiasis, DI, sickle cell anemia, pyelonephritis, hypercalcemia and hypokalemia.
- In chronic renal disease BUN correlates better with symptoms of uremia than serum creatinine. BUN of 50-150 mg/dL indicates a serious renal impairment.
- BUN is also useful as an evidence of hemorrhage within GI tract and also in nutritional management and monitoring of catabolic patients of cancer and burns.
- BUN/creatinine ratio of >20 in a patient of impaired renal functions may mean increased tissue catabolism (infection, fever, cachexia, thyrotoxicosis, some drug intake), or a patient with reduced muscle mass.
- Ratio may rise in a patient of renal disease when prerenal azotemia is superadded (congestive heart failure, salt/water depletion, shock)
- Estimation of creatinine clearance is also important in patients who need treatment with a nephrotoxic drug.
- The concentration tests are not reliable in the presence of severe water and electrolyte abnormality, low protein/salt diet, chronic liver disease, adrenal insufficiency and pregnancy.

❑

Part IV

Important changes in laboratory results in pregnancy by term, except when stated otherwise

- BUN and serum creatinine decrease by 25% mostly in the first half of pregnancy. Serum uric acid decreases by 35% in first trimester and returns to normal by term.
- Proteinuria (in about 20%), glycosuria (there is also reduced glucose tolerance) and lactosuria are common.
- Serum iron ($\downarrow$) by 40%; transferrin ($\uparrow$) by 40% and percent saturation ($\downarrow$) upto 70%.
- Serum protein ($\downarrow$) by 1g/dL in first trimester (same at term); albumin ($\downarrow$) by 0.5 g/dL in first trimester ($\downarrow$) by 0.75g/dL at term. Globulins ($\uparrow$) by 0.5g/dL (maximum ($\uparrow$) in β-globulin).
- Serum TAG ($\uparrow$) by 100-200% and cholesterol ($\uparrow$) by 30-50% (also see chapter 9).
- ($\uparrow$) of serum ceruloplasmin by 70% and ($\uparrow$) of serum copper
- Serum folate ($\downarrow$) by 50%, serum B_{12} by 20%.
- Serum ALP increases by 200-300%; CK decreases by 15% by 20 weeks to normalize at term: no changes in AST, ALT, LD, acid phosphatase.
- Urinary ketosteroids increase to upper normal limit.
- TBG is increased: Serum T_4 increases (from 4-8ug/dL at 12th week to 10-12ug/dL at term; normalizes by 6 weeks postpartum): RUT_3 is decreased: FT_4I is not changed: hCG can cross react in TSH assay; TSH by sensitive TSH assay (iimunometric) is normal: TRH response unchanged.
- Serum Ca and Mg decreases by 10% and no change in phosphate.
- Serum aldosterone is increased
- Fasting blood glucose decreases by 5-10 mg/dL by the end of 1st trimester.
  During glucose tolerance test, peak glucose increases and remains elevated longer, especially in later half of pregnancy.
- No response to GnRH.
- Cortisol response to ACTH infusion increases.

❑

Part V

The test groups useful for different clinical situations.

Common patient management tests (CPMT): Na^+: K^+: Cl^-: HCO_3^-: Glucose: BUN: Creatinine: *Different anemias:* Clinical blood counts with indices, reticulocyte count and microscopic examination (CBC etc.)
Liver disorders: Bilirubin (total and direct); ALP: γ-GT: AST: ALT: Total protein and albumin: PT: *Cardiac damage*: CK: CK-MB: Myoglobin: Troponin-I: *Acute pancreatitis*: Amylase: Lipase: Glucose: Ca: TAG: *Renal disorders*: CPMT: CBC etc: Creatinine clearance: Ca: PO_4: Mg: Albumin and total protein: 24h urine protein: *Fluid, electrolyte disorders*: CPMT: plasma and urine osmolality: Creatinine clearance: Anion gap: Urine conc. and dilution tests: *Acid base and blood gas disordes*: pH: pO_2: O_2 saturation: CO_2 content: pCO_2: Alveolar-arterial pO_2 difference: *Diabetes mellitus management*: CPMT: Hb1c: Anion gap: Lipid profile: *Lipid profile:* Total-C: LDL-C: HDL-C: TAG: *Hypertension*: CPMT: Renin: Urinary free cortisol: Urinary metanephrines: Urinalysis: fT_4 and TSH (for thyroid status). *Microcytic anemia*: CBC etc.: Serum iron: TIBC: % saturation: Ferritin (for iron status): ESR: *Macrocytic anemia*: CBC etc.: B_{12}: Folate: TSH: *Normocytic anemia*: CBC etc.: Bilirubin: Haptoglobin: Free Hb in plasma and urine: LD: Antiglobulin test, direct and indirect: Reticulocyte count (for hemolysis): ESR: *Parathyroid disorders*: Ca: Total proten and albumin: ALP: PO_4: Mg: Creatinine: Urinary Ca^{++}: PTH: *Bone disorders*: Ca: PO_4: ALP: Protein total and albumin: Osteocalcin: Uric acid: *Coagulation screening*: PT: TT: PTT: BT: Platelet count: *DIC:* Platelet count: TT: PT: PTT: Fibrinogen: Fibrin split products: CBC etc.: *COMA*: CPMT: Arterial pH and blood gas profile: Toxicology screen (see Chapter 12): Ammonia: Anion gap: Alochol: Lactic acid: Ca^{2+} and albumin: Serum osmolality: *Collagen disease/SLE*: ESR: C-reactive protein: C_3 and C_4: ANA: Anti-DNA: ANCA: *Arthritis*: ESR: C-reactive protein: Rheumatoid factor: Uric acid: ANA: *Acute Hepatitis (serology)* IgM anti-HAV: HBsAg: IgM anti-HBc: Anti HCV: *Chronic Hepatitis (serology)*: HBeAg: Anti-HBe: HBsAg: Anti-HCV: *Enteral/Parenteral nutritional management*: CPMT: CBC etc.: Ca: Mg: PO_4: ALP: Total protein and albumin: Prealbumin: TAG: *Newborn screening*: The actual selection of diseases for screening will depend upon the country and the state: Hypothyroidism: Phenylketonuria: Sickle cell disorders (Hb electrophoresis), Galactosemia, Homocystinuria, Maple syrup urine disease, CAH, Cystic fibrosis, Biotinidase deficiency, Duchenne's muscular dystrophy, G6PD deficiency and Hypercholesterolemia are important conditions. *Prenatal screening*: CBC etc.: Uric acid: BUN: Creatinine: Glucose: fT_4: Urinalysis: Urine culture: Cervical culture (for GC, Chlamydia, group B Streptococci): Cervical Pap smear: ABO and Rh typing: VDRL: HBsAg: Screening for CMV, toxoplasmosis, rubella and Herpes simplex.

- Source of information for Appndix B is ref. Nos. 1, 3, 4, 41, 49 & 59; the information in Part V is from ref. no. 1.
- In part V, all or a few tests, from a group may be needed, depending upon the clinical situation.

Books and Monographs for Reference and Further Reading

1. Henry JB (ed) (1996) Clinical Diagnosis and Management by Laboratory Methods. 19th ed. Philadelphia: Saunders.
2. Burtis CA Ashwood ER (1996) Fundamentals of Clinical Chemistry. 4th ed. Philadelphia: Saunders.
3. Jacques W (1996) Interpretation of Diagnostic Tests. 6th ed. Boston: Little Brown.
4. Gowenlock AH (ed) (1988) Varley's Practical Clinical Biochemistry 6th ed. London: Heinmann.
5. Davidson I Henry JB (eds) (1974) Todd-sanford Clinical Diagnosis by Laboratory Methods. 15th ed. Philadelphia: Saunders.
6. Sox HC Jr (ed) (1990) Common diagnostic Tests: Use and Interpretation. 2nd ed. Philadelphia: American College of Physicians.
7. Tietz NW (1993) Textbook of Clinical Chemistry. Philadelphia: Saunders.
8. Mayne PD (1994) Clinical Chemistry in Diagnosis and Treatment. 6th ed. Great Britain (ELBS): Churchill Livingstone.
9. Marshall WJ (1995) Clinical Chemistry. 3rd ed. London: Grower Medical Publishing.
10. Fraser GC (1986) Interpretation of Clinical Laboratory Data. Oxford: Blackwell.
11. Ransohoff DF, Fienstein AR (1978). Problems of spectrum and bias in evaluating the efficacy of diagnostic tests and procedures. N Engl J Med; 299: 926-30.
12. Ross DL Neely AE (1983) Textbook of Urinalysis and Body Fluids. Norwalk: Appleton-Century-Croft.
13. Arieff AI, DeFronzo RA (eds) (1995) Fluids Electrolyte and Acid-Base Disorders, 2nd ed. New York: Churchill Livingstone.
14. Narins RG (ed) (1994) Clinical Disorders of Fluid and Electrolyte Metabolism. 5th ed. New York: McGraw-Hill.
15. Cogan MG (ed) (1991) Fluid and Electrolytes. Norwalk: Appleton and Lange.
16. Brenner BM (ed) (1996) The Kidney. 5th ed. Philadelphia: Saunders.
17. Seldin DW Giebisch G (eds) (1992) The Kidney: Physiology and Pathophysiology. 2nd ed. New York: Raven Press.
18. Lloyd MN (ed) (1997) Mastery of Surgery. 3rd ed. New York: Little Brown.
19. Ritzmann SE Daniels JC (eds) (1975) Serum Protein Abnormalities. Diagnostic and Clinical Aspects. Boston: Little Brown.
20. Hunninghake D (ed) (1994) Lipid Disorders. Med Clin North Am 78; 1.
21. Hardman JG et al (eds) (1996) Goodman and Gilmans The Pharmacological Basis of Therapeutics. 9th ed. New York: McGraw-Hill.
22. Paul WE (1993) Fundamentals of Immunology. 3rd ed. New York: Raven Press.
23. Sherlock S Dooley J (1993) Diseases of Liver and Biliary System. 9th ed. Oxford: Blackwell.

24. Silen W (1991) Cope's Early Diagnosis of the Acute Abdomen. 18th ed. London: Oxford.
25. Sleisenger MH Fordtran (eds) ((1993) Gastrointestinal Diseases. 5th ed. Philadelphia: Saunders.
26. Moore MR et al (eds) (1987) Disorders of Prophyrin Metabolism. New York: Plenum.
27. Wyngaarden JB Kelly WN (1976) Gout and hyperuricemia. New York: Grune and Stratton.
28. Schuckit MA (1995) Drug and alcohol abuse: A clinical Guide to Diagnosis and Treatment. New York: Plenum.
29. Amdur MO et al (eds) (1996) Casarett and Doull's Toxicology: The Basic Science of Poisons. 5th ed. New York: McGraw-Hill.
30. Ellenhorn MJ Barcelous DG (1988) Medical Toxicology: Diagnosis and Treatment of Human Poisoning. New York: Elsevier.
31. Dreisbach RH Robertson WO (1987) Handbook of Poisoning. Norwalk: Appleton and Lange.
32. Plum F Posner J (1980) The diagnosis of Stupor and Coma. 3rd. ed. Philadelphia: Davis.
33. Shils ME et al (eds) (1994) Modern Nutrition in Health and Disease. Philadelphia: Lea and Febiger.
34. Waterlow JC (1992) Protein Energy Malnutrition. London: Edward Arnold.
35. Alleyne GAO et al (1997) Protein Energy Malnutrition. London: Butler and Tanner.
36. Linden MC (1991) Nutritional Biochemistry and Metabolism. New York: Elsevier.
37. Combs GF Jr (1992) The Vitamins. San Diego: Academic Press.
38. Brock J et al (1994) Iron Metabolism in Health and Disease. London: Saunders.
39. Wilson JD Foster DW (eds) (1992) Williams Textbook of Endocrinology. 8th ed. Philadelphia: Saunders.
40. DeGroot LT et al (eds) (1994) Endocrinology. 3rd ed. Philadelphia: Saunders.
41. Greenspan FS Baxter JD (eds) (1994) Basic and Clinical Endocrinology. 4th ed. Norwalk: Appleton and Lange.
42. Yen SSC Jaffe RB (eds) (1991). Reproductive Endocrinology. 8th ed. Philadelphia: Saunders.
43. Braverman LE Utiger RD (eds) (1997) The Thyroid. 7th ed. Philadelphia: Lippincott.
44. Speroff L et al (eds) (1989) Clinical Gynecological Endocrinology and Infertility. London: Williams and Wilkins.
45. Queenan JT (ed) (1994) Management of High Risk Pregnancy. London: Blackwell.
46. Avioli LV, Krane SM (eds) (1990) Metabolic Bone Disease and Clinically Related Disorders. Philadelphia: Saunders.
47. Krishna Menon MK et al (1982) Postgraduate Obstetrics and Gynecology. Hyderabad: Orient Longman.
48. Pritchard JA et al (eds) (1985) Williams obstetrics. 17th ed. Norwalk: Appleton. Century-Croft.
49. Levene MI Tudehope D (1993) Essentials of Neonatal medicine. 2nd ed. Oxford: Blackwell.
50. Srivastava et al (1990) Pediatric and Neonatal Emergencies. New Delhi: Indian Pediatrics.
51. Gardner RJM Sutherland GR (1996) Chromosome abnormalities and Genetic Counseling. 2nd ed. New York: Oxford University Press.
52. Darnell J et al (1995) Molecular Cell Biology. 3rd ed. New York: Scientific American Books.
53. Thompson MW et al (1993) Genetics in Medicine. Philadelphia: Saunders.
54. Simpson JL Elias S (1993) Essentials of Prenatal Diagnosis. Vol 1. New York: Churchill-Livingstone.
55. Harrison MR et al (1991) The Unborn Patient: Prenatal Diagnosis and Treatment. 2nd ed. Philadelphia: Saunders.
56. Royce PM Steinmann B (eds) (1993) Connective Tissue and its Heritable Disorders. New York: Wiley-Liss.
57. Bondy PK Roenberg LE (eds) (1976) Duncan's Diseases of Metabolism. 7th ed. Philadelphia: Saunders.
58. Scriver CR et al (eds) (1995) The Metabolic and Molecular Basis of inherited Disease. 7th ed. New York: McGraw-Hill.
59. Fauci AS et al (eds) (1998) Harrisons Principles of Internal Medicine. 14th ed. New York: McGraw-Hill.
60. Stanbury JB et al (eds) (1983) The metabolic Basis of Inherited Disease. 5th. ed. New York: McGraw-Hill.

Index

t following a page no. means a table entry: f following a page no. means a figure entry.